The Silent Revolution in Cancer and AIDS Medicine

Note from the Author

The knowledge that this book conveys may revolutionize cancer and AIDS therapy in the coming years. After having read this book, no responsible doctor should continue to provide such harmful therapy to the patients in his/her care and trust. This book will inform them about the fatal mistakes of their previous therapies, of which until now they were the unwitting victims.

Additionally, this book is indispensable reading for the patient afflicted with cancer or AIDS. Herein for the first time, the exact reasons are revealed to the world why neither cancer nor AIDS must inevitably result in death. These two illnesses are the natural result of a systemic imbalance, which not only can be halted, but can also be healed.

The Silent Revolution in Cancer and AIDS Medicine

New fundamental insights into the real causes of illness and death confirm the effectiveness of biological compensation therapy.

Heinrich Kremer

Library of Congress Control Number		2008905475
ISBN:	Hardcover	978-1-4363-5084-6
	Softcover	978-1-4363-5083-9

Editor: Felix A. de Fries, Zürich, Study Group AIDS Therapy, Zürich (Switzerland)
E-mail: felix.defries@tele2.ch
Translator: Jamie Mc Intosh, Freiburg (Germany)
Proofreading: David Lowenfels and Dorion Sagan, San Francisco (USA)

German edition: Heinrich Kremer: Die stille Revolution der Krebs—und AIDS—Medizin Ehlers Verlag, Wolfratshausen (Germany) 2001

Italien edition: Heinrich Kremer: La Rivoluzione Silenziosa della Medicina del Cancro e dell' AIDS, Macroedizioni, Diegaro di Cesena (Italy) 2003

We would like to thank Monique Altmann, Benglen (Switzerland) for her sponsoring of the English edition of this book and the Macroedizioni Publishing House for permission to use the illustrations made for the Italian edition.

This book was printed in the United States of America.

To order additional copies of this book, contact:
Xlibris Corporation
1-888-795-4274
www.Xlibris.com
Orders@Xlibris.com
38692

Dedicated to the memory of my teacher and friend:

Prof. Dr. med. Alfred HÄSSIG (1921-1999)

As a long-standing head of the central laboratory of the Swiss Red Cross, Professor of Immunology at Berne, Advisor to the World Health Organization in all continents, President of the International Society for Blood Transfusion, and Chairman of the Study Group for Nutrition and Immunity, Alfred Hässig was an eminent pioneer in the field of hematology, immunology and stress-medicine.

With an exemplary medical ethic, he tirelessly and courageously made clear the uncertainty of the so-called HIV test and the fatal consequences of toxic AIDS and cancer therapy. In spite of legal persecution up until his death, he imparted the practical alternatives of biological regulation therapy.

Patients around the world will owe their survival to the doctor and researcher Alfred Hässig, who has liberated them from the fatal mistakes of HIV/AIDS medicine. His impressive reminder—that the service to health must always take priority over profit from illness—remains a lasting legacy and lesson, not only for his friends and colleagues but also for his opponents, who are as skilled and resourceful as they are stubbornly misinformed.

Contents

Chapter I A Disastrous Decision 19
20 years of abusing nitric gases for sexual enhancement—the seemingly mysterious consequences

Chapter II The Sensational Discovery 29
Gaseous Nitrogen Monoxide as bioenergetic regulator within and between living cells—the gas war between humans and microbes

Chapter III The AIDS Mystery 41
Why the AIDS diseases were misinterpreted—inhibition of the gaseous defense is the cause of acquired immune cell weakness

Chapter IV AIDS is not a Contagious Disease 59
Opportunistic infections and Kaposi's sarcoma were well known long before the AIDS era—a variety of causes trigger the same immune response, as programmed by biological evolution.

Chapter V Challenging the Previously Valid Immunity Theories 103
How acquired immune cell impairment actually develops

Chapter VI The Most Successful Fusion in the History of Evolution 141
How the micro-Gaian milieu functions—the vital role of the mitochondria

Chapter VII Collective Tunnel Vision 183
Why "HIV characteristics" are the outcome of evolutionary biological programming, and are not specific causes of strong and/or continuous immune stress—what the "HIV test" really measures.

Chapter VIII The Solution to the Cancer Puzzle 219
Why normal cells become cancerous—the degeneration of cancer cells back to an embryonic state is programmed by evolutionary biology, and is the result of mitochondrial inactivation.

Chapter IX HIV/AIDS Medicine run Amok 269
Why AIDS drugs cause cancer, degenerative changes in muscular and nervous cells, and even AIDS itself-the explanation of how AZT, Bactrim/Septra, and their ilk actually work.

Chapter X The Daunting Task of Reconsideration 313
The fundamental malpractices of AIDS and cancer medicine—why patients die by chemotherapeutic poisoning

Chapter XI The Lifesaving Knowledge of Healing 393
On the practice of diagnosing, preventing, and treating AIDS, cancer, and other systemic diseases—rebalancing instead of eradication

Chapter XII Resistance against Mass Poisoning in Africa 459
The international initiative of President Mbeki—answers from the South African government's open discussion: on the causes of AIDS in the West and developing nations, on the nontoxic prevention and therapy for AIDS, on AZT's true mechanism of action, and the global terror epidemic spread by physicians and the media—the international HIV cartel's refusal to join the discussion, and the disinformation campaign it launched.

The Secret of Cancer and the Concept of Cell Symbiosis Therapy 501-508
The Secret of Cancer "short-circuit" in the photon switch.—
Change in the medical world-view of tumorology,
The Concept of Cell Symbiosis Therapy—The Way Out of the Therapeutic Dead End.

David Lowenfels:
The Dual Strategy of the Immune Response 517
A Review of Heinrich Kremer's Research on the Pathophysiology of AIDS, Cancer, and Other Chronic Immune Imbalances

Bibliography: 539

Tables 635

Tables

Chapter 8:

Chapter 10:

Illustrations

Chapter I

A Disastrous Decision

20 years of abusing nitric gases for sexual enhancement—the seemingly mysterious consequences

In 1960, the Food and Drug Administration (FDA), the U.S. authority responsible for the admission and surveillance of food, medicine and cosmetics, made a fateful decision that resulted in a disastrous course of events; the FDA cancelled the prescription requirement for the gaseous organic nitrite compound with the biochemical name "amyl nitrite." This policy change would bring grave consequences, which later in the 1980s would indirectly lead modern medicine to an even more devastating decision: the propagation of the allegedly viral origin of the "most frightening epidemic illness of the 20th Century, which we call today AIDS" (Gallo 1991).

Nothing can clarify better how closely the glamour and gloom of modern medicine lie together, than the simultaneous research results of one field that would eventually refute the calamitous mistakes of another. The gradual illumination of the working mechanisms of the amyl nitrites, as well as other nitrogen derivates in human cell systems, has led to a quiet revolution of the medical worldview; meanwhile the AIDS orthodoxy, vociferously controlled by retrovirus cancer researchers, has unleashed an unmitigated fiasco.

Over 140 years ago, nitrites and nitrates were known to affect the circulatory system

The dawn of modern medicine began in the middle of the 19th century, when chemists and physicians introduced the methods of experimental physiology and pharmacology into medical research. At that time, chemists had recently synthesized amyl nitrite and nitroglycerin (triglycerine-nitrate). In 1860, a physician named Richardson demonstrated the effect of gaseous amyl nitrite by inviting the audience attending his lectures to inhale it. He determined that "amyl nitrite, when inhaled, produced an immediate action on the heart, increasing the action of the organ more powerfully than any other known agent." Richardson did not recommend the use of amyl nitrite in medical treatment, however, as he felt the intensity of its effect was too strong (Fye 1986).

In 1867, Brunton published the first comprehensive medical report on the use of amyl nitrite for angina pectoris, a sudden attack of pain in the chest area due to a constriction of the coronary blood vessels (Brunton 1867). In 1871, Brunton correctly recognized that after inhalation of amyl nitrite, the induced lowering of blood pressure takes place "not due to a weakening of the heart's action, but to a dilation of the vessels, and that this depends on the action of the nitrite on the walls of the vessels themselves. Whether this is due to its action on the muscular walls themselves, or the nerve-ends in them, cannot at present be said" (Brunton 1867, Fye 1986, Berlin 1987).

This fundamental question in cardio-circulatory research would not be definitively answered until the next century. In fact, it was only in the last 20 years that this research gap was filled. In the past two decades, the findings of numerous research groups have led to the discovery of nitrogen oxides as essential mediators and modulators of all cellular life on Earth, humans included.

In 1879, Murell published several works on the effects of amyl nitrite and nitroglycerin, although he only recommended the latter for the treatment of angina pectoris (Murell 1879). Alfred Nobel, who made his fortune in the late 19th-century by packaging volatile nitroglycerin into the stable form of dynamite, wrote in a letter to a friend: "It sounds like the irony of fate that I should be ordered by my doctor to take nitroglycerin internally" (Snyder 1992). Nobel could not have guessed that one century later, his eponymous prize would be awarded for the discovery of the mechanism of this organic nitrate, leading to major discoveries regarding the physiological and pathophysiological roles of nitrogen oxides (nitrogen monoxide = nitric oxide = NO) in human cell systems.

It has been known for 50 years that nitrites and nitrates in food, industrial products, and pharmaceuticals can be transformed into carcinogenic nitrosamine.

For thousands of years, nitrites and nitrates played yet another important role: namely the preservation of meats, sausage and ham. Nitrites occur as natural impurities in salts. Many foods are enriched with nitrate, which can be transformed by bacteria into nitrite. Both nitrites and nitrates kill *Clostridium botulinum*, the bacterium that causes the dreaded botulism poisoning.

Research interest into the working mechanism by which nitrites kill bacteria, however, was only aroused when it was proven that the food additive sodium nitrite could produce carcinogenic nitrosamine. Nitrites and the related N-nitroso compounds can bond with amines and amides in numerous configurations (overview Magee 1976, Lijinsky 1992, Loeppky 1994 a). In 1954, the research group of Barnes and Magee (Barnes 1954) first published the discovery of the toxic characteristics of nitrites, from which nitrosamine had formed. Two years later, the same research group proved that ingestion of dimethylnitrosamine caused primary liver cancer in animals (Magee 1956). After this innovative work by Barnes and Magee, hundreds of N-nitroso compounds were examined for their toxic and carcinogenic characteristics. Carcinogenicity has been confirmed in 252 of these substances. In experimental comparisons of the metabolism of N-nitrosamines in animal and human tissues, identical pathways of metabolic activation have been conclusively proven (Bogovski 1981). Cancerous tumors were induced by nitrosamine in 39 different animal species, with no species resistant to these substances (Preussmann 1983). In 1937, it was reported that two laboratory scientists had died after exposure to dimethylnitrosamine (Freund 1937). Since the 50s, autopsy findings have revealed cellular and genetic changes similar to those produced by N-nitrosamine in animal experiments (Magee 1956). In the USA and Germany, patients with fatal nitrosamine poisoning exhibited genotypic mutations and base-pair methylation errors in the DNA, similar to animals treated with nitrosamines (Cooper 1980, Herron 1980).

A 1964 report caused considerable attention: the lethal poisoning of sheep that had eaten feed containing fishmeal, with amines and nitrites added as preservatives. It was shown that both the fishmeal fodder and the sheep meat contained nitrosamine, and that long-term consumption might well prove carcinogenic in the human consumer of mutton (Ender 1964).

However, nitrosamines are to be found in many places in the human environment: in food and beverages, cosmetics, cigarettes and tobacco smoke, at jobs in the rubber and tire industry, in metallurgy, in powdered milk, and elsewhere (overview Loeppky 1994 a). In addition, certain groups of medicines—analgesics, antibiotics and chemotherapeutic agents—exhibit a carcinogenic potential by inducing the production of N-nitrosamines. Lijinsky proved in 1972 that the painkiller aminopyrine could form dimethylnitrosamine in the human organism very rapidly when reacted with nitric acid (Lijinsky 1973). Likewise, Amdinocillin, an amidine-containing antibiotic, and Hexetidine, a frequently used antimicrobial substance, also produce nitrosamine in the body (Loeppky 1994 b). Cancer chemotherapy treatments such as Gemustine (CNU), a nitrosourea product, increased the rate of the appearance of leukemia in stomach cancer patients (Boice 1983). Procarbazine, used in the so-called MOPP treatment scheme in combination with vincristine sulfate, nitrogen mustard, and prednisone—all used extensively for cancer therapy—led to the increased development of cancerous neoplasia of lymphatic cells in the immune system. The International Agency for Research on Cancer (IARC) declared the MOPP combination a human carcinogen, due to its ability for nitrosamine formation (Magee 1996). The carcinogenic effect of the MOPP treatment has been confirmed by animal experiments, (Fong 1992, Souliotis 1994).

40 years ago, the lifting of the prescription requirement for the immunotoxic and carcinogenic nitrogen gas led to its epidemic abuse as a recreational sex-drug.

In light of the fact that it was known since the fifties that organic nitrites in humans can be converted into nitrosamine—a toxic and carcinogenic substance—the FDA's 1960 decision to exclude amyl nitrite from obligatory prescription is baffling. Aside from the weighty carcinogenic effect, this decision had even greater consequences, as was shown earlier in human and animal experiments, in that more specific damage occurred after inhalation of organic nitrites, affecting the circulatory and central nervous systems, the lung epithelium, and hemoglobin (Pearlman 1970).

The introduction of the birth control pill (1961) marked the dawn of an era publicized by the media as the "sexual revolution." The atmosphere of sexual liberation, combined with the new over-the-counter availability of amyl nitrite, led to the heavy abuse of amyl nitrite as a recreational sex-drug in young American adults. This nitrogen inhalant was originally sold in glass ampoules that caused a popping sound when crushed between the fingers, leading to the colloquial slang "poppers." The poppers craze spread quickly, and in 1963 the first report was published on the inhalation of amyl nitrite as a recreational drug (Israelstam 1978). At the same time, the synthetic opiate methadone was imported to the USA as a substitution therapy for heroin addiction; in response to the drop in heroin use, black-market cocaine production was increased. Since this point in time, statistics show that cocaine use in the US rose dramatically. Cocaine spread through the hard drug scene and quickly caught on as a sexual performance-boosting drug, often used in combination with poppers. Compared to the heavy problems associated with the use of hard drugs, and the enormously repressive war against them, poppers seemed like relatively harmless sexual stimulants. It later became apparent, that the complex medical misinterpretation of syndromes at first induced by nitrites, and the mistaken generalized diagnoses of similar immune disturbances from other causes, have claimed just as many victims, at least worldwide, directly and indirectly, as the consumption of hard drugs has to this day. The history of this "confusing" medical interrelation will be covered in detail in subsequent chapters.

In 1964, the first acute symptoms and deaths attributed to poppers were documented in the USA (Lubell 1964). The leading pharmaceutical manufacturer, Burroughs-Wellcome, feared legal consequences and intervened with the FDA, which under pressure ordered the reinstatement of obligatory prescriptions for amyl nitrite in 1969.

However, this belated countermeasure could not prevent the uncontrolled availability of amyl nitrite (Newell et al. 1984, 1988). Furthermore, the recreational drug market was inundated with products containing organic nitrites in the form of butyl and isobutyl nitrites, which cause similar effects as amyl nitrite. These copycat substances had a different FDA classification to amyl nitrite; while not to be used for medicine or cosmetics, they could be sold freely for commercial purposes, e.g. as intermediate products during perfume manufacture or even as antifreeze. Usually they were offered under imaginative trade names such as room odorizers. The sales volume was considerable; in only one US city, annual proceeds were estimated at 50 million dollars (Sigell 1978). In 1979, an estimated 5 million Americans used poppers more than once a week (Mayer 1983). By a conservative estimate, recreational consumption of nitrites was placed at 250 million bottles per year (Lowry 1980). Between 1979 and 1985, studies showed that more than 10% of college students had tried poppers, and 0.5% of them used them daily (Johnston 1986, Lange 1988). However, surveys of teenagers and students in the US at the end of the 1970s and beginning of the 1980s reflect only a narrow slice of the murky problem of nitrite abuse, which inevitably resulted in chronic nitrite poisonings in the Western world (Schwartz 1988).

The effects of nitrite intoxication as desired by homosexuals

In the summer of 1969, a milestone event in gay history occurred: the infamous street fight between homosexual men and the police in front of the Stonewall Inn at Christopher Street in New York City. To this day, gays and lesbians around the world celebrate this event annually as Christopher

Street Day, or Gay Pride. This event marked the beginning of a decade in which a minor subset of homosexual and bisexual men saw an explosive increase in promiscuity, accompanied by the excessive supply of nitrite-containing sexual doping agents (Young 1995, overview Lauritsen 1986, Haverkos 1988, Root-Bernstein 1993). Authentic reports documenting the type and number of homosexual sex-acts show that the normal physical and psychological capacity for psychosexual stress was exceeded, in many cases on a long-term basis, by means of nitrite-containing doping agents and multiple performance-enhancing drugs, not to mention substantial antibiotic abuse (Levine 1982, Root-Bernstein 1993). Such accumulation of multiple stressors was unprecedented in medical history.

In 1975, it was reported in an overview work titled "Amyl Nitrite ('poppers') as an Aphrodisiacum" that some homosexual nitrite abusers could not experience normal sexual performance without the regular inhalation of organic nitrites (Everett 1975, Sigell 1978). This realization of the potentially addictive character of the uncontrolled use of organic nitrites as psychosexual doping agents, in accordance with the addiction criteria by the Diagnostic and Statistical Manual (DSM III) of the American

Psychiatric Association was acknowledged during a 1978 clinical-psychiatric investigation (overview Haverkos 1988).

All of the organic nitrite mixtures available on the Western recreational drug market produce the same effects; some of these effects are desirable, while others are not (Nickerson 1979, Pryor 1980).

The acute dose-dependent effects, particularly desirable among some homosexual men include:

- Relaxation of the smooth muscle, facilitating the opening of the anal sphincter during intercourse,
- Vasodilation of the penile blood vessels, resulting in stronger erection,
- Euphoric "high" by increase of the intracranial pressure, via dilation of cerebral blood vessels,
- A feeling of warmth,
- Reduced pain threshold in the receptive partner during anal sex,
- Enhancement of sexual pleasure (thought to prolong orgasm),
- Reduction of social and sexual inhibitions.

The acute, dose-dependent unwanted effects include:

- Abrupt drop in blood pressure (flushing),
- Tachychardia (abrupt increase of the heartbeat for the maintenance of the blood supply to vital organs),
- Rapid pulse rate and pounding sensations,
- Heat loss and chills
- Skin irritation upon direct contact to lip, nose, penis, scrotum and elsewhere,
- Allergic reactions,
- Tracheobronchitis with cough, fever, coughing up blood (hemoptysis), difficulty in breathing,
- Dizziness, headache, nausea,
- Disturbances in oxygen transport of the red blood cells methaemoglobinemia) (Bruckner 1977, Jackson 1979, Haley 1980).

The first diagnosed homosexual AIDS patients, 20 years ago, were chronic nitrite consumers.

The high point of the ubiquitous saturation of the US gay scene with habitual use of amyl, butyl and isobutyl nitrites, which were frequently contaminated with chemical impurities, can be dated from 1974-1977 (Newell 1988). Similarly, this behavior peaked in the European gay centers between 1977 and 1980. At this time, a systematic mass-poisoning by organic nitrites occurred within the majority of the gay scene; remarkably, there were hardly any clinical studies regarding the chronic and cumulative post-effects of long-term and high-dose intoxication by organic nitrites. In particular, the annals of medical history had never witnessed nor investigated the mass consumption of organic nitrites in connection with multiple infectiosity, abuse of a multiplicity of antimicrobial substances, the promiscuous ingestion of substantial quantities of strongly oxidizing semen, unprotected anal intercourse, the consumption of a variety of psychotropic drugs with immunosuppressive effects, the disturbance of sleep cycles as a function of the party lifestyle, etc. Almost zero usable research data was available to estimate the primary and secondary effects on the particularly nitrite-sensitive cells of the endothelial blood vessels, immune system, and brain, under concommitant burden of multiple stressors.

Starting in 1978, unusual medical symptoms began to appear in US homosexual patients. Of note were malignant cancers of the endothelial cells, the flat cells that thinly line the walls of the blood and lymph vessels. The first cases of this illness were officially identified in the middle of 1981, when a brief report was published regarding five cases of illness in homosexual men, who suffered from an opportunistic lung infection which in some cases resulted in death; all of these homosexual patients were nitrite abusers (CDC 1981 a, CDC 1981 b). The attending physicians were helpless against this disease that occurred in "previously healthy homosexual men" (Gottlieb 1981), and assumed that a viral infection must have weakened the immune defense. The fact that these homosexual patients were habitual nitrite abusers was only mentioned casually, and not initially discussed in further detail. Since the middle of 1982, when increasing numbers of homosexual patients were diagnosed with Karposi's sarcoma (KS) and Pneumocystis carinii pneumonia (PCP), as the two diseases are medically termed, these medical cases were generalized as "acquired immune deficiency syndrome" (AIDS) for the purpose of epidemiological accounting. To this day, PCP and KS remain the most frequently diagnosed clinical manifestations of AIDS in homosexual patients.

Background to the "politically correct" misinterpretation of the toxic and pharmacotoxic causes of cancer and immune weakness as a viral infection.

The fact that the attending physicians first attributed the disturbance of the immune response in homosexual patients, as demonstrated by the cases of PCP and KS, to a microbial infection, shows the mental attitude of modern medicine, which has dominated many important disease theories since the discovery of microbes by Louis Pasteur in the middle of the 19th century (overview Wangensteen 1979). This approach is based on the idea that microbes, organisms with extraordinary abilities to mutate, repeatedly attack the integrity of the human organism in incalculable ways. The crucial historical question of medicine is more elementary: which is more important, the milieu of the human organism or the microbes which settle in it? The AIDS doctors, imprinted with the predominance of microbes in all etiology by prevailing medical thought, rashly answered with the frightening vision: that a previously unknown agent, probably a new type of sexually-transmitted virus, infected and progressively destroyed certain immune cells of the AIDS patients, inevitably resulting in death by normally harmless pathogens (Friedman-Kein 1984, Haverkos 1982). The circumstances of this "tragic premature consensus" (Root-Bernstein 1993) regarding the cause of these AIDS indicating diseases are extraordinarily complex and multi-layered. The most important factor, however, is the political climate of cancer research in the US and other Western countries.

In 1971, the US Congress announced a new research priority: the hunt for cancer-causing retroviruses. Nixon, the Republican President at that time, compared the new retrovirus cancer research project to the landing of US astronauts on the moon, and the Manhattan Project which built the atom bomb during WWII. This "War on Cancer" became a national priority, and was anticipated to succeed within ten years. Record amounts numbering billions of dollars were invested in retrovirus and cancer research at the expense of other research activities (Duesberg 1996, De Harven 1998 c).

By 1981, at exactly the same time that the retrovirus cancer project had run its course, and was deemed a failure, the first AIDS cases were diagnosed. The horrific idea of a deadly retroviral infection, transmittable to anyone by sex and blood, was forced by the now penniless retrovirus cancer researchers, whose high-tech job skills were now most conveniently available for retrovirus-AIDS research (De Harven 1998 c).

In 1992, the American Chemical Society (ACS) lamented that "research emphasis has also been impacted by governmental policy decisions and funding priorities . . . Beginning in 1980 significant policy and regulatory philosophy changes in the U.S. toward hazardous contaminants, such as nitrosamines, have resulted in very little information on nitrosamine occurrence during the intervening period. A great deal of work on the chemistry and biochemistry of nitrosamines as it relates to their occurrence and carcinogenic properties has been done in Germany, however. The German government sponsored a *Schwerpunkt* program under the direction of Rudolph Preussmann of the German Federal Cancer Research Institute. This program was very successful in revealing and eliminating many of the hazards due to volatile nitrosamines in that country and had a world-wide impact. The program, however, ended in 1982 and the general level of research in this area has also diminished considerably" (Leoppky 1994 c).

As the ACS was quoted, 1980 marked the change of political power in the US, and a similar regime change in Germany occurred in 1982. 1980 saw the election of the Republican Governor and former Hollywood actor, Ronald Reagan, as President of the USA. His Vice President was the former CIA boss, George Bush, who in 1977 had become the director of Eli Lilly Pharmaceutical Co. Bush succeeded Reagan to become President himself, between 1988-1992. In 1982, Helmut Kohl, who began his professional career with the chemical industry lobbyist group "Verband der Chemischen Industrie," became Federal Chancellor of Germany (1982-1998). Political pressure from the food and agriculture industry, tobacco, pharmaceuticals, chemical, metal, rubber, and other industries, was a definite hindrance to research funding and progress. However, independent of these politics, research on nitrite and nitrosamine had a crucial handicap. It was known since the 50's that exposure to nitrites and nitrosamine produced unique toxic and carcinogenic effects in numerous mammals, including humans (Barnes 1954, Magee 1956, Magee 1976). It was also known that organic nitrites in the body are converted into free-radical nitrite ions (Sutton 1963). Yet scientists did not have a sufficient understanding of the biochemical and bioenergetic transformation of these materials in living cell systems, despite a substantial improvement in detection procedures for gaseous and non-gaseous nitrogen compounds.

Above all, it was not yet known that gaseous nitric oxide and its metabolites are produced within all living cells including the cells of the human body, and play a central role in both physiological and pathophsysiological metabolic processes. This crucial research gap explains why many laboratory scientists and physicians, not understanding the underlying processes in diseases like AIDS, traced the cause of cancer and numerous other local and systemic illnesses back to virtually nonexistent viruses. The presence of these phantom pathogens was deduced from metabolic products, the proof of which the medical profession tried to explain with untenable laboratory jargon. The medical and scientific community, as well as the patients, readily swallowed these cryptic explanatory models as fact, since they corresponded to the familiar pattern of thinking: that the insidious lap of nature continually gives birth to dangerous germs; and not rather that mankind is responsible for the risk of disease, through unawareness of, or disregard for the laws of co-evolution between microbes and humans.

Fortunately, parallel to the generously funded retrovirus cancer and retrovirus-AIDS research, innovative scientific realizations flourished between 1978, the year of the first AIDS diagnoses, all the way through 1998, when the Nobel Prize for Medicine was awarded for the discovery of the bioregulation of human cell systems by gaseous nitrogen oxides. These new insights not only led to the revision of many previously valid disease theories, but also revolutionized the foundations of elementary human biology.

Chapter II

The Sensational Discovery

Gaseous nitrogen monoxide as a bioenergetic regulator within and between living cells—the gas war between humans and microbes

In scientific research, the following principle applies: a theory enables valid claims only if it describes as many model observations as possible (using as few unproven assumptions as possible) and makes verifiable predictions regarding future observations. Reproducible - mutually verifiable

The lengthy and late proof of the existence and function of nitrogen oxides in human blood vessels, immune cells, and nerves

In 1916, the biochemist Mitchell observed that humans excrete more nitrites and nitrates than they could have ingested from food. However, Mitchell and his colleagues could not locate the source of nitrite and nitrate excretion in the human body. Mitchell made an astute statement, the validity of which would only be acknowledged 70 years later: "The problem is of peculiar theoretical interest, since the production of an oxidized radicle [sic] by animal tissues would be unique" (Mitchell 1916). Mitchell's prediction regarding the "uniqueness" referred to the fundamental acceptance that nitrogen oxides could not be formed in the environment of mammalian cells. This belief remained unquestioned for decades.

In 1978, the synthesis of nitrites and nitrates was thought to be explained by the activities of microbes in the human small intestine (Tannenbaum 1978). Soon thereafter, the same research group corrected this interpretation, using evidence that rats purged of gut bacteria still produced nitrates in the small intestine. From this finding it was concluded that nitrites and nitrates are actually synthesized in mammalian cells in their own unique metabolic pathway (Green 1981). Thus it was for the first time demonstrated, in opposition to a long-held dogma, that nitrites and nitrates are actually created internally (endogenously) by mammalian cells, independent of the exogenous supply of organic nitrites and nitrates, that is, from outside the body, (i.e. from food, medicine, or "Poppers").

At the same time, important realizations were made regarding the biological action of exogenous nitrites and nitrates. In 1973, the action of orally ingested organic nitrates was tested; they could not be found in the bloodstream after consumption, so it was assumed that they were rapidly metabolized. Beginning in 1976, however, the US research groups of Diamond and Murad showed that the vasodilatory effect of organic nitrates was based on the activation of ferrous enzymes (Diamond 1976, Murad 1978). In this context, Murad first hypothesized that the endothelial cells of the blood vessels release nitric oxide (NO). Ignarro's research group confirmed this by demonstrating that NO bound with iron in the enzyme guanylate cyclase. This in turn activates the production of a messenger substance, cyclic guanosine phosphate, in the vascular smooth muscle cells. In this way the blood vessel is relaxed, thus lowering the blood pressure (Gruetter 1979). Ignarro and his colleagues also made the pivotal connection that organic nitrites must be metabolized into gaseous NO, in order to create the vasodilatory effect. They showed that molecules of NO bind with sulfur-containing molecules in the cellular metabolism, to create nitrosothiols (Ignarro 1981). This finding would later turn out to be extremely relevant to AIDS research; the exhaustion of thiol by nitroso-bonding, for example, caused by a continual surplus of exogenous nitrite/NO (Poppers!) and/or endogenous NO (chronic infectiosity), would lead to extreme reactions and counter-reactions in the immune cells, in addition to other consequences. Unfortunately, at the time of the first publicized clinical cases of AIDS in 1981, the research of Murad and Ignarro was not yet acknowledged; prominent cardiac researchers were still quite convinced that NO could not be synthesized in mammalian cells (Ignarro 1992). It was not until 1998 that, together with Furchgott, they were awarded the Nobel Prize for Medicine for the discovery of the biological role of NO (Ignarro 1992).

The Furchgott research group got lucky when, somewhat accidentally, they discovered further crucial findings in 1980. The pharmacologists found that the smooth muscle relaxation of blood vessels in response to vasodilatory nitrogen compounds is dependent on intact endothelial cells. Some of the endothelial cells were accidentally damaged in preparation, which prevented vasodilation from occurring. This accidental damage led to the conclusion that only intact endothelial cells were able to deliver the vasodilatory signalling chemical to the neighboring smooth muscle cells. This messenger compound was dubbed endothelium-derived relaxing factor (EDRF) (Furchgott 1980). Finally, in 1986 Ignarro and Furchgott independently postulated that EDRF was identical to gaseous NO. In 1987, the laboratories of Ignarro and Moncada furnished the first direct biochemical proof that NO is formed by the endothelial cells, and diffuses through the cellular membrane into the nearby smooth muscle cells (Ignarro 1987, Palmer 1987).

This time the skeptical researchers finally suspended their disbelief, because research in immunology had already proven that mammals could actually synthesize endogenous nitric oxide. The same research group that in 1981 proved the biosynthesis of nitrates in mammalian intestinal mucosa detected very high quantities of nitrate in the urine of an experimental subject with diarrhea. The researchers concluded correctly that the nitrate had formed from inflammatory reactions caused by the diarrhea. This was verified by injecting rats with bacterial proteins called endotoxins, which are biochemical lipopolysaccharides (LPS) composed of fat and sugar. The rats exhibited increased quantities of nitrate in their urine (Wagner 1983). Thus fortuitously the researchers had come to discover one of the most important immune-cell reactions: the production of nitrogen compounds in immune cells after stimulation by toxic microbial proteins. In 1985, American laboratory researchers furnished the unique proof in studies with mice; they found that macrophages (cells which digest foreign matter), present all throughout the body, exercise a central function for the non-specific immune defense; in response to contact with bacterial LPS, the cells form a gas cloud of nitrites and nitrates, which penetrates the bacterial membrane and disrupts its metabolic processes. The cell-killing (cytotoxic) effect of nitrogen compounds, as a defensive weapon of mammalian cells against bacteria, had been discovered at last (Stuehr 1985). In subsequent studies, other researchers demonstrated that the amino acid L-arginine, present in every cell of the body as a building block for protein synthesis, was also necessary for the synthesis of the cytotoxic nitrogen compounds used by macrophages (Hibbs 1987).

A short while later it was published that macrophages, if activated by special cellular communication proteins synthesized by all immune cells and other bodily cells, oxidize L-arginine into nitrite and nitrate, forming NO gas as an intermediary product (Marletta 1988). These communication proteins are called cytokines, since they act within and between cells to precisely regulate important cellular functions. Currently, about a dozen cellular proteins are recognized as members of the cytokine family. Later that year, Moncada et al. proved that endothelial cells in walls of the blood vessels also synthesize NO gas from L-arginine (Palmer 1988).

The crucial questions that AIDS researchers failed to ask

Because of the research findings secured in 1988, a crucial question arose as to whether the functional disturbances that the AIDS patients demonstrated (among certain immune cells, resulting in "opportunistic infections"; and within endothelial cells in the walls of blood and lymph vessels, resulting in the cancer-like Kaposi's sarcoma and lymphoma) could be triggered by plausible nonviral causes.

AIDS researchers failed to ask the following crucial questions :

1. Whether the long-term inhalation of organic nitrites in combination with the intake of medicines that enhance the formation of NO and nitrosamine could lead to supra-elevated production of NO or its decay product nitrosamine?
2. Whether exposure to microbial toxins through chronic infection could lead to increased NO and nitrosamine production?
3. Whether an imbalance in cytokine synthesis as the net effect of exogenous and endogenous stimulation could result in production of NO gas and its biochemical decay products?
4. Whether the binding of overproduced NO to nitrosamine and/or sulfonamide detoxification metabolites to form nitrosothiol could result in the long-term exhaustion of the thiol pool?

These precise biochemical and bioenergetic crucial questions were not asked by the experimental and clinical AIDS researchers. The "tragic premature consensus" (Root-Bernstein 1993) blocked these plausible questions in favor of the consequence-fraught disease theory of a "new infectious agent" (Haverkos 1982).

The discovery of the archaic enzyme used for the biosynthesis of NO gas

Parallel to the realizations in immunological and cardiac research, NO gas was shown to be a neurotransmitter in the central and peripheral nervous system. In 1982, a research group found that the activation of cyclic guanosine monophosphate mediated the inhibition of impulses between nerves and muscles—similar to the processes between the endothelial cells and the smooth muscle fibers in the blood vessels (Bowman 1982). This inhibitor was identified as NO in 1988 (Martin 1988); the same year, published findings showed that if certain neurons in the brain were stimulated by the excitatory neurotransmitter glutamate, they delivered a messenger substance to nearby cells, which as in the muscle cells activated the ferrous enzyme guanylate cyclase, causing the formation of the important secondary messenger substance cyclic guanosine monophosphate (Garthwaite 1988). One year later, it was proven that nitrite and nitrate were synthesized from L arginine in brain cells from cattle (Schmidt 1989). This finding was corroborated by evidence that NO is synthesized from L-arginine in the brain cells of rats (Garthwaite 1989). A further important discovery was made by American brain researchers, who in 1990 established for the first time in mammalian brain cells, the enzyme which uses molecular oxygen (O_2) to liberate gaseous NO from L-arginine. This process also requires the presence of calcium (Ca^{2+}). The calcium ion, when bound to a protein called calmodulin, was found to control the activity of this newly discovered enzyme called NO synthase (NOS) (Bredt 1990).

A short time later came the proof of an NO synthase in endothelial cells, which is also regulated by Ca^{2+} and calmodulin. The NOS enzyme of the endothelial cells was found to have a slightly different structure than the NOS enzyme of the nerve cells (Pollock 1991).

At the same time, a third NO synthase was isolated in activated macrophages (Stuehr 1991). This NOS enzyme is fundamentally different from the Ca^{2+}-dependent NO synthases in the endothelial and neuronal cells; it can produce NO gas in large quantities and for a longer time, as long as the stimulation persists and the supply of L-arginine and other factors are provided.

The pioneering work of NO researchers in immunology, cardiology, and neurology released an unparalleled explosion of research (overview Lincoln 1997). In 1992, the prominent research journal "Science" named NO as the molecule of the decade. In 1998, the Nobel Prize was awarded to the American physician Murad and the American pharmacologists Ignarro and Furchgott, for their innovative discoveries in nitric oxide (NO) research. The Nobel Prize committee spoke of a "sensation."

The regulation of electron flows and proton gradients (redox equilibrium) by NO and its derivatives

Why were the discovery of the existence, and the various functions of gaseous nitrogen monoxide (NO) in mammalian cells systems, including humans, so sensational?

Nitrogen monoxide = nitric oxide = NO is one of the smallest molecules found in nature. It consists of a nitrogen and an oxygen atom. From this molecular combination, an unpaired electron results. NO is thus a radical: it can snatch away an electron from other atoms and molecules, thereby oxidizing them. The uptake of an electron (as well as a positively charged hydrogen ion, a.k.a. proton) by a receiving molecule is called reduction; conversely, the donation of an electron (as well as a hydrogen ion) is called oxidation. In living cells, the effective proportion of reduced substances to oxidized substances is called the redox balance. The redox potential can be measured in millivolts, for instance at the membrane of cells or their organelles.

A distinguishing feature of living cells is the dynamic maintenance of energy flows away from thermodynamic equilibrium. This is done via constant electron transfer, which at the same time produces proton gradients to increase or decrease the electromotive force.

A fundamental principle of evolutionary biology states that the more complex an organism has evolved, the more reduced it must be. In order to ensure the necessary predominance of the reduction status, any oxidation of a molecule or an atom (in each case by other molecules which can deliver electrons and protons) must quickly be reduced again. In living cells, this takes place particularly by means of sulfur-containing amino acids, sulfurous peptides with low molecular weight, and other sulfurous molecules. These sulfur molecules, biochemically termed thiols, together form a bodily reservoir known as the thiol pool. Thiols possess sulfur-hydrogen bonds, which contain an unpaired electron. This gives them a reductive capacity, in which they can exchange protons and electrons with other atoms and molecules. In this manner thiols can neutralize oxygen radicals and NO radicals. If the thiols are consumed by strong formation of oxygen and/or NO radicals, and free radicals can be no longer sufficiently controlled and neutralized, substantial shifts in the redox status will occur either in the entire cell or its component structures. Vital molecules such as proteins, nucleic acids, fatty acids and many other biological substances are damaged by reactive oxygen species (ROS) and reactive nitrogen species (RNS), which are created by oxidative and nitrosative stress reactions. Too much damage can give rise to mutations and under certain conditions lead to cell death. Between these extreme responses to pro-oxidation (oxidative and/or nitrosative stress), various pathophysiological states can occur; dependent on the cell type, the extracellular environment, and a variety of counterregulations. These counterregulations, called into action by thiol deficiency resulting from strong ROS and RNS production, can occur temporarily or on a long-term basis. Knowledge of the regulation and counterregulations, controlled by the thiol-depletion sensor, is critical in solving the mystery of AIDS and cancer.

Since an unpaired electron develops during the formation of NO from L-arginine and molecular O_2, NO is a paramagnetic monoxide radical (NO^0). In addition, it can also assume other redox statuses yielding different characteristics and reactivity: NO^+ (nitrosium) and NO^-(nitrosyl anion). This free-radical characteristic enables NO to bind to metals such as iron in metallic enzymes and in other proteins (metalloproteins). Many enzymes in living cells contain such metalloproteins. Because of this, NO was already used more than 50 years ago to demonstrate metalloenzymes by means of Electron Paramagnetic Resonance (EPR) spectroscopy; in 1983, this procedure demonstrated that bacteria release NO after they come into contact with nitrites. The NO then binds to bacterial metalloenzymes and in this way causes their death (Lancaster 1992). However at that point in time, it did not occur to check whether nitrites and the NO formed from them are also produced in human immune cells as a diffusive gas for microbial defense. The mental block still existed that nitrogen oxides were not formed in mammalian cells. Thus the window of opportunity was missed by a few years in light of the mass poisoning of millions by organic nitrites as a sexual doping agent (poppers), to realize that the provocation of NO synthesis not only inhibits bacterial metalloenzymes, but with excessive and long-term inhalation of poppers also results in substantial regulation and counterregulation of the human immune and other cell systems (acquired immunodeficiency syndrome). Experiments with mice and rats were executed, by fumigation with organic nitrites or nitrosamine supplied via intranasal drip. It would have been possible to prove unique toxic effects in a variety of immune cell types after exposure to nitrites via animal experimentation or small groups of volunteer subjects, but the actual biochemical mechanism had not yet been recognized (overview Haverkos 1988).

NO gas as a soluble and diffusive messaging substance, which does not need target receptors

NO is not the most reactive of free-radicals, since it cannot react with itself. In the aqueous solution of biological cell systems, in presence of O_2, it has a half-life of less than 30 seconds. Since NO is electrically neutral however, it can disperse freely within and between cells, and diffuse unhindered across the membranes of cells and their organelles. These characteristics led to the long-held assumption that NO was not a suitable candidate for an intracellular messaging substance.

Until the end of the 80s, it was assumed that only complex molecular structures, emitted by precisely controlled mechanisms, could relay messages to complementary receptive target structures. In this manner a large distance between the message source and the receptor cells can be overcome, as is the case with hormones in the bloodstream. It was also known that transmission pathways of a very short range existed, as is the case with biochemical signal transmission between nerve cells (neurotransmitters). For hormonal messengers, special receptors on the cell membrane are not necessarily needed, as they can also penetrate into the target cell and interact with internal receptors (e.g. the hormone cortisol). In contrast, neurotransmitters do their work at receptor sites on the target cell. In both cases, the messenger molecule must make contact with a specific receptor. Therefore only specialized target systems should be able to synthesize the compatible messenger materials. Yet some exceptions to this biological rule are known. For example, prostaglandins occurring in many cell types, and adenosine triphosphate (ATP), the key molecule for energy metabolism synthesized in all living cells; both act as functional messengers between different cell types. Thus, molecules can play an important role in the metabolism of individual cells, as well as fulfil highly specialized functions between different cell types. A prerequisite, however, is that these molecules, active throughout the cells, once outside the cell boundaries find specific receptors on or in the recipient cells.

So far unique throughout evolutionary biology however, is the fact that NO, after synthesis and release from the originating cell to the adjoining cells, can cause a specific modification of the redox processes—without having to bind, for this purpose, to highly complex receptor molecules. These neighboring cells can be normally differentiated body cells, red blood corpuscles, tumor cells or any kind of microbial cells. The effects which NO produces in living cells, either within or between them, depend therefore not on the molecular shape, but solely on the characteristic of being a paramagnetic radical (Snyder 1992).

The NO synthesis enzymes have been evolutionarily conserved

Contrary to the simple structure of NO, three isoforms of the NO-synthesizing enzyme, NO-synthase (NOS), were discovered, the first one in 1991. Close examination showed that these enzymes had a unique structure never before seen in mammalian cells. It was demonstrated that these enzymes are actually a combination of two different enzymes. This assertion applies both to the calcium-dependent isoforms, nNOS (first discovered in nerve cells) and eNOS (first discovered in endothelial cells), and to the calcium-independent isoform, iNOS (first discovered in phagocytes). One half of the NOS enzymes supplies the electrons for the synthesis of NO by means of O_2 from arginine, while the other half carries out the actual synthesis. A comparable enzyme that donates electrons has so far only been found in bacteria (Marletta 1993).

Comparative investigations of the three isoforms of NOS show a 50% commonality between the structures of the NOS subtypes. Furthermore, a comparison of these NOS isoforms in various mammalian species demonstrated a 90% structural equality. Thus, from an evolutionary-biological perspective, the structure of the NOS enzymes has been highly conserved (Knowles 1994, Nathan 1994, Sessa 1994).

Nitrogen oxides are an ancient principle for communication within and between cells, which interact with metal ions and sulfur-hydrogen bonds, in order to adjust the redox potentials

The central findings of NO research can be summarized as follows:

- The unique function of the NO molecule in all living cells, from bacteria to humans.
- The uniqueness of the NO-synthesizing enzyme among thousands of enzymes in mammalian cells, human cells included, with the only occurrence of a similar enzyme being found in bacterial cells.
- The high degree of structural equality between the isoforms of the NO-synthesizing enzyme throughout evolution favors the perspective that NO gases and their synthesizing enzymes are an age-old communication principle within and b between single-celled organisms, a principle which was retained by multi-cellular organisms and has thus been evolutionary and biologically conserved. This regulatory strategy works via the short-term modification of redox statuses, as NO is a paramagnetic radical which can, as an uncharged molecule, diffuse freely within and between cells; it binds with metalloproteins, especially ferrous enzymes. The bioenergetic modification of the redox potentials caused by this process are counter-regulated by sulfurous bonds (nitrosothiol), especially by high concentrations of low-molecular weight sulfur bonds, for example glutathione and cysteine, which together with other thiols form an anti-oxidative resevoir against ROS and RNS.

NO and its descendants are indispensable for the killing or restraint of intracellular pathogens

Over the course of the evolution, two strategies of NO production developed:

- Synthesis of small amounts, dependent on the level of intracellular calcium, has been proven in practically all human cell systems and is involved in a multiplicity of physiological and pathophysiological processes (Moncada 1991).
- The inducible large-quantity and long-lasting NO production, which is carried out by activation of the calcium-independent enzyme iNOS. The iNOS enzyme and the corresponding high output of NO gas clouds were proven in numerous non-specific and specific cell types of the human immune cell network, especially in macrophages and monocytes, microglial cells of the brain, Kupffer's cells, spleen cells, neutrophilic leukocytes and T-cells (overview Kroencke 1995, Lincoln 1997).

Due to the realization that immune cells produce cytotoxic (cell-restraining or cell-killing) NO gas, the question of crucial interest was whether an elimination of NO synthesis within mammalian immune cells would cause a measurable reduction of the immune defense against microbial agents. This question, central to infectious-disease medicine, was tested in numerous cleverly devised experiments.

For example, a research group working with knock-out mice blocked the gene responsible for the protein biosynthesis (expression) of the inducible NOS enzyme. These mice could no longer produce cytotoxic NO gas in the appropriate immune cells. In other experiments, the cytotoxic NO synthesis in immune cells was prevented by iNOS inhibitors. These types of experiments all showed the same thing: that without sufficient production of cytotoxic NO gas, the ability of the immune cells to restrain or kill microbial agents was heavily suppressed. These particular knock-out mice were shown to be extremely susceptible to bacterial and parasitic infections, since due to NO inhibition their activated macrophages could no longer kill bacteria (Wei 1995 a, MacMicking 1995, overview Lincoln 1997). Such experiments led to another important realization: macrophages of knock-out mice in which iNOS synthesis was blocked could no longer restrain the growth and uncontrolled cell division of lymphomas (= rampant cancerous growth of lymphocytes, among other things an AIDS-indicating illness). Likewise, macrophages with blocked iNOS synthesis cannot restrain tumor cells in co-cultivated cell cultures (MacMicking 1995). On the other hand, the expression of iNOS in tumor cells from a multiplicity of cancerous human tissues was demonstrated, for example in ovary, uterine, and breast cancer (Henry 1993, Nussler 1993, Bani 1995, Thomsen 1995).

Many non-immune cells also produce cytotoxic NO gas, and are involved in the inhibition of fungi, parasites, viruses, bacteria and cancer cells

These findings and many others (overview Kroencke 1995, Lincoln 1997) were supplemented by the proof that the following cell systems, including mobile immune cells, can produce cytotoxic NO gas:

- Mucous membrane cells (stomach, intestine, kidney, lung, and many others),
- Endothelial cells,
- Vascular smooth muscle cells,
- Cardiac muscle cells,
- Cartilage cells,
- Bone cells (osteoblasts),
- Fibroblasts of the connective tissue,
- Keratinocytes of the skin,
- Liver cells,
- Pancreatic cells,
- Astrocytes in the brain,
- Peripheral nerve cells (overview Kroencke 1995, Lincoln 1997).

Within a few years it could be demonstrated to the world that in practically all cell systems of the human organism, with appropriate stimulation, the universal diffusive messenger gas NO plays a crucial role in the regulation of the redox potentials, both within cells and between neighboring cells, e.g.: between immune cells and microbes, local mucous membrane cells and microbes, normally differentiated cells and cancerously transformed cells.

The research explosion of experimental and clinical NO research leads to the revision of disease theories and treatment strategies in many important areas of medicine

Since that time, experimental and clinical study of gaseous nitrogen monoxide and its biochemical descendants in human cell systems has had a profound impact on the understanding of elementary disease processes. Below is a partial list, with some references, of the medical fields affected by the new nitrogen research:

- Immunology (von Rooijen 1997, MacMicking 1997, Zidek 1998, Kolb 1998),
- Infectious disease (Clark 1996, 1997; Alexander 1997, Mayers 1997, Liew 1997, Peterhans 1997, Akaike 1998),
- Hematology (Yonetani 1998),
- Oncology (Tamir 1996. Xie 1996, Chinje 1997),
- Cardiology (Habib 1996, Birks 1997, Dewanjee 1997, Matsumori 1997, McQuaid 1997, Wever 1998),
- Diabetes research (McDaniel 1996, Rabinovitch 1998, Sjoeholm 1998),
- Hepatology (Suematsu 1996, Stadler 1996, Ceppi 1997, Taylor 1998, Khatsenko 1998),
- Sepsis research (Beizhuizen 1998, Ketteler 1998, Kirkeboen 1999),
- Lung research (Singh 1997, Sanders 1999),
- Tuberculosis research (Kwon 1997),
- Organ transplantation research (Krenger 1996),
- Rheumatology (Mijasaka 1997, Ralston 1997, Amin 1998),
- Brain and nerve research (Bolanas 1997, Leist 1998, Vincent 1998, Minghetti 1998, Murayama 1998),
- Multiple Sclerosis research (Parkinson 1998, Santiago 1998),
- Stress and hormone research (McCann 1998 a, 1998 b; Rivier 1998),
- Sleep research (Liew 1995 b),
- Sexual medicine (Guiliano 1997).

The universal function of the cytotoxic NO gasification and of the metabolites derived from this pervasive bio-molecule, as an archaic regulatory principle in human cell systems, has placed into question all previous disease theories—particularly those of AIDS and cancer. However, in light of a dynamic evolutionary view of these disease phenomena, an abundance of findings can be integrated into a revised holistic conceptual understanding.

Chapter III

The AIDS Mystery

Why the AIDS diseases were falsely interpreted—the inhibition of the gas defense is the cause of the acquired immune cell weakness

On June 5, 1981, the first medical report regarding lethal opportunistic infections in US homosexual men was published by the supervising authority for diseases, the Center for Disease Control (CDC), in the weekly report on morbidity and mortality (CDC 1981 a). Of note were five "active homosexuals" between the ages of 29 and 36, who were treated in two Los Angeles hospitals between October 1980 and May 1981. These five patients had no sexual contact with each other. They all suffered from a fungal infection of the lung, which led to a rare form of pneumonia called *Pneumocystis carinii* pneumonia (PCP), as well as previous or current infections with cytomegalovirus (CMV) and a fungal infection of the mucous membranes called candidiasis. Two of the patients had died.

The clinical and immunological findings of the first historically diagnosed AIDS patients

In three of the five patients, tests were run to determine the quantity and reactivity of the immune cells in their blood serum. "All three patients had profoundly depressed *in vitro* [in the test tube] proliferative responses [inhibited maturation] to mitogens [substances which energize the cell division] and antigens [substances which activate the T-helper immune cells]" (CDC 1981 a).

The report did not give any details of prior consumption of antibiotics, antifungals, antiparasitics, antivirals, chemotherapeutic agents, or corticosteroids. It was only stated succinctly that "the 5 did not have comparable histories of sexually transmitted disease." The complete oversight or inadequate investigation of the prior use of antibiotics, etc. (whether medically or self-prescribed), would become an unfortunate hallmark of subsequent AIDS medicine and corresponding clinical publications.

In the case of the five patients in Los Angeles, four of them previously had hepatitis B, as determined by serological investigation, but had no current hepatitis S surface antigens. Without any further explanation or discussion, it was casually noted in one sentence that "*all 5 reported using inhalant drugs*, and 1 reported parenteral drug abuse."

Half a year after this historic medical report on AIDS-indicating illnesses in homosexual patients, the attending physicians of the UCLA clinic published a follow-up report on four of the original five patients (Gottlieb 1981). This second report had more specific detail regarding immunological data and clinical procedures.

"These patients presented a distinct and unusual clinical syndrome. All were exclusively homosexual and had been in excellent health before late 1980. Their medical histories did not suggest preexisting immunodeficiency. All were anergic and had infections in which cell-mediated immunity plays the major part in host defense. *P. carinii* pneumonia, extensive mucosal candida infections, and chronic viral shedding were uniformly present .... The most striking abnormalities were the nearly total elimination of Leu-3+ [CD4+] helper/inducer cells and an abnormally increased percentage of Leu-2+ [CD8+] suppressor/cytotoxic cells .... The absolute numbers of cells in both subsets were decreased .... The virtual absence of the Leu-3+ subset was undoubtedly the major contributing factor to the severe immune deficiency observed in our patients. The mechanism of this differential effect on the Leu-3+ subset is still unclear, since cytomegalovirus has not been shown to infect subpopulations of lymphocytes directly .... We acknowledge the possibility that cytomegalovirus infection was a result rather than a cause of the T-cell defect, and that some other exposure to an undetected microorganism, drug, or toxin made these patients susceptible to infection with opportunistic organisms, including cytomegalovirus .... The explanation for the elevated IgA levels in these patients remains unclear" (Gottlieb 1981).

In summary the University physicians observed: "All patients were anergic and lymphopenic; they had no lymphocyte proliferative responses to soluble antigens, and their responses to phytohemagglutinin [a mitogen] were markedly reduced" (Gottlieb 1981).

At the same time, these clinical and immunological findings were acknowledged by several medical centers in New York in sexually active homosexual patients with AIDS-indicating diseases: "None of the patients had cutaneous reactivity to any of the antigens tested. This anergy was present during the acute illness, and it persisted in the patients who were tested for delayed hypersensitivity [DTH, a routine test for the reactivity of the immune cells in the skin, tested by means of a variety of microbial toxins and other substances] more than two weeks after the *P. carinii* pneumonia had clinically resolved . . . . The patients had lower proliferative responses [of the T-helper cells] to various mitogens, antigens, and allogeneic cells [all of which are materials that energize the activation and division of lymphocytes] than did a simultaneously tested age-matched control group. These responses represent the maximal lymphocyte proliferation that could be elicited with a range of concentrations of stimulating substances and cells. Since only pooled normal human serum was used to supplement the lymphocyte-culture mediums, it is not possible that serum suppressor factors had a role in these abnormally low responses. An impaired cellular immune response in the patients, as compared with the controls, was observed in *in vitro* studies of lymphocytes cultured with non-specific inducers of T-lymphocyte activation: phytohemagglutinin, concanavalin A, and the T-cell-dependent inducer of mitosis in B-cells, pokeweed mitogen. Lymphocyte responses to the microbial activators *C. albicans, Staph. aureus, Esch. coli,* and purified protein derivative of tuberculin were also depressed . . . . These tests of lymphocyte proliferation were performed when the patients were not acutely ill. In addition, repeated evaluation more than one month after the first evaluation confirmed the same type of abnormally depressed responses" (Masur 1981).

In 1981, doctors and immunologists did not yet know that there exist both NO-producing and non-NO-producing T-helper immune cells

These historic medical reports clearly show the lack of knowledge in the fields of immunology and clinical infectious medicine in the early 80's; the fact that the T-helper immune cells in AIDS patients were drastically diminished in number and could not be stimulated, was incongruent with the fact that simultaneously the production of certain antibodies was increased. According to the then-valid immune theory, B-cells (B for bone), which mature in the bone marrow, need to receive an activation signal from the T-helper lymph cells which mature in the thymus (T for thymus) in order to produce antibodies against a microbial antigen detected by the T-cells; therefore the designation "helper."

What immunologists and clinicians did not yet know in 1981 was the fact that there are two kinds of T-helper cells: type 1 and type 2, defined accordingly as Th1 and Th2. These two kinds of T-cells behave in markedly different ways:

- Th1 cells are produced and stimulated, compared with Th2, by a different profile of signal and communication proteins from the large family of cytokines. The cytokine profiles of type 1 have the particular characteristic that they stimulate production of cytotoxic NO gas in the Th1-immune cells, as a defense against intracellular microbes. In contrast, the type 2 cytokines cause T-cells to mature into Th2 cells, which produce no cytotoxic NO gas but rather take on the actual helper function, to activate the B-cells and thereby stimulate anti-body production. The type 2 cytokines of the Th2 cells even inhibit the protein expression (biosynthesis) of the enzyme for inducible NO synthesis (overview Lincoln 1997).
- The central study of cytokines only intersected with NO research at the beginning of the 1990s. Unaware of the basic facts regarding the existence of the type 1 and type 2 cytokine-producing T-cells, AIDS doctors were inevitably perplexed by the immunological and clinical findings of their homosexual patients. In the context of this medical helplessness, it can be understood why a hypothetical retrovirus, whose existence was maintained solely as a result of indirect laboratory markers, was so readily accepted as the cause of AIDS.

The biological evolution of a dual strategy for the human immune defense

Now the crucial question to be asked is why does this dual strategy for immune defense exist? This question can only be answered in the context of evolutionary biology, namely the development of the immune defense in invertebrate and vertebrate organisms.

The equivalent of T-cells are first seen in primitive invertebrate animals, for example the sponges, evolving more than 500 million years ago (Roitt 1985). Upon contact with bacterial toxins, T-cells form a cloud of NO gas that diffuses across the bacterial membrane and binds to metalloenzymes or thiol-peptides, paralyzing the energetic metabolism of the invaders and thus rendering them lame or dead. A similar process occurs when macrophages or other special cells present fragments of protein chains (peptides) to the T-cells, as molecular antigen signals. These peptide fragments come from intracellular bacteria, viruses, parasites, or fungi, which were cleaved by protein-splitting enzymes in the antigen-presenting cells. After activation by the antigen signal, the T-cells produce specific cytokines, mature and propagate identically (as clones), and under influence of type 1 cytokines continuously synthesize large amounts of cytotoxic NO. The NO gas diffuses into the antigen-containing cells, which die along with their intracellular passengers. The mouth-like cells of the immune system, the macrophages, usually devour the remaining cellular debris.

When vertebrate animals developed from invertebrates after a long evolutionary epoch, they needed more than just the singular immune response against bacteria, viruses, parasites, and fungi as they were themselves invaded by invertebrate animals, namely worms. Such invaders could not be captured by the macrophages and presented to the T-cells as "fillets." Compared to the single-celled microbes and the smaller multi-cellular parasites, the invertebrate parasites are enormous. Such quantities of the gas-cocktail would have been required from the gas-producing T-cells that the integrity of the defending organism's own cellular systems would be compromised. The host animals would have been damaged and destroyed by their own gas defense.

Thus arose the need for a more modern immune response, and so the immune defense was retrofitted by evolution with the (specific and non-specific) cell-mediated defense, known as the humoral immunity (from the Latin: *humor* = liquid). The humoral immune response has both a specific and nonspecific component. The nonspecific part is called the complement system, which involves a series of proteins occurring in the blood plasma and intracellular fluids, and can be activated in different ways via an intricate cascade of chain reactions. In a very complex way, the complement system is counterregulated by inhibitors and control proteins. The end result of the activated complement cascade is the perforation (opsonization) of cellular membranes, for example those of bacteria, resulting in their destruction. The non-specific complement system is closely coupled to the specific humoral defense system by immunoglobulins: glycoprotein antibodies that are custom manufactured by a special class of lymph cells called the B-cells. As they mature, the B-cells go through a complicated developmental sequence. On their surface, mature B-cells carry cell-bound immunoglobulin (antibody). If a soluble antigen (for example a protein molecule from microbes or the host, or a non-protein molecule) binds to a corresponding antibody-mature B-cell, this antigen is recognized as abnormal and an activation signal is released to other B-cells. Under the influence of the nonspecific (by macrophages) and specific (by T-cells) immune responses, the B-cells divide (by clonal expansion) and mature into antibody-producing plasma cells, which can set their immunoglobulins free as soluble antibodies.

Human antibodies are differentiated into five immunoglobulin (Ig) classes: IgM, IgG, IgA, IgD and IgE. Formation of IgM is the initial response in a humoral immune reaction; IgG and the other sub-classes are formed as a secondary response. Only IgG can cross the placental barrier, conveying protection to the newborn child in the first phase of its life until the development of its own antibodies. The antibodies of the IgA class are found in the serum, and in secretions, for instance in the breathing passages, the digestive tract, and breast milk. IgD is used as receptors on the surface of B-cells in their early maturation phase. IgE plays an important role in parasitic worm infections and allergic reactions.

The plasma cells can manufacture an extraordinary variety of custom-made immunoglobulin proteins, using a relatively small number of genes for synthesis by aggregate combination and rearrangement; these proteins can selectively react with as many abnormal foreign and self proteins and with other molecules. However, due to sophisticated surface properties, specific antibodies can also bind non-specifically with divergent antigens (foreign or self molecules), and conversely the same antigen can interact with many different antibodies (cross-reactivity).

In invertebrate animals, humoral immune factors are called antisomes, and resemble the enzymes of the complement system. With more highly developed invertebrates such as crabs and spiders, these humoral complement factors are already substantially evolved. However, antibody-producing lymphocytes are only possible with the development of bone marrow and a sophisticated circulatory system, which can be traced back to the first amphibians (anurans) and fish (Roitt 1985).

Control over the balance between NO gas defense and antibody immunity

Thus through different stages of biological development, the human immunity evolved different components that require precise coordination. The harmonization between the T-cell system and the antibody-producing B-cells is regulated via cytokine patterns. Like genetic expression (protein biosynthesis), cytokine expression is also redox-dependent (Senn 1996). If the redox status changes, so does the cytokine pattern. If the expressed pattern leans towards type 2 cytokine dominance, more Th2 cells are produced. The consequence is increased antibody formation by the B-cells, since the stimulating relationship between T-helper lymph cells and B-cells is predominantly controlled via the Th2 cells; Th1 cells control only a small branch of antibody production.

Excessive and prolonged NO gas production exhausts the detoxification molecules and prepares the way for AIDS

In the context of evolutionary biology, the development of the complement system and B-cell antibody production are to be regarded as extracellular assistance for the T-cell network (which is responsible for intracellular disposal). Historically in research, however, certain T-cells were regarded as helper cells for the B-cells and therefore were named accordingly. The control circuit behind the cellular immune network, and within the network of organ cells enabled for NO synthesis is, however, far more complex.

Over the course of evolution, the autopoietic (from the Greek: *auto* = self + *poiein* = make, meaning: self-organizing) maintenance of the reduction potential potency, apart from states of scarcity and hunger, naturally proved to be threatened by too great a load of microbial antigens. The unique diffusivity of NO within cells, for the short-term modification of the redox status by means of binding to metalloproteins, could additionally be used as a cell-penetrating cytotoxic defense. NO gas is a double-edged molecular sword: under excessive and/or prolonged antigen presentation, the T-cells are substantially stimulated and produce too many type 1 cytokines. These in turn further energize the cytotoxic NO synthesis, namely by interferon-γ. At the same time, especially by the production of type 1 cytokines, tumor necrosis factor is increased, which in turn increases the formation of oxygen radicals in the mitochondrial respiration chain. The reactive oxygen species (ROS) include, among other things, the superoxide anion (O_2^*), peroxides (hydrogen peroxide (H_2O_2), lipoperoxides) and hydroxyl groups (OH); together the NO radical and the superoxide anion form peroxynitrite, which in large quantities is more toxic than NO.

Excessive production of nitrogen oxides and ROS must be counterregulated against, in order to protect the organism from serious cellular damage due to loss of the reductive potency by hyperoxidization. Thus at this critical juncture, multiple counterregulation programs will intervene. The pivotal control variable is the thiol pool. Since sulfur and oxygen are in the same series of the Periodic Table of Elements [have the same number of valence electrons], reduced thiol electrons (and at the same time protons) can transfer to the radical oxides (NO, CO_2^{*-}). In this way, the redox equilibrium is adjusted within the cell in cooperation with antioxidative enzymes, vitamins and certain coenzymes.

Since the more complex cells of mammals and humans exhibit a greater antioxidative reduction potency than microbes, they can usually adjust to the state of oxidative emergency caused by the chain reaction of antigen stimulation. However, the cells that are directly bombarded with large quantities of NO gas by T-cells suffer programmed cell death, bringing down with them the microbes settled inside. Crucial, however, is the circumstance that the oxidized thiols are brought back to a reduced state by certain enzymes and coenzymes in order to maintain their function as redox regulators. However, if this rebalancing does not occur (perhaps, because the ratio of reduced to oxidized thiols shifted too much towards oxidization; or the supply of available reduced thiol was exhausted, for example by heavy nitrosothiol binding; or due to an insufficient exogenous supply of sulfurous amino acids such as methionine and cysteine, or other thiols) then the low level of thiol pool antioxidants will trigger counterregulations in the particularly redox-sensitive immature T-helper cells. This T-cell sensor, now below a critical threshold, triggers genetic counterregulations that switch the expression of cytokines from type 1 to type 2. The consequence is that the natural equilibrium between the type 1 cytokine T-cells (Th1) and the type 2 cytokine T-cells (Th2), shifts in favor of increased Th2 cells. This means that the immune reaction is relocated predominantly into the extracellular sphere, to the detriment of the intracellular microbial defense. Not enough of the NO-synthesizing Th1 cells are available, and the intracellular microbial defense is weakened. By the increase of the Th2 cells, whose type 2 cytokines suppress NO synthesis, antibody production is increased in the B-cells. Just like the Th1 cells, Th2 cells become activated after antigen stimulation by antigen-presenting cells (APCs, e.g. the ubiquitous dendritic APCs and the macrophages). The difference lies in the fact that unlike Th1 cells, the Th2 immune cells do not spray cytotoxic NO gas, but rather set the antibody synthesis into motion by cytokine signalling to the B-cells. Put casually, the immune defense thus switches from an ancient NO gas war, to the subsequently evolved biological missile attack of the antibodies.

The pros and cons of the dualistic strategy of the immune defense

This dualistic strategy, however, has pros and cons for the infected organism. On one hand, cell systems are protected against heavy nitrogenous and oxidative stress in the case of excessive and/or prolonged burden by antigens and microbial toxins. On the other hand, the complement and antibody defense are not sufficient against a multiplicity of microbes. Bacteria (with the exception of mycobacteria, the agent of leprosy, tuberculosis and other infections) are held relatively well in check by the complement antibody reaction, since their cell membranes are vulnerable to antibodies. However, fungi and parasites possess a more complex cell wall and often have developed their own molecular defense. In mammals and humans they must, just as with mycobacteria and intracellular viruses, be restrained or killed by sufficient NO gasification by the Th1 immune cells, the neutrophilic leukocytes, the macrophages, microglial cells in the brain (which act there as mouth-like cells), and others.

The crucial matter, which thus gives the "opportunity" of infectious seeding to the fungi, parasites, mycobacteria, and intracellular viruses which cause opportunistic infections in AIDS patients, is to determine the cause of the switching from a Th1 response to a predominant Th2 response. This switch is almost certainly related to a suppression of the cytotoxic NO gasification for lack of type 1 cytokines. Additionally, the production of type 2 cytokines further attenuates NO synthesis, and results in increased antibody levels in the blood serum and extracellular fluids.

A rational solution to the apparent AIDS mystery

The immunological observations (anergy and strong reduction in number of T-cells, combined with elevated antibody levels) in the homosexual patients with opportunistic infections in Los Angeles and New York, first published in 1981 (CDC 1981 a, Gottlieb 1981, Masur 1981) must be interpreted retrospectively as the Th1-Th2 switch. The acquired immune deficiency syndrome (AIDS) is the consequence of an acquired exhaustion of the antioxidative thiol pool in the T-helper immune cells and other cell systems. Immunologically, this thiol deficiency syndrome manifests itself by the type 2 cytokine pattern (Th1-Th2 switch), and clinically by opportunistic fungal and parasitic infections, due to reduced production of cytotoxic NO gas by the T-helper immune cells and by increased antibody formation due to successful inhibition of bacterial infections (with the exception of mycobacteria). The cause is an unusually excessive and prolonged nitrogenous and oxidative stress load from:

- nitrite inhalation
- microbial antigen and toxin stimulation
- immunotoxic medicines
- many other stress factors (outline to the pathophysiological stressors of homosexual patients with Root-Bernstein 1993, Haverkos 1988).

For the understanding of AIDS-indicating diseases, it is crucial to realize that the evolutionary and biologically programmed flipping of the cytokine switch is caused by depletion of the thiol pool, independent of the source of NO gas hyperproduction. Thiol exhaustion—as both a sign of excessive and/or prolonged nitrogenous and oxidative stress, and a sensor for the protection of the cell systems by modification of the redox status—switches the pattern of cytokine expression in all cases identically. This occurs, for example, due to excessive and/or prolonged NO production after stimulation with microbial antigens and toxins, and likewise after inhalation of nitrites. The latter is metabolized in the bloodstream into nitrate, and intracellularly as NO. NO can further be bound as nitrosothiol, and stored stably in special cell organelles called lysosomes (Ignarro 1992).

Thus long-term nitrite inhalation simulates the same net effect on the T-helper immune cells as NO gas hyperproduction in response to microbial antigens or toxin exposure. Starting from a critical threshold value in the particularly redox-sensitive and short-lived immature T-helper cells, the predominant cytokine synthesis pattern is adjusted in response to the changed redox environment, and the Th1-Th2 switch flips towards Th2 cell dominance.

This process happens in two phases: a preliminary phase of NO gas hyperproduction with corresponding antioxidative thiol consumption, followed by a phase of the restriction of NO gas production by type 1 cytokine inhibition in the T-helper immune cells and other cell systems. The result is a partial weakness of the cell-mediated immunity, which can be temporary or long lasting.

As to the AIDS clinicians who in 1981 diagnosed the first homosexual AIDS patients with immunological anomalies, the lack of T-helper cells and their anergy is thus plausibly explained by an imbalance of the Th1/Th2 immune cells favoring the type 2 cytokine pattern. The stimulation of the T-helper cells by the usual mitogens and antigens presupposes the presence of certain type 1 cytokines, namely interleukin-2. Anergy is thus primarily based on interleukin-2 insufficiency. The relative total number of T-helper cells, measured only in a sample of blood serum by means of monoclonal antibodies, can be misleading as to the quantity of T-helper cells actually available in the organism. The quantity of T-cells in the blood serum depends on many factors, and is not constant over time. For example, the cortisol level explains the fact that T-cell counts in the morning can be up to 100% lower than in the evening and night hours. This explains the well-known fact that inflammatory illnesses can worsen at night because of the higher Th1 cell quantity and thus higher NO synthesis, which is central to inflammatory processes. Usually only 2-4% of the T-helper cells circulate in the bloodstream; within 24 hours they progress through the lymph fluids in a dormant state (so long as they are not activated to function as effector cells), and flow back into the bloodstream. With a Th1-Th2 switch, the T-cell count in the bloodstream changes. The function of the Th2 lymphocytes is the cytokine-supported stimulation of B-cells for antibody production. Thus they are predominantly outside the bloodstream at their actual work place in the neighborhood of the B-cells, instead of uselessly roaming the bloodstream. The ratio of the B-cells to the T Helper lymphocytes in the bloodstream amounts to 1:6, even though in adults, more B-cells are produced in the marrow than T-helper cells are in the thymus, an organ which usually deteriorates continuously starting from the first year of life.

The AIDS medical profession falsely interpreted, albeit unwittingly, the clinical and immunological findings of:

- The cytotoxic NO synthesis of the Th1 helper cells,
- the inhibition of the cytotoxic NO synthesis by the switch from Th1-Th2 dominance,
- the change of the cytokine pattern from type 1 to type 2,
- the migration of Th2 helper cells into the domain of the B-cells, and
- the evolutionary-biological program of the Th1-Th2 switch controlled by the thiol pool as redox regulator.

Based on the level of knowledge at that time, they believed that the snapshot of a depleted T-helper cell count in circulating blood, combined with anergic reactions in both the DTH skin test and test tube stimulation, was a sign of a T-helper cell defect. As possible reasons for the assumed immune cell defect they considered:

- an unknown microorganism,
- drugs (pharmaceutical or recreational), or
- a toxin (Gottlieb 1981, Masur 1981).

Yet a serious difference exists between an immune cell defect and an immune cell imbalance as the consequence of a systemic functional adjustment of the cellular immune network in response to a changed redox environment. If the cause of the postulated immune cell defect is, for example, an unknown microorganism in the form of a virus that infected the T-helper cells, then this virus would also propagate with each natural cell division of the T-cells, and the subsequently matured T-cells would be defective as well. Additionally, the danger exists that the viruses will migrate from the defective T-helper cells and infect healthy T-cells. The result will be difficult-to-treat opportunistic infections by fungi and parasites. The healing of this progressive immune defect can only occur if one succeeds in medically restraining or killing the assumed viruses in the T-helper cells without destroying the immune cells themselves. If one assumes that the carriers of virus-infected T-helper cells can transfer these through sexual intercourse by means of semen to a sexual partner, or by transfer of blood and blood products to recipients, or from virus-infected pregnant women to their children, then this logic induces the existence of a potentially deadly mass epidemic with unpredictable consequences.

However something important could not be explained by this scenario of a T-cell defect induced by a hypothetical virus: the increased antibody production of the B-cells. In the early 1980s, the dominant paradigm of immunology rightfully held that such defective and decimated T-helper cells could not possibly activate B-cells. Thus the hypothesis of a virally induced T-cell defect resulted in an unsolvable contradiction, which was labelled with the term: "intriguing AIDS puzzle" (Friedman-Kein 1984).

Yet if an imbalance of the immune cells is postulated to be the cause of the clinical and immunological anomalies, then the findings can be explained without contradiction: the cell-mediated immune response of the T-helper cells involving NO synthesis is restrained by the *acquired lack of thiol*, thus the cytokine patterns are reprogrammed and the resulting Th2 dominance stimulates B-lymphocyte activity for increased antibody production; this acquired immune cell imbalance is not contagious, and thus gives no massive viral epidemic transmitted by sex or blood. What can be transferred however, are fungi, parasites, viruses, and bacteria, which in humans with a preexisting immune cell imbalance can lead to opportunistic infections.

We have encountered these illnesses since the beginning of mankind, since the Th1-to-Th2 switch represents an ancient evolutionary-biological mechanism for adjustment to extreme nitrogenous and oxidative stress. Modern medicine only relabelled these symptoms as AIDS, when a subset of homosexual men experimented with a previously unknown combination of nitrite inhalation, consumption of immunotoxic medicines and drugs, as well as multi-infectious antigen and toxin exposure, causing immune cell imbalance as the inevitable outcome. It was the unusual provocation of the immune system that was new, not its response according to evolutionary-biological principles.

If the crucial connection between the role of NO gas, the cytokine patterns, the immune cell switch, and the sulfur detoxification molecules in human cell types, had already been investigated 15 years ago, the alleged "most frightening epidemic illness of the 20th Century" (Gallo 1991) would never have occurred as such. The diagnosis and treatment of Acquired Immuno-Dysbalance Syndrome in place of an Acquired Immuno-Deficiency Syndrome would not have necessitated the presumption of an "undetected microorganism" as cause of the disease (Gottlieb 1981).

Fig. 1) Diagram of some of the important interactions of nitric oxide (NO) and the effects of NO as a physiological messenger and cytotoxic agent.

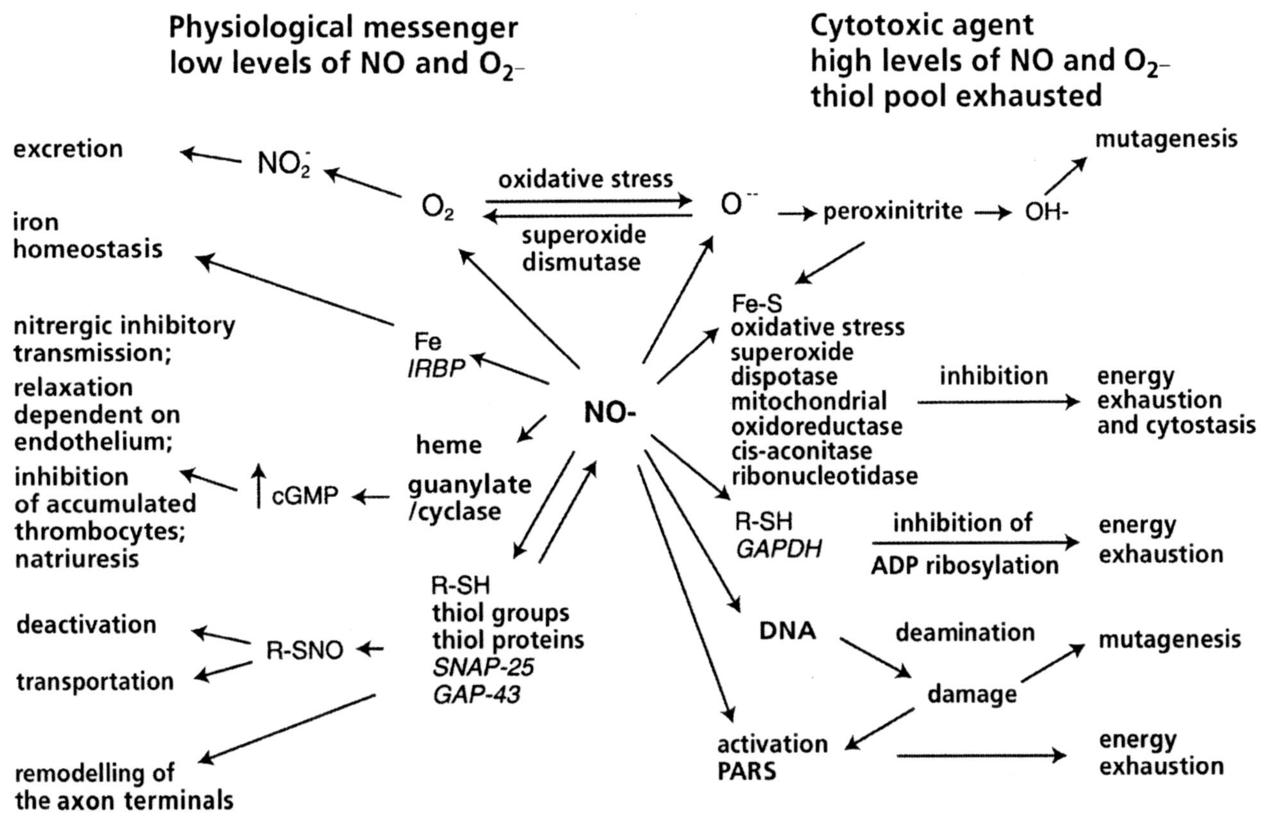
Physiological messenger
low levels of NO and O_2^-
Cytotoxic agent
high levels of NO and O_2^-
thiol pool exhausted
excretion
NO_2^-
O_2
oxidative stress
superoxide dismutase
$O^{\cdot-}$
peroxinitrite
OH-
mutagenesis
iron homeostasis
Fe
IRBP
nitrergic inhibitory transmission;
relaxation dependent on endothelium;
inhibition of accumulated thrombocytes;
natriuresis
NO-
heme
guanylate /cyclase
↑ cGMP
Fe-S
oxidative stress
superoxide
dispotase
mitochondrial
oxidoreductase
cis-aconitase
ribonucleotidase
inhibition
energy exhaustion and cytostasis
R-SH
GAPDH
inhibition of
ADP ribosylation
energy exhaustion
R-SH
thiol groups
thiol proteins
SNAP-25
GAP-43
R-SNO
deactivation
transportation
remodelling of the axon terminals
DNA
deamination
damage
mutagenesis
activation PARS
energy exhaustion

Fig. 2) Immune cells and non-immune cells that synthesize cytotoxic NO gas

A. Immune cells

Macrophages/monocytes (blood *, spinal cord, lungs, peritoneum*)
Kupffer cells
Mesangial cells*
Microglial cells*
Splenocytes
Neutrophiles*
T-lymphocytes including:
Natural killer cells*
Th1 cells (not Th2 cells)

B. Non-immune cells

Epithelial cells (gastric mucosa, intestinal, kidney, lung*)
Endothelial cells (aorta, brain)
Vascular smooth muscle cells
Cardiac myocytes
Chondrocytes*
Osteoblasts*
Fibroblasts
Keratinocytes*
Hepatocytes*
Pancreatic B-cells
Astrocytes*
Neuronal cells

---

*indicates that cytotoxic NO has been found in human cells

Fig. 3) Type-1 and Type-2 Cytokines and other factors that activate or inhibit NO synthesis

Activators/Promoters

- Lipopolysaccharides (LPS)
- Tumor necrosis factor α (TNF-α)
- Interferon-γ (IFN-γ)
- Interleukin-1
- Interleukin-12
- Granulocyte-macrophage colony-stimulating factor (GMCSF)
- Platelet-activating factor (PAF)
- Tumor-derived recognition factor (TDRF)
- Prostaglandins (low concentrations)
- NO (low concentrations)
- Leucotriene B_4
- Cisplatin
- Taxol
- "HIV" proteins
- Heat shock
- Hypoxia

Inhibitors

- Transforming growth factors β
- Glucocorticoids
- Interleukin-4
- Interleukin-6
- Interleukin-8
- Interleukin-10
- Epidermal growth factor (EGF)
- Platelet derived growth factor (PDRF)
- Prostaglandins (high concentrations)
- NO (high concentrations)
- Thrombin
- Noradrenaline
- ATP (via P2Y)
- Nicotinamide
- Glibenclamide
- NF-KB activation inhibitor
- Serine/cysteine protease inhibitor
- BH4 synthesis inhibitor
- Tyrosine kinase inhibitor

Fig. 4) Pathogens and cellular targets of NO

Virus
- Herpes simplex
- Coxsackie virus
- Vaccina virus
- Ectromelia virus

Bacteria
- Francisella tularensis
- Mycobacterium tuberculosis
- Mycobacterium bovis
- Mycobacterium leprae
- Mycobacterium avium
- Listeria monocytogenes
- Chlamydia trachomatis

Fungi
- Cryptococcus neoformans
- Histoplasma capsulatum

Parasites
- Leishmania species
- Trypanosoma, cruci, musculi and brucei
- Plasmodium falciparum, chabaudi
- Toxoplasma gondii
- Schistosoma mansoni
- Entamoeba histolytica

Mammalian cells
- Tumor cells

Fig. 5) Mechanisms of NO gas attack on tumor cells.

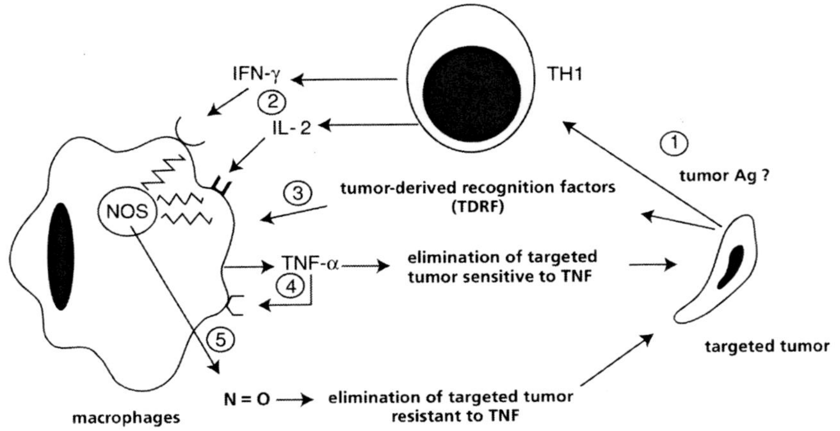
IFN-γ
TH1
②
IL-2
①
tumor Ag ?
③
tumor-derived recognition factors
(TDRF)
NOS
TNF-α
elimination of targeted
tumor sensitive to TNF
④
⑤
targeted tumor
N = O
elimination of targeted tumor
resistant to TNF
macrophages

Fig. 6) NO attack of an immune cell (macrophage or phagocyte) mitochondrium on the nucleus of a tumor cell.

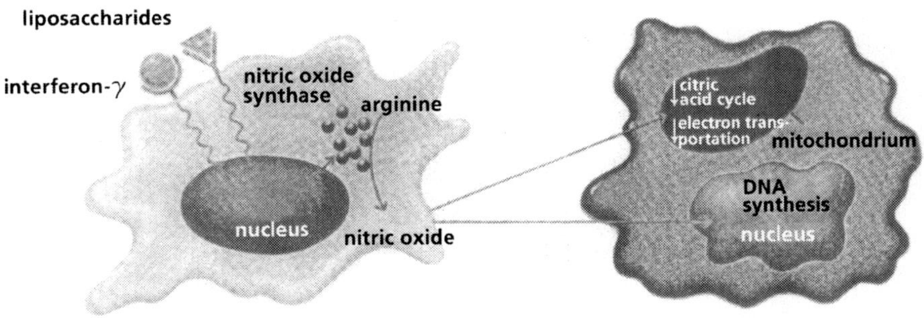
liposaccharides
interferon-γ
nitric oxide
synthase
arginine
nucleus
nitric oxide
citric
acid cycle
electron trans-
portation
mitochondrium
DNA
synthesis
nucleus

Chapter IV

AIDS is not a Contagious Disease

Opportunistic infections and Kaposi's sarcoma were well known before the AIDS era—a variety of causes trigger the same immune response, as programmed by biological evolution

In 1909, the Brazilian microbiologist Chagas published his findings about a particular parasite in the lungs of an infant and termed it *trypanosoma* infection. Trypanosomes are, among other things, the pathogens of sleeping sickness. Research on animals initially substantiated the diagnosis. In 1912 the Italian microbiologist Carini defined a similar pathogen in the lungs of rats as *Trypanosoma lewisi.* The husband and wife team Delanoe in Paris compared the findings of Carini with the results of research on the lungs of sewer rats and proved that they were not trypanosomes but an independent pathogen, which they named *Pneumocystis carinii* (Cantwell 1984, Armengol 1995).

Pneumocystis carinii pneumonia (PCP) is the most frequent AIDS-indicating illness in Western countries, and was seen more than 60 years ago after the use of sulphonamides on premature infants.

It took almost a generation until this pathogen was recognized as clinically relevant in non-bacterial (atypical) pneumonia in premature babies and newborn infants with dystrophy. The latter denotes a protein-energy deficiency syndrome, frequently combined with vitamin deficiencies. The first published reports of cases of *Pneumocystis carinii* pneumonia (PCP, also known as pneumocystis of the lungs) in infants appeared in Germany (Ammich 1938, Benecke 1938). Before the introduction of sulphonamides as anti-bacterial chemotherapy by Domagk (Nobel Prize for Medicine 1939), most of the premature and dystrophic infants died of bacterial infections within the first weeks of life. However, the pharmaceutical containment of the bacterial sepsis precipitated the development of pneumocystis, which was especially prevalent in orphanages. Between the years 1941 and 1948, alone in Switzerland, more than 700 cases of infant pneumocystis were reported, in Hamburg between 1950 and 1954 it was more than 190. This was mainly due to epidemics in orphanages, which began to end around 1960 as a result of considerable improvements in nourishment. Individual cases of PCP, however, were reported from all countries carrying out systematic autopsies on deaths of premature and newborn infants, except the USA (Vanec 1952, 1953, Deamer 1953, Weller 1956, Gajdusek 1957, Dutz 1970, Pifer 1978, Cantwell 1984, Armengol 1995). A Canadian pathologist stated: "PCP is much more common in this country than we thought, we just have to open our eyes to see it" (Berdnikov 1970). In 1970, PCP in newborn infants was classified differently than PCP in older children and adults.

PCP in patients treated with immunotoxic substances and in those with disturbances of antibody binding and formation

- Diffuse and bronchial PCP was diagnosed in premature and newborn infants in overcrowded paediatric wards and orphanages. Immunological analysis showed a pronounced immune imbalance, mostly between the first 10 to 28 weeks of life, as a result of prematurity, starvation or inadequate nutrition, frequent intermittent debilitative infections with antibiotic therapy, and recurrent diarrhoea in conjunction with artificial feeding and vitamin resorption deficiencies.
- PCP occurred with a congenital immunity imbalance in older children, as a result of insufficient T-cell ripening in the thymus and an underproduction of the immunoglobulin Ig class G.

PCP developed in children and adults in three forms of acquired immunodeficiency (AID):

1. In cancer and organ transplant patients treated with immunotoxins.
2. After long term treatment with corticosteroid hormones for patients with rheumatoid arthritis, connective tissue diseases, dermatosis, allergies, haemolytic anaemia, organ transplants and cancer diseases.
3. In patients with disorders of immunoglobulin formation, especially immunoglobulin class G, malignant degeneration of the B-cells (multiple myeloma and all forms of lymphoma), tissue macrophages (histiocytoma) and white blood cells (all forms of leukaemia).

It must be emphasized that PCP, whether caused by congenital or acquired immunity deficiency, very often appears in conjunction with fungal and viral infections (Dutz 1970, Pifer 1978).

Experimentally induced PCP in immunosuppressed animals

Extensive animal experiments have been carried out since the 1950s. Experiments on rats, dosed with antibiotics after corticosteroid treatment, demonstrated that pneumocystis could be provoked. Sterile rats in isolators did not develop PCP after corticosteroid and tetracycline treatment, but with the same treatment plus a protein-free diet the animals displayed signs of a pneumonitis, like PCP, but no PCP pathogens were found in the lungs after death. However, when the immunosuppressed animals, under corticosteroid treatment, came into contact with non-sterile animals they developed a pronounced pneumocystis with evidence of PCP pathogens. The PCP pathogens were carried through the air from animal to animal without affecting the non-immunosuppressed animals (Weller 1956, Sheldon 1959, Frenkel 1966).

PCP in the Third World, as a result of starvation and malnutrition, has been well known for centuries

In Western countries, pneumocystis diagnoses among dystrophic infants (as a result of starvation or malnutrition) point to the millions of statistically unmeasured illnesses and deaths in the Third World through acute or chronic protein-energy malnutrition syndromes (PEM): "In the tropical developing countries very frequent and socially highly significant, nutritional diseases emerge—a distinction is made between *marasmus* (caloric undernourishment corresponding to infant dystrophy) and *kwashiorkor* (protein deficiency syndrome corresponding to a flour-based nutritional disturbance). Hybrids and combinations of vitamin deficiency are frequent, only a fraction of the nutritional disturbances become clinically manifest. They account indirectly for a sharp increase in infant and child mortality, in that they weaken resistance against acute infectious diseases. Therapy: Introduction of a diet with sufficient energy and proteins. Prophylaxis: improvement of the social situation, improvement in farming and nutritional counselling" (Pschyrembel 1990).

This definition of PEM stems from the Klinisches Wörterbuch (Clinical Dictionary) commonly used by German-speaking doctors. Apart from the inept therapy recommendations (which from the viewpoint of affluent Western society gives the impression that people from the Third World are starving as a result of ignorance), there is no reference, whatsoever, to concrete opportunistic infections as a result of PEM. They are the typical AIDS-indicator diseases like PCP, other fungal infections, mycobacterioses like miliary tuberculosis, and viral infections inclusive of cytomegalo and herpes viral infections with concurrent thymus atrophy as a result of a cell-mediated T-cell immunity dysbalance

(Purtilo 1975). Significantly, this form of thiol deficiency syndrome resulting from the absence of the sulfurous amino acids, methionine and cysteine is extensively referred to as "nutritional AIDS" (Beisel 1992, 1996).

According to long-term statistics of the WHO, which are based on incomprehensible estimates, 90% of the AIDS sufferers worldwide live in the African countries south of the Sahara. Scandalously, the cause of this is not considered to be the "very frequent and socially highly significant, nutritional diseases" due to protein and vitamin deficiencies, but a new retrovirus that is presumed to have been transmitted to humans by apes. Since the 1980s, this virus is now supposed to have triggered the opportunistic infections that have been observed for centuries.

PCP and Kaposi's sarcoma (AIDS) seen in chemoimmunosuppressed organ transplant patients since the 60's

Patients having undergone an organ transplant are of special interest. Since the 1960s patients have been treated with immunotoxic substances in order to prevent rejection of the transplanted organs through cell-mediated immunity. Some of the patients developed a distinct immunity dysbalance, opportunistic infections like PCP, fungal and viral infections, and Kaposi's sarcoma and lymphoma, in particular of the central nervous system. The clinical symptoms were identical to the AIDS-indicating illnesses of homosexual men that were diagnosed since 1978 and published since 1981. To inhibit the reaction of the immune system, three groups of substances were deployed:

- Azathioprine
- Corticosteroids
- Cyclosporine A

In the 1940s, biochemists focused on how the biosynthesis of the basic structure of nucleic acids could be medicinally altered to inhibit or block the growth and proliferation of microbes or tumor cells. The genes contained in the human cell nucleus are assembled from nucleic acids, biochemically synthesized as deoxyribonucleic acid (DNA). Within certain genetic sections, transcripts are produced as coded building blocks for the synthesis of amino acids into protein molecules, which is carried out in the cytoplasm. This transcript moves from the nucleus to specialized protein synthesis structures (ribosomes) as messenger RNA (mRNA). RNA is a modified form of DNA. Other forms of RNA are used for protein and other biosyntheses.

The idea back then was to attack one of the nucleic acid's building blocks, biochemically termed bases, by substituting a false or analogue molecule. The nucleic acid of the DNA contains four different bases, which combine in the DNA chain to produce the alphabet of the DNA code. There are two purine bases (adenine and guanine) and two pyrimidine bases (cytosine and thymine). A fifth pyrimidine base, uracil, is only present in RNA.

In addition to the obligatory base, the individual building blocks of nucleic acids contain ribose sugar, and are coupled to each other by phosphate. Such a macromolecule is called a nucleotide. These nucleotides also play an essential role in co-enzymes for many biosyntheses, e.g. NO synthesis in T-cells and in all other cell systems.

It is important to have a basic understanding of the role of nucleotides in NO synthesis, in order to comprehend what happens to patients with organ transplants, opportunistic infections, and certain forms of cancer; immunotoxic interventions on such patients with excessive NO constitutes the model for the development of AIDS in homosexuals and other patients, without the primary cause of a hypothetical virus.

In his acceptance speech for the 1988 Nobel Prize in Medicine, the American biochemist Hitchings, whose team among other things developed the immunotoxic drug Azathioprine, spoke of synthetic nucleotide analogues for introduction into the nucleus instead of natural nucleotides: "Now we have the chemotherapeutic agents; we need only to find the diseases in which they will be active" (Hitchings 1989).

One such chemotherapeutic analogue, Azathioprine, inhibits the synthesis of the purine bases, adenosine and guanine, rendering them ineffective and thereby disrupting the synthesis of DNA, RNA and the nucleotides. Azathioprine is called a purine blocker as it's mercaptopurine metabolite blocks the body's natural amino purines. Even though Hitchings had already stated, in 1989, that this mechanism could transform certain cells into cancer cells, Azathioprine was prescribed to patients whom had undergone kidney, heart, liver or bone marrow transplants. 6% of the kidney-transplant patients developed Kaposi's sarcoma and T-cell lymphoma, as well as lymphomas of the central nervous system. The malignant cell mutation appeared after 30 months on average, with a variability between a few weeks and 13 years. The average patient age was 40.

Opportunistic infections like PCP, fungal and viral infections including cytomegalic infections were common. The immunologic function of T-helper cells was drastically reduced: the DTH skin reaction after antigenic stimulation, as well as mitogenic and antigenic stimulation in vitro, was strongly anergic (overview Penn 1979, Penn 1981 Zisbrod 1980, Schooley 1982, Harwood 1984, Levine 1984, Friedman-Kein 1984). These patients developed an immunotoxically-induced immune dysbalance with typical indicator illnesses, fully analogous to homosexual patients, whose illnesses would just a few years later be called AIDS.

The fact remains unexplained why the tumors of some patients regressed after discontinuing the immunotoxic Azathioprine:

"Malignancies have been occurring with astonishing frequency in patients receiving grafts of kidneys and hearts in recent years, and the only plausible explanation for this is the routine, mandatory use of immune suppressive drugs. It became clear that a substantial number of brand new cancers were occurring in the course of the intensive treatment of not only graft recipients with immune suppressive drugs, but also in patients treated with the same drugs for other reasons. The cancers have been of all types: Kaposi's sarcoma, lymphomas and carcinomas. Some have appeared in or near the graft areas, others at distant sites. The most remarkable feature of the phenomena, apart from the cancers themselves, has been that a few of these spontaneous tumors regressed when the immune suppressive drugs were discontinued. On a few occasions, malignant growths the size of a hen's egg or larger, some with already established lymph node metastases, some of them Kaposi's have been reported to melt away after stopping the drugs. Transplant patients who developed neoplasms were routinely maintained on immune suppressive drugs, usually a combination of Azathioprine and prednisone. Krikorian summarized the results of Stanford experience with heart transplants three years ago. Out of the 143 transplanted patients who survived for three months or longer, 10 developed cancer, 6 lymphomas, 3 carcinomas and 1 acute leukaemia. All of these patients were under forty which indicates that the incidence of *de novo* cancer was really extraordinarily high" (Thomas 1984, Krikorian 1978).

Azathioprine (a.k.a. Imuran), when administered experimentally to research animals in combination with exogenous antigenic stimuli, caused a high occurrence of lymphomas. When Azathioprine was administered to mice bred for autoimmune dysfunction, a high rate of lymphomas was also seen.

First World Congress on AIDS in New York denies the extreme immunotoxic burden of the first AIDS patients and instead postulates a "new illness" by a "new AIDS agent."

The findings of the simultaneous provocation of opportunistic infections and cancer cell transformations by medically administered immune cell-inhibiting substances were presented at a historically decisive conference. In March 1983 more than 500 specialists from the USA, Canada, Europe and Africa discussed: "AIDS: The Epidemic of Kaposi's sarcoma and Opportunistic Infections." The conference was organized by the New York University Medical Center and in the words of the organizers, was to, "present a broad overview of the disease as it is currently understood." At this point in time in the USA there were just over 1,200 patients, mostly homosexuals, who had been clinically diagnosed with AIDS; worldwide there were also some 500 further AIDS patients, again mostly homosexuals. The organizers pointed out that "the world was witnessing the emergence of a new disease—a devastating disease which within two years would reach epidemic proportions in the United States" (Fernandez 1984).

However this "profound, unexplained impairment of cell-mediated immunity" was not a uniform disease, in that Kaposi's sarcoma was diagnosed solely in homosexual men, with and without opportunistic infections. Most homosexual AIDS patients suffered however not from Kaposi's sarcoma but had developed opportunistic infections, predominantly PCP. But other patients with anomalies in their immune cells together with one or more opportunistic infections (even those without PCP but with, for instance, candida infections) were also counted as AIDS patients: "Haitians, hemophiliacs, intravenous drug users, blood transfusion recipients, and female sexual partners of men with this disease" (Fernandez 1984). This listing of the patient groups shows the power of suggestion of the implicit assumption that every anomaly in the immunocells associated with one or more opportunistic fungal or parasitical infections, must always be caused by "this presumably contagious illness" (Fernandez 1984).

We are not talking about a "new disease" (Fernandez 1984), but well-known anomalies of cell-mediated immune response and its resulting symptoms. These could arise from a number of root causes as supported by the quoted medical examples. What was new was the possibility, with technical advances, to differentiate between the T-helper cells and other T-cells in blood samples using monoclonal antibodies. To take such laboratory findings and then to claim that all opportunistic illnesses must be caused by this "presumably contagious illness" was arbitrary and digressive as the immune cell network and other cell networks respond to every toxic, traumatic, infectious, nutritive, psychological or other stress related overload with an evolutionary biologically programmed counterregulation.

Forms of Kaposi's sarcoma in Africa have been well known for centuries

Kaposi's sarcoma (KS) also was not new. The disease symptoms have been familiar in Africa for centuries, particularly among the Bantu tribes in South Africa and an endemic belt located in equatorial Africa (overview Freidman-Kein 1984 a). KS was rarely found in people of European or Asian descent, even in areas of Africa where KS was relatively common among the indigenous population. In Uganda, for example, 9% of all tumors were diagnosed as KS (Taylor 1971). In Africa, KS is most common in adults between the ages of 25 and 45 with a male to female ratio of 17:1, the benign nodular form being more common. There is also an extremely malignant form with a high mortality rate affecting African children between the ages of two and 15, with a male to female predominance of 3:1. This is seldom linked with the otherwise common skin lesions, but rather with pronounced lymph nodes involvement and KS tumors in the visceral organs (Templeton 1976). No causative relation to a particular pathogen was proven; differentiated research has yet to be published (Olweny 1984).

Kaposi's sarcoma in Europe was already clinically defined 130 years ago by the Hungarian dermatologist Moritz Kaposi

Sarcoma idiopathicum multiplex haemorrhagicum, as KS is known medically, was first described in medical journals in 1872 by the Hungarian dermatologist Moritz Kaposi. Seen were made up of multiple, hyperpigmented, vascular cutaneous nodules on the lower extremities of elderly males (Kaposi 1872). Later on KS, "a fascinating curiosity" (Friedman-Kein 1984 a), was seen in a benign and malignant progression. Publications about most of the KS cases were in Europe and North America. On the one hand the cases concerned white males over fifty of Italian, Jewish or African extraction but on the other occurred in younger patients of differing ethnical backgrounds (Rothman 1962). Two progressions became apparent; multifocal brownish-red to blue nodules, primarily on the lower extremities, and in a later stage systemic or disseminated manifestations above all in the visceral organs and the lungs. Massive disruption to cell-mediated immunity was detected (Dubozy 1973). What was striking was the incidence of particular tissue antigens in KS patients of specific ethnic extraction. Such tissue antigens are found on the cell membranes of all human cells and as they are especially well pronounced on white cells, are termed HLA systems (human leucocyte antigens). The genes for the biosynthesis of these tissue proteins are consolidated in the major histocompatibility complex (MHC). As a result of the extraordinary diversity of expression of these genes an enormous number of HLA antigens are present on cell surfaces. These HLA antigens play an important part in the presentation of irregular proteins (antigens) for activation of T-helper cells. As a consequence it is crucial to ensure before tissue or organ transplantations, that there is as much compatibility of the HLA types as possible between the donor and recipient. Specific illnesses are associated with specific variations of the HLA types. In the HLA gene complex (MHC) four main areas are differentiated (A, B, C, D). The HLA proteins in area D appear, above all, on activated T-lymph cells (specific cell-mediated immunity), T-helper cells (specific humoral immunity) and macrophages (unspecific cell-mediated immunity). KS patients belong, conspicuously often, to the HLA-DR5 group (O'Hara 1982). From these findings it is concluded that people with this HLA variant, after treatment with immunotoxics, react more sensitively to an immune cell dysbalance and could develop AIDS-indicating illnesses. The findings, however, do not exclude the possibility that patients not displaying signs of this HLA variant, but taking high dosages of immunotoxic substances, or over a long time span, also develop an immunity dysbalance and the associated AIDS-indicating illnesses (Levine1984).

All antibiotics have more or less immunosuppressive effects

As a result of the findings of organ transplant patients who developed immune cell dysbalances, opportunistic infections, Kaposi's sarcoma, lymphoma, as well as other cancer types after Azathioprine medication, it became absolutely crucial to search for substances with analogous immunotoxic potency in the medical histories of homosexual AIDS patients. Antibiotics, chemotherapeutics, antiparasitics, fungistatics (fungal suppressive drugs), virustatics (viral suppressive drugs), recreational drugs or combinations thereof, all came into the question. The exceptional strain on a promiscuous minority of homosexuals through long-term medication with antimicrobial substances was clinically sufficiently well documented (overview Root-Bernstein 1993). Firstly, all participating doctors were aware of the principal immunotoxicity of all antimicrobial substances and recreational drugs (Descotes 1988). Azathioprine, as was realized, also acts repressively and antimicrobially on cell-mediated immunity.

The hypotheses that were brought forth at the First World Congress on AIDS regarding the causes of AIDS and cancer are in unsolvable contradiction to the clinical reality. A "planned series of human experiments" on AIDS patients is explained as necessary, in order to observe whether cancer develops or progresses after direct pharmaceutical blockade of the cellular immune defense.

The historic conference in March 1983 reflected a completely different realm of interest than its name might imply:

Of the 44 lectures held over the three days the leading specialists covered the following focal points:

- 12 lectures about Kaposi's sarcoma (20% of the diagnosed AIDS cases at that time).
- 1 lecture on PCP (80% of the diagnosed AIDS cases at that time).
- 3 lectures on the hypothetical viral cause of AIDS and cancer.
- 9 lectures on immunological problems and cytokine research.
- 2 lectures on lymphadenopathy (swelling of the lymph nodes).
- 5 lectures on clinical specific problems.
- 4 lectures on epidemiological questions.
- 1 lecture on macaque monkeys.
- 1 lecture on changes in the sexual lifestyle of homosexual men since the end of the 1960s.
- 1 lecture on changing patterns of sexually transmitted diseases since the end of the 1960s.
- 1 lecture on the sexual practices of homosexual men and Kaposi's sarcoma.
- 1 lecture about the challenge to the public of AIDS.
- 1 lecture on the psychosocial support in AIDS.

Not one of the specialists gave a lecture about the immunotoxic and carcinogenic effects of nitrites, nitrosamines, antibiotics etc. The main focus of the conference was clearly concentrated on Kaposi's sarcoma and viruses as the hypothetical cause of the onset of cancer. The medical professor and cancer researcher Dr. Lewis Thomas, director of the Memorial Sloan-Kettering Cancer Center in New York, one of the most important cancer research centers in the USA, held the opening lecture. He clearly outlined the dominant direction of research, which has prevailed until today: "Whatever we learn about the mechanisms releasing Kaposi's sarcoma in AIDS will be useful information for the study of cancer in general, and whatever we can discover about the role of immunity in cancer will turn out to be a piece of applied science for the AIDS problem .... What is needed, of course, is a series of human experiments, planned and executed in order to answer the sort of question which automatically raises itself: what would happen if you were to remove the putative defense mechanism of cellular immunity in human beings? Would this affect either the incidence or clinical course of cancer? As it happens, unplanned experiments have already been done .... It seems to me that there are two alternative explanations for the high incidence of cancer in AIDS patients, and the same alternatives exist for the patients with organ homografts treated with immune suppressive drugs. One is that the impairment of cellular immunity has allowed an oncogenic virus to invade and proliferate, and what we are seeing is a human cancer running wild. This would seem plausible enough for the AIDS patients with Kaposi's sarcoma if this were the only neoplasm, but these patients are developing other types of neoplasm as well, including the same lymphomas with a special predilection for invading the central nervous system, which are seen in the homograft [tissue transplant] patients. The second possible explanation, which I favor, is that the AIDS agent, whatever its nature, is not a cancer virus, but has as its sole action the suppression of cellular immunity. This action opens the way for a multitude of opportunistic pathogens and at the same time releases any clone of transformed, neoplastic cells that happen to turn up" (Thomas 1984).

Both of the rendered hypotheses about the origins of cancer are inextricably in opposition to the clinical reality:

1. The cellular immunity (T-helper cells) can only recognize intracellular viruses once they have infiltrated the cell, they cannot prevent infiltration. "The impairment of cellular immunity" cannot "allow an oncogenic virus to invade and proliferate" (Thomas 1984).
2. The speaker states that: "AIDS patients are developing other types of neoplasm as well, including the same lymphomas with a special predilection for invading the central nervous system, which are seen in the homograft patients" (Thomas 1984). The same speaker also stated: "The most remarkable feature of the phenomenon, apart from the cancers themselves, has been that a few of these spontaneous tumors have regressed when the immune suppressive drugs were discontinued. On a few occasions, malignant growths the size of a hen's egg or larger, some with already established lymph node metastases, some of them Kaposi's, have been reported to melt away after stopping the drugs" (Thomas 1984).

So the speaker ascertains that the tumors of homosexual AIDS patients, identical to those of graft patients, regressed. He diagnosed a clear causative connection between the growth of the tumors after medication and regression after discontinuation of Azathioprine. The "regression when immune suppressive drugs were discontinued" (Thomas 1984) in no way means that the cellular immunity, gathering momentum, had finally discovered the hypothetical viruses in the cancer cells and destroyed them. The immunosuppressive drugs were in actuality not removed, but rather exchanged for corticosteroids and other substances, in order to prevent a potential rejection of the transplanted organs of these patients (Penn 1979, 1981). So the cellular immunity remained suppressed, but still the tumor regressed. The cause of the growth and regression of the tumors was solely the effect and cessation of Azathioprine. The cause of tumors in organ transplant AIDS patients and homosexual AIDS patients could not in any way be "a clone of transformed, neoplastic cells" (Thomas 1984).

3. The second hypothesis, that "it is not itself a cancer virus, but has as its sole action the suppression of cellular immunity . . . at the same time releasing any clone of transformed neoplastic cells" (Thomas 1984) is incongruous because the cellular immunity does not identify cancer cells as long as firstly, the T-helper cells have not been activated by cells representing the antigens and secondly, the cytotoxic T-cells (including nonspecific macrophages), activated by Th1 helper cells, recognize and attack the presented antigens of the cancer cells. The presentation of cancer cell antigens takes place only after the unprogrammed cell death of cancer cells via necrosis. From this it follows that the primary growth of the cancer cells cannot be caused by immunosuppression, but as in the case of blocked purine metabolism in organ recipients, by Azathioprine. This same substance also negatively affects the immune cells (suppression of the T-helper cells), endothelial cells (Kaposi's sarcoma), T-helper cells (lymphoma), as well as other cell systems (carcinoma), although under differing circumstances.

   Like most of his colleagues, the oncologist ignored the objective fact that Azathioprine is absorbed not only by T-cells, but also in principle by all human cells. Azathioprine is preferentially absorbed by the immune cells only because the metabolism is especially active in transplant patients and has a special affinity to the substance. Depending on the dosage and duration of the prescription, as well as the disposition of the patient (for instance variance of the HLA type), the purine metabolism of other cells can be critically disrupted; for instance, as a result of a provoked immune cell imbalance, the uptake of Azathioprine by the immune cells decreases, and instead the substance is relatively strongly taken in by the other cell systems, thereby systemically disrupting the purine metabolism.

4. In the same context the prominent cancer researcher spoke, as if it were self-evident, of "an AIDS agent, whatever its nature" obviously with the consensus of his colleagues. Although he had established that the AIDS-indicating diseases of organ recipients were clinically completely identical to those of homosexual AIDS patients and that the former are clearly caused by the immunotoxic drug Azathioprine, he postulated in the same

context a possible viral source for the AIDS-indicating illnesses of organ transplant patients both for the suppression of the cellular immunity and for the development of cancer tumors: “There are two alternative explanations for the high incidence of cancer in AIDS patients, and the same alternatives exist for the patients with organ homografts treated with immune suppressive drugs . . . the second possible explanation, which I favor, is that the AIDS agent, whatever its nature, is not itself a cancer virus, but has as its sole action the suppression of cellular immunity” (Thomas 1984). This speculative premise, including the organ recipients, is inextricably in opposition to the factual assertions made in the same lecture: “Malignancies have been occurring with astonishing frequency in patients receiving grafts of kidneys and hearts in recent years, and the only plausible explanation is the routine, mandatory use of immune suppressive drugs” (Thomas 1984).

In 1983, the viral cancer researchers arbitrarily called the Kaposi's sarcoma seen in homosexual nitrite users a "mystery" and an "intriguing puzzle" although by 1982 animal experiments had already demonstrated that even short-term nitrite use unleashes immunotoxic and carcinogenic effects

It is undeniably evident that the disease hypothesis of an “AIDS agent” and an “immune suppressive virus” was from the outset introduced as a speculative construct lacking any substantial proof. In order to add substance irrefutable medical historical facts were arbitrarily re-evaluated. Urgent and necessary immunotoxicological studies were either not carried out, or their methods were insufficient, as medical interest had been narrowly confined to the construction of the hypothetical “AIDS agent.”

After the above-quoted lecture, two dermatologists and microbiologists from the New York University Medical Center gave a lecture entitled: “An Overview of Classical and Epidemic Kaposi’s Sarcoma.” “Some unexplained, profound, acquired disorders of cell-mediated immunity that predisposes the afflicted host to a variety of unusual and often lethal opportunistic infections as well as a disseminated form of Kaposi’s sarcoma . . . The cause of this new disease entity remains a mystery. It is most unlikely that Kaposi could have imagined that the neoplasm that bears his name would become linked 100 years later to one of the most devastating epidemics in modern history. The sudden increased occurrence of this rare tumor and its association with specific epidemiologic, immunologic, and clinical findings has focused the attention of the medical community to explore the intriguing puzzle of how these factors may be directly involved in the pathogenesis of AIDS and especially this particular neoplasm” (Friedman-Kein 1984 a).

Nobody in the past had described the fully identical illnesses of organ transplant patients as "a mystery" and "an intriguing puzzle," as the causative relation between chemotherapeutic immunosuppression and growth and regression of "this particular neoplasm" (namely Kaposi's sarcoma), was blatantly obvious! Why were these illnesses considered "new disease entities" although identical illnesses were well known in organ transplant patients? Why was there talk of a "sudden increased occurrence of this rare tumor," although it was documented that practically all KS patients were homosexuals with a preference for anal intercourse, with long-standing use of nitrites, antibiotics, and chemotherapeutic substances?

"Probably the immune deficiency precedes KS. The various drugs, such as amyl nitrite and butyl nitrite, which have been used excessively by many homosexual KS patients, should be tested in animals for their immunosuppressive, mutagenic, and oncogenic potential. Aggressive chemotherapy and persistent infections, such as CMV, Epstein-Barr virus, hepatitis B, pneumocystis, and amebiasis, likely contribute to the final degree of immunologic incompetence" (De Wys 1982). These carefully chosen but explicit formulations were published by, among others, researchers at the American National Institutes of Health and the CDC.

In 1982 a clinical study by the CDC demonstrated that the amount of T-helper cells in the blood of nitrite users was lower than those in the blood of non-nitrite users (Goedert 1982). In a further study at the Cancer Prevention and Control Research Center of the University of Texas, it was shown in human cell cultures that the quantity of T-helper cells was reduced by nitrite, even at low concentrations that did not kill lymph cells. Nitrite retards the synthesis of type 1 cytokines, such that a two-hour contact of moderate amounts of nitrite with human immune cells is sufficient to induce immunosuppression. "The results suggested that prolonged exposure [to nitrites] may not be necessary [for immunosuppressive and carcinogenic effects] .... and their use should be condemned by those physicians who treat patients who use these drugs regularly" (Hersh 1983, Newell 1984, Newell 1988).

The causative connection between nitrate use (Mayer 1983), "aggressive chemotherapy," (De Wys 1982) and acute, concurrent, and chronic antigenic stress through a variety of infections (overview Root-Bernstein 1993) has been amply covered. The fact that this substance induces immune cell dysbalance, both in organ transplant patients and homosexual AIDS patients, preceding the emergence of KS in most cases, has been conclusively established by researchers from the CDC and other governmental research institutes (Jaffe 1983).

Why did the cancer researchers at the historic conference in March 1983 claim, against better knowledge, that an apparently "new disease" was a "mystery" and a "intriguing puzzle" which in turn led to the arbitrary construction of an "AIDS agent" and an "immunosuppressive virus"?

The background of research politics (1971-1984) leading to the misinterpretation of indiscriminate test tube creations as "HIV characteristics"

In 1981, the financial backing for research into retroviruses and cancer, instigated by the republican president Nixon in 1971 as "The War on Cancer," was withdrawn due to the lack of concrete success. At that time it was, by far, the largest capital investment in medical research. One of those who had profited from the Nixon project was the research scientist Robert Gallo, leader of the Laboratory of Tumor Cell Biology at the National Cancer Institute in the USA. Gallo reported, along with some of his colleagues, at the conference in March 1983, that the team had identified a retrovirus in T-helper cells from blood samples of two homosexual AIDS patients. Gallo and his colleagues had published the first reports about proof of such a retrovirus in human blood cells in 1981. It was concerned with a virus that appeared in an unusual form of leukaemia in Japan and the Caribbean in the leukaemia cells of a small percentage of affected patients. This hypothetical proof of a retrovirus in a few human leukaemia cells, shortly before the termination of the Nixon project with its billions of dollars of investment, was the only meager return from the whole retrovirus cancer research program.

It became later apparent that the Gallo team could by no means produce evidence of the isolation of a retrovirus but only the "fingerprint" of a hypothetical virus, in reality only a partial "fingerprint" of a retrovirus in leukaemia cells. By comparison, it was as if a part of a fingerprint had been discovered and from this a photofit picture was made from which a clear-cut case was being made against the suspect. Likewise, the Gallo team had then apparently located this "photofit" retrovirus in the T-helper cells of two AIDS patients. In doing so there is, however, a trick involved—the T-helper cells from the blood samples of the AIDS patients were incubated together with leukaemia cells to which were added massive amounts of type 1 cytokine as a growth stimulator. Additionally the cell mixture was aggressively treated with highly oxidative maturation stimulators. Often with such cell culture procedures, tiny, virus-like, membrane-encased particles can be observed, which contain cellular debris ejected from the cells. The standard rule in virology is that such particles are only recognized as real viruses once the proteins and nucleic acids have been shown to take on a certain structure, making it possible for the virus to identically copy its RNA/DNA in the DNA strand of a host cell. The Gallo team could not produce such evidence, although it is demanded by routine laboratory practice. It was also unclear whether the particle originated from the T-helper cells or the leukaemia cells. Instead of this, the Gallo team produced the previously mentioned "partial fingerprint." Such viruses are supposed to be retroviruses, when their genetic make-up is coded by RNA structures, rather than the DNA forms found in most viruses and eukaryotes (single—and multi-celled organisms with nuclei). The RNA make-up of this hypothetical retrovirus is supposed to be transcribed into DNA form in the host cells by means of a virus-specific enzyme. The term retrovirus (from the Latin: *retro* = reverse), comes from the notion that these tiny particles, contrary to the usual practice, are transcribed from RNA into DNA and then from the DNA matrix back to RNA copies, with the help of the host cell DNA mechanisms. These RNA structures are then encased by membranes, and bud out of the host cell in order to colonize other cells. That is the theoretical concept, anyway; but how exactly these hypothetical retroviruses are thought to trigger cancer during this process is highly speculative. As proof for the existence of these retroviruses, Gallo and his colleagues offered a "partial fingerprint" as supposed evidence of the transcription enzyme of the hypothetical retrovirus (Gelmann 1984).

Such reverse transcription processes, from RNA into DNA rather than the usual way from DNA to mobile messenger RNA, were observed in animal cells since 1970. Instead of the old dogma (DNA to messenger RNA), a new dogma was formulated, namely, that the deviating transcription was exclusively confined to the hypothetical retroviruses (Temin 1970, 1972). By the mid-seventies, researchers reported that reverse transcription had been observed in a variety of cells, not just virus-infected cells, and that this was a repair procedure, principally in embryonic cells and in cancer cells (overview Temin 1975, 1985, Baltimore 1985). The enzyme that supposedly enabled this transcription to take place was termed reverse transcriptase. In laboratory jargon this is shortened to RT. The Gallo team wanted this RT enzyme proven. *However, as RTs appear in cancer cells such as leukaemia, and as the lymph culture was incubated together with leukaemia cells to prove the existence of the supposed retrovirus in T-helper cells of AIDS patients, the RT itself was not convincing proof for the existence of a retrovirus in these T-helper cells.* Furthermore, evidence in human immune cells, even if the retrovirus had been precisely isolated, in no way means that it had to have a pathological influence. Similar such RNA sequences, termed endogenous retroviruses, have been observed in many animal cells as stowaways and have exercised no pathological influence whatsoever (overview Duesberg 1987, Teng 1996).

The only evidence of a supposed retrovirus in the T-helper cells of AIDS patients that the Gallo team could offer was merely a virus-like particle without documentation of protein and nucleic acid structures within this particle to enable infection, and the RT effects of proteins in a centrifuged culture soup (Gelmann 1984).

Just over a year after the historic conference of March 1983, something unique in the history of medicine took place. The Health and Human Services Secretary of the Reagan Administration, Margaret Heckler, together with Gallo announced at an international press conference in April 1984 that the Gallo team had discovered the "probable cause of AIDS" and had developed a blood test, which could detect evidence of the newly found retrovirus in everyone. Within two years a vaccine would probably be developed. Gallo was hailed by the world's press as the saviour of mankind from one of the "most devastating epidemics in modern history" (Friedman-Kein 1984 a).

Since then, everyone knows the hysteria in the mass media and medical journals about "Plague! Sex! Sensation!" Without any critical counteranalysis, most doctors throughout the world adopted the construct of the disease theory "HIV causes AIDS." The State doctrine that the "lethal AIDS agent" could be passed to anyone through sex and blood became the collective obsession that has claimed the lives of countless people.

The prediction of the oncologist Prof. Thomas in the opening paper of the conference of March 1983 served the ideological conversion from "War on Cancer" (President Nixon) to "War against Public Enemy Number One" (namely the "AIDS agent"), as President Reagan declared in the year of his re-election, but this prediction had not met the expectations of the HIV/AIDS researchers. "Whatever we learn about the mechanisms releasing Kaposi's sarcoma in AIDS will be useful information for the study of cancer in general, and whatever we can discover about the role of immunity in cancer will turn out to be a piece of applied science for the AIDS problem" (Thomas 1984).

25 years after the one-sided promotion of retrovirus cancer research, the "War on Cancer" in the USA is declared to be a failure, after proof is furnished that in fact only nitrite-inhaling homosexual AIDS patients fell ill with Kaposi's cancer, and retrovirus-AIDS researchers declared they were perplexed in solving the AIDS puzzle

The opportunity to learn something from the well-known AIDS illnesses, which had been diagnosed before it was called AIDS, had been lost. "A president of the USA 25 years ago declared a War on Cancer, confident that it was winnable. It has been judged, so far, lost. With the exception of advances in the treatment of haematological cancers, and a few others, 25 years has seen little progress" (editorial in the British medical journal The Lancet on July 6th, 1996). This concise statement documents that retrovirus AIDS research had contributed nothing decisive to the advancement of knowledge about cancer and vice versa. Clinical data merely confirmed what has already been known since 1981: KS as a "particular neoplasm" (Friedman-Kein 1984 a) is not "a new disease entity" and not "one of the most devastating epidemics in modern history." In Germany, for example, in the 15 years from 1982 to 1997, 2,736 cases of KS had been officially reported. Of those officially diagnosed, 2,505 were men of homosexual preference (92% of all KS cases). There remain, on average, 15 KS cases per year, which in the official reports cannot be labelled as relating to homosexuals or bisexuals (8% of all KS cases) (Harmouda 1997). A 10-year study in Chicago re-checked all male AIDS patients over the age of 18 who had described themselves as non-homosexual. 50% of these AIDS patients turned out to be homosexual after all (Murphy 1997). Correspondingly, with regard to sexual preference, the official annual average of 15 KS cases can be assumed to be a diagnostic contortion and as a result almost all KS AIDS patients could be considered as homosexual. This does not exclude the possibility that on rare occasions, patients other than homosexuals became affected with KS, for instance, from pharmacotoxic sources (excluding organ transplant patients and patients with malignant illnesses who had been treated with immunotoxic substances).

Consequently KS as a "particular neoplasm" and as a toxic/pharmacotoxic illness can be considered to be an illness exclusively confined to homosexual men, at least in Western countries. In sharp contrast to the official announcements KS, even within the male homosexual community, is a rare disease form and in Germany, for example, the annual incidence of KS cases affects one in 10,000 homosexual men.

So what was new about this "new disease entity" manifested by immune dysbalance, opportunistic infections and/or Kaposi's sarcoma/lymphoma? What was new was the appearance of a combination of diseases in homosexual males, which had previously been confined to organ transplant recipients after treatment with Azathioprine. The conclusion arises that toxic factors which cannot be explained by a retroviral "AIDS agent" must have been originally operative for the complete syndrome of acquired immune deficiency, including the fact that KS practically only appears in homosexual males.

The "complete" syndrome of AIDS illnesses in organ transplant patients proves that the phantom-like retroviruses are neither necessary nor sufficient in order to be able to understand the genesis and the interaction of immune dysbalance, opportunistic infections and cancer.

Nitrosamine research had irrefutably proven that nitrosamines are extremely potent carcinogenic substances in the human cell system. It was proven that these carcinogens are intermediate by-products of industrial processes, also present in agricultural products, pesticide residues, in tobacco, in cosmetics and in a diversity of other contamination sources of modern life (Magee 1976, Preussmann 1984). But they have also demonstrated that pharmaceutical products including analgesics, antibiotics, chemotherapeutics, and cancer drugs lead to the development of nitrosamines in human metabolism and are potential carcinogens (Lijinsky 1973, Preussmann 1984, 1986, Loeppky 1994 a). There were also no longer any biochemical doubts that nitrites could be converted to nitrosamines in the human metabolism, and could as a result also have carcinogenic effects (Doyle 1983, Loeppky 1994 a. Lijinsky 1994, Bartsch 1987, Haverkos 1988).

Why did the clear carcinogenic effect of nitrosamine-forming nitrites and nitrosamine-forming drugs have to be shrouded as a "new disease entity" in the etiological context of toxic AIDS effects? Why did the great minds describe the damage to the cellular immunity and the appearance of KS in habitual nitrite users and long-term consumers of nitrosamine-forming antibiotics and chemotherapeutics as a "particular neoplasm"? Why the "mystery" and the "intriguing puzzle"? Why were "only around 1,200 cases, all told between 1980 and early 1983—not many in a population exceeding 200 million" (Thomas 1984) sold to the mass media at that point in time as "one of the most devastating epidemics in modern history" (Friedman-Kein 1984)?

The financial backing for nitrosamine research, as the American Chemical Association established, had been drastically reduced as a result of pressure from the industry lobby, from 1980 in the US and from 1982 in Germany (Loeppky 1994 a). The competing billion-dollar project of the retrovirus/cancer research of Nixon's "War on Cancer" ceased to be financed in 1981, due to lack of success (Gallo 1999). The highly tuned laboratory machinery began to falter. It was in this context that the oncologist Thomas, chancellor of the Memorial Sloan-Kettering Cancer Center in New York (which together with the Laboratory of Tumor Cell Biology of the National Cancer Institute under the directorship of the laboratory researcher Gallo, had profited enormously from the billion dollar retrovirus/cancer project), seized the opportunity to reanimate retrovirus research.

Nitrosamine cancer research had a fundamental handicap: research had clearly proven that nitrosamines, formed from both exogenous and endogenous sources, damaged immune cells and triggered cancer. At that time and even today, the prevailing theory is that cancer develops in the nucleus of cells, through a random genetic mutation of the DNA. Nitrosamine researchers could demonstrate displacements and losses in the DNA sequence in the coding mechanisms of the genomes, which is the sum of the 100,000 genes in human nuclei. What could not be conclusively demonstrated, however, was how the random dispersion of defects and mutations in the DNA sequence coding were supposed to alter the transcription (from DNA to messenger RNA) and the subsequent translation (biosynthesis of amino acid proteins from messenger RNA outside of the nucleus), so that the cell mechanisms did not actually stop, but rather switched to an ongoing cancerous cell division program.

Besides this, some of the cancer cells also developed without any detectable mutation to the DNA of the nucleus of the cells (Lijinsky 1994). The retrovirus cancer researchers tried to solve this problem by postulating that the supposedly isolated retroviruses, after their transcription from RNA to DNA, docked onto a particular location on the DNA strand near the oncogenes of the host cell so that they could activate the oncogenes which up until that point had been inactive, in order to start the ongoing cell division process. But cell division is a highly complex interplay requiring many genes to synthesise the necessary proteins and protein enzymes. This can by no means be considered a "human cancer virus running wild" (Thomas 1984). The cancer cells are highly efficient, active cells, which after a very complex program produce cell energy and organize their proliferation. The difference of normal differentiated cells is, in essence, that cancer cells after transformation no longer attune their activity to neighboring cells and in relation to the organism as a whole become cell parasites. Neither the nitrosamine researchers nor the retrovirus/cancer researcher have managed to convincingly solve the complicated problem of this transformation to cancer cells.

The "particular neoplasm" of Kaposi's sarcoma in homosexual AIDS patients through "unplanned experiments" (Thomas 1984) now brought Thomas, Gallo and their colleagues the fateful idea of circumventing the unsolved problem of the origin of cancer cell transformation, by relocating the "scene of the crime" of their phantom retroviruses to the T-helper cells. "The second possible explanation, which I favor, is that the AIDS agent, whatever its nature is not a cancer virus, but has as its sole action the suppression of cellular immunity. This action opens the way for a multitude of opportunistic pathogens and at the same time releases any clone of transformed, neoplastic cells that happen to turn up" (Thomas 1984). The critical logical question as to the cause of the initial growth of the "clones of transformed, neoplastic cells" is no longer posed. The original research question of the primary cause for the transformation of the tumor cells, which actually was supposed to be explained by the hypothetical existence of retroviruses in the transformed cells, had suddenly become a secondary issue. The "human cancer virus running wild" (Thomas 1984) had been reinvented as the "AIDS agent" running wild among T-helper cells. The existence of "clones of transformed, neoplastic cells that happen to turn up" (Thomas 1984) is simply presented as a biological fact.

The thought processes of the assistants at the birth of the retrovirus HIV (human immunodeficiency virus), behind this decisive step, have to be made rationally clear in order to understand the implications of this construct and its grave consequences for the whole world.

Gallo who had hitherto localized his hypothetical retrovirus as activator of oncogenes inside the leukaemia cells (as transformed cancer cells), transplanted his retrovirus artefact, in March 1983, for the sake of simplicity into the T-helper cells as an "AIDS agent." A "cancer virus running wild" (Thomas 1984) becomes with the wave of a hand a "T-helper cell virus" which now, instead of transforming T-helper cells, is supposed to destroy them.

Indeed, Gallo and his colleagues knew since the mid-seventies that in organ recipients and other patients treated with corticosteroids for immune suppression, of whom a certain percentage developed KS, lymphoma and carcinoma, the T-helper cells were not destroyed but under the influence of cortisol moved out of the circulatory system to the bone marrow and other areas (Fauci 1974, 1975, Cupps 1982). The assumption that a destruction of the T-helper cells as the cause of an immune cell dysbalance (a decrease in the T-helper cells circulating in the bloodstream) was by no means compelling. As long as the corticosteroid hormone treated patients developed differing types of cancer then the origin of the cancer could not have been from the T-helper cells as they had drifted out of the bloodstream and so could not be detected in blood samples.

The theory of an "AIDS agent" destroying immune cells and subsequently, as a result of a failure of the immunity surveillance, a "clone of transformed, neoplastic cells" (Thomas 1984) plucked out of thin air, rests solely on the assumption that the number of T-helper cells circulating in the bloodstream is reduced because the T-helper cells have been destroyed beforehand. However, it has been shown that there were homosexual patients with Kaposi's sarcoma without a reduction of T-helper cells in their blood plasma and without clinical syndromes of opportunistic infections (CDC 1981 b, Haverkos 1982).

Thus the development of Kaposi's sarcoma does not have to be caused by a reduction in immune cells. In Central Africa, in research on indigenous KS patients, it was also shown that Kaposi's sarcoma appeared without destroying the immune cells (Kestens 1985). Such cases of KS could, for instance, be triggered by drinking water contaminated by nitrite-forming bacteria. The nitrites are converted to nitrates by hydrochloric acids in the stomach and subsequently enter the bloodstream. Here the nitrates come into close contact with endothelial cells which form NO and its derivatives. These can cause KS, if a long-term NO surplus exhausts the thiol pool and specific counter regulatory measures occur in the endothelial cells.

The postulated pathophysiological sequence—first, suppression of the cellular immunity, and then proliferation of cancer—is the crucial premise for the construction of the "AIDS agent." "The second possible explanation, which I favor, is that the AIDS agent, whatever its nature is not a cancer virus, but has as its sole action the suppression of cellular immunity. This action opens the way for a multitude of opportunistic pathogens and at the same time releases any clone of transformed, neoplastic cells that happen to turn up" (Thomas 1984).

The assumption of an AIDS agent in the fundamental theory of the immune cell destruction as a prerequisite for the origin of Kaposi's sarcoma could have objectively been recognized as wrong from the outset. Gallo, in his presentation of a wrong theory deduced from misinterpreted findings, at no point in time actually isolated a retrovirus. The tragedy of this fateful blunder was that the world believed that a high-flying doctor had discovered the right causes, the right theory, at the right time. Gallo had given the world what it wanted, and profited handsomely as a result. In fact the cancer researchers had not solved the problem of transformation to cancer cells, and they had deliberately ignored all available clinical, immunological, biochemical and toxological data about identical AIDS-indicating illnesses, against the better knowledge of researchers in the pre-AIDS era. They sacrificed scientific accuracy and protocol for a timely and "politically correct" theory of a "lethal AIDS agent." The "mystery" and "intriguing puzzle" is not the supposed "new disease," but the fact that the so-called "invisible hand of the market" managed to override the fundaments of scientific medical ethics with barely a peep of opposition.

More than 14 years after the historic conference of March 1983, when the idea of the "new agent" came into existence, the most prominent minds in the international community of retrovirus researchers met for another conference. They wanted to take stock of all the knowledge that had in the meantime been gathered as to how the "AIDS agent," according to the doctrine championed by these researchers that "HIV causes AIDS," destroyed the T-helper cells. In the meantime more than 200,000 scientific publications about HIV/AIDS had been published and more than *200 billion* dollars had been invested. The result of this stocktaking was a remarkable—and remarkably unpublicized—scientific admission of defeat: "The riddle of CD4 cell loss (from the bloodstream) remains unresolved. We are still very confused about the mechanisms that lead to CD4 depletion . . . but at least we are now confused at a higher level of understanding" (Balter 1997).

In plain language, this meant that the retrovirus-AIDS/cancer theory, elaborated since 1983 from the retrovirus cancer theory, had flopped! The "phantom" retroviruses did not cause cancer directly, by infecting organ cells and creating "human cancer running wild" (Thomas 1983). Nor did they cause cancer indirectly, by destroying the cell-mediated immunity which monitors cancer cells, thereby releasing a "clone of transformed, neoplastic cells" (Thomas 1983).

Furthermore, the depletion of T-helper cells from the bloodstream was not a result of progressive destruction following viral infection. The retrovirus researchers could provide no evidence to support this theory. Rather the stem (progenitor) cells of the T-helper cells undergo a functional shift (Th1-to-Th2 switch) and drift out of the bloodstream to other organ areas where they carry out their special function of supporting the B-cells in the production of antibodies. Just because there is a depletion of T-helper cells in the blood circulation (demonstrated by the so-called T4 or CD4 cell counts) does not necessarily mean that these T-helper cells must have been destroyed by a retrovirus. This conclusion also cannot be reached by the observation of premature extinction of T-helper cells in a test tube after they have been stimulated by certain oxidizing substances. There is a perfectly plausible explanation for this observation, which will be covered later in this text.

The concept of the Non-Retroviral disease model

The "new disease entity AIDS" had been explicitly defined on the basis of three patterns of findings:

1. Anomalies within the T-helper cells (AID) based on three criteria—depleted counts in the bloodstream, inhibited maturity and division after stimulation in a test-tube, and negative (anergic) reaction in DTH test.
2. Development of opportunistic infections (OI).
3. Development of Kaposi's sarcoma (KS).

All three patterns lead back to a single hypothetical origin: a progressive infection and destruction ofT-helper cells through a "new agent," a hypothetical retrovirus (see Table 1. Disease Model of the Retrovirus AIDS Theory).

In reality, the immunological, clinical, and epidemiological data showed a considerably different picture of the symptoms (see Table 2. Disease Model of the Non-Retrovirus AIDS Theory).

While all five symptomatic constellations were seen in cases of homosexual patients, the constellations AID+OI+KS, AID+KS and KS applied almost exclusively to this group. The Retrovirus Theory crucially demands that KS cannot appear without a retroviral infection of the T-helper cells. It is contrary to every biological probability, that a retroviral infection of the T-helper cells simultaneously triggers KS in some homosexual patients, but not in others. Conversely, one or more factors must have a direct effect on both the endothelial cells and/or the T-helper cells. This factor cannot be a retrovirus as, according to the Retrovirus Theory, it does not have any effect on endothelial cells. Furthermore, despite all the efforts of research, no hypothetical retroviruses were found in KS cells (Beral 1990).

The alternative explanation accounts for all five constellations in homosexuals who had been diagnosed (AID, AID+OI, AID+OI+KS, AID+KS, KS), in that, dependent on the intensity and duration of the affecting factors and/or the disposition of the patient, the T-helper cells and/or the endothelial cells could be affected to differing degrees.

Transplantation AIDS by inhibition of the cytotoxic NO synthesis supports the Non-Retroviral Concept

This is the same situation as with organ recipients, for whom without any reasonable doubt, Azathioprine had a causal effect both on the T-helper cells and the endothelial cells and in a certain percentage induced AID, OI and/or KS.

Azathioprine inhibits the synthesis of the purine bases, which effects a disruption of the DNA and RNA synthesis and thereby the biosynthesis of enzyme proteins. It also affects the synthesis of enzyme proteins in the NO synthase, which produces the immunological defense gas NO. However, the NO-forming enzymes need pyridine nucleotides for NO production. These nucleotides contain the purine base adenine, whose synthesis is inhibited by Azathioprine. This involves NAD^+ (nicotinamide adenine dinucleotide) as co-enzyme, and both FAD (flavin adenine dinucleotide) and FMN (flavin mononucleotide) as co-factors for NO synthase. These pyridine nucleotides play an essential role as hydrogen donors and acceptors in many biosyntheses, above all in cellular respiration (Bredt 1992, Marletta 1993, Knowles 1994, Richter 1996, Schweizer 1996, Lincoln 1997).

Corticosteroids, frequently deployed for immunosuppression in organ recipients, which also in some cases triggered KS and carcinoma (Hoshaw 1980), also attack the biosynthesis of NO in the T-helper cells in that they penetrate the cells and combine with factors that are important for the transcription (from DNA to mRNA). In this way, the corticosteroids inhibit the biosynthesis of proteins, among others the communication proteins (type 1 and type 2 cytokines), as well as the NO-forming NO synthases. Type 1 cytokines are potent stimulators of NO production (Cupps 1982, Colosanti 1995, Brattsand 1996, Kunz 1996, Lincoln 1997).

Cyclosporine A (CSA) is an important substance introduced in 1983 for the immunosuppression of organ transplant patients. It was isolated from the fungus *Tolypocladium inflatum*. CSA has an effect on the type 1 cytokine interleukin-2 (IL-2), a growth factor for T-helper cells, in that it indirectly inhibits its synthesis. CSA binds to proteins, the cyclophilins, which are present in many cells and participate in important regulatory processes. CSA medication also inhibits the synthesis and function of NO and its derivatives such as peroxinitrite. CSA medication had also triggered KS, lymphoma and various carcinomas in transplant patients (Kahan 1984, Penn 1991, Schreiber 1992, Richter 1996, Lincoln 1997). The mode of action of the fungitoxin Cyclosporine A, illustrates important aspects of the genesis of cancer, and will be discussed later in this text.

Counterarguments against NO inhibition as the cause of AIDS, in attempts to salvage the Retrovirus AIDS Theory, are totally illogical

The similarity of the various inhibitory mechanisms on the NO syntheses by immunosuppressive drugs, and the cellular counter-regulation, in high dosage long-term exogenous nitrite usage, endogenous NO stimulation in high and long-term antigen exposure and endogenous nitrosamine formation through long-term consumption of antibiotics, chemotherapeutics and analgesics with a secondary depletion to the thiol pool, has not been discussed by the AIDS researchers. Two illogical arguments are submitted by the nitrosamine researchers, when discussing nitrite inhalation by homosexuals (poppers) as a possible cause factor for AID, OI, and KS:

1. Amyl nitrite and nitroglycerin have been used for many years as treatment for angina pectoris (a narrowing of coronary vessels due to deficiencies in NO synthesis), without carcinogenic effects (Mirvish 1986).
   This argument compares the long-term, high dosage abuse of inhaled nitrites, with the equalization of impaired calcium-dependant NO synthesis in the coronary arteries via short-term treatment with nitrites or nitrates. Nitrite abusers initially have a normal physiological NO production, but simultaneously subject the NO metabolism and the antioxidant thiol pool to other stress factors. In a similar fashion, the risk of lung cancer to a chain smoker could be argued away by equating their habits to those of an occasional smoker. As Paracelsus said, "The poison is the dose." However nitrites can indeed have a double-edged effect, for instance in cases of dilated cardiomyopathy. The type 1 cytokine, tumor necrosis factor α, is produced in the endothelial cells of the coronary arteries, which suppresses the calcium-dependent NO synthesis and causes the painful symptoms of angina pectoris. However, the induced NO is increased in the cardiomuscular cells, which leads to a slowing down of the heart's action (negative ionotropic effect) (Habib 1996). An NO balance in the already NO-suppressed endothelial cells cannot trigger KS in the coronary arteries. But the cardiomuscular cells, which cannot develop cancer as they can no longer proliferate, can still be degeneratively damaged.
2. The appearance of KS in heterosexuals in Africa is, in all likelihood, not associated with poppers abuse (Mirvish 1986). Although the researchers confirm that nitrites can be transformed inside the human cell system to become carcinogenic nitrosamines, and that amyl nitrite and isobutyl nitrite both have a high carcinogenic potential in humans, they do not consider the possibility that African KS without AID (Kestens 1985) or

> with AID (Marquart 1986) could be caused by other nitrite nitrosamine sources—for instance, nitrite-contaminated drinking water and nitrite-preserved foodstuffs stored under the tropical hygienic conditions that are a fact of life in the poorer countries. On account of the frequency of Kaposi's sarcoma in Africa long before the AIDS era, found in all its various benign and malignant forms with and without AID, the restriction of causal research for KS in Africa to possible poppers consumption is obviously absurd. The association of KS in Africa with leprosy and anti-leprosy therapy, likewise points to a destroyed NO synthesis (Oettle 1962, Olweny 1984). As leprosy medication attacks the folic acid metabolism, the purine synthesis is also affected; additionally the homocysteine production is inhibited, and thus the thiol pool more rapidly expended and the NO synthesis suppressed by counterregulation. In this context, there may exist similar predisposing factors as seen with organ transplant patients, e.g. genetic HLA type of the affected person.

Contrary to the predictions of the Retrovirus AIDS Theory, the fact that there has been no higher incidence of other common cancer forms in homosexuals over the last twenty years (with the exception of lymphoma after AZT treatment) also disproves the assumption that retroviruses indirectly provoke cancer by destroying the immune cells. It was inevitable that this prognosis would be made by the retrovirologists as there was no biological reason to suppose that "a release of clones of transformed, neoplastic cells" (Thomas 1984), and other cancer cell forms such as KS, would occur after depletion of the postulated T-cell surveillance of cancer cells. Incidentally, it had already been demonstrated before the advent of the retrovirus infection theory (supposedly transmitted by sex and blood) that the transformation and growth of cancer cell clones was not dependent on immune surveillance (Kinlen 1982). The fact is, that after the decline of the "poppers craze" among homosexuals, the number of cases of KS in the USA and other Western countries also declined (Haverkos 1990). This clinical finding conforms to the fact that after legal restrictions on nitrite preservation in meat and sausages, together with increased use of refrigeration, the only cancer form to decline was stomach cancer; meanwhile, for instance, the incidence of lung cancer, due among other things to the creation of nitrosamines in tobacco during the drying process, had greatly increased (Hoel 1992, Burton 1994, Djordjevic 1994).

The given data proves that the hypothetical chain of causes—T-helper cell loss leading to provocation of KS cell clones—does not exist biologically.

As a result, the "new disease entity" (AID-OI-KS) is not a new syndrome describing a causal disease entity, but rather comprises two separate disease forms in separate cell types: AID (with or without OI) as a disease form of the T-helper cells, and KS as a disease form of the endothelial cells, independent of AID but appearing within the same time-span as AID.

So when we refer to an AID syndrome (AIDS) we must factor out KS as an independent disease form. If we wanted to be more precise we could talk about an *Azathioprine syndrome* or a *nitrite syndrome*, in which the term syndrome relates to the appearance of AID and/or KS with the same cause in different cell types. AID can only trigger OI: AID+OI = AID syndrome = AIDS. It is correct that both AID (as anomaly of the T-helper cells) and KS (as anomaly of the endothelial cells) can be triggered by the same causal factor(s), but both disease forms could develop in these cases independently of one another at the same time or at different times in the same patients. There remain pathological changes in two different cell types without the changes in the one cell type being initially responsible for the changes in the other. By analogy, it would mean that if "smoker's leg" and a lung carcinoma were diagnosed in a single patient, smoking could be seen as the common cause, but the damage to the arteries in the leg could not be blamed on the lung cancer.

On the other hand, AID or AID+OI (= AIDS) can have many different singular causes, or a combination of causes, in that the immune cell network is evolutionary-biologically programmed to react uniformly once a critical threshold has been crossed. The cause of AIDS (without KS), in homosexuals, does not have to be traced back to inhalation of nitrites alone. There has always been AID and AID+OI in homosexuals (overview Root-Bernstein 1993). The most frequent AID+OI disease in homosexuals, PCP, was not diagnosed much before 1980 because the diagnostic techniques were complex and risky. A long needle had to be inserted into the lung tissues and cell material drawn out for analysis (a transbronchial biopsy).

An improvement in diagnosis was made possible after advances in bronchial lavage techniques, for the purpose of extracting cell material for the microbiological determination of the PCP pathogen (Blumenfeld 1984, Broaddus 1985). PCP, however, was a very well known AID+OI syndrome, seen after multiple applications of chemotherapeutics and immunosuppressives in cancer patients, organ recipients and patients with autoimmune illnesses (Young 1984). Patients without specifically-named illnesses were mostly treated pragmatically and the PCP was not identified: "Young men presenting with interstitial pneumonia without an underlying disorder may not have received a definite diagnosis or specific therapy for *P. carinii* pneumonia; others may have received empirical therapy with trimethoprim-sulfamethoxazole [Septra or Bactrim]" (Auerbach 1982). The "sudden appearance of PCP in homosexuals" was inevitable as a result of improvements in PCP diagnosis. The sophisticated agent-specific diagnostic process supported the statement of the Canadian pathologist some 20 years ago. "PCP is much more common in this country than we thought, we just have to open our eyes to see it" (Berdnikoff 1959).

The rush to implicate a sexually transmitted infection

Before 1981, there were no medical statistics to show the separate development of atypical non-bacterial lung inflammations specifically in homosexual patients. From the later-published initial diagnosis of KS in a homosexual patient in 1978 until the historic conference of March 1983, a number of important factors acted together to facilitate the (facile) hypothesis of a "new disease entity":

- 1978: first assignation of a subgroup of T-helper cells (T4 cells) as AID was reported
- Discovery of T4 cell depletion in many other illnesses (Reinherz 1979,1981 a, 1981 b, Huzzell 1982)
- 1978-1981: first diagnosis in homosexual patients of KS and PCP combined with T4 cell depletion
- After improvements in diagnosis, PCP was now more frequently recognized, while earlier it had often been overlooked
- Homosexual patients report the practice of sexual doping via inhalation of nitrite gases (CDC 1981 a, CDC 1981 b, Gottlieb 1981, Masur 1981, Durack 1981, Haverkos 1982, Auerbach 1982, De Wys 1982, Marmor 1982, Goedert 1982)
- In 1980 the American Chemical Association speaks of a change in the "political philosophy" concerning nitrite and nitrosamines as the toxic causes for cancer and immune disruption—research funding was restricted after conservative government regime change (Loeppky 1994 a)
- 1980-83: First publications from researchers from the National Cancer Institute regarding the so-called retrovirus particle in human cancer cells (leukaemia and lymphoma cells) and of antibodies in blood serum against proteins from these particles—a connection between these particles and the origins of cancer can not be proved—funding for retrovirus cancer research, in existence since 1971, is discontinued in 1981 (Poiesz 1980, Kalyanaraman 1981 a, Kalyanaraman 1981 b, 1982, Gallo 1986, 1991, 1999, Duesberg 1987)

- 1982: The unproven theory that the development and growth of cancer cells is dependent on destroyed immune cells is questioned but supported by most researchers (Spector 1978, Kinlen 1982).

Under the prevailing political circumstances the original explanation of the "new disease entity" in homosexuals as a result of intoxication by industrial products (excessive consumption of nitrites, exogenous nitrosamines, antibiotics, chemotherapeutics) was not considered fashionable. "The only reason for preferring the explanation that an 'undefined' infectious factor relating to sexual behaviour appears to be the cause, and not the alternative, appears to be a predisposition to favor a sexually transmitted infection. In fact in homosexuals evidence exists that the variable most strongly associated with KS is the consumption of more than four 'hits' of nitrites per night of use" (Papadopulos-Eleopulos 1992).

The obvious intoxication of the patients had somehow now to be turned into an infection by an "unknown agent." The pathogen must have the capacity to infect T-helper cells in order to explain their depletion in blood serum. However, a new pathogen is not needed to explain the depletion of T-helper cells in many other illnesses. In these cases, the disappearance of T-helper cells can be regarded as a secondary consequence of the primary disease processes. In the case of a "new disease entity," however, a new rationale had to be found because the toxic damage of the immune and/or endothelial cells was not accepted as the primary cause of the illness and at the same time the appearance of the "intriguing puzzle" of Kaposi's sarcoma was not allowed to be explained by the use of toxic/pharmacotoxic substances, as it was in the case of KS in graft (transplant) patients.

Homosexual men have the highest rates of infectious disease of all other risk groups in North America or Europe

Type B hepatitis (HBV) was regarded as the model for a viral infection transmitted through sexual intercourse as well as blood and blood products, and urban homosexuals were very often diagnosed as HBV-positive (Schreeder 1981). Acute and chronic HBV infections also cause a depletion of T-helper cells and a decline in cell-mediated immune functions (Klingenstein 1981).

At the end of the seventies, the first vaccine against Hepatitis B was developed in the USA; beginning in November 1978, it was tested on 549 homosexual men in New York, while a further 534 homosexual men were injected with a placebo as a control (Szmuness 1979). The vaccine was licensed in 1981 in the USA and in 1982 in Germany. At the time of the vaccine trials, there were no longer any doubts about the extremely high antigenic stress in urban homosexual men. "Homosexual men have the highest disease load of any North American or European risk group" (Root-Bernstein 1993)

This extreme antigenic stress could indeed adequately explain, as it does in other patient groups, the depletion of T-helper cells, but the rationale of a "new disease entity" demanded a connection between T-helper suppression and the development of Kaposi's sarcoma. Such a coincidence between immunosuppression and KS was only known among graft patients and others, who had been treated with toxic, immunosuppressive substances. A sexually-transmitted agent was sought as a possible link between immunosuppression and KS—an agent of a new type, which not only suppressed T-helper cells but also destroyed them—because then the disappearance of the T-helper cells from the bloodstream could be attributed to their destruction. A pathogen that was simultaneously an immune cell eradicator and also an indirect KS trigger was unknown. The logical question would have been to ask whether the extremely high antigenic stress along with the disappearance of T-helper cells, was enough to trigger KS, because during this same time, the theory was being promoted that cancer was actually dependent on immunosuppression (Gatti 1971, Waldmann 1972, Spector 1978). It is significant in the light of this theory that children with a congenital malformation of the thymus who suffer from a T-helper cell deficiency, develop fungal, parasitic and viral infections; however, they do not suffer from high-grade bacterial infections, as the function of the B-cells is completely intact. This syndrome matches the symptoms of AIDS patients who can also develop opportunistic infections, but who have an intact or even increased antibody production of B-cells. As a rule AIDS patients do not become ill from bacterial infections, with the exception of mycobacterial infections, as long as toxins do not inhibit the maturation of the B-cells. Even more significant is the fact that children with Di George syndrome (a failure of development of the third and fourth pharyngeal pouches at the embryonic stage) did not have a heightened risk of KS or any other cancer forms (Di George 1968, Lischner 1975). This fact is in opposition to the Retrovirus-AIDS Theory, which states that the depletion of T-helper cells is the causal factor for both Kaposi's sarcoma and lymphoma.

This evident contradiction was interpreted at the historic conference of 1983 by stating that the Di George children would not grow old enough to develop cancer, and that some factors associated with puberty might be necessary for the development of Kaposi's sarcoma (Levine 1984). This assumption, however, is in opposition to the development of lymphomas and leukemias in children with combined T and B-lymph cell defects (severe combined immunodeficiency, SCID). These children also develop opportunistic infections and additional high-grade bacterial infections (Gatti 1971, Spector 1978).

The sole presence of congenital or acquired cellular immune weaknesses is not directly implicated as a cancer cause

The second hypothesis as to why there was no KS in Di George syndrome cases was that the genetic variants of HLA types which are detectable in 50% of classical KS cases, were underrepresented in this group of children (Levine 1984). The discrepancy in this hypothesis is that, particularly in younger patients with classic KS, this HLA variant was also not detected (Rothman 1962).

The fact remains that neither congenital nor acquired T-helper deficits have been traced as an indirect trigger for cancer.

A "new agent" was not needed in order to explain this "new disease entity;" already present was a massive and diverse blend of microbial and toxic contaminations, which were virtually unknown to medicine before the era of excessive promiscuity. No one in his right mind should assume that an organism, even a young adult, can limitlessly manage industrial and microbial toxins without specific symptoms being manifested. All the evidence summarized thus far, and to be put forth subsequently, suggests that AIDS is the systemic result of such cumulative toxic stress, and not a retrovirus-caused syndrome. This environmental question was, however, treated as a taboo because then the cumulative effect of all toxins in the years preceding the disease (nitrites, antibiotics, chemotherapeutics, recreational drugs, etc.) would have to be included in the diagnostic calculations. As a result of this diagnostic censorship, there came a blanket explanation that all infectious and toxic contaminations of promiscuous homosexual men were insufficient for immunosuppression and the triggering of Kaposi's sarcoma. At the very most, there was talk of nebulous "co-factors."

The apparent proof of "HIV" in the T-helper immune cells of AIDS patients was based on the provocation of cellular products that signify the evolutionary-biologically programmed immune response (experimental laboratory AID).

At the historic conference in March 1983, Gallo and his colleagues reported that they had found, in the T-helper cells of two AIDS patients, evidence of an infection of the human T-cell leukaemia virus (HTLV) discovered in his laboratory. The evidence, however, turns out to be rather odd: The Gallo team had mixed human leukaemia cells with T-helper cells and stimulated their growth with oxidizing substances and type 1 cytokine. Finally, the residue of this "culture soup" was placed in a high-speed centrifuge, and the proteins from this amorphous mixture were made to react with antibodies from the blood serum of AIDS patients. The team then claimed this antibody reactivity as evidence of infection with a hypothetical leukaemia virus.

Such procedures cannot be accepted as evidence for real virus isolation, let alone an infection of the patient. The extracted proteins, which reacted to the antibodies in the serum of patients, could have originated from the co-cultivated leukaemia cells and/or the T-helper cells—not necessarily the hypothetical leukaemia virus. First of all, the supposed virus has to be isolated; it must be separated from any other cell material. The core of the selected virus particle would have had to have been examined, the proteins and nucleic acids documented. Only once it had been established that it was a stable virus capable of spreading infections, the proteins from the real isolated virus would be put into contact with human serum.

Yet even if all the preconditions of proper viral isolation had been followed according to the standard rules of virology, the antibody reaction in the serum of a human being to a precisely identified viral protein would still not be evidence of a prior infection with this virus. In every human's serum there are millions of antibodies of varying kinds that were originally formed to act against a totally different protein, but are similar enough to react against new, previously unseen viral proteins. Every immunologist knows this process—it is called a "cross-reaction."

The laboratory stunts of the Gallo team were, however, accepted without any criticism by the gathering of over 500 specialists at the conference. A virologist from the National Institutes of Health also gave a lecture at the conference with the suggestive title: "Viruses, Immune Dysregulation, and Oncogenesis: Inferences Regarding the Cause and Evolution of AIDS." Among other things he stated: "Retroviruses are also distinctive in that they cause prolonged immune suppression in the presence of neutralizing antibodies, and this has again been found in the case of the recently isolated and characterized human T-cell leukaemia virus (HTLV) . . . Here, then, is an example of a virus specifically and primarily interacting with the T-helper population" (Levine 1984).

In support of his contentions, the lecturer quoted six publications from the Gallo team and one publication from a Japanese research group (Popvic 1983, Popvic 1982, Poiesz 1980, Manzari 1983, Gallo 1982; Miyoshi 1981 b). The Japanese researchers had incubated leukaemia cells together with leukocytes from a human umbilical cord and used the same laboratory techniques as the Gallo team. None of the studies tested whether the same effects using the same laboratory techniques would be demonstrated without the co-cultivation of T-helper cells with leukaemia/lymphoma cells (or in the case of the Japanese team, umbilical cord leukocytes without co-cultivation with leukaemia cells).

In his lecture, the virologist Levine had proposed his reasoning of the existence of an exemplary virus, but he did so using an unproven argument that presumably confirmed his rationale. The quoted studies of the Gallo team and the Japanese researchers by no means assume that human retroviruses cause a long-term immunosuppression in the presence of neutralising antibodies. The Gallo team had in 1981 merely demonstrated that a structural protein (p24), extracted from a cell culture and centrifuged with human lymphoma cells, had reacted to antibodies from human serum. Without precisely following the standard isolation procedures (proving whether the proteins actually originated from the studied particle, and whether the particle actually encased structural proteins and RNA of a hypothetical retrovirus), it would be arbitrary to claim that a retroviral protein had reacted to human antibodies, and thus that the person with these antibodies in his serum must have been infected by a retrovirus. As these structural proteins could just as well be structural proteins that were extracted from lymphoma cells during the laboratory process, the reaction with an antibody in human serum proves nothing. Such antibodies are able to react to all proteins from human cells, once the protein is no longer protected by the cell membrane. The biological function of antibodies is such that they react equally to microbial or allergenic proteins, as well as with all the body's own proteins. These bodily proteins are leaked into the plasma upon cell death if they have not already been dispersed to their individual building blocks. Antibodies only react to proteins above a certain molecular size. Therefore it is also fundamentally absurd to state that retroviruses could cause long-term immunosuppression in immune cells in the presence of neutralising antibodies. Virus particles, whether hidden in immune or other cells, cannot be identified by antibodies. This can only take place in the plasma outside of the cells, once the virus particles bud out of the infected cells, or when viruses have infiltrated an organism but not yet colonized the cells. In order to cause a long-term suppression of immune cells, the retroviruses (if they exist at all) would have had to continuously mature and bud out of the short-lived T-helper cells, in order to colonize newly formed T-helper cells. However, when neutralizing antibodies are already present, they will impede the viruses exiting the immune cells from colonizing new immune cells, thereby *neutralizing* the infection.

The publications of the Gallo team and the Japanese researchers cited by Levine only demonstrate the following:

- When human cancer cells (leukaemia or lymphoma cells) are treated under certain laboratory conditions with certain biochemicals then particles mature out of these cells that after inspection with an electron microscope could either be viral particles or non-viral particles.
- When leukaemia or lymphoma cells and T-cells which have not transformed to cancer cells are treated in the same way, then particles mature out of the leukaemia or lymphoma cells but likewise out of the T-cells that after studying with an electron microscope could either be viral particles or non-viral particles.
- When the supernatant residue of the co-cultivated cancer and T-cells has been centrifuged a protein mixture is obtained that could contain proteins from cancer cells, T-cells and matured particles. If one were to select a protein from this mixture and put it into contact with antibodies from human serum which displays an antigen-antibody reaction to this protein, then it is not possible to tell from this procedure whether the cause of the reaction was a protein from a cancer cell, lymphoma cell, viral particle, or non-viral particle. This differentiation would only be possible after proper viral isolation following the standard procedures of virology: the viral particles in question—having been cleared of all other cell components, proteins and other molecules—are shown to be composed of specific viral proteins, and contain viral RNA capable of replication.
- When leukaemia cells are co-cultivated with T-cells under the same laboratory conditions and particles mature from both cell types, then the assumption that either viral or non-viral particles from the leukaemia cells have colonized the T-cells is logically inconclusive. Under the same laboratory conditions particles could have matured from either cell types. The counterclaim that lymph cell particles colonized the leukaemia cells is equally inconclusive. Similarly under the same conditions, when lymphoma cells are co-cultivated with T-cells, or leukaemia cells with umbilical cord leukocytes, or umbilical cord cells with T-cells, then the assumption remains inconclusive. The maturation of particles in co-cultivated cell cultures does not prove that the particle will be transferred as an infection from one cell type to another.
- When, under the same laboratory conditions, particles mature in non-transformed T-cells without co-cultivation with cancer cells or other cell types, this does not mean that they are viral particles; proteins in the supernatant which react to human serum does not prove viral origin of the proteins. Such a statement could only be verified if the particle had been truly isolated from other cell components, the contents of said particle had been clearly identified as both structural and enzymatic proteins, the viral RNA was capable of being replicated, and finally that proteins from these

pure and proven retroviral particles had reacted to the antibodies in human serum. To this day no one has published these would-be conclusive pieces of evidence (Papadopulos-Eleopulos 2000 a).

- But notwithstanding the grossly inconclusive evidence of the applied laboratory techniques even if the particle had been properly identified as a real retrovirus particle, this finding in itself would not be enough proof to show a pathological infection.

One of the most famous retrovirologists in the USA, the German-American molecular biologist Duesberg, professor at the University of California-Berkeley, (whom Gallo had described in 1985 as the retrovirologist with the sharpest wits) submitted a fundamental analysis of the entire retrovirus species just four years after the memorable birth of the "AIDS agent." Duesberg came to the conclusion that all retroviral particles were nothing more than benign passengers in the genetic make-up of humans, and by no means were able to cause infections. Duesberg expanded his statement by classifying the cancer genes as unusual re-combinations of DNA instead of activated oncogenes (Duesberg 1987).

"An example of a virus specifically and primarily interacting with the T-helper population" (Levine 1984), which in 1983 was introduced as the prize candidate for the "AIDS agent," had only attained special scientific attention for a short period of time. In the diagnosis and therapy of cancer diseases it has remained insignificant. A good year later, however, a newer prototype of such a tailor-made retrovirus in the serum of AIDS patients surfaced in publications from the Gallo team. Gallo had created a new variant in his retroviral family with the classification HTLV-III. The product also came from the co-incubation of T-helper cells from the serum of AIDS patients and a leukaemia cell line. Using the same dubious laboratory techniques as with his prototype HTLV, Gallo distilled a protein mixture from the supernatant of co-cultivated hybrid cell culture, which he then used as the substrate for his antibody test.

Again Gallo failed to produce evidence as to whether the proteins in question were the body's own proteins from the incubated T-helper cells and/or leukaemia cells, or whether they were in fact real retroviral proteins. But this time the "invisible hand of the market" was in play before Gallo introduced the new retrovirus variant and the antibody test to scientific discussion. He patented the test first, and then subsequently announced (together with the then-current US Health Secretary, Margaret Heckler) in front of the international press that he had discovered the "probable" AIDS agent, that he had developed a blood test capable of supplying evidence of HTLV-III, and that in two years a vaccine against this retrovirus would be ready for the market. Since this announcement, the techniques used in producing this HIV test have been protected by patent rights. HTLV-I and HTLV-II, again in the blood serum of AIDS patients, re-emerged in ensuing publications. Later, this supposed leukaemia virus was no longer mentioned, as it had somehow mutated into a phantom-like immune-weakening virus. Evidently the AIDS/leukemia virus was a laboratory artefact, as no AIDS patient ever suffered from it. Rational questioning—why these hypothetical leukaemia viruses suddenly stopped triggering leukaemia and instead (even though only for a short time until it was ousted by its successor), destroyed immune cells and puzzlingly indirectly effected Kaposi's sarcoma only in the gay community—was thrust aside in the midst of the mass hysteria that the "AIDS agent HIV," (as the successful laboratory product was termed) has lamentably and scandalously caused until today.

The simple but decisive trick that Gallo used to sell to the world his former leukaemia agent (which had received little acclaim among oncologists), as the AIDS agent similar to the one he had used for HTLV-I and HTLV-II. Gallo now claimed that during co-cultivation of the T-helper cell lines from AIDS patients with the transformed T-cells from leukaemia patients, the retrovirus jumped from the T-helper cells to the leukaemia cells. Correspondingly, Gallo simply repackaged the classification from Human T-cell Leukaemia Virus to Human T-cell Lymphotropic Virus (both HTLV). The jump from the T-cells to the leukaemia cells, according to Gallo, was the proof that the retrovirus had to be the much-sought "AIDS agent." Thus the cancer agent that transforms lymph cells into uninhibited and growing leukaemia cells became the "AIDS agent" that kills T-cells. Why Gallo had to co-incubate T-helper cells with leukaemia cells in order to elicit the supposed retrovirus from the T-helper cells was explained by stating that the retroviruses develop better in leukaemia cells. In reality, Gallo needed the leukaemia cells to stimulate the repair enzyme, reverse transcriptase (RT). This RT enzyme repairs the last part of the DNA strand in cancer cells (which with every division becomes a little shorter), so that the division frequency of the cancer cells remains stable. Citing as evidence the presence of the RT enzymes (which transcribe RNA sections into the DNA sequence), in his "cell culture soup," Gallo decisively concluded the existence of a new retrovirus in T-helper immune cells. However, this sequence of reverse transcription (Temin 1985, Baltimore 1985, Greider 1996, Boeke 1996, Teng 1996, Teng 1997, Strahl 1996, Yegorov 1996, Hässig 1998, 1998 a) had long been established in many animal and human cell types (Temin 1970, 1972. 1985, Varmus 1987, 1988), as had the transcription of genetic information from RNA to DNA, which was demonstrated by the American microbiologists Temin and Baltimore (both Nobel prize winners in 1975).

Evidence of reverse transcription after co-cultivation of T-helper immune cells with leukemic cancer cells cannot be considered as proof that the retro-transcription must be due solely to a retrovirus in the T-helper cells. Such an assumption is not only arbitrary, but also contrary to the established biological facts.

The "HIV antibody" test was calibrated so that a positive result will occur in a person with particularly high levels of polyspecific antibodies (not HIV antibodies) in the blood serum

Gallo again decanted the cell liquids from his culture mixture, filtered out a mixture of proteins and let them react to the serum of AIDS patients. The expected protein/antibody reaction in these AIDS patients was again proclaimed as a retroviral infection. Gallo had as evidence of a retroviral presence in the T-helper cells of donors with clinical AIDS symptoms, nothing more in his culture than a RT reaction and in the sera of the AIDS patients, nothing more than an antibody reaction to the test proteins from his "cell culture soup." When Gallo, who also wanted to sell his patented test to the blood donor services, brought his test proteins into contact with the sera of healthy donors, 10% of these healthy sera also reacted! Because a test that turns evidently healthy blood donors into doomed men is unmarketable, Gallo altered the sensitivity of the measuring reaction. This meant that with fewer antibodies in the serum, the test now read negative; correspondingly, with more antibodies there was a positive reading. The arbitrary measuring threshold decides whether a subject will be labelled HIV-positive or HIV-negative (Popovic 1984, Gallo 1984, Schüpbach 1984, Samgadharan 1984, Gallo 1991).

The apparently astounding correlation between those testing HIV-positive and a certain percentage of the target group—antigen-stressed homosexuals, intravenous drug addicts, hemophiliacs with substituted high antigen-contaminated coagulation proteins, multi-transfusion recipients, children of drug-dependent mothers, people from poor countries, etc.—is not surprising (Giraldo 1999 a). Long after the "discovery of the AIDS agent," a better understanding of the relationship between T4 cell analysis, HIV seropositivity, AIDS-indicating illnesses, cancer, AIDS therapy, etc., is uncovered in light of important newer research findings.

The "HIV positive" laboratory result is based on circular logic

The "predisposition to favor a sexually transmitted infection" (Papadopulos-Eleopulos 1992) set the stage to blindly trust the laboratory stunts of the failed retrovirus cancer researchers who had mutated, so to speak, to retrovirus-AIDS researchers. As there was no other "AIDS agent" in the offing from the laboratory researchers, the phantom-like retroviruses made the grade. With fear of the "lethal virus" infecting the global population, free reign was given to previously muted irrational fantasies. The dictatorially stage-managed fear of a plague became taken as a real plague. US virologists and specialists from varying disciplines had accomplished the task of blaming well-known opportunistic infections and cancer forms on a laboratory construction and then sold it to the mass media as one of the "most devastating epidemics in modern history" (Friedman-Kein 1984 a).

The most terrifying thing about this fateful failure of modern medicine, was the fact that scientists from around the world, with very few exceptions, swallowed whole this transparent construction without critically analyzing the published data.

A glance at the relevant medical journals of the sixties would have been enough. At that point in time, over a decade before the "sudden appearance" of a supposedly new retrovirus, the manifestation of the most common AIDS-indicating illness, *Pneumocystis carinii* pneumonia (PCP), was clearly known as an immunodeficiency disease and the causes given were clearly of an immunotoxic nature. PCP fungal infections were confirmed not only in children, but also in adults after autopsies. Outbreaks of PCP after chemotherapy were demonstrated in animal experiments. After 1964, there were publications about PCP in graft and cancer patients who had been treated with immunotoxins and chemotherapy (Schmid 1964, Hill 1964, Frenkel 1966, Esterly 1967, Robbins 1967, 1968, Harrlin 1968). Opportunistic infections caused either by missing or malfunctioning T-helper immune cells were often classified as immunological deficiency diseases (IDD) (Bergsma 1968). IDD developed into acquired immunodeficiency (AID) so as to distinguish between AID and congenital immunodeficiency (CID). AID then became acquired immunodeficiency syndrome (AIDS) starting in 1982.

Initially there was only the need to state the clinical fact that AID+OI appeared simultaneously in some patients as KS, but by no means stipulate that AID was the cause of KS. At the historic conference of March 1983 the described disease definition became a causal disease definition: it was postulated that the "new agent" was the cause of AID and that AID was the cause of KS. The coincidence of the appearance of two disease phenomena in different cell types became a causal link between two different cell types. From the very beginning, as initiator for the postulated causal link, a virus as a "new agent" was constructed which was supposed to have infected the helper immune cells, triggered AID, and as a result precipitated KS. This construction of a "new disease entity" of a "retrovirus AID syndrome" (HIV/AIDS) facilitated with a greater variability than AID, for whatever reasons, to re-interpret AID plus selected disease symptoms as AIDS. Real symptoms with actual and differing causes were distorted to a virtual disease entity. Mass-psychological stage-managed plague fears were stoked by a laboratory construction. It was the moment of birth of a phantom medicine, which engineered a universal lethal threat from real diseases and by these means created a global market for itself. The "planned experiments on humans" (Thomas 1984) mentioned at the historic conference in 1983 were ready to begin.

Even medical knowledge 20 years ago could have correctly diagnosed the immunotoxic causes of AIDS without the presumption of a "new agent"

It does not take a lot of diagnostic shrewdness to identify the causes of AID indicator diseases, which were diagnosed since 1978 and publicized since 1981, and to see through and rebut the supposed rationale of a "new disease entity" which supposedly could only be caused by a "new agent." It merely needed a thorough review of the medical facts to avoid millions of people being frightened to death by being "HIV stigmatized" and abandoned to the "clean torture" of AIDS treatment with highly toxic drugs which had been proven to trigger AIDS and cancer.

The published declarations of the University researchers of 1981 that the people suffering from AIDS had been "previously healthy" patients (Gottlieb 1981) can only be taken as unprofessional sophistry, as every patient feels healthy up to the first symptoms of illness. Long-term abuse of prescribed and unprescribed antibiotics and chemotherapeutics, long-term nitrite inhalation, long-term injections of highly contaminated coagulation proteins for hemophiliacs, long-term intravenous drug consumption under the conditions of the street scene, multitransfusions of on average 35 transfusions for grave primary illnesses along with the corresponding medications, extreme antigen stress even in the womb (overview Root-Bernstein 1993)—all of these would provoke any "previously healthy" organisms into counter-regulation without the need to construct a "new agent" for this "intriguing puzzle" (Friedman-Kein 1984 a).

But the engineers of the "AIDS agent," in addition to the distortion of biological facts, profited from another ominous development. Since 1977 in the USA and in Great Britain discoveries in the laboratory could, like other inventions, be patented. This break in research culture caused a division within the medical research community. Some researchers, whose planned research projects were oriented to marketing possibilities, allowed pharmaceutical companies to finance their research work (either to a large extent or completely), or allowed them options to buy shares in biotechnological companies at below-market prices. Gallo's "AIDS test" patent was sold to five pharmaceutical concerns, and he is making money to this day from the royalties. For others it is ethically a matter of course to deepen the understanding of healing. These researchers lay open their research work without the using a shroud of secrecy for patents like Gallo and his colleagues. Happily, groups of ethical researchers who are prepared to question and re-evaluate fixed dogmas of medical research have brought fundamental insights that have profoundly changed the concepts of the medical world. But the work of these ethical medics and researchers, although important and welcome, comes tragically too late for the countless victims of the "*Virus Hunting*" (Gallo 1991).

Fig. 7) Cover of the German Journal *Deutsches Ärzteblatt*.

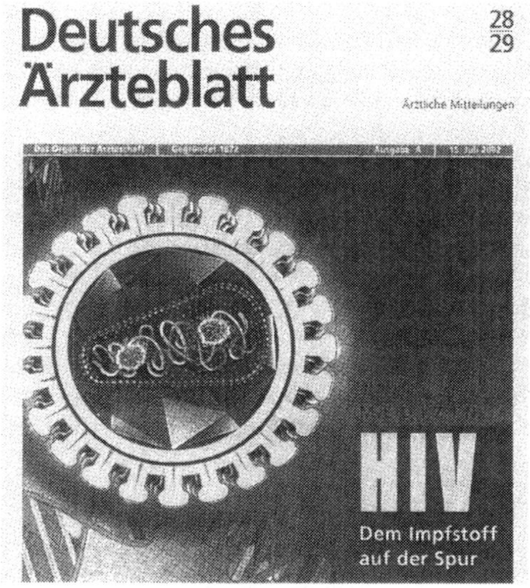
Deutsches Ärzteblatt
28
29
Ärztliche Mitteilungen
HIV
Dem Impfstoff auf der Spur

20 years after the supposed isolation of "HIV" a computer-designed picture was shown on the cover of the July issue of the German medical journal *Deutsches Ärzteblatt*, one week before the World AIDS Conference. This picture is the work of imagination and claimed to be a depiction of "HIV". The specialist magazine is the official organ of the German Medical Association to which all qualified German physicians belong.

Fig. 8) Type C RNA tumor virus isolated from cultured human acute myelogenous leukemia cells.
(Gallagher, Gallo, 1975 Science 187 pp. 350-353)

"Today nobody, not even Gallo, considers HL23V as being the first human retrovirus or even a retrovirus"

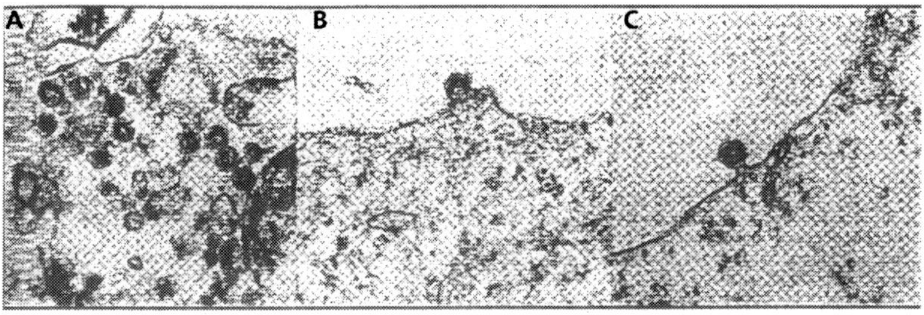
A
B
C

A. "HL23V" banded (band 1.16 gm/ml) and purified **B. Early viral budding** **C. Full viral budding**

Fig. 9)

Beginning in the 50's, so-called retroviruses have been isolated in sarcoma cells (tumor cells of the connective tissue) of guinea-pigs and birds with electron microscopes. Despite strenuous efforts by researchers, it has never been possible to confirm the presence of analogous retroviruses in human tumor cells. For this reason some researchers proposed so-called indirect markers to provide additional proof of the presence of retroviruses in human cells. These markers are also composed of fragments of cells that under highly oxidative stress conditions are produced in vitro by several types of cells. Since these fragments called vesicles look similar to real retroviral particles, standard rules were established in 1972 for the purification of these vesicles, for their reproduction with electron microscopes and for their biochemical preparation, in order to avoid mistaking them for the human retroviruses. In 1975 Gallo, the American physician, published the alleged additional proof of retroviruses in a line of human leukemic cells. From the verification of his findings it became apparent that Gallo had not applied the standard rules. Gallo was compelled to acknowledge his "error", and the presumed isolation of retroviruses in accordance with the standard rules could not be confirmed (see Chapter IV fig. 8).
In 1983 Gallo and his French colleague Montaigner stated simultaneously that they had furnished documentary evidence for the presence of retroviruses in the T4 immune cells of AIDS patients. Both groups of researchers had not applied the standard rules for the isolation of retroviruses (see Chapter IV, fig. 10).
Only 14 years later, after the "HIV causes AIDS" theory had become established, two groups of researchers, one French and one German, published the first pictures of the "HIV" vesicles with electron microscopes: the pictures showed "purified vesicles", whose size and shape did not correspond to those assumed for "HIV" up to that time. However, the pictures of the "purified vesicles" with the electron microscope chiefly reproduced fragments of cells. The substrata for the "anti-HIV" antibody tests are drawn from this "cellular soup" [Montaigner, 1997]. That is why we are actually dealing with proteinic dregs of cultivations of human cells and not with "HIV proteins" that are used as proteinic antigenes to confirm the "HIV infection" (see Chapter IV, figs. 11 and 12).
On adopting the standard method of purification for cellular vesicles of suspicious viral origin, electron microscope photographs always show a homogeneous picture in the presence of real retroviruses
(see Chapter IV, fig. 13; purified retroviruses of guinea-pig sarcoma).

Fig. 10) Electron microscope photo of banded and purified HIV.

Never published in scientific literature

Fig. 11 HIV banded and purified, 1997

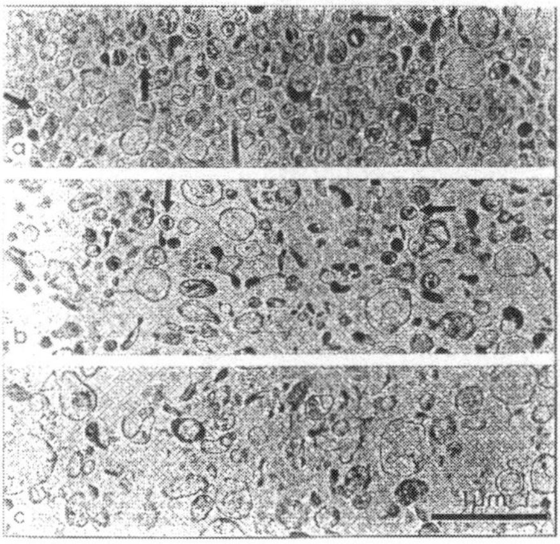
a
b
c

Gluschankof et al. Cell membrane vesicles are a major contaminant of gradient-enriched human immunodeficiency virus type-1 preparations.
Virology, 1997, n. 230, pp. 125-133

"Purified HIV-1 preparations of are contaminated by cellular vesicles. Purified vesicles from infected H9 cells (a) and activated PBMC (b) ... non-infected H9 cells (c)"

NB: The authors do not claim that photos a and b represent purified "HIV" but just "purified vesicles".

Fig. 12)

"The photos show that most of the material in the density gradient is of cellular origin"

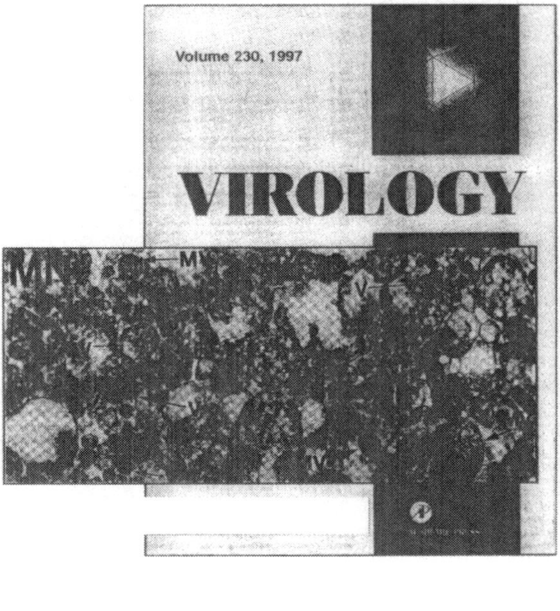
Volume 230, 1997
VIROLOGY

Fig. 13)

Purification of retroviral particles ultracentrifugation of the density gradient.

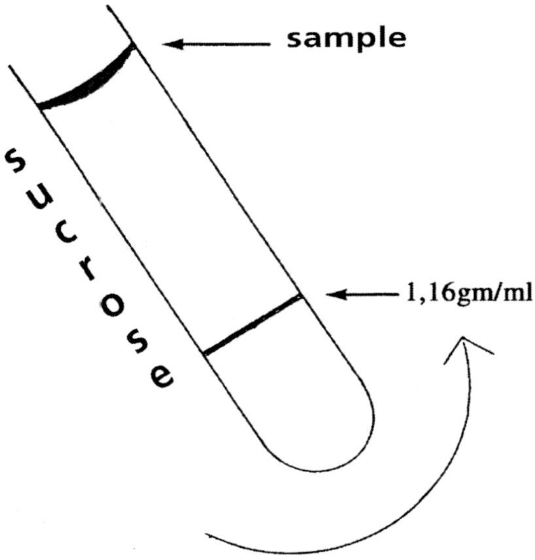
sample
sucrose
1,16gm/ml

Murine sarcoma virus banded and purified, 1973
Sinoussi, F., Mendiola, L., Cherman, J.C., (1973)

Purification and partial differentiation of the murine sarcoma virus (MMSV) based on the sedimentation rates of the density gradients of sucrose. *Spectra 2000, 4: 237-43*

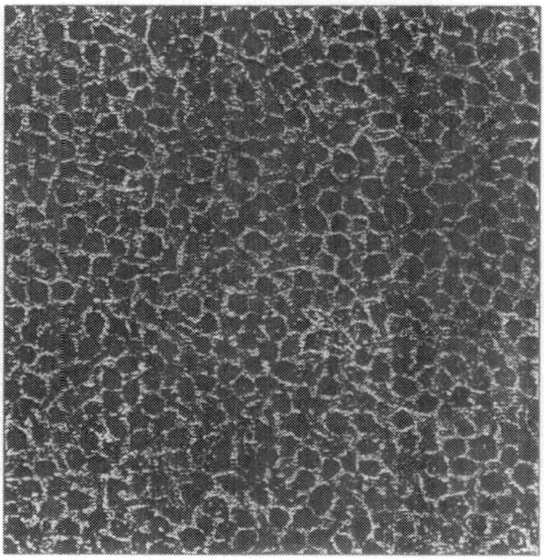

Chapter V

Challenging the Previously Valid Immune Theories

How acquired immune cell impairments actually develop

The clinicians and immunologists could not explain three decisive findings of the immune response of the T-helper cells of their patients who came down with massive fungal lung infections and other opportunistic infections:

1. The depletion of the T-helper cells in the blood serum of the patients while at the same time an increase in certain classes of antibodies
2. The unsuccessful or unsatisfactory maturing response to stimulation with antigens and/or proliferation factors (concanavalin A, a.k.a. con A; phytohaemagglutin, a.k.a. PHA)
3. The anergic response of the immune cells in the skin after provocation with recall antigens in delayed-type hypersensitivity (DTH) tests (Gottlieb 1981, Mazur 1981).

The laboratory construct "retrovirus HIV" also could not be used to explain these immunological anomalies as the cause of opportunistic infections or as an indirect cause of Kaposi's sarcomas and lymphomas (Balter 1997).

The discovery of the opposing subtypes of T-helper immune cells (T4 cells type-I and type-II = Th1 and Th2)

In 1986, the research group of Mosmann and Coffman identified in experimental research on T-helper clone cells (identically duplicated T-cells) two sub-groups of T-helper cells. They varied in the profile of their communication proteins, the cytokines (still in those days termed lymphokines), which were produced after stimulation.

The T-helper cells with a type 1 cytokine profile were termed Th1 and those with a type 2 cytokine profile were termed Th2. A decisive factor that became apparent as the researchers stimulated the T-helper cell culture with different antigens was that there was a shift in the balance between Th1 and Th2 related to the type, dosage and duration of the antigens applied. If the balance tipped towards Th1 then there was an increase in production of the type 1 cytokine profile and the synthesis of type 2 cytokines was inhibited, and vice versa if the balance shifted in the other direction. So it was found that there was a reciprocally inhibiting regulation between the sub-groups Th1 and Th2 and their synthesized cytokines.

The researchers concluded that:

- Th1 cells principally interacted with the nonspecific macrophages, reciprocally to type 2 cytokines.
- Th2 cells principally perform helper functions for the antibody-producing B-cells (with the exception of a sub-group of B-cells which is activated by Th1 and produces antibodies of a sub-group of immunoglobulin class G).
- A shift in balance to Th1 produced a very marked DTH reaction and, vice versa, a dysbalance towards Th2 led to a weak DTH or no response at all (Mosmann 1986, 1988, 1989).

The DTH skin test used in clinical sepsis research as a diagnostic for the Th1/Th2 immune cell balance

The DTH response was a phenomenon that has been recognized for 200 years and was first described by Jenner in 1798. He observed redness, hardening and blistering at the location where he had injected the vaccine (cow pox) reaching a peak after 24 to 72 hours. In 1890 Robert Koch described a similar reaction to live tubercle bacilli injected into the skin of guinea pigs which had previously been infected with the TBC bacillus, but not in animals that were not infected. In 1942, Chase and Landsteiner demonstrated the interconnection between the DTH reaction and sensitized lymph cells. In addition to cell-mediated immunity the non-specific immune response of the macrophages and the coagulatory systems are chiefly active in the DTH reaction.

Since the mid-1970s, surgeons considered how an improvement could be made in prognosis of the dreaded sepsis after heavy traumata, burns or operations. Sepsis (blood poisoning) is a general infection with constant or periodical dispersion of microbes (bacteria, fungi) spreading from the source of infection into the bloodstream. With this purpose in mind a surgical team in Montreal recorded the DTH reaction of all patients between 1975 and 1985 before and after surgery. Every trained nurse can conduct and record the DTH reaction. The Canadian surgeons categorically stated: "Nearly two centuries following Jenner, and a century following Pasteur, Koch, Lister, Metchnikoff and others, the leading cause of morbidity and mortality after major surgery is sepsis . . . Despite better surgical techniques, and increased choice of powerful life support systems, sepsis continues to be a major cause of morbidity and mortality in the surgical patient" (Christou 1986).

The DTH reaction of 202 patients was tested before surgery. 3-5% of all the surgical patients tested developed a sepsis; for patients in post-operative intensive care the proportion was one third. Of the patients with positive skin reactivity, 50% were anergic on the third day after the operation and by the seventh post-operative day most of them had recovered reactivity. Patients who subsequently remained anergic had a higher rate of sepsis in 32% of cases. When the skin test failed to normalize, a subsequent sepsis was associated with a higher level of mortality. Of all the patients that were DTH positive upon hospital admission, 8% developed sepsis and 4% died; of those who were DTH negative (relatively anergic), 21% developed sepsis and 15% died; of those who were DTH negative (anergic), 33% developed sepsis and 31% died.

The surgeons established that many of the immunological parameters of sepsis patients had altered in comparison to the non-sepsis patients. In particular the type 1 cytokine interleukin-2 (IL-2), a growth factor protein for T-helper cells, was heavily inhibited in sepsis patients. Certain antibody classes (IgG and IgA) considerably increased while other antibody classes and the complementary reaction decreased. Additionally, many inhibitors formed in the serum of sepsis patients: "These inhibitors have a profound effect on T-helper lymph cells and polymorphonuclear leukocytes. Teleogically, there is a suggestion that this inhibition postinjury may be a normal response related to the 'healing processes' and the prevention of autoimmune reactions to self-denatured proteins. The host is, therefore, caught in a dichotomy between healing and sepsis, in the midst of breached defenses" (Christou 1986).

After severe damage and attacks to the self-regulation of organisms, highly complex and diverse regulations and counterregulations occur, countless mediators and compensating modulators intervene, and cells are thereby activated or suppressed. This total response of the bioenergy, biochemistry and cell biology of the organism to the utmost of stress has until now not been adequately understood, and depends on many predisposing factors (Calvano 1986, Cerami 1992, Jochum 1992, Waydhas 1992, Nast-Kolb 1996). However, the core statement of the Canadian surgeons is worth repeating. They reported that an anergic DTH reaction as an expression of the inhibited cell-mediated immune competence before admission to the hospital was significantly linked to the sepsis results, which, despite massive use of antibiotics, led in a high percentage of cases to the patient's death. A decade later surgeons at McGill University confirmed that the strong correlation remained between a reduced DTH response and mortality after sepsis of heavily traumatized patients in intensive care, despite a reduction in overall mortality (Christou 1995).

The Canadian surgeons had recognized the evolutionary, biologically programmed dual strategy of the immune response: 50% of the surgical patients responded to the profound stress to the system with a T-helper cell dysbalance up to the seventh post-operative day, and a certain percentage of patients, especially those who had already shown signs of an immune dysbalance before the operation, had a long-standing T-helper cell dysbalance until death or upon overcoming the aftermath of the operation. Whether the surviving anergic patients remained anergic after leaving the hospital was not recorded.

The significant fact still remains that a long-lasting T-helper cell dysbalance under pressure from heavy stress is not altogether uncommon in the population as a whole: anyhow 24% of the surgical patients were anergic on admission, 14% relatively anergic. Conversely, data from the findings also express that not every patient with a T-helper cell dysbalance was threatened by a lethal infection, as 67% of the pre-operative anergic and 79% of the relatively anergic patients did not develop a sepsis. (Christou1986). This fact is just as significant as the correlation between anergy, sepsis and mortality. It indicates a high variability of the regulation of the immune response between the cell-mediated and humoral immunity manifested either in a stable immune cell balance, a flexible immune balance, or a fixed immune cell dysbalance with or without ensuing sepsis. A long-lasting immune cell dysbalance under profound stress loads (acquired immunodeficiency = AID) with or without infectious syndrome is by no means a rare or "puzzling" occurrence.

Experimental and clinical evidence for the causal relation between Th1/Th2 immune cell balance, dominance of the type 2 cytokine profile, and anergy of the DTH skin reaction in chronic infections

The clinical and immunological data from surgical sepsis research before the discovery of type 1 cytokine—type 2 cytokine dysbalance of the T-helper immune cells, concurred with the experimental data of Mosmann and Coffman on T-helper clone cells of infected mice. The researchers could prove a definitive shift to a type 2 cytokine profile with a preponderance of Th2 cells in the spleen lymph cells and lymph node cells of mice that had been infected with the parasite *Nippostrongylus brasiliensis*. The type 1 cytokines interleukin 2 (IL2) and interferon-γ (IFN-γ) were below normal readings and the amounts of the type 2 cytokines, interleukin-4 (IL-4) and interleukin-5 (IL-5) had greatly increased. As IL-2 was also greatly reduced in surgical sepsis patients and IL-4 and IL-2 inhibit each other reciprocally, it can be assumed that a systemic shift to Th2 dominance had taken place in surgical sepsis patients with an anergic DTH reaction. The clinical and immunological findings were induced by the Th1-Th2 shift.

In a further experiment the researchers infected mice with the parasite *Leishmania major* (Lm). They chose one strain of mice that was susceptible to an Lm infection and one that was resistant. The susceptible mice developed heavy and advanced infections and died. Like surgical sepsis patients, immunologically they displayed all the features of Th2 activation: anergic DTH skin reaction, high antibody levels, reduced type 1 cytokines and increased type 2 cytokines. The resistant mice on the other hand merely showed signs of a local infection and fully recovered. Their DTH skin reaction was highly developed, the antibody production low and conversely type 1 cytokine syntheses increased and type 2 cytokine syntheses reduced. Lm is an intracellular parasite of the macrophages, so it was clearly demonstrated that an intact Th1 response with type 1 cytokine production is necessary for the elimination of an intracellular pathogen. The reverse was also shown, in that the susceptibility to an intracellular infection leading to a progressive illness and death is dependent on a predominant shift to a Th2 response with type 2 cytokine production; which in fact leads to an increased antibody production and protection from extracellular pathogen attacks but cannot prevent intracellular microorganisms from proliferating (Mosmann 1989).

The fundamental perceptions about the dualistic strategy of the immune response have been substantiated in countless experiments and research on animals and humans. For instance, researchers prepared Th1 and Th2 cell lines and clone cells specifically for Lm antigens. When these cells were re-injected into Lm-infected mice, the Th1 cell lines completely recovered from infection while the Th2 cell lines deteriorated during the course of the infection (Scott 1986). Humans can also become infected by *Leishmania* parasites with two alternative progressions of the immune response: either a strong DTH reaction leading to a local confinement of the parasitic infection and the elimination of the *Leishmania* agent, or an increased antibody production with little or no DTH reaction (anergy) and a heavy dispersion of the parasites. In tropical countries like India, this disease is called *Kala-azar* (Sacks 1987).

The Th1-Th2 switch has been intensively studied in mycobacterial infections like leprosy and tuberculosis. In leprosy, there are two polar disease types, the tuberculoid and the lepromatous forms, with manifestations of a spectrum of transitional forms. The tubercular form is characterized by a strong cell-mediated immunity and few pathogens. A type 1 cytokine profile was found in Th1 clone cells cultivated from the blood serum of tuberculoid leprosy sufferers (Haanen 1991). Th1 helper immune cells are dominant in the damaged skin. Conversely in the lepromatous form, the pathogens are numerous and the cell-mediated immunity of the Th1 helper cells is greatly reduced. A type 2 cytokine profile is dominant in the skin lesion (Modlin 1993).

In cases of human tuberculosis (TBC) the counter-controls primarily come from the type 1 cytokines of the Th1 immune cells although TBC sufferers produce plenty of antibodies against the tubercular bacilli. These antibodies, however, have no protective function against the development of tuberculosis in humans (Des Prez 1990). A strong type 2 cytokine production has been shown in active tuberculosis (Surcel 1994). On the other hand a strong Th1 reaction (DTH reaction) can be responsible for both eliminating the agent and for the tissue damage (Dannenberg 1991). Whether type 1 cytokine plays a beneficial or detrimental role depends on the relative Th1-Th2 balance. In a type 2 cytokine milieu or a mixed type 1/type 2 cytokine milieu, the type 1 cytokines interferon-γ (IFN-γ) and tumor necrosis factor α (TNF-α) are more likely to destroy tissue cells than attack the tubercular agents (Hernandez-Pando 1994).

The third important mycobacterium, *M. avium complex*, is an opportunistic agent above all in AIDS patients. It appears in a Th1-Th2 switch and type 2 cytokine dominance (Holland 1994, Newman 1994).

Cytokine production and the T-helper cell status in human worm infections are of special interest in that worms played an important role as parasites in the transition from invertebrates to vertebrates, and the humoral antibody immunity developed at the beginning of the evolution of vertebrates. As a consequence, the immune strategy against worm infections should concentrate on the switch to Th2 status with a type 2 cytokine production. With worm infections, there is a pronounced production of antibodies of immunoglobulin class E, and simultaneously a marked increase of a certain type of white blood cells, the eosinophilic leukocytes, known as eosinophilia. The two main groups of worm infections, filariasis and schistosomiasis, which cover numerous sub-groups of human worm infections, are important. With filariasis the Th2 cells in peripheral blood are distinctly increased, the type 2 cytokines boosted with simultaneous increase of antibody production. Among the antibodies the immunoglobulin class E is strongly elevated with a simultaneously strong eosinophilia. The eosinophilic blood cells mainly produce type 2 cytokines. The type 2 cytokines and the antibody production (IgE and IgG) have been experimentally inhibited by type 1 cytokine and interleukin-12, a product of macrophages, which among other things stimulates type 1 cytokine in the Th1 cells (Mahanty 1993, King 1993, 1995). Worms are, however, under certain conditions attacked by Th1 cells, and under other conditions by Th2 controlled antibodies and special eosinophiles. Worm eggs, in contrast, generally provoke a Th2 response. In humans a type 2 cytokine response rather than type 1 cytokine production is associated with immunity against worms from the genus *Schistosoma:* antibodies of the immunoglobulin class E and type 2 cytokine IL-5 inhibited a re-infection (Capron 1994). A Th2 status generally heals or protects against worm infections (Mosmann 1996).

There are only a handful of studies regarding the cytokine profile in fungal infections in humans. These studies fundamentally support similar research on animals. They show that advanced forms of fungal infections are associated with a type 2 cytokine dominance, for instance in aspergillosis of the lungs and bronchii, candidiasis, cryptococcosis, paracoccidioidomycosis, coccidioidomycosis, blastomycosis and histoplasmosis. Conversely, protection from fungal infections comes principally from Th1 immunity. Also in cases of fungal infections the polarity of the immune response can be beneficial or detrimental: if the cell-mediated immunity was only slightly inhibited then the number of fungal microbes was also small; if the Th1 response was heavily impaired then the number of fungal pathogens was large (Mosmann 1996, Lucey 1996).

In the meantime, of the human protistan infections, only *Leishmania* infections have been more intensively researched. In all studies the infections with an intact Th1 status and type 1 cytokine production resolved, while an increased type 2 cytokine level was accountable for a lack of protection against these parasitic infections (Bloom 1993). Differing cytokine activities, however, were shown to be dependent on the infestation of the individual organs

(Karp 1993). Extracellular bacterial infections (excluding mycobacteria) in humans, with differing cell and organ systems have in relation to the cytokine profile been little researched. There is, however, the tendency in the findings that in acute intracellular infections the Th1 response is decisive, while in cases of chronic infection a Th1-to-Th2 switch with a weak DTH reaction was observed. A comparison between syphilis and leprosy is illuminating. Latent and secondary syphilis is similar in progression to transitional leprosy between the tuberculoid and lepromatous forms. Overcoming syphilis with a strong DTH reaction and an increase in type 1 cytokine profile showed an analogy to the tuberculoid form with few syphilis pathogens. The tertiary stage was analogous to lepromatous leprosy, exhibiting a strong drift towards type Th2, increased type 2 cytokine production and a weak DTH reaction (Sell 1993).

In cases of acute viral infections the stage at which the cytokine readings are taken is decisive. A good example of this is measles: type 1 cytokines increased during and shortly after the appearance of the skin rash. After the acute phase there is an increase in formation of type 2 cytokines, a decrease in type 1 cytokines and a weakened DTH reaction (Griffin 1993). The duration of the Th2 dysbalance or the re-establishment of the Th1-Th2 balance after resolution of the measles infection was not researched.

T-helper cells from liver tissues of patients with chronic active hepatitis B display a type 1 cytokine profile (Barnaba 1994). In test subjects who did not react to the vaccine by forming antibodies (so-called non-responders), the peripheral blood cells after stimulation with the specific antigens HbsAg did not react by cytokine synthesis. The same peripheral blood cells from test subjects who showed a strong reaction to vaccination formed increased amounts of type 1 cytokines. It was concluded that hepatitis B vaccine antigens induced a Th1 response (Vingerhoets 1994).

Experimental and clinical data indicate a clear conclusion:

DTH skin reactivity is an indicator for the competence of the cell-mediated immune response of the Th1 immune cells. If the DTH reaction is positive then a successful defense and elimination of all intracellular microorganisms (bacteria, viruses, fungi, protozoa) can be expected. If the DTH reaction is negative then a successful elimination of intracellular pathogens is less probable. Chronic, opportunistic or highly acute infections could develop.

An anergic DTH reaction indicates a re-arrangement of cytokine synthesis in the stem cells of the T-helper cells mainly towards a type 2 cytokine profile (DTH immune cell status). The type 2 cytokines inhibit the synthesis of type 1 cytokines leading to a diminished capacity to stimulate T-helper cells in the blood serum. Type 2 cytokines activate antibody production. Antibodies, as a preventative barrier to entry, can only attack pathogens outside the cell. During massive bacterial dispersion after heavy traumata, burns, and serious operative invasions, it is possible that the previously existing or incurred Th2 immune cell status is not sufficient for the extracellular inhibition of bacterial or fungal agents. thereby a sepsis develops with a high mortality rate (see Dualistic Strategy of the Immune Response, Table III).

The immune cell balance of "HIV positives" is already disturbed prior to exhibiting "HIV characteristics"

The immunological findings from AIDS clinics in 1981:

- Anergic skin reaction
- Decrease in the number and the capacity for stimulation of T-helper cells in blood serum
- Increased B-cell activity and specific antibody production (Gottlieb 1981, Masur 1981, Mildvan 1982)

The above are clear expressions of a predominant type 2 cytokine synthesis with a Th2 immune cell dominance, the diagnosed opportunistic fungal infections (PCP, candida, etc.), protozoal infections (toxoplasmosis etc.), mycobacteria (*M. tuberculosis, M. avium intracellulare*) and cytomegaloviral infections are characteristic manifestations of prolonged toxic, medicamentous, and microbial stress. The development of a specific immune cell status and the specific resulting diseases in promiscuous anally receptive homosexual patients was, with the same conclusive certainty, as predictable as the appearance of sepsis in anergic surgical patients.

The decisive correlation of the DTH reaction as indicator of the dominance of the cell-mediated immunity or the dominance of humoral immunity, were amply documented in medical literature before the laboratory product "HIV" as a "new agent" was imposed, and as a result of groundbreaking work from Mosmann and Coffman the differentiations in type 1/type 2 cytokine functions of the T-helper cells and other immune and non-immune cells were recognized (Zinsser 1921, Landsteiner 1942, Chase

1945, Alexander 1972, Vadas 1976, Hurd 1977, Meakins 1977, Christou 1979, Dvorak 1979, Platt 1982, Poulter 1982, Rode 1982, Van Dijk 1982, Razzaque-Ahmed 1983, Oppenheim 1983, Asano 1983, Van Loveren 1984, Wood 1984).

In contrast to the surgical patients, there was hardly any systematic research carried out on DTH skin reactions in the so-called HIV/AIDS risk groups. Such a study, with very little cost, could have indicated the status of the immune cell deficiency of those affected both in Western and Third World countries, and could have led to a corresponding risk education without the stigma that became associated with a deadly HIV infection. There were, however, numerous studies on patients at risk regarding the T-helper cell status and the antibody status after the introduction of the "anti-HIV antibody tests," which have clearly proven a significant increase in dysfunctions of cell-mediated immunity in members of the risk groups. After the introduction of the "AIDS test" further cross-sectional and longer-running studies were carried out with HIV-negative and HIV-stigmatized probands from risk groups, which distinctly indicated that both stigmatized and non-stigmatized people from risk groups have a higher frequency of acquired immunodeficiency (AID) than test subjects from non-risk groups (overview Root-Bernstein 1993). In plain language, this means that within comparable risk groups, AID existed before the invention of "HIV-positivity." Thus "HIV" cannot be the cause of AID, but rather the laboratory result of "HIV-positivity" *must be the effect of some other primary cause.*

A "positive HIV test" merely discloses whether the test subject has formed, at a particular point in time, enough antibodies in the blood serum to react to the presented protein antigens in the test substrate. As the sensitivity of the HIV tests is set at a certain high level; probands could have the same antibodies in their blood serum but come up either positive or negative. The decisive factor for a negative test result is not the fact that a proband has antibodies in their blood serum that have reacted to the test proteins, but whether the *amount* of antibodies capable of reacting had reached or exceeded the preset threshold of the "HIV test." By analogy, a driver who has been drinking is considered capable of driving if during a control the prescribed legal alcohol limits have not been exceeded. A driver who has been drinking can register a positive or a negative result. If the level exceeds the prescribed limits, then the result is positive. In relation to the HIV theory this means that one who has fewer antibodies is negative, and one with more and is positive. In terms of the retrovirus theory, however, *both* could be "HIV infected". The test thresholds for "HIV-negative" or "HIV-positive" in the case of an actual

"HIV infection" would be totally arbitrary, as the presence of viruses does not depend on an artificially set number of antibodies.

The number of reactive antibodies says very little about the actual capacity of the proband's T-helper cells to eliminate intracellular agents. *The quantity and quality of antibodies play no decisive role in the inhibition and elimination of intracellular agents*, as countless studies of cell-mediated immunity have proven. The "HIV test" can, however, give clues about previous events in the immune cell network of test subjects, albeit for different reasons than those claimed by the HIV researchers. Analogous to surgical patients with anergic DTH tests, of whom only a third actually developed a sepsis, a "positive HIV test" does not allow for individual predictions of an unavoidable deadly disease. The "positive HIV test" also reveals nothing about a contagious "retroviral infection." The "HIV test" can only give general indications of the possible formation of antibodies against cell proteins in test subjects or against certain alloantigens or microbial antigens. Such cell proteins could be released by (among other things) the body's own cells, for the same reasons as was emulated in the laboratory in the extraction of test proteins from human cell cultures. The antibodies could have been formed against proteins released by an increase in necrosis (unprogrammed cell death), which then reacted after the blood serum of the test subjects made contact with the test proteins derived from human cell cultures.

In this context, it would be of interest to know whether the immunological findings of people at risk detected a type 2 cytokine profile indicating a Th1-Th2 dysbalance (AID). Such an assumption is likely, as the Th1 and Th2 cells are defined after their cytokine synthesis and the immunological findings of the first diagnosed AIDS patients showed characteristic signs of a Th2 dominance. In that case, the basic supposition of the HIV/AIDS theory, namely the destruction of the T-helper cells by a new retrovirus, would no longer be necessary as an explanation for Th2 dominance. Th2 dominance with increased B-cell activity can indeed be activated by a temporary or long-lasting viral infection, but without the necessity of the destruction of T-helper cells. The number of short-living Th1 cells in blood serum automatically decreases in Th2 dominance, in that the stem cells of the T-helper cells are predominantly adapted to the synthesis of type 2 cytokines and the Th2 cells circulate to a lesser degree in the blood serum as their helper function is performed where the B-cells are to be found. The Th2 cells do not produce cytotoxic NO gas with which to target the intracellular pathogens. The Th2 cells do not patrol the bloodstream and the lymph vessels like the Th1 cells—the much quoted "police of the immune system." By analogy, the situation would be like police officers on the beat being given desk jobs and anyone with a bit of imagination thinking that since the police were no longer to be seen patrolling the streets, they must have all been killed by gangsters.

As immunologists like to use somewhat graphic terminology ("killer cells", "killer viruses") this comparison suits the retrovirus AIDS researchers' explanation that T-helper cells are terminated en masse by "HIV." The fact that the Th2 cells are able to survive this supposed immune cell destruction, evident by the intact function of antibody production by the B-cells, like so many other facts, cannot be explained by the HIV theorists. This fact led the surveillance authority, the CDC, to emphatically exclude bacterial diseases from the definition of AIDS-indicating illnesses (CDC 1993). Massive bacterial illnesses only appeared in AIDS patients after highly toxic cell poisons adopted to combat the "HI-viral infection," had systemically damaged the maturation of the B-cells in the bone marrow of patients.

The primary problem of AIDS patients then is not the production of antibodies by the B-cells, which in turn were stimulated by the type 2 cytokines of the Th2 cells. What is decisive for the development of intracellular opportunistic pathogens (fungi and parasites), is the lack of cytotoxic NO gas due to the missing synthesis of type 1 cytokines in T-helper cells. As the Th1 and Th2 cells in the blood serum cannot be distinguished by the protein types on their cell membrane, the differentiation between whether a proband had formed mainly Th1 or Th2 cells is only possible by determination of cytokine synthesis in the T-helper cells. Such experiments were carried out on the T-helper cells of asymptomatic "HIV-positive" subjects and on AIDS patients with obvious symptoms. The results showed that the maturation and proliferation of T-helper cells was severely impaired even in the probands of those without symptoms who were "HIV-positive" and who had a nearly average amount of T-helper cells in their blood serum (Shearer 1986, Giorgio 1987, Miedema 1988, Clerici 1989 a, 1989 b).

"It was suggested that cytokine imbalance contributed significantly to AIDS progression and was associated with a switch or shift from a dominant Th1-like to a dominant Th2-like cytokine profile" (Lucey 1996; Salk 1993, Clerici 1993, 1994, Pinto 1995, Shearer 1996). There were, however, no publications about the desperately needed control experiments on the cytokine synthesis in the blood serum of "HIV-negative" risk group test subjects who also had a nearly average or reduced number of T-helper cells and simultaneously an inhibited maturation after stimulation with recall antigens, alloantigens or mitogens. There have been, since the introduction of the "HIV tests" in 1984, numerous experiments that have proven that "HIV-negative" immunosuppressed homosexual patients, drug addicts, hemophiliacs, heterosexuals and children have a reduction and proliferation inhibition of T-helper cells in the blood serum identical to "HIV-positive" patients from the same groups. In comparative clinical studies from 1982 on "HIV-negative" and "HIV-positive" homosexuals, for instance, it transpired that 30% of the "HIV-negative" homosexual men had anergic T-helper cells after stimulation. This anergy has been shown to remain constant (Weber 1986).

This finding conspicuously concurs with the percentage of anergic surgical patients on admission to clinics before operations in the Canadian study (Christou 1986). A comprehensive study in New York showed that almost 75% of homosexual men had an active infection with cytomegalovirus, Epstein-Barr virus, *Herpes simplex* virus or Hepatitis B infection, fully independent of whether they had reacted positive or negative to the "HIV test." These findings are in sharp contrast to heterosexual control patients, a mere 6% of whom are actively infected, and then only with a single virus type in semen, saliva or blood. None of the heterosexual control patients had multiple infections whereas 20% of the homosexuals had more than one infection (Buimovici-Klein 1988).

Similar immunological and clinical findings have been made in numerous studies with patients from all risk groups. The criteria for a T-helper switch were apparent in all these patient groups, independent of a negative or positive "HIV status" and the development of opportunistic AIDS-indicating diseases (overview Root-Bernstein 1993). It is then even more astounding that research on cytokine synthesis in the T-helper cells of these patients could apparently only be carried out once the patients had registered positive in the "HIV test" (Lucey 1996, Abbas 1996). This failure must be judged as grave malpractice. Logically an anergy of the T-helper cells (indicator of a switch of the cytokine profile to Th2) of homosexual patients who at first register "HIV-negative" and then a year later "HIV-positive" cannot be retroactively traced to an "HIV retrovirus infection." *A positive reaction to an "HIV test" merely indicates that at a certain point in time there was a gradual shift in the amount of certain antibodies.* Whether this increase in antibody production took place at an earlier time or was taking place at the time of the test cannot be determined by the test results, given that antibodies once produced can be detected in blood serum for years, and sometimes for life. The "HIV-positive" test results also cannot give any indication as to whether or not opportunistic illnesses will develop. Such a probabilistic prediction depends on a completely different set of factors including the kind of medical intervention.

"HIV characteristics" occur predominantly in the T4 cells associated with type 2 cytokine patterns

It is especially striking that the researchers discovered that the laboratory products, which in the T-helper clone cells were interpreted as indirect evidence of a "retrovirus HIV," could be found primarily in Th2 clone cells but not in Th1 clone cells (Maggi 1994, Chehimi 1995, Abbas 1996, Lucey 1996). These laboratory findings presented the HIV/AIDS theory with an unsolvable paradox. Since 1981, a causal factor was sought that was supposed to destroy those T-cells that were responsible for the elimination of intracellular opportunistic fungal microbes (*Pneumocystis carinii*, candida), protoctista (toxoplasma, etc.) and viruses (cytomegalovirus, etc.). But these T-helper effector cells are Th1 cells. If the Th1 cells, according to the laboratory experiments were not colonized by the hypothetical "retrovirus HIV," then they certainly cannot be destroyed by it. Whoever is not at the scene of the crime, cannot have committed it. On the other hand, the number of Th1 cells depends on how many stem cells of the T-helper cells were trained in the synthesis of type 1 cytokine profile (Mosmann 1996). So HIV must colonize and destroy the stem cells. In that case there would not be any Th2 cells, which are imprinted on the type 2 cytokine profile and stimulate the B-cells to produce antibodies. The patients therefore should have developed massive bacterial infections analogous to those seen with Burton syndrome (lack of gamma globulins) or SCID (combined T—and B-lymph cell destruction). In fact, the contrary was the case: a hypergammaglobulinaemia was observed (Lucey 1996) and in contrast to the imposing opportunistic infections, there were no conspicuous bacterial infections (CDC 1993). The hypothetical colonization of the Th2 cells by a hypothetical "HIV" had zero medical consequences.

However, the type 2 cytokines of the Th2 cells do not inhibit the Th1 cells indirectly with their cytokines, but rather the biosynthesis of the cytokine profile is inhibited or promoted by influencing the genetic expression in the stem cells (Mosmann 1996). The genetic expression of the cytokine proteins is dependent, like all genetic expression, on the redox milieu which inhibits or promotes the transcription factors. The redox milieu is, however, governed by a complex multiplicity of extracellular and intracellular factors. But if particular patterns of the cytokine proteins are expressed, they engage the redox milieu in a regulatory fashion—both in their own expression and in the cytokine proteins and enzyme proteins such as, for instance the NO synthases and many other protein enzymes. If a non-expressed cytokine is added to a culture of peripheral blood cells from "HIV-positives," the Th2 cells suddenly respond to the recall antigens and exhibit proliferation (Clerici 1993 b). Thus the redox-dependent expression of the cytokine mixture determines the human immune response. A "new agent" is by no means necessary to explain this elementary process. which has functioned in redox-dependent self-organization for millions of years.

The HIV/AIDS theory is a priori false, because the fundamental self/foreign concept of immunology is incorrect

The HIV laboratory researchers have tied themselves in a logical knot with their contrived test-tube experiments on T-cell clones, and therefore must continually develop ever more complicated rescue hypotheses in an attempt to justify the existence of HIV (Shearer 1995). Thus they increasingly lose sight of the biological reality, namely the conditions the strategy depends on, which the immune response adopts as partial regulation for the balance as a whole. This question touches on a fundamental dogma of immunology, namely the assumption that immune cells can "recognize" foreign proteins and other foreign molecules and can differentiate between the body's own 55,000 odd proteins and other molecules, and foreign molecules such as microbial proteins. This perception largely contributed to the seemingly plausible (for the layman) theory that a new sophisticated virus had infiltrated the central recognition base of T-immune cells during sexual intercourse or blood transfusions and had disabled the native defense network of "HIV-positives" and AIDS sufferers.

Unresolved discrepancies in the self/foreign theory

This immunological dogma has, in the last decade, been severely shaken. The "self/non-self theory" has at no point in time been able to explain certain contradictions, e.g.:

- Why do T-helper cells and antibodies, under certain conditions, attack the body's own proteins (autoimmune reaction)?
- Why are cancer cells not recognized by immune cells as being foreign?
- During pregnancy, why don't immune cells attack the embryo, whose cells contain foreign genes and thus synthesize foreign proteins?
- Why are intestinal bacteria not regarded as foreign?

The basic rules of inactivity of T and B-cells against the body's own proteins ("self-tolerance")

The decisive assessment is that the T-helper cells cannot differentiate between "self" and "non-self" molecules but in principle can inter-react with all molecules. T-cells mature in the thymus. They are produced in the millions by random genetic recombination. Every negatively-charged T-lymph cell is programmed to a suitably charged profile on proteins or other molecules. Most of the T-cells already hook up with the suitable molecule at the location of maturation in the thymus. This contact causes the death of the T-cells. The encounter with the suitable proteins or other molecules, termed antigens, is not enough to activate the T-cells for their ultimate function as effector cells. Only a very small proportion, namely those that cannot find a suitable antigen in the thymus, leave the thymus and move into the bloodstream and lymph vessels (positive selection).

There are essentially three kinds of T-cells:

The T-helper cells, which as Th1 cells can activate cytotoxic T-cells and macrophages,

1. The T-suppressor lymph cells,
2. The cytotoxic T-cells, a.k.a. killer cells, which after activation bind directly on cells but do not absorb them like the macrophages do.

The virgin T-helper cells become experienced T-helper cells once they encounter their antigen for the first time. After this initial contact, they either die off or survive as resting cells in a dormant state. Once they have received a specific double signal, the experienced but dormant T-helper cells become effector cells. Signal 1 is offered by special antigen-presenting cells (APCs), which for example present a fragment of a protein molecule. This takes place in the middle of the receptor molecules (MHC II). Signal 2 comes from co-stimulatory molecules of the same APCs, which are mainly termed dendritic cells. The second signal is not only picked up by experienced T-helper cells, but also by macrophages and B-cells; however it cannot be received by virgin T-helper cells.

The basic rule for virgin T-helper cells is as follows:

– If signal 1 is received without signal 2, then die off or wait; but if both signals are received from dendritic cells, B-cells or macrophages, then activate.

The relatively simple, but biologically quite successful principle, of why T-helper cells do not (or very rarely) respond to the presentation of the cell's native proteins, is a question of statistical proportionality: the few T-helper cells that are programmed to recognize cell native proteins and have not already encountered their protein antigen in the thymus, have an extremely high chance of encountering their molecular partner in the bloodstream, lymph vessels, lymph nodes, or spleen, before they encounter an APC. Relative to the billions of bodily cells and remaining soluble proteins and other molecules, the APCs are quite rare; therefore a virgin T-helper cell, programmed to native antigens, has an extremely low chance of finding its matching molecular partner together with signal 2 on an APC.

The same basic rule also applies to the B-cells, which mature in the bone marrow. Roughly 25% of mature B-cells are sensitive enough to be able to produce antibodies (negative selection). Again the basic rule applies:

- Die if only the antigen signal is received.
- Activate if the second signal comes from activated T-helper cells (Th2 cells).

For the experienced/activated effector T-helper cells and effector B-cells, the basic rule is:

- Perform effector function if signal 1 (antigen contact) has been given irrespective of the presence or absence of signal 2.
- Die or revert to resting state if signal 1 is not received (overview Matzinger 1994).

This simplified representation is enough for a basic understanding of why B—and T-helper lymphocytes, in cooperation with antigen-presenting cells, are able to recognize a viral infection even when a virus particle has colonized some T-helper cells. In the case of the destruction of T-helper cells, these viral proteins will be trapped by APCs and presented along with the necessary additional signals to the T-helper cells (of which only a few would be colonized at the start of such an infection). Therefore, it makes no difference to the T-helper activity whether the virus infected T-helper cells or other cell types.

T-helper immune cells do not detect "foreign" and "self," but rather are particularly sensitive to redox state; as such they act as sensor and effector cells, in the regulation and counterregulation of various disturbances of the redox equilibrium

In the case of the hypothetical "HIV infection," however, there must be other reasons for a systemic switch from Th1 cell types to mainly Th2 cell types. When followed over a number of years, patients with the same risk factors and identical results of a Th1-Th2 deficiency (AID), but without an "HIV-positive" test result, only experienced seroconversion (a flipping of test results from "HIV-negative" to "HIV-positive") in a minority of cases (Weber 1986, Root-Bernstein 1993). *While both variants exhibit identical anomalies of the immune status (AID with or without "HIV-positivity"), they simply differ in individual proclivity to antibody production.*

According to the laws of logic, factor B cannot be the cause of factor A if factor A precedes factor B. As about 2 million new T-cells and 20 million B-cells are formed every day (George 1996, Osmand 1993), the general dominance of type 2 cytokines measured at an early stage of seroconversion in asymptomatic risk-group patients, cannot be traced back to a singular virus, which selectively infects a minority of the T-helper immune cells. *Consequently, this means that the impairment of cell-mediated immunity, acquired through a Th1-Th2 switch, is not a reflection of a "retroviral infection" but the expression of a pre-existing long-term prooxidative (oxidative and/or nitrosative) stress.*

The T-helper cells do not operate in isolation, but are programmed as particularly redox-sensitive cells with a specialized mission to react to signals of oxidative/nitrosative danger. Such signals are conveyed to them by the change in intracellular redox caused by antigen presentation with its associated co-stimulatory signals, as well as by exposure to toxins. The result of this interaction is the activation of the genetic expression for type 1 cytokine synthesis, which in turn activates the biosynthesis of enzymes which produce cytotoxic NO. With no additional signalling necessary, Th1 cells which have thus been activated to become effector cells will emit an NO gas cloud the next time they encounter the antigen on an infected cell. The gas infiltrates the infected cells and oxidizes essential metalloenzymes of the microbes, leading to the inhibition or death of the pathogen.

The dilemma of self-defense versus self-preservation

Not only T-helper cells, but also countless other immune and non-immune cells are capable of cytokine synthesis and cytotoxic NO gas formation. The triggers are not only antigens, but also toxic and other oxidative and nitrosative stress factors (Lincoln 1997). After a critical level of NO production has been reached through continuous stimulation, the looming threat of systemic antioxidative depletion gives rise to a dilemma between self-defense and self-preservation. A strategic decision has to be made at a genetic and non-genetic level. In these cases a braking effect happens in T-helper cells by redirecting the genetic expression of the cytokine synthesis and the induced NO syntheses. A Th1-Th2 switch occurs, which leads to an immune dysbalance (AID). The thiol pool is then the critical sensor and modulator of this switching effect; thiol depletion triggers a multidimensional network of regulations and counterregulations. Severe cases of acute infection, serious injuries and burns, operative invasions and poisonings (acute AID) can lead to an emergency polarization between "healing and sepsis" (Christou 1986). Insidious assimilation series with variable intermediary stages can also develop, until the final faulty adjustment of the interconnected regulatory systems to a set level occurs; this happens through protracted fungal, protozoal, viral and mycobacterial infections with a long-term antigenic burden, chronic intoxication (including cytotoxic drugs), malnutrition, starvation, aging processes, and many other prooxidative states of stress (long-term AID). Whether the net effect is primarily a Th1 or Th2 dominance (locally, organ-specifically, or systemically), depends on many internal and external factors. A particularly important external factor is the course of medical intervention, which is influenced by the dominant theories, and supported consciously or subconsciously by non-medical interests.

The experimental findings of the feedback system between polarized T-helper cells and cytokine patterns, as well as the cytotoxic NO synthesis

Since 1990, the paths of cytokine researchers and NO researchers have crossed. Shortly after Furchgott and Ignarro provided fundamental evidence that exogenous nitrate and nitrite in the endothelial cells metabolized into NO (Furchtgott and Ignarro independently of one another in 1986), Marletta reported for the first time about evidence of NO as an oxidation product of arginine in macrophages (Marletta 1988). When Gillespie published in 1989 that NO gas in nerve cells inhibited the transmission of nerve impulses (Gillespie 1989), an unforeseen research boom began. Within a few years it was recognized that NO, from molluscs (Franchini 1995, Johanson 1995, Octaviani 1998) to humans, controlled basic biological functions in all cell systems via oxidation—of metallic compounds such as ferrous proteins and enzymes (e.g. the iron-sulfur centers in the respiratory chain of the mitochondria), and of the sulfur-hydrogen (thiol) groups in the amino acids methionine and cysteine, and the proteins and enzymes which contain them (Moncada 1991). These basic discoveries laid the foundation for a profound change in the understanding of the AIDS and cancer puzzle.

Research on the production and function of cytotoxic NO gases in T-helper cells concentrated on three key areas:

- The significance of cytotoxic NO gases for the inhibition and elimination of microorganisms by the T-helper cells.
- The interplay between the syntheses of the cytokine profile and the inducible NO synthesis in T-helper cells.
- The counterregulation of the cytokine synthesis and the long-term NO synthesis in the context of the Th1-Th2 switch (immune cell dysbalance = AID).

The consequences of the discovery of NO synthesis in the immune cells were recognized at an earlier stage. Had it been apparent that the capacity of the cell-mediated immunity (Th1 cells) and the switching to a mainly humoral immune status (Th2 cell dominance and over-activation of antibody production) were dependent on cytotoxic NO synthesis—then the Th1 immune cell deficiency would not have been a puzzle at all. All factors involved with a long-term functional inhibition of the NO synthesis (nitrite consumption, cell toxic drugs, high and/or long-term antigen and alloantigen loads, oxidizing influences, protein malnutrition, etc.) could potentially trigger immune anomalies and opportunistic infections. An explanation of the Th1-Th2 switch from "HIV-negative" to "HIV-positive" in risk group patients no longer requires a "new agent." The causes of such diseases could be found in the dysbalance of the cytotoxic NO synthesis. In order to be effective, AIDS therapy would have to treat the causes of the cytotoxic NO blockade.

In 1990, NO production was demonstrated for the first time in the T-lymph cell cultures of rats that had been stimulated with the mitogen, phytohaemaglutinin (PHA). When a substance that inhibits NO production was added to the T-lymph cell cultures, there was a strong increase in the maturation and proliferation of the T-cells (Hoffman 1990). Since then, these findings have been confirmed in numerous T-lymph cell cultures of mice, as well as in living mice. Bacterial infections in mice lead to greatly increased NO levels and a subsequent inhibition of lymphocyte proliferation, resulting in a reduced T-helper cell immune response (Gregory 1993). When the T-cells from the spleen of mice infected with the malaria parasite (Plasmodium) were cultivated with malarial antigens, a significant production of type 1 cytokines (interferon-γ, interleukin-2) was observed. The synthesis of these cytokines was considerably increased when the mice were treated with an NO synthesis-inhibiting substance (Taylor-Robinson 1994). The researchers could also demonstrate these effects when the Th1 clone cells, which specifically had reacted to malaria antigens, were brought into contact with NO synthesis inhibitors; there was a substantial increase in the syntheses of interferon-γ and interleukin-2. Vice versa in the same Th1 clone cells, the same type 1 cytokine synthesis was much reduced when an NO-donating substance was added; above all the synthesis of the growth factors for the proliferation of Th1 cells, interleukin-2, was reduced in proportion to the amount of NO-donating substance added. The inhibition on proliferation of Th1 cells could be reversed by adding interleukin-2 to the cell culture of Th1 clones (Liew 1995). These experiments showed that NO in the Th1 clone cells inhibited the secretion of the type 1 cytokine IL-2. Further experiments with the mitogen concanavalin (Con A) confirmed that the Th1 cells were activated to NO synthesis when stimulated (Kirk 1990). In other experiments with T-helper cells from mammals and humans it was demonstrated that bacteriotoxic lipopolysaccharide (LPS) stimulates type 1 cytokines in Th1 cells, which in turn activate the production of cytotoxic NO gases (Kröncke 1995).

NO gas has two important functions:

- First, NO diffuses from activated Th1 effector cells into infected target cells, in order to inhibit or eliminate intracellular pathogens. This effector function applies in response to all intracellular microorganisms (bacteria, viruses, fungi, parasites). In the same way, cytotoxic NO gas also diffuses into extracellular microorganisms, for instance worms, fungi and parasites. The Th1 cells are supported in this task by the macrophages, which also produce NO gas (van Rooijen 1997, MacMicking 1997). Between macrophages and the Th1 cells, a mutual stimulation occurs through the exchange of type 1 cytokines and interleukin-2.
- Secondly, cytotoxic NO modulates the immune response of the Th1 cells by inhibiting further production of type 1 cytokine synthesis and by doing so, hinders an excessive proliferation of Th1 cells. At the same time, the synthesis of NO gas is inhibited because type 1 cytokines are its strongest stimulators. Hereby a negative feedback loop exists between the NO synthesis and type 1 cytokine synthesis. In cases of acute infection, this braking mechanism can prevent tissue damage from excessive amounts of NO. In cases of chronic infections, this self-inhibition of the NO synthesis can develop into a vicious circle and sustain the infection. NO gas acts simultaneously as a cytotoxin and as an immune regulator (Lincoln 1997).

When the gene for the expression of the protein for the synthesis enzyme of NO was blocked in mice, the inducible NO synthase (iNOS) in these "knock-out" mice displayed exactly this double-edged sword effect. The mice showed a substantially stronger immune response of Th1 cells, as the type 1 cytokines were no longer braked by the NO gas. Simultaneously, they were considerably more susceptible to infections than control mice. They could no longer form NO gas clouds to disable the metabolism and growth of intra—and extracellular agents (Wei 1995). These mice suffered from a special form of AIDS: an acquired immunodeficiency due to lack of effector gas with over-stimulated Th1 cells.

Of special significance was the question of whether the Th2 helper cells can synthesize cytotoxic NO. When the Th2 cell clones were treated in the same way as Th1 clones—with NO synthesis inhibitors, NO donor substances, or type 1 cytokines—they showed no signs of cytotoxic NO production, nor differences in proliferation performance (Taylor-Robinson 1994). Th2 cells differ from Th1 cells in that they do not produce cytotoxic NO (but they do regulate small amounts of calcium-dependent NO for internal modulation of numerous other cell biological processes, as do other cells). Thus, Th2 cells do not participate in the intracellular elimination of intracellular agents (Sher 1992, Kröncke 1995, James 1995, Barnes 1995, Vodovetz 1997 O'Garra 1998, Morel 1998).

The clinical consequences of the T-helper cell status, the associated cytokine synthesis and the inhibition of the overproduction of the cytotoxic NO gas during AIDS, sepsis and autoimmune reactions

A switch to Th2 predominance additionally inhibits the synthesis of cytotoxic NO, as type 2 cytokines are released which suppress the production of cytokines in macrophages. For example, type 2 cytokines inhibit the interleukin-12 of the macrophages, which normally stimulate type 1 cytokines in Th1 cells, and in turn activate the cytotoxic NO synthesis. It is not surprising then, that if a Th2 dominance exists in people with an intact antibody production, irregardless of "HIV status," opportunistic pathogens (fungi, parasites, mycobacteria, several virus types) will be able to colonize and proliferate within cells—as an effective NO gas attack cannot be mounted against them. This process becomes further complicated due to the fact that fungi and parasites, if they remain unchallenged, can themselves secrete substances that decelerate the NO synthesis in macrophages, and probably also in Th1 cells (Liew 1994, 1997, Green 1994, James 1995, Remick 1996,

Lucey 1996, Clark 1996, de Waal 1997, Leit-de-Moraes 1997, Ramshaw 1997, Akaike 1998, Karupiah 1998, Murphy 1998, Cobbold 1998).

Conversely, the danger exists that with a strong NO production for self-defense, localized chronic inflammations could be triggered and/or serious tissue damage could occur (Nussier 1993). Inflammatory processes develop in various organs which are difficult to control (overview Lincoln 1997). Sepsis as a systemic inflammatory process does benefit from a Th2 dominance, however as a result of the massive bacterial dispersion, excessive microbial endotoxins (lipopolysaccharides, a.k.a. LPS, etc.) are formed which stimulate a strengthened NO production in various cell systems, since with the exception ofTh1 cells, many other immune and non-immune cells (macrophages, Kupfer cells, mesangial cells, microglial cells, splenic cells, neutrophilic leukocytes, natural killer cells, epithelial cells, endothelial cells, vascular smooth muscle cells, heart muscle cells, liver cells, pancreatic cells, chondrocytes, osteoblasts, fibroblasts, keratinocytes, astrocytes, peripheral nerve cells, etc.) carry the enzymes for inducible NO synthesis, and therefore can produce surplus amounts of cytotoxic NO when under massive provocation from endotoxin. With septic shock, a malignant drop in blood pressure occurs which can lead to impaired circulation in the vital organs. The elevated quantity of NO oxidizes the ferrous enzyme, guanylate cyclase, in the endothelial cells. Through formation of cyclic guanosine monophosphate (cGMP), the vascular smooth muscles become continuously relaxed. The mortality rate of septic shock remains high even today. Promising findings in animal experiments with NO-inhibiting substances are problematic in humans, as it is difficult to attain a selective and organ-specific balance (Petros 1993, Kettler 1998, Kirkeboen 1999).

One of the principal dangers of the inflammatory process, as a result of extreme NO production, is the increase in cell death. The increased type 1 cytokine synthesis leads to an increase in the formation of interferon-γ and tumor necrosis factors, which in turn activates the production of oxygen radicals. These in turn can trigger programmed cell death (apoptosis) or unprogrammed cell death (necrosis), via a cascade of reactions. Unlike programmed cell death, if the cell contents, after the bursting of the cell membrane by necrosis, have not been previously recycled, proteins and other molecules will be released into the extracellular milieu. These are then processed as "foreign substances" by APCs (in this case primarily the dendritic cells and macrophages) and subsequently offered to virgin T-helper cells, as well as being captured by membrane-bound antibodies.

Compatible Th1 cells are similarly activated by a double signal, as with other proteins not originating from native cells, and produce cytotoxic NO clouds once they re-encounter activated cell proteins. The subsequent attacks against cell proteins proceed similarly as with intracellular microbial proteins. The Th2 cells activated by antigen signals from B-cells pass on stimulating signals to the B-cells, which then secrete soluble antibodies. Not only can these antibodies inter-react with the necrotic proteins they were produced against, but just as equally they can cross-react with other native proteins having analogous binding sites on the polymorphic protein structure. Following this model of interaction, autoimmune reactions are thereby geared towards "self" cells (Nicholson 1996, Vergani 1996, Rocken 1997, O'Grady 1997, Heurtier 1997, Weigle 1997. Lafaille 1998, Del Prete 1998, Pearson 1999).

The role of type 2 cytokines and self-tolerance of the T- and B-cells in cancer cell transformation

Cancer cells, on the other hand, are tolerated as "self" cells, as long as they do not yield antigens to the APCs. Cancer cell antigens cannot be presented, and therefore T-helper cells and B-cells cannot be activated, until necrotic cell death occurs. In their intact state, the cancer cells are too large for assimilation by macrophages (Matzinger 1994). Cells that are able to divide, shift to enzymatic production of the universal energy carrier adenosine triphosphate (ATP) outside of the specialized cell organelles (mitochondria in which normally 90% of the ATP production is gained by oxidative phosphorylation), and transform into cancer cells. Research up until now suggests that cancer cells are associated with type 2 cytokine synthesis (Lucey 1996).

The self-tolerance of anaerobic colonies of the intestinal flora as an exosymbiotic discharge of the immune balance of the entire organism

Intestinal bacteria on the other hand, 99% anaerobes, likewise obtain ATP energy enzymatically instead of with the aid of oxidative phosphorylation of adenosine diphosphate (ADP). Not only do these anaerobes have the task of digesting food remains, but they also line the lower intestines, forming an exosymbiosis with the intestinal mucosa. They are an integral part of the immune defense, in that they supply the organism with sulfurous reducing substances by means of their complex metabolism, and in this way strengthen the reductive powers of the host. Additionally, the anaerobes produce from the amino acid tryptophan the vitamin niacin, essential as the building block of the co-enzyme NAD^+, which is irreplaceable in many biosyntheses as a carrier and receptor of hydrogen ions. It is striking that in the polymorphic cell composition of the intestinal wall and its mucous membrane, which represents the largest exchange and contact area in the human organism with the outside world and its manifold contaminations, the concentration of T-cells is relatively small, although 85% of all T-cells are found in the intestinal tissue. Clearly the anaerobe colonies, which produce more bacterial cells than the total number of body cells, relieve and strengthen the type 1 / type 2 cytokine balance of the entire organism. There is still too little research into the exact biodiversity and metabolic performance of the anaerobic intestinal flora, but a dyssymbiosis can lead to an increase in Th1 cell activity and the production of cytotoxic NO. Clinically, this reactive local Th1 dominance manifests itself as inflammatory intestinal diseases such as ulcerative colitis, Crohn's disease, or in both "HIV-negative" and "HIV-positive" homosexuals, the not uncommon inflammatory bowel syndrome (Tomita 1998, Guslandi 1998, Perner 1999, Murad 1999).

A successful pregnancy is possible only under the protection of Th2 dominance, with type 2 cytokine status and the inhibition of cytotoxic NO

The question why during pregnancy the embryonic cells are not recognized as being "foreign" by T-helper cells and then attacked, has been sufficiently explained. During pregnancy the maternal T-helper cells in the region of the placenta (retroplacentary blood lymphocytes) increase the synthesis of type 2 cytokines, most likely governed by elevated progesterone levels. As researchers in animal experiments and with human pregnancies have demonstrated, a Th1 dominance does in fact lead to termination of pregnancy. A successful pregnancy is only possible with the protection of the local synthesis of type 2 cytokines (Lin 1993, Wegmann 1993, Mosmann 1996, Raghupathy 1997, Kasakura 1998).

The force that controls the immune balance

The questions asked earlier about contradictions in the self/non-self concept dominant in immunology can plausibly be answered in light of the type 1 / type 2 cytokine balance and the related stimulation or inhibition of cytotoxic NO synthesis. But a far-reaching question arises from this knowledge: if the reaction to self and non-self identification is not the special function of the immune cell network, then what is the self-regulatory control for the adjustment of the balance between cell-mediated and humoral immunity? The strongest criticism of the self/non-self paradigm was formulated by the American immunologist Matzinger from the National Institutes of Health (NIH), the highest research authority for health matters in the USA. Matzinger, through analysis of a great many immunological research findings, reached the viewpoint that it is not the recognition of self and non-self molecules, but rather the realization of a danger to the organism in the form of tissue destruction that alerts the immune cell networks:

"Looking from the perspective that the driving force behind immunity is the need to recognize danger, we are led to the notion that the immune system itself does not stand alone. It is not simply a collection of specialized cells that patrol the rest of the body, but an extended and intricately connected family of cell types involving almost every bodily tissue. Tolerance no longer resides solely with deletion vs persistence of single lymphocytes; rather it is seen to be a cooperative endeavor among lymphocytes, APCs, and other tissues. Memory no longer resides with long-lived lymphocytes but in their interactions with antibodies, antigen, and follicular dendritic cells. Immune response modes are governed by interactions between lymphocytes, APCs, basophils, mast cells, and all of their lymphokines (and perhaps themselves, as they try to influence the immune system). By these networks of co-operating cells, the immune system can be alerted to danger and destruction without ever needing to consider the question of self vs non-self. It can contain myriads of auto and foreign reactive lymphocytes, each ready to respond and each ready to be tolerized if necessary. In this way it has the strength to destroy the things it needs to destroy, the tolerance to leave others alone, and the ability to tell the difference" (Matzinger 1994).

The danger theory explains the rules that are followed by the immune cell network when responding to active and passive stress factors. It does not explain the common elements within such apparently heterogeneous conditions as, for instance, protein energy malnutrition, organ transplants, sepses, chronic fungal or parasitic infections, chronic tuberculosis and lepromatous leprosy, AIDS, pregnancy or the aging process. In all of these conditions, the immune cell network switches, partially or systemically, to a type 2 cytokine synthesis and a limitation of cytotoxic NO production. The organism then tries to avert a particular danger, and in doing so takes other risks into account. In dangerous situations the organism has to make decisions as to how it can maintain balance, temporarily or long-term, in the individual compartments of the body, or for the body as a whole. This continuous balancing act can sometimes lead to an overcompensation in one or the other direction, and possibly to self-damage—either through inflammatory processes and autoimmune reactions, as a result of a too high, unchecked cytotoxic NO production (Th1 dominance); or through the deactivation of cytotoxic NO production and the switching of the immune response to an extracellular humoral defense, resulting in an immune cell dysbalance (Th2 dominance). The immune cell network can give too much gas or brake too hard. With acquired immunodeficiency syndrome (AIDS), the organism seems, after a phase of excessive NO activation, to be too exhausted to brake NO production. In the case of pregnancies, for reasons of the physiological cell division frequency, there is no possibility of choice. Not only do the T-helper cells of pregnant women switch to Th2 dominance between mother and embryo in the contact areas of the placenta, but the T-helper cells of the newborn child are imprinted with the Th2 type. After birth, a regulated Th1/Th2 balance has to be trained (Delepesse 1998).

Worldwide increase of allergies, atopy and AIDS are indicators of the civilization-dependent shift of the immune cell balance towards Th2 dominance

The fact of the type 2 cytokine imprint of foetal T-helper cells in the womb has been linked to other significant clinical phenomena. Worldwide epidemiological studies in many countries have revealed that the prevalence of atopy, including allergic rhinitis, asthma, eczema, and atopic skin diseases have continuously increased since WWII. This increase in susceptibility to allergic reactions is correlated with a Th2 immune cell dominance, an increase in antibody production of immunoglobulin E and certain immunoglobulin G antibodies, an increase in eosinophils and a relatively anergic DTH skin reaction. The immunological findings of atopic patients are analogous to the immune response to worm infections. It can be assumed that there is a cross-reaction between allergy-causing antigens (allergens) and worm antigens, as the immune cell network reacts exactly as it would to a worm infection. That means that the immune cell network, as sensor for internal and external environmental dangers in atopic patients, is adjusted to danger in much the same way as the early developmental stage of vertebrates, when worm parasites made necessary the evolutionary biological innovation of the double strategy of cell-mediated (Th1 cells and cytotoxic NO production) and humoral (Th2 cells and a broad antibody repertoire) immune response (Fedyk 1997, Holt 1997, Romagnani 1998, Paronchi 1999). However, there is an important difference: it has been established that early childhood bacterial infections have a negative correlation with the later development of atopy, so it seems that the lack of childhood infectious incidents encourages atopy and the Th2 dominance promotes susceptibility to atopic reactions. It is hypothesized that the reduction of infections during childhood due to vaccinations and antibiotics contributes to atopic disposition. Also intrauterine conditions, for instance nutritional factors which force the Th2 status and IgE synthesis, have also been discussed as causes (Howarth 1998). What is difficult to understand, is why the exposure of mothers to drugs, foodstuff and drinking water contamination (nitrosamines, pesticides, hormones, antibiotic residues, etc.), cigarette consumption, environmental poisons, exposure to natural and artificial radiation, heavy metals, contraception pills, and so on, have not been discussed.

In this context, it is striking that homosexual AIDS patients who are affected were predominantly born after WWII (average age, mid-30s) although it would be reasonable to assume that precisely older homosexuals could have inhaled nitrite as a means of sustaining erections, comparable to heterosexuals using Viagra for a similar purpose. Nitrites expand the blood vessels in the penis by releasing NO, which in turn activates the ferrous enzyme, guanylyl cyclase, which stimulates cyclic guanosine monophosphate (cGMP), which relaxes the smooth muscle fibers of the blood vessels. Viagra hinders the rapid reduction of cGMP and in this way produces an effect similar to nitrite inhalation. Homosexual AIDS patients, during the progression from asymptomatic AID (anergic DTH skin reaction, Th2 dominance) to opportunistic infections (AID-S), often developed atopic symptoms and allergic reactions to drugs, greatly increased IgE antibody production, and eosinophils with significantly increased amounts of eosinophilic cationic proteins in the blood serum (Parkin 1987, Grieko 1989, Wright 1990, Lucey 1990, Paganelli 1991, Isreal-Biet 1992, Small 1993, Smith 1994, Drabick 1994, Vigano 1995 a, 1995 b, Paganelli 1995).

Immune cell dysbalance in old age

In general, when compared to younger people, the elderly have a higher prevalence of bacterial, viral and opportunistic infections and cancer. However, this pathology is not associated with AIDS. T-cells of older people exhibit a reduced proliferation after induction with mitogens; and a reduced type 1 cytokine synthesis, while type 2 cytokine synthesis is increased. This Th2 dominance is also typical of healthy elderly people. During stimulation of leukocytes with bacterial endotoxins (LPS), however, records show an increased synthesis of interleukin 1, 6 and 8 as well as tumor necrosis factors in older people as compared to younger people (Rink 1998, Shearer 1997). In T-lymph cell experiments on mice, with increasing age there was a clear shift of the Th1-Th2 profiles, a reduction of natural killer cell activity, and disruption of the B-lymphocyte functions (Doria 1997).

Th2 dominance in newborn children indicates that the T-helper cell activity with cytotoxic NO synthesis cannot be imprinted during foetal development. The increased predisposition in old age for infections and neoplasia demonstrates that the cytokine balance is no longer maintained.

The reasons for these immunological findings at the beginning and end of life, as well as for the symptomatic immune dysbalances due to specific stressors with varying causes are of a profound nature. They are determined by the evolutionary biological fact that all human cells, as with all multi-cellular organisms and most protista, in reality comprise a cell colony formed by intracellular symbiosis. All influences in the course of a lifetime, from embryonic development until death, affect the vital function of this cell symbiosis. The dynamics of acquired immunodeficiency are a special case of regulatory and counterregulatory disruption of this highly complex symbiosis in specific cell systems. This evolutionary medical fact has until now been sparsely contemplated, if at all, in practical medical science; in the HIV/AIDS field it has been repressed by an obsession with a hypothetical retroviral infection.

Independent of specific causes, all immune weaknesses are governed by the same evolutionary-biological rules

Recapitulating, the causes of "acquired immune cell deficiency" can be explained: We are dealing with an evolutionary-biologically programmed switching of the immune cell network and other cell systems, acting to protect the cell symbiosis. Dependent on whether the changes to the redox milieu are temporary or long-term, the T-helper cell populations, influenced by the cytokine profile, are imprinted with a Th2 dominance with increased antibody activity. The cytotoxic NO production, reliant on type 1 cytokines, is suffocated, as is the production of reactive oxygen species (ROS), The price of this inflammatory blockade is a weakness in the elimination of intracellular pathogens. This can lead to opportunistic infections (AIDS), as the intracellular opportunistic microbes can only be fought off by an adequate NO synthesis. Very often, the pathophysiological type 2 cytokine dominance follows a short-term and excessive, or a long-term and continual, switching of the NO synthesis and the type 1 cytokine synthesis of the counterregulation to a type 2 cytokine profile. In this sense, the inhalation of nitrites for sex-doping is a special factor in increasing the NO formation in certain cell systems. The results are inflammatory processes, higher local or systemic cell death, necrosis (with antibody formation and tissue damage through autoimmune reaction) and/or apoptosis (without autoantibody formation). Such processes could develop, also in phases and at certain stages of illness, parallel to a Th2 dominance of the immune response.

In extreme cases, the counterregulations for the protection of cell symbiosis could become overcompensatory and lead to malignant cancer cell transformation; i.e. enzymatic ATP fermentation as an emergency backup plan for cellular survival when mitochondria are malfunctioning. The triggering stressors are of a diverse nature; toxic (including pharmacotoxic), traumatic, nutritional, microbial, alloantigenic (including intake of oxidizing semen during anal intercourse as well as highly contaminated blood products), environmental, psychoemotional, and age-related. Individually or in combination, such stress factors could exert an influence on life expectancy. In relation to dosage, duration, type and combination of the prooxidative stress burden, together with the predisposition of the individual (influenced by genetic, intrauterine, and early childhood imprinting) a latent AID state can shift to manifest AID syndrome (AIDS). This can occur with or without a positive result from an "HIV antibody test." As a logical consequence, the US surveillance authority (CDC) has since 1987 diagnosed AIDS by the most frequent AIDS-indicating diseases in a catalogue of 29 disease forms, without the laboratory construct of "HIV-positive" (CDC 1987): the laboratory construct "HIV-positive" merely proves the presence of adequate amounts of antibodies and autoantibodies to reach the measuring thresholds of the "anti-HIV antibody test." Conclusions as to the origins of an acquired immune cell deficiency cannot be drawn from an "HIV test," because the origin of the proteins used in the testing procedure as evidence of antibodies has not been identified, but merely attributed by virtue of inadequate evidence to a "retrovirus." A "retroviral" infection of T-helper cells would be neither necessary nor sufficient to explain a Th2 dominance. Only in the context of other clinical and laboratory parameters, can the "HIV test" indirectly give nonspecific clues about the existence of a Th2 dominance and the disintegration of cell symbiosis. There are some 70-odd different conditions in which an "HIV test" comes up positive and even HIV dogmatists recognize that these have nothing to do with having "retroviral" infections (Giraldo 1999).

The "HIV-associated" AIDS cases represent, in stark contrast to the official propaganda, only a small section of the total spectrum of acquired immune dysbalances.

It is a fact that only 0.1% of the total population of Germany show signs of the quantitative and qualitative antibody and autoantibody combinations that could lead to the laboratory construct of "HIV-positivity." The majority of these cases are members of the "risk groups": a minority of anally receptive homosexuals, a minority of intravenous drug addicts, half of the hemophiliacs, and some multi-transfusion recipients. This must be compared to the fact that within a general surgical patient population, roughly 30% featured an anergic Th2 dominance (Christou, 1986).

Independent of their respective specific causes, all of these AIDS forms comply with the same evolutionary-biological rules. Causal research can only be of use when considering all of the "risky" events in an individual's life. The actual meaning of Th2 dominance concerning AIDS is dependent on whether the affected patient recognizes and learns to avoid the actual risks, whether the given bioenergetic and biochemical deficit for protecting cell symbiosis can be balanced, and whether medical intervention does not cause more harm than good. Knowledge of the self-organization of cell symbioses, in existence for some 2 billion years, is indispensable in order to reach this curative objective.

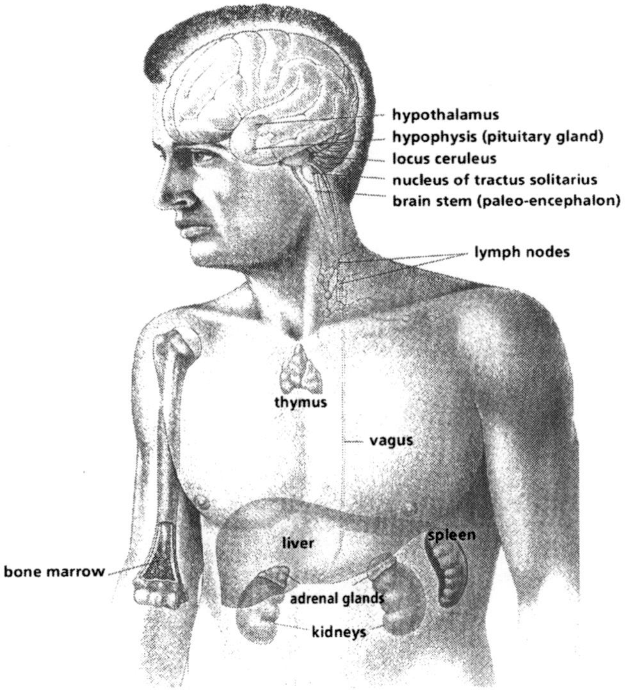
hypothalamus
hypophysis (pituitary gland)
locus ceruleus
nucleus of tractus solitarius
brain stem (paleo-encephalon)
lymph nodes
thymus
vagus
liver
spleen
bone marrow
adrenal glands
kidneys

Fig. 14)

Many doctors, through a high degree of specialization, have lost the holistic approach. However, well-being and health depend on the balance between body and mind. There is a close link between stress and the immune system.Both exchange numerous biochemical signals and thus cooperate especially to the outcome of pathologies. The body reacts to each threat or exposure with a stress response that starts from the brain, which is linked with all the organs and tissues and receives information from them. In cases of stress, the hypothalamus, the pituitary and the locus ceruleus as well as the sympathetic nervous system and the suprarenal glands activate the body and stimulate a response. At this stage the messages to the immune system begin, which unlike the nervous system, represent a network without a base, and with a capacity to react in different ways to dangerous substances, penetrating microorganisms and damaged or degenerated body cells. The immune cells develop in the spinal cord, the lymph nodes, the spleen and the thymus. They communicate amongst themselves by means of small proteins that are able to convey messages even to the brain. This takes place via the bloodstream or via nerves, like the vagus (part of the intestinal nervous system), and the nucleus of the solitary tract.

Fig. 15) Diagram of hematic and immune cells.

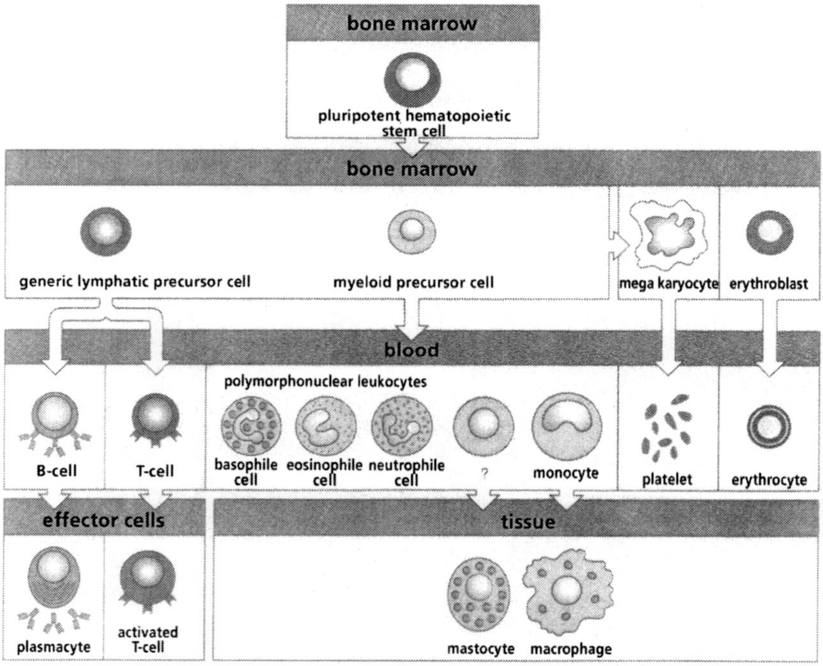
bone marrow
pluripotent hematopoietic stem cell
bone marrow
generic lymphatic precursor cell
myeloid precursor cell
mega karyocyte
erythroblast
blood
polymorphonuclear leukocytes
B-cell
T-cell
basophile cell
eosinophile cell
neutrophile cell
?
monocyte
platelet
erythrocyte
effector cells
tissue
plasmacyte
activated T-cell
mastocyte
macrophage

Fig. 16)

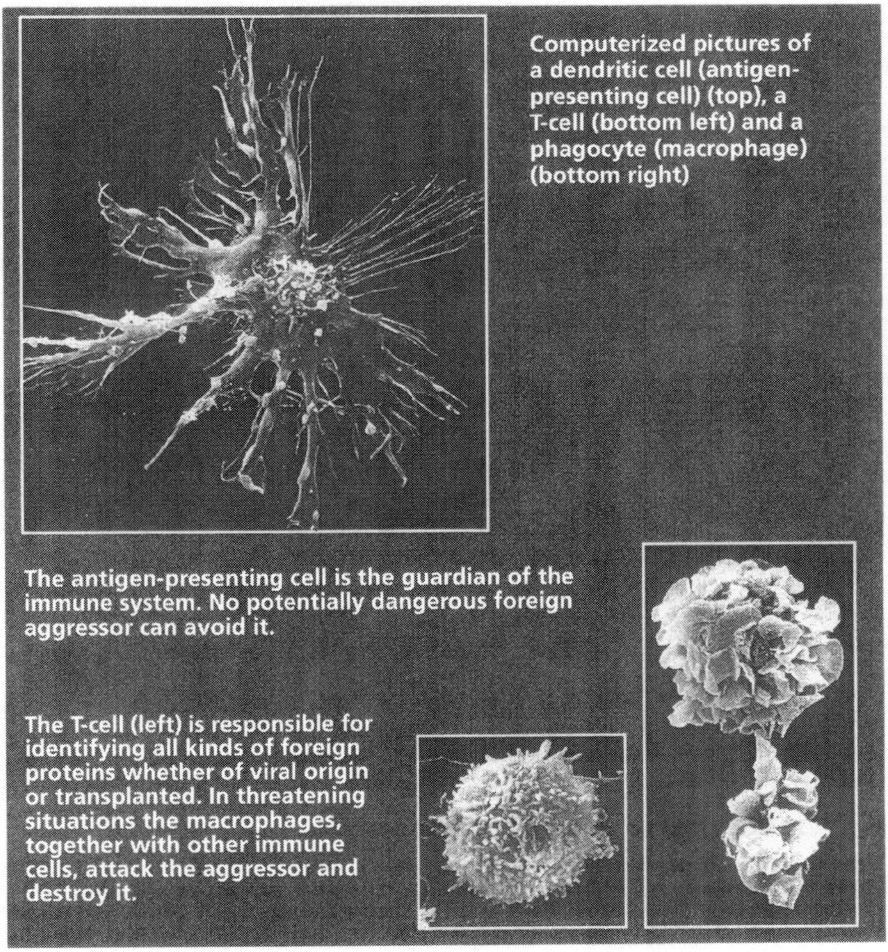
Computerized pictures of a dendritic cell (antigen-presenting cell) (top), a T-cell (bottom left) and a phagocyte (macrophage) (bottom right)
The antigen-presenting cell is the guardian of the immune system. No potentially dangerous foreign aggressor can avoid it.
The T-cell (left) is responsible for identifying all kinds of foreign proteins whether of viral origin or transplanted. In threatening situations the macrophages, together with other immune cells, attack the aggressor and destroy it.

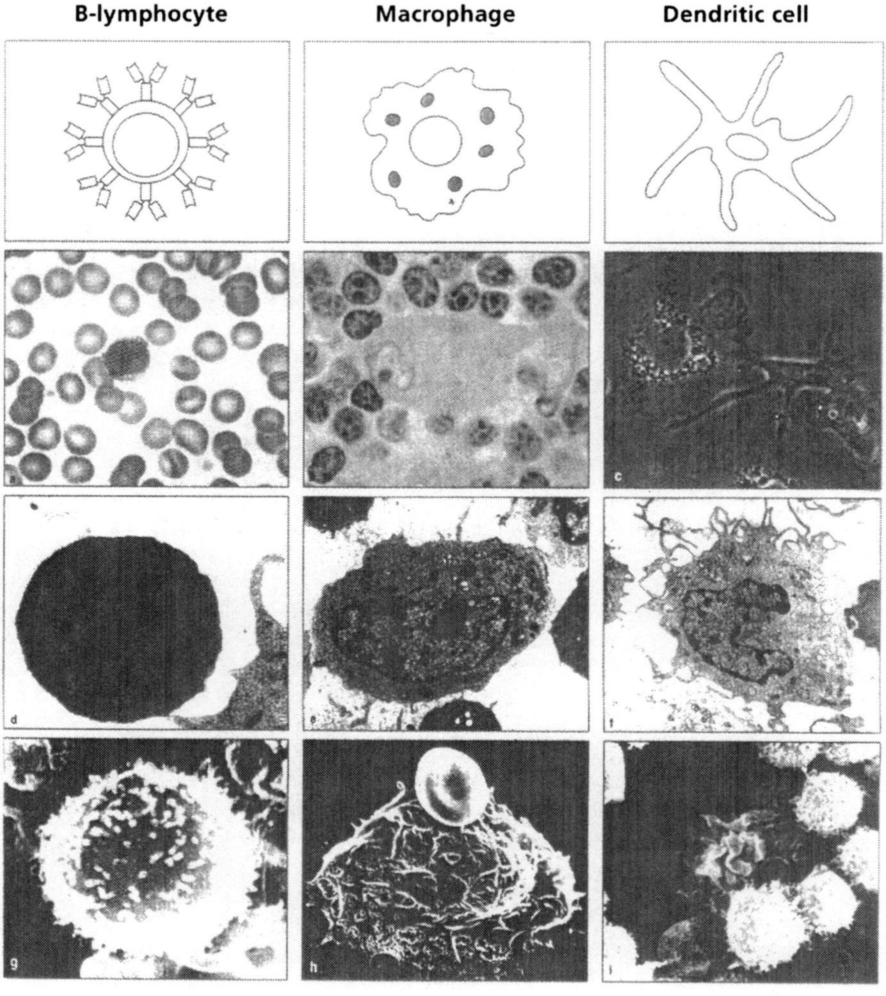

B-lymphocyte
Macrophage
Dendritic cell

Fig. 17) Professional cells that expose antigens

Three kinds of cells are shown in the illustration, by means of a schematic picture (first row), an optical microscope (second row), a transmission electron microscope and a scanning electron microscope (fourth row). The B lymphocytes are endowed with specific receivers for the antigens represented by superficial immunoglobulins. These immunoglobulins permit the cells to display a recognised antigen in high concentrations. They can be stimulated to carry out a co-stimulation. Macrophages are specialized in capturing and exposing antigens in the form of particles. If macrophages are stimulated they are able to carry out co-stimulation. Dendritic cells are present both in lymphatic and in other kinds of tissue. Due to their make-up they are co-stimulating and are probably important for antiviral immunity.

Fig. 18) Diagram of the T immunocyte population:

CD4 immune cells or T4 cells: subgroup T4 inflammatory cells or type 1 T helper cells = TH1 or Th1, subgroup T4 helper cells or type 2 T helper cells= TH2 or Th2 CD8 immune cells or T8 = cytotoxic T cells or killer T cells = type 1 Tc cells (Tc1) or type 2 Tc cells (Tc 2).
The maturation and role of the T immunocytes is controlled by polar profiles of cytokines and is balanced by means of mutual inhibition.
These polar profiles of cytokines also control activation or inhibition of cytotoxic NO gas production and the interaction with antigen presenting cells.
In AIDS and cancer patients, the balance of cytokines and T cells is always shifted towards a type 2 profile.

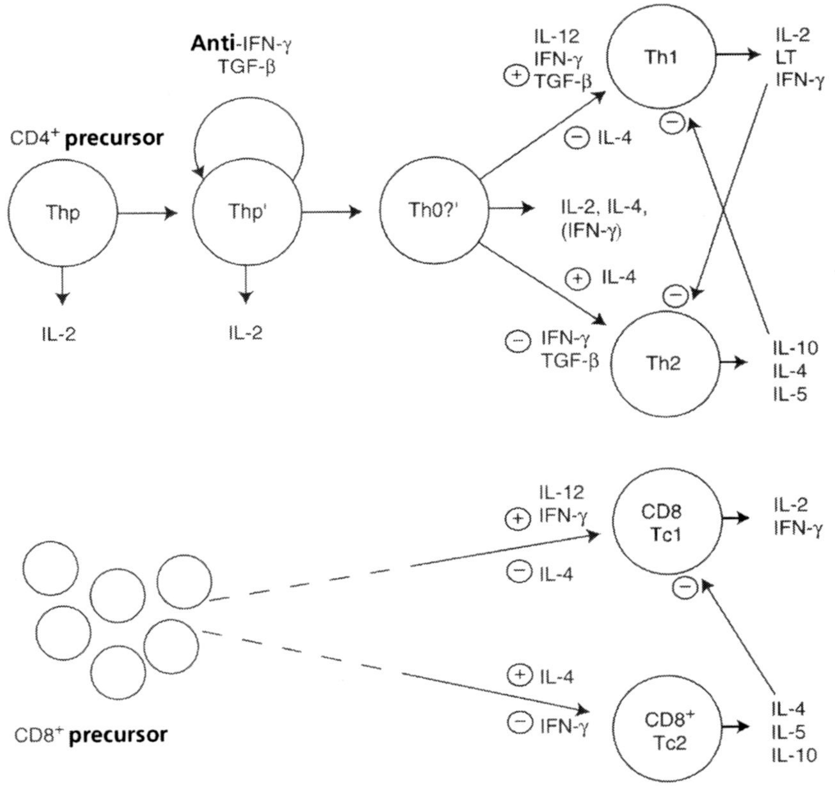

Anti-IFN-γ
TGF-β
CD4⁺ precursor
Thp
Thp'
Th0?'
IL-2
IL-2
IL-12
IFN-γ
+ TGF-β
Th1
IL-2
LT
IFN-γ
− IL-4
IL-2, IL-4,
(IFN-γ)
+ IL-4
− IFN-γ
TGF-β
Th2
IL-10
IL-4
IL-5
IL-12
+ IFN-γ
CD8
Tc1
IL-2
IFN-γ
− IL-4
+ IL-4
− IFN-γ
CD8⁺
Tc2
IL-4
IL-5
IL-10
CD8⁺ precursor

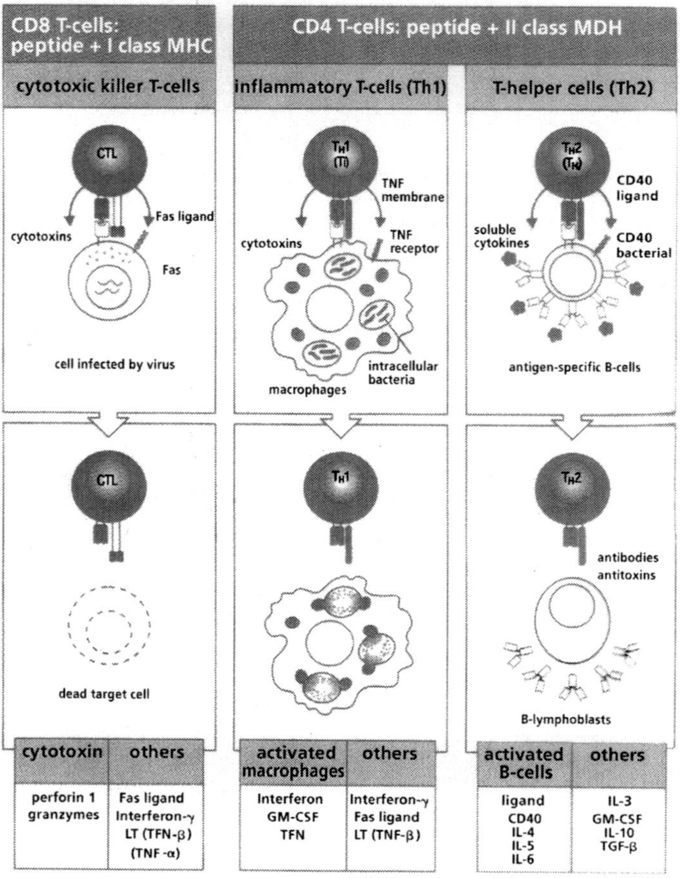
CD8 T-cells:
peptide + I class MHC
CD4 T-cells: peptide + II class MDH
cytotoxic killer T-cells
inflammatory T-cells (Th1)
T-helper cells (Th2)
CTL
Fas ligand
cytotoxins
Fas
cell infected by virus
TNF
membrane
TNF
receptor
cytotoxins
intracellular
bacteria
macrophages
CD40
ligand
soluble
cytokines
CD40
bacterial
antigen-specific B-cells
CTL
dead target cell
antibodies
antitoxins
B-lymphoblasts

cytotoxin	others
perforin 1 granzymes	Fas ligand Interferon-γ LT (TFN-β) (TNF-α)

activated macrophages	others
Interferon GM-CSF TFN	Interferon-γ Fas ligand LT (TNF-β)

activated B-cells	others
ligand CD40 IL-4 IL-5 IL-6	IL-3 GM-CSF IL-10 TGF-β

Fig.19) The three principle effector T-cells produce several effector molecules.

The CD8 T-cells are mainly killer cells that recognize the pathogens peptides of the cytosol linked to class 1 MHC. These molecules produce perforin 1 that damage the membrane of the targeted cells. They also produce granzymes, e.g. proteases and often Interferon-γ. The effector molecule linked to the membrane in CD8 T-cells is probably the ligand for Fas, a receptor whose activation provokes apoptosis. The CD4 T-cells recognize the peptides linked to class II MHC molecules. There are two functional types: Inflammatory CD4 T-cells (Th1) specializing in the activation of macrophages that contain or absorb pathogens. They secrete Interferon-γ and other effector molecules and they are thought to express the TNF linked to the membrane. The CD4 T-helper cells (Th2) specialize in activating B-cells and secrete growth factors IL-4, IL-5 and IL-6 that play a role in the activation and differentiation of B-cells. They also express CD40 ligand, which is an effector molecule linked to the CD40 membrane in the B-cell and induces its proliferation.

Fig.20) Interaction between T4 cells and B-cells or dendritic cells.

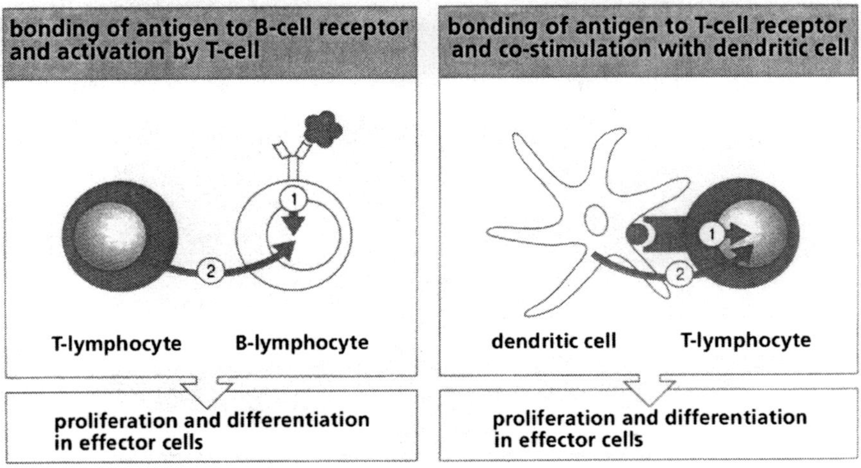

bonding of antigen to B-cell receptor and activation by T-cell
1
2
T-lymphocyte
B-lymphocyte
proliferation and differentiation in effector cells
bonding of antigen to T-cell receptor and co-stimulation with dendritic cell
1
2
dendritic cell
T-lymphocyte
proliferation and differentiation in effector cells

Fig. 21) Diagram of the interaction between a macrophage and a T4 activator cell (Th1) or a T4 inhibitor cell (Th2) and the polar cytokines. With clear cases of AIDS this mutual interaction becomes highly unstable. In tumors macrophages, as a rule, undergo a functional inhibition.

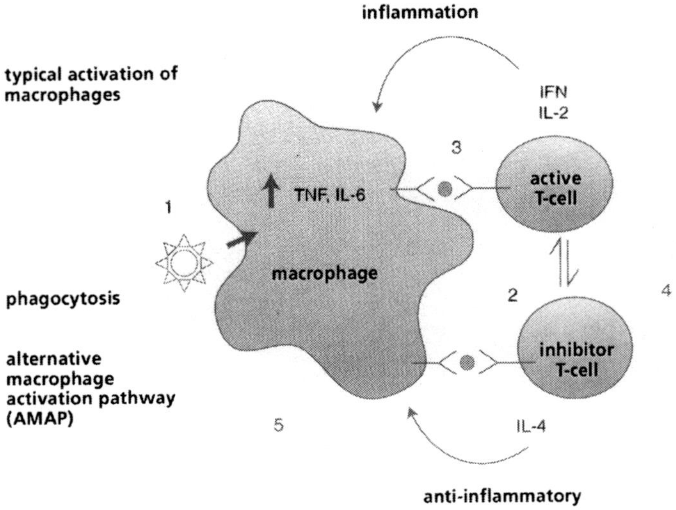

inflammation
typical activation of macrophages
IFN
IL-2
3
TNF, IL-6
active T-cell
1
macrophage
phagocytosis
2
4
alternative macrophage activation pathway (AMAP)
inhibitor T-cell
5
IL-4
anti-inflammatory

Fig. 22)
Typical antibody molecules, composed of four peptidic chains that together create the shape and structure of a Y. The trunk is composed of two heavy chains which spread up the 'branches' of the Y while the two light chains are restricted to the 'branches'. Each polypeptide has constant and variable domains. All antibodies of a certain type have the same constant domains, while the variable domains differentiate between one clone or another of B cells. At the end of each 'branch' the variable domains of both heavy and light chains are folded to form a coupling point for antigens.

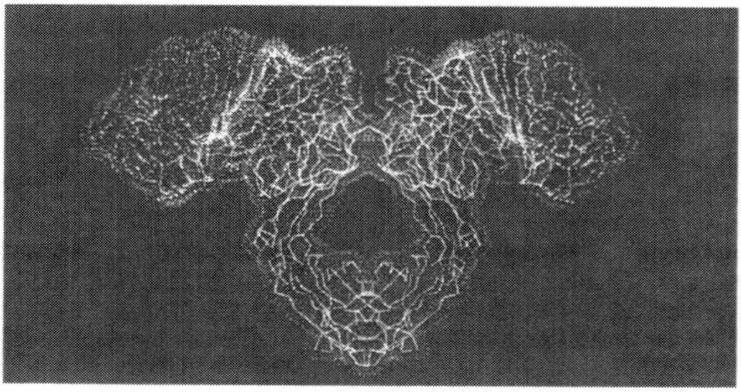

Fig. 23)
An antibody is composed of repeated domains, i.e., of separate units of folds of polypeptidic chains. A light chain is composed of two of these domains, whereas the heavy ones shown here have four. The polypeptide chain in the domain is folded in a typical way, some sections form a so-called beta folding structure. The variable area of each chain has only one domain at the amino end. Here there are three spirals (hypervariable domains) that help the coupling point of the antigen. The domain structure is represented here with a diagram but actually the chain is more complex. Similar domains are present in T cell receptors and in proteins of the major histocompatibility complex (MHC) that characterize the cells of the body. The three groups of molecules probably go back to the same common ancestor.

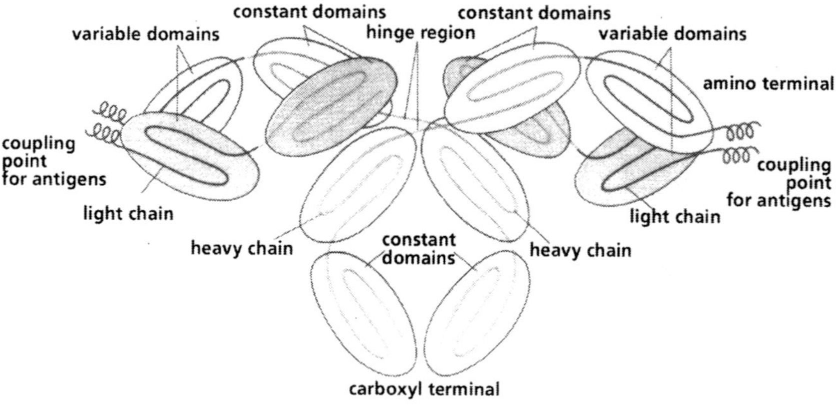
constant domains
constant domains
variable domains
hinge region
variable domains
amino terminal
coupling point for antigens
coupling point for antigens
light chain
light chain
heavy chain
constant domains
heavy chain
carboxyl terminal

Chapter VI

The Most Successful Fusion in the History of Evolution

How the micro-Gaian milieu functions—the vital role of the mitochondria

Over the course of the 19th Century, cell biologists discovered a series of living structures in the cells of vertebrates and invertebrates. In 1856 Kolliker discovered rounded forms along the transverse muscle fiber. Later he noticed that these granula became swollen in water and evidently had a membrane. Altmann conducted the first systematic studies of these membrane-coated cell granula. He named these intracellular forms "bioblasts" (from the Greek: *bios* = life + *blastos* = grain) or "elementary organisms." He believed that they were similar to bacteria, and demonstrated that bioblasts could survive as free-living structures when not living in colonies within the cells. Altmann also developed the first methods for the isolation of nucleic acids free from protein, but what he could not have known at the time was that bioblasts themselves also contained small amounts of nucleic acids and genes (Altmann 1894). This discovery was made seventy years later, and confirmed Altmann's earlier speculation that the cell organelle, known since 1898 as mitochondria (from the Greek: *mitos* = thread + *chondros* = granule), originated from former bacteria. By the end of WWI, many cell researchers had described the existence, number, form, and distribution of mitochondria in a multitude of cells: in nuclear protista, fungi, parasites, invertebrates and vertebrates, as well as in human cells (Cowdry 1918). There was much speculation about the function of mitochondria. Altmann had already implied that mitochondria could be a part of the cellular respiration process, but it was not until 1912 that this hypothesis was explicitly established (Ernster 1981). During the first two decades of the 20th Century, there were competing theories as to the process of oxidation in live tissues and cells. The German chemists Wieland

and Thunberg had demonstrated that large numbers of organic bonds could be oxidized when brought into contact with small amounts of metal catalysts that could both absorb and emit hydrogen. This reaction supported the hypothesis that biological oxidation was based on previous processes which supply hydrogen, and then release it via substrates as the hydrogen atoms react with the molecular oxide (O_2). Wieland showed that an inhibition of cellular respiration with cyanide led to a blockade of the enzyme, catalase, which neutralizes hydrogen peroxide (H_2O_2). However, no significant increase of H_2O_2 was observed in living cells when treated with cyanide (Tyler 1992).

The gigantic energy supply in the respiratory chain of the mitochondria

The German biochemist and later Nobel Prize winner, Warburg, believed that the key process in tissue and cell respiration was the activation of oxygen. He demonstrated that the oxygen was activated by a ferrous enzyme that he termed "atmungsferment," (breathing enzyme) a term that is used to this day in English medical literature. The ferrous components of an "atmungsferment" are reduced by metabolites to bivalent iron (Fe^{2+}, ferrous state) or oxidized by O_2 to trivalent iron (Fe^{3+}, ferric state). This reaction could be inhibited by either carbon dioxide or cyanide (Warburg 1949).

Researchers had already recognized that the respiratory process was linked to a special cell structure that served as a catalyzing surface for the reduction/oxidation (redox) process. In 1925, Keilin published a report on the respiratory pigment, cytochrome, in plant cells. He was able to prove that the competing theories about respiratory procedures were two sides of the same coin, and that the activation of hydrogen and oxygen, mediated by cytochromes, interacted as the essential partners in respiration. Cytochrome pigments in muscle fibers had already been discovered 40 years previously, but their function and chemical structure had not been clearly resolved. In the ensuing four decades, the work of Keilin (Keilin 1933) would be the starting point for a gradual clarification of the central function of mitochondria in energy metabolism of all animals, fungi and plants, and nearly all protista (Tyler 1992). In humans, as a general rule, every cell is colonized by approximately several hundred to several thousand mitochondria (with the exception of red blood corpuscles, which have neither cell nucleus nor mitochondria, and obtain their energy enzymatically). If the numbers are extrapolated to the 2 trillion odd body cells, then there are some 2,000 trillion active mitochondria in humans.

The mitochondria are identifiable as solid bodies in a light-optical microscope with a resolution of 0.2-0.4 microns. Their actual structure could only be clarified by analysis with electron microscopes in the 1950s. Mitochondria possess an outer and inner membrane typical of bacteria. The latter is folded as cristae (from the Latin: *crista* = crest) into the matrix. A mitochondrion can vary its inner and outer form depending on its functional status. The molecular complexes for the respiratory chain are embedded in the inner membrane and comprised of four complexes: Complex I (NADH-ubiquinone reductase), complex II (succinate-ubiquinone reductase), complex III (ubiquinol-cytochrome-c reductase), complex IV (cytochrome c oxidase). These four complexes are linked by ubiquinone (Q) and cytochrome c, which can diffuse through the membrane. Q acts as a transport molecule for electrons from complexes I and II to complex III. Similarly, cytochrome c transports electrons from complex III to complex IV. This transportation of electrons serves to power the hydrogen pumps in complex I, II and IV with energy. The hydrogen ions are channelled through canals in the inner membrane, and concentrate in the gap between the inner and outer membrane. The hydrogen ion gradients, powered by electrons, activate the coupling of adenosine diphosphate (ADP) with inorganic phosphorus (P_i) to form adenosine triphosphate (ATP) in a fifth complex (F1 ADP-synthase). Complex V is situated in the cristae of the mitochondria. The ATP exits the mitochondria into the cytoplasm, via a special transport protein complex, in exchange for ADP and P_i.

The electrons are absorbed by molecular oxygen (O_2) at the end of the respiratory chain of complex IV, and subsequently immediately reduced to water. This bioenergetic and biochemical process is termed oxidative phosphorylation (OXPHOS). In human cells almost 90% of the energy-bearing molecule ATP is produced in the mitochondria. ATP serves as a source of energy in countless biosyntheses; as the phosphate bonds of the ATP molecules are split by the absorption of water, and the energy released becomes available for biochemical metabolic processes. As ATP cannot be stored in an organism, it must be continuously produced. In humans, it is estimated that daily 70 kilograms of ATP have to be produced, released and re-produced. Even a short interruption in ATP production can lead to an energetic deficiency. Some 90% of an organism's absorbed oxygen is used by the OXPHOS system in the mitochondria. Only about 10% of the necessary ATP is produced enzymatically (substrate level phosphorylation) via metabolites from glucose metabolism, occurring in the cytoplasm outside of the mitochondria (Tyler 1992). These data show the immense capacity of the mitochondria, upon whose vital functions all cells, tissues, organs and the entire organism as a whole are dependent for all internal and external activities.

While the OXPHOS system can be fueled by oxidation of a number of different nutrients, it is mainly carbohydrates and fats that are oxidized.

Glucose is reduced to pyruvate by a metabolic chain with the participation of a series of enzymes and co-enzymes a number of which are supplied by vitamins, and then infiltrates the mitochondria. The metabolic path from oxidation of the glucose to pyruvate is termed glycolysis. The end product, two molecules of pyruvate, is fed into the citric acid cycle of the mitochondria and completely oxidized to form six molecules of carbon dioxide (CO_2). In this process the co-enzymes NAD^+ (nicotinamide adenine dinucleotide) and FAD (flavin adenine dinucleotide) are reduced and afterwards deliver their hydrogen ions for the respiratory chain (oxidation). NAD^+ contains the vitamin niacin from tryptophane and FAD the vitamin riboflavin. There are four metabolic pathways that intermesh during the oxidative process of gaining ATP from glucose: glycolysis in the cytoplasm, the citric acid cycle in the mitochondria, the respiratory chain and the OXPHOS system. Beforehand NAD has to be synthesized in an auxiliary metabolic path of glucose and $NADH^+H^+$ has to be formed by means of a special enzyme reaction. The latter cannot, however, take place in the inner membrane of the mitochondria. For this purpose shuttle molecules act as ferries taking on the hydrogen in reduced form from the $NADH^+H^+$ which they then transport into the mitochondria. The shuttle molecules are converted and return to the cytoplasm to recommence the transport cycle. But the respiratory chain and ATP production are kept going by $NADH^+H^+$ and $FADH_2$.

This simplified representation serves to demonstrate the tightly regulated import/export system that takes place between the mitochondria and the cytoplasm. If the transport or production pathways are interrupted at any point in the chain then the entire cell is affected. This interrelationship could be compared to the modern just-in-time system between suppliers and a production company, but with the crucial difference that in living cells, the flows of energy and biosyntheses occur according to the principles of self-organization (autopoiesis). The cycle outlined above, however, only describes one of the many functions of the thousands of mitochondria in every cell. Numerous interconnected import and export paths exist between the mitochondria and the cytoplasm, the nucleus, other cell organelles and the cell membrane.

The coordinated interaction of DNA, mitochondria and the cell nucleus

In the 1960s, observations with electron microscopes made it evident mitochondria had their own DNA and a circular, double-stranded genome (Tandler 1972). It turned out that mitochondrial DNA governed, to some extent, the protein synthesis for the respiratory chain complexes and for the ATP synthase complex. The biogenesis (biological manufacture) of mitochondria is a coordinated interplay of different genetic systems—the genome in the nucleus controlling the synthesis of the majority of mitochondrial proteins, and the remaining mitochondrial genomes controlling the synthesis of their own proteins—all of which are crucial for the proper bioenergetic function of mitochondria. Mitochondria, above all, synthesize a proportion of the proteins for the four complexes of the respiratory chain as well as complex V, the ATP synthase. This is the case in all eukaryotic organisms. Despite the considerable contribution of mitochondrial DNA for the biosynthesis of proteins, the majority of genetic information for the formation and function of the mitochondria is encoded in the genome of the cell nucleus (Schatz 1974, Gray 1999, Saraste 1999).

All in all, the mitochondria import over 1,000 proteins that are coded by DNA in the nucleus and synthesized in the cytoplasm. These findings have encouraged discussions about the origin of mitochondria and the role of endosymbiosis (from the Greek: *endo* = inner + *symbiosis* = coexist) between a larger unicellular host organism and smaller unicellular cell symbionts, as the forerunners of the evolution of all multicellular organisms, humans included. Today, the fact is generally accepted that all eukaryotic unicellular protista and all multicellular eukaryotic organisms have developed via the integration of various prokaryotic organisms lacking cell nuclei (De Duve 1991). There are, however, different scenarios as to how this endosymbiosis has developed over the course of evolution. These ideas are of crucial importance in understanding human disease processes, including AIDS and cancer.

The Gaian hypothesis and the theory of endosymbiosis

A popular scenario is the serial endosymbiosis theory enthusiastically propagated by the American microbiologist Lynn Margulis (Margulis 1970, 1988). This theory posits that initially two prokaryotes (from the Latin: *pro* = before, and Greek: *karyon* = kernel, meaning before the formation of the nucleus) from the two unicellular domains of cell life—bacteria and archaea—merged and formed a primary cell nucleus. This new cell type—the eukaryon (from the Greek: *eu* = right + *karyon* = kernel, meaning with the right nucleus)—developed roughly 2.1 billion years ago. Margulis deduced this concept in part from the fact that there are primitive protista with nuclei that contain no mitochondria or endosymbionts. The necessity of nuclear formation is explained by the Gaia hypothesis of the British chemist Lovelock (Lovelock 1972, Lenton 1998). In the 1960s, Lovelock contracted with the American space agency, NASA, researching whether life could exist on Mars.

Lovelock recognized that the atmosphere on Earth differed from those of the neighboring planets Venus and Mars, due to its high content of oxygen. He postulated that the biosphere of the Earth is a global gas exchange system that had been formed by the bioenergetic activities of prokaryotes, which still today produce 80% of the active biomass in the oceans, on land, and in the air. Lovelock described the biosphere as the outcome of the combined metabolic activities of the prokaryotes, and termed this circulatory, self-regulating, homeostatic system "Gaia." Together with Margulis, Lovelock further refined this elementary perception by the notion that life on Earth had created its own conditions as massive amounts of oxygen, which had accumulated as the metabolic product of cyanobacteria in the oceans and later in the atmosphere over an immense period of time, created the evolutionary biological conditions for prokaryotes to evolve. Cyanobacteria and other prokaryotes had developed the ability to split water (H_2O) with the help of photonic energy from sunlight, in order to utilize the hydrogen together with carbon dioxide for the composition of energy-stimulated sugar molecules. This photosynthetic process in cyanobacteria, algae and plants to this day forms the basis for the organic substrate of the food chain of the unicellular protista (falsely termed protozoa from the Greek: *protos* = first + *zoon* = animal), and the multicellular fungi, animals and humans. According to the serial endosymbiosis theory of Margulis, nucleus formation of the primary endosymbiosis protects the DNA from the corrosive effects of oxygen (Margulis 1988). A further decisive act of integration, according to Margulis and other researchers, was implemented by a targeted attack of proto-mitochondria that could already use molecular oxygen as a source of energy. This predatory parasite is thought to have been domesticated by anaerobic host cells that already had nuclei, with the advantage of the mutual utilization of ATP production of the OXPHOS system of the mitochondria (Margulis 1981). The argument against this scenario was that an aerobic robber and its anaerobic booty could not have met at that point in time as there were hardly any oxygen-free niches in the biological ecosystem and yet the host cell and the proto-mitochondrion must have lived in the same environment. This implies that the host cells could also utilize oxygen, or at least protect themselves from its poisonous effects (De Duve 1991).

The genetic information inside the cell nucleus of all eukaryotic organisms, humans included, descended from the DNA fusion of several singled-celled organisms

In recent years, however, this alternative scenario, together with the serial endosymbiosis theory, have been seriously challenged. In systematic genetic comparative studies in countless cell systems the long-held perception of the endosymbiosis model, that the host cells introduced the already developed nucleus for the integration of proto-mitochondria in the cell combination, has been shaken. It has, however, been confirmed that the nucleus does not originate from a sole unicellular progenitor. The nucleus contains many more DNA components from at least two precursor cells. The eukaryotic genome is thus a chimera: the primary components originate from both an archaeum and a bacterium. The informational genes are mainly archaean, whilst the operational genes are primarily of bacterial origin. The eubacterial portion of the nuclear genome, which until then had been attributed to the gene transfer from the protomitochondria, are not transmitted from the mitochondria, so what we are talking about here are genes that participate in the biogenesis and function of mitochondria.

The colonization of proto-mitochondria in evolution history, as bioreactors for all multicellular life

One surprising finding was the fact that primitive eukaryotes lacking mitochondria also provided evidence of genes coding for typical mitochondrial proteins. In some cases these "mitochondrial proteins" have been found in special cell organelles of these eukaryotes without mitochondria. These cell organelles were called hydrogenosomes, and produce ATP in the absence of molecular oxygen (and are thus anaerobic). In this process, hydrogen is formed as the reduced end product of the energy metabolism of the cell organelles. This finding posits that the hydrogenosomes and the mitochondria had a common evolutionary-biological source—one that had probably relinquished its genes to the genome of the host cell. The revolutionary conclusion drawn from these genetic analyses was that all eukaryotic cell systems, with or without mitochondria (amitochondrial protista and certain types of animal, plant and fungal cells have lost their mitochondria) owe their existence to a single event. This means that both the eukaryotic formation of the nuclei and the proto-mitochondrial formation took place at the same point in time. The "hydrogenosome hypothesis" explains this primary act of creation in the genealogy of all eukaryotes as a union of eubacteria (α-Proteobacteria) with archaea. The archaebacterium profited from the diffusion of hydrogen through the membrane of the α-Proteobacteria into the cytoplasm of the archaebacterium. They were able to utilize this hydrogen, produced as the end product of the energy metabolism of the eubacterium, as a reductive agent thus increasing their bioenergetic reduction ability. This energetic boost was used to simultaneously merge parts of the genome of the reproducing eubacteria with the genome of the archaea, to form a nucleus with its own membrane (overview Gray 1999). The packaging of genes from both bacterial species into one membrane-coated nucleus, enabled the functional division of transcription within the nucleus (the transcription of DNA information into mobile messenger RNA) and translation outside of the nucleus (translation of the RNA message) onto special structures of ribosomes, which assemble amino acids into proteins according to the coded instructions of the messenger RNA. The result was much improved protein and enzyme syntheses. These "fused" cells were able to increase in size and differentiate (see illustration: model of the fusion of an archaebacterium with proteobacteria for formation of the nucleus and for the development of proto-mitochondria (cell symbiosis) 1.5-2 billion years ago (Gray 1999) (see table IV)).

This interpretation facilitated the notion that the conversion of a part of the eubacterial hydrogen and gene-donating proteobacteria into mitochondria was performed in a second, nearly simultaneous developmental act. The fused cell structure's opportunity for improved energetic yield was due to the combustion of the end product of the enzymatic ATP synthesis of the archaeal host cell—the still energy-rich pyruvate—by further oxidation stages within the eubacterial symbionts, and to make the gained energy available to increase the ATP production for the entire cell. To achieve this aim, however, the hydrogen from the hydrogenosomes must no longer diffuse through the membrane into the cytoplasm during the ATP production phase in the eubacterial symbionts, but rather concentrate in the intermembrane space so that it can serve as the kindling source for ATP synthesis. In order to achieve this, the membrane potential of the symbionts had to be built in such a way that the diffusion of the hydrogen ions (protons) was no longer possible. An electron transport link had to be developed as energy consolidators for the hydrogen ion pumps which in controlled steps could harness the energy flows in these bioreactors which are now termed mitochondria (Gray 1999, Saraste 1999).

The gas-controlled import/export membranes of the mitochondrial colony are reminders of the early developmental period of cellular symbiosis

This model—the reversal of the original hydrogen donation processes of the symbionts for optimal energetic yield, by using a respiratory chain with molecular oxygen as the final electron recipient—explains certain phenomena of cell symbiosis much better than the previously held beliefs. Above all, changes and disruptions to the membrane potential of the mitochondria in physiological and pathophysiological conditions become more clearly understood. The workings of the mitochondrial membranes as import and export facilitators for the complicated relationship among the cell symbionts (as well as the cytoplasm, the nucleus, other cell organelles, the cytoskeleton and the cell membrane) still show characteristics of the most successful fusion in the early history of evolution. These processes are also gas-driven and can get out of control in situations of extreme stress, or as a result of certain deficiencies.

Unexplained for more than 70 years, the Warburg Phenomenon of aerobic glucose decomposition in cancer cells (fermentative ATP production in the cell plasma without the use of oxygen) also appears in T-helper immune cells after stimulation during mitosis

Energy metabolism during stimulation of these cell types is of interest in view of the performance of T-helper cells. It was demonstrated that during maturation and proliferation, T-cells exhibited behavioural patterns similar to tumor cells (Wang 1976, McKeehan 1982, Ardawi 1982, Brand 1986, Dröge 1987).

As early as 1924, Warburg described the phenomenon that carcinoma cells predominantly do not produce ATP in the mitochondria, but enzymatically from glucose metabolites in the cytoplasm in the presence of oxygen. The same "Warburg Phenomenon"—aerobic glycolysis with a strong simultaneous increase in the synthesis of the enzymes needed to produce sufficient ATP without the mitochondrial OXPHOS system and in the presence of O_2- was also observed in T-cells during the division phase (Tollefsbol 1985, Marjanovic 1988, 1993). Two crucial questions could not be plausibly answered:

1. How is the transition from predominantly oxidative to mainly glycolytic glucose decomposition switched to lactate and pyruvate in the cells that have not transformed into cancer cells in the division cycle?
2. How could the cells synthesize sufficient ATP in this division phase without an increased ATP production of the mitochondria? In other words, why do the dividing cells maintain a high rate of glycolytic enzyme synthesis, even though the energy yield is considerably smaller than ATP synthesis via the OXPHOS system?

During glycolytic ATP synthesis from the decomposed products of sugar in the cytoplasm, 1-2 ATP molecules are obtained using the energy of 1 molecule of glucose, whilst the oxidative ATP yield in the mitochondria from 1 glucose molecule is a total of 38 ATP molecules. The formidable difference in balance of energy yields exists, thanks to an archaic fusion of two prokaryotes during the evolutionary biological "big bang" of eukaryotes.

Experimental evidence for the physiological toggle-switch of the oxidative energy supply between cellular respiration in the mitochondria and the predominantly fermentative ATP synthesis inside the cell plasma (Warburg Phenomenon) in the presence of oxygen during the late phase of cell division

The German research team under Brand looked into these questions using the latest laboratory techniques. The researchers studied thymus cells of rats as a model for the changes in the energy metabolism of these cells during the transition from dormant state (quiescence) to division cycle (mitosis, or cell proliferation). A complete division cycle took between 72-84 hours, climaxing with the so-called S-phase(the late cell division phase) after 44-48 hours. This peak is determined by measuring the point of maximum incorporation of labelled thymidines (as the molecular building blocks) in synthesized DNA, the maximum DNA and protein content of the cells, the cellular volume, the number of newly formed cells, and by electron photomicroscopy.

The thymus cells were stimulated with the mitogen concanavalin (Con A). Con A is a glycoprotein of the jack bean and belongs to the phytohemagglutins (PHAs). PHAs are extracts from plants or plant seeds and are used, among other things, for the differentiation of subgroups of blood groups A and AB. Con A and PHA are deployed in laboratories as stimulators (mitogens) for the division of cultivated cells in test tubes. Immunologists in 1981, for example, tried to stimulate the anergic lymph cells, matured in the thymus, of AIDS patients with Con A and PHA. The same mitogens were used by Gallo and his colleagues in 1984 during the supposed isolation of hypothetical retroviruses from thymus-matured T-helper cells from AIDS patients in co-cultivation with leukaemia cells and in the production of the reputedly retroviral proteins as the basis for the "anti HIV antibody test."

The findings of Brand's research group and numerous others are important in understanding what really happens in mitogen- and antigen-stimulated cells, as molecules similar to Con A and PHA are also found in the cell membrane of bacteria and all eukaryotic cell membranes (e.g. polysaccharides, glycoproteins, glycolipids). In the case of the mitogen-stimulated thymus cells it transpired that glucose consumption through outright oxidation in the proliferating and in the dormant cells was roughly the same. The total consumption of glucose in proliferating cells, however, was 19 times higher than in the dormant cells. The considerable increase of glucose consumption seen in the proliferating cells is due to the extra-mitochondrial, anaerobic, cytoplasmic synthesis of ATP via glycolytic enzymes. The switch from primarily oxidative glucose reduction. to primarily enzymatic glucose reduction took place during the transition from the dormant to the proliferation state. The heightened energy requirement for the increased biosyntheses related to cell division is met exclusively by the aerobic glycolysis, without the involvement of mitochondria. The total consumption of oxygen, however, remains the same in both proliferating and dormant cells. Taking the balance as a whole, it follows that 86% of the total ATP production in proliferating cells was generated by glycolytic enzymes. In this process glucose is reduced to form pyruvate and lactate. 14% of the ATP production continued to be obtained from the mitochondria. In the dormant cells, the proportions are precisely reversed: 86% of the ATP of these non-stimulated dormant cells is obtained through the OXPHOS system in the mitochondria, and 14% through glycolytic glucose reduction in the cytoplasm.

In order to clarify the question of why eukaryotic thymus cells switch to aerobic glycolysis to obtain energy during cell division, the researchers investigated the formation of reactive oxygen species (ROS) in the proliferating and dormant thymus cells, and in other cells. The hydrogen peroxide formation of Con A-stimulated and non-stimulated cells was measured after 46 hours (S-phase). There was a clear-cut difference: practically no hydrogen peroxide (H_2O_2) was found in the mitogenically stimulated cells, whilst the non-stimulated cells produced a clear H_2O_2 reaction. In order to demonstrate that these findings were dependent on mitosis, the non-stimulated cells were, 46 hours after the beginning of cultivation, also stimulated with Con A. 48 to 72 hours after the start of mitogen stimulation, the previously non-stimulated cells also displayed no signs of H_2O_2 formation. Additionally, a similar experiment was carried out regarding the formation of superoxide radicals (O_2^-). O_2- and H_2O_2 are byproducts of molecular oxygen in the respiratory chain. Some 2% of the spent O_2 in the respiratory chain is channelled off for production of O_2^-, H_2O_2 and hydroxyl radicals (HO°).

Such ROS are formed when oxygen reacts with ferrous proteins, as for example in the mitochondrial respiratory complexes. If not intercepted at the proper time by antioxidative molecules, ROS can oxidatively damage cellular macromolecules (DNA, proteins) and lipids. Superoxide radicals are neutralized by the enzyme superoxide dismutase (SOD). SOD in the cytoplasm contains copper and zinc, whereas mitochondrial SOD contains manganese. No superoxide radicals were found in the analyzed proliferating thymocytes which consume SOD, however nor were they found in the non-stimulated cells which form H_2O_2.

The researchers came to the following conclusions: since pyruvate is an effective antioxidant, the ROS were quenched by the pyruvate formed by aerobic glycolysis; at the same time, by minimizing oxidative glucose reduction in the mitochondria (during the critical phase of increased biosynthesis and cell division), the DNA and proteins are protected from damage by radicals and the membrane lipids are protected from peroxidation (Brand 1997 a, 1997 b). The counterargument to this concept was that in T-cells, the expression of genes for the type 1 cytokine, interleukin-2, and its transcription factors, require ROS production for genetic activation; thus the target molecule for T-lymph cell activation needs oxidative signals (Los 1995). However, Brand's research group demonstrated that the redox status in the gene expression of quiescent and proliferating cells are different: oxidative signals are necessary in the early division phases, whilst reductive signals are needed in the later phases (Schäfer 1996). The researchers concluded that their data showed that the long-known, but until then unexplained, switching of ATP production during cell proliferation—from mitochondrial OXPHOS to a predominant aerobic glycolysis, enzymatically facilitated in the cytoplasm—is an ingeniously simple yet effective strategy to minimize the oxidative stress on proliferating cells (Brand 1997 a, 1997 b).

These research findings demonstrated that the redox-dependent alternating switch of energy production exists as a protective mechanism between the mitochondrial cell symbionts and the dividing host cell during the later stage of cell division. However, it is worth questioning whether this antioxidative protection similarly applies to the mitochondria themselves. If an extended energy requirement for increased biosyntheses during cell division has to be met primarily by escalation of mitochondrial ATP production, the unavoidable increase in ROS formation would damage the macromolecules of the mitochondria. Mitochondrial DNA is ten times more sensitive to oxidative stress than nuclear DNA. Mitochondrial DNA, unlike the DNA in the nucleus, is neither protected by histone proteins nor has any effective repair mechanisms (Tyler 1992, Yakes 1997). Dröge's research group at the Deutsches Krebsforschungszentrum (The German Cancer Research Center) had shown that in cultures of Con A-stimulated T-cells, the division readiness of these cells was facilitated by the antioxidative sulfur molecules (thiols), cysteine and glutathione, and the addition of H_2O_2 to the Con A-stimulated T-lymph cell cultures inhibited DNA synthesis (Dröge 1994). H_2O_2 formed in the mitochondria is neutralized mainly by the selenium-dependent enzyme, glutathione peroxidase, which receives the necessary hydrogen ions from reduced glutathione. Glutathione is oxidized in the radical quenching process, and must be reduced by the glutathione reductase enzyme, with the help of the hydrogen-donating co-enzyme NADPH. As, according to the findings of Brand et al., pyruvate assumes the role of principal antioxidant in the later division phase, it is worth asking whether the thiol pool is the decisive sensor for initiating the protective switch between the mitochondria and the host cell, in the earlier phases of cell division and redox-dependent DNA biosynthesis.

The switching between predominantly aerobic glycolysis and OXPHOS in fetal cells after birth

The alternating relationship between the mitochondria and the host cell, which raises many unanswered questions, has been intensively studied in the liver cells of developing embryos. With the exception of the later division phase, mature liver cells produce their metabolic energy through oxidation of substrates via the mitochondrial OXPHOS system. Remarkably, however, the embryonic liver cells, and probably all embryonic cells, obtain their ATP energy almost entirely from glycolysis in the cytoplasm. In such cells, the quantity and bioenergetic activity of the mitochondria are quite limited in comparison to the symbiont of mature cells. Correspondingly, the enzymes for the oxidation of pyruvate and fatty acids in the mitochondria are not very active, nor are the regulatory enzymes for the specialized metabolic activities of the liver. In contrast, the glycolytic enzymes in the cytoplasm are more active than in mature liver cells, and therefore more lactate is formed. The necessary amounts of glucose are delivered, without restriction, by the maternal circulation, and the produced lactates are re-processed into glucose by the mother's liver.

The astonishing thing, however, is the fact that within only an hour of birth, the infant's mitochondria become fully active, and glycolysis is to a large extent reduced. In a rapid process of transformation the mitochondria of the newborn change, not only in their structure and enzymatic activity, but also in that directly after birth the proton leak for diffusion of H^+ across the inner membrane is sealed. Adenine nucleotides accumulate which interact with special protein complexes in the inner membrane—the adenine nucleotide translocator. The mitochondrial membrane loses its uniform permeability and instead becomes a controlled export/import channel. Simultaneously, the messenger RNA transcripts (which have already been prefabricated in the fetal cells of the DNA in the nucleus and are "waiting in the wings", so to speak) are in a concerted action between the nuclear genome and the mitochondria, converted to the synthesis of the necessary proteins for the OXPHOS system. This program of rapid maturation into fully effective mitochondria, recapitulates in fast-forward motion the synergistic events that in the earliest of days made cell symbiosis possible. The H^+ leak is a clear evolutionary-biological remnant of the hydrogenosomes, as it was the sealing of the mitochondrial membrane which allowed for the build-up of the electron transport chain as a proton-driven power source for the hydrogen ion pumps, and the use of the sealed hydrogen ions as the driving force for ATP synthesis in the mitochondrial OXPHOS system.

The proliferation phase of the mitochondria occurs in parallel to the rapid differentiation program. This longer-lasting phase leads to an increase in mitochondrial population, and a functional homeostasis in relation to the development of the cell as a whole. In this final phase of maturation, the cooperation between the mitochondria and the whole cell is regulated on all levels of genetic expression: the promotion of genes by transcription factors, the transcription of coded DNA sequences into messenger RNA, and the translation of messenger RNA for protein synthesis (overview Cuezva 1997).

The temporary switching of oxidative ATP production in the mitochondria to enzyme-controlled ATP production from glucose in the cytoplasm, is the model for a flexible transition from OXPHOS to glycolysis. The extreme endpoint of this model is illustrated by tumor cells, which are predominantly focused on aerobic glycolysis and remain trapped in the division cycle.

Pathophysiological (re)fetalization

The converse model, of the switch from aerobic glycolysis to OXPHOS, is the fetal cell. The triggering of the OXPHOS machinery remains on hold until the first breath is taken, even though the messenger RNA for the proteins of the four complexes of the respiratory chain (and complex V for ATP synthesis) have already been transcribed in increasing amounts. Tumor cells, which can no longer manage to switch back to OXPHOS, also display this apparently paradoxical phenomenon. That is one reason, although there are others, why the term “re-fetalization” is used in regard to the formation of tumor cells (Cuezva 1997).

The other extreme model is the programmed cell death that can occur in cases of overregulation of OXPHOS activities, as a result of the exhaustion of the thiol pool following a state of extreme prooxidative stress (See illustration: Toggle-switch between OXPHOS and aerobic glycolysis, (Table V)).

The system of calcium exchange between the cytoplasm and the mitochondrial symbionts regulates a multitude of energetic and metabolic processes

The physiological and pathophysiological cell models demonstrate that cell symbiosis, between the mitochondrial cell symbionts and the cell as a whole, is bioenergetically regulated and counterregulated. Calcium balance plays an important role here. Intracellular calcium (Ca^{2+}) regulates numerous metabolic processes and energy flows. When T-helper immune cells are stimulated by the appropriate antigen presentation with co-stimulating signals, the calcium levels change. Simultaneously, the synthesis of cytokines and diffusible NO gas is triggered; therefore type 1 cytokines like the tumor necrosis factor (TNF-α), as well as NO° and its metabolites like peroxinitrite ($ONOO^-$), can exert an influence on Ca^{2+} levels and Ca^{2+} circulation. The mitochondria are an important balancing pool for the Ca^{2+} concentrations in the cytoplasm as they attach Ca^{2+} to proteins that are not membrane-bound. Within the mitochondria, Ca^{2+} regulates the nucleic acid synthesis for DNA assembly, protein synthesis, the indispensable enzymes for dehydrogenation—(dehydrogenases), and the enzymes for ATP synthesis(Ca^{2+}-ATPases). In order to protect the cytoplasm from toxic surges of Ca, the mitochondria can absorb large amounts of Ca^{2+} and later release it through various pathways. The releasing and re-absorption of Ca^{2+}, termed the "Ca^{2+} cycle," is crucially relevant to the fate of cells under both physiological and pathophysiological conditions.

In principal, Ca^{2+} can leave the mitochondria in three ways. Ca^{2+} is released non-specifically when the membrane potential (voltage) of the mitochondria drastically falls (for example through disruption to the respiratory chain), and Ca^{2+} leaks out of the inner membrane. Ca^{2+} is also released from the mitochondria by high membrane potentials, assisted by oxidizing co-enzymes like NAD^+. This occurs on the one hand in a sodium-dependent way, and on the other hand in a sodium-independent way. In the Ca^{2+} exchange, both reactive oxygen species (ROS) and NO and its derivatives can attack. The mitochondria are the richest production source of the physiological metabolites of oxygen (superoxide radicals, hydrogen peroxide, hydroxyl radicals, singlet oxygen), as 90% of oxygen consumption happens in the OXPHOS system. As long as ROS production can be neutralized by the thiol pool and other antioxidants, physiological Ca^{2+} cycling is not threatened. If, however, the ROS production is over-stimulated, perhaps by type 1 cytokines (TNF-α), certain pharmaceutical substances, or oxygen restriction through a sudden deficiency in blood supplies followed by recirculation(hypoxia-reperfusion e.g. cardiac infarction), then excessive Ca^{2+} cycling can be induced. The consequence is a mutual build-up of both Ca^{2+} and ROS. The mitochondrial membrane becomes energetically destabilized, the enzymatic activities of the respiratory chain diminished, and ATP production curbed. A deficiency in the counterregulation will initiate programmed cell death, as a drastic ATP decline leads to the bursting of the cell (overview Richter 1996).

The interactions between NO and calcium act to switch the cellular symbiosis between OXPHOS and aerobic glycolysis (Warburg Phenomenon)

The interactions between NO and Ca^{2+} regulation in mitochondria are complicated, as NO can adopt various redox states (NO radical: NO°, NO anion: NO^-, nitrosium: NO^+); NO° can bind with the ROS superoxide radical (O_2^-) to form peroxinitrite ($ONOO^-$), and NO can form covalent bonds with metalloproteins, thiols, and thiol-proteins with sulfhydryl groups (R-SH). Research findings indicate that a calcium-dependent enzyme for NO production is also located in the mitochondria. Ca^{2+} absorption in the mitochondria activates the enzyme for NO synthesis. In competition with O_2, NO binds with the respiratory chain enzyme, cytochrome oxidase, and thus inhibits the entire OXPHOS system. In actual fact, the NO concentrations that were measured in a series of biological systems, are similar to those that have been conclusively demonstrated to inhibit the cytochrome oxidase and choke the mitochondrial respiration. Conversely, in many cell systems the experimental inhibition of NO synthesis leads to stimulation of the respiratory chain. From these findings, some researchers have deduced that NO° exercises considerable physiological and pathophysiological effects on the inhibition of cytochrome oxidase in the mitochondrial respiratory chain (overview Richter 1996. Schweizer 1996, Lincoln 1997). NO° could also act as a switch in Ca^{2+} cycling for the toggling between the OXPHOS system and aerobic glycolysis.

The interaction of NO and calcium inside the mitochondria during programmed cell death (apoptosis) and sudden cell death (necrosis)

Then again NO° promotes Ca^{2+} release and re-absorption reducing the membrane potential of mitochondria by bonding with cytochrome oxidase. The consequence is a loss of energy, which occurs temporarily in low concentrations of NO, but is long-term with higher NO concentrations. In cell cultures, the collapse and re-constitution of the mitochondrial membrane potential relative to NO levels was accompanied by a corresponding rise and fall of cytoplasmic Ca^{2+}. From these findings, the researchers drew the following conclusion: "Apparently NO can kill cells by releasing Ca^{2+} from mitochondria and thereby flooding the cytosol with Ca^{2+}" (Richter 1996).

The consequence of the oxidative and nitrosative stress from an excess of NO can become aggravated when, for example, type 1 cytokine synthesis is stimulated by simultaneous high and long-term antigen and alloantigen loads. The type 1 cytokine, tumor necrosis factor, can lead to cell death by either apoptosis or necrosis—triggered by increased stimulation of ROS production and subsequent Ca^{2+} cycling. In both cases, the decline in mitochondrial enzymatic activities and ATP production precedes the consequences of prooxidative stress. Both forms of bioenergetic stress are termed prooxidative stress, but as nitrosative stress when NO and its derivatives bind to thiol or to thiol containing proteins. "On the basis of these and other findings, it was suggested that a pro-oxidant-induced Ca^{2+} release from mitochondria, followed by Ca^{2+} cycling and ATP depletion, is a common cause of apoptosis" (Richter 1996).

The double-edged sword of peroxynitrite in the control of cellular symbiosis

Under certain conditions, NO can paradoxically perform a protective function, counteracting programmed cell death or necrosis. This occurs when NO interacts with the superoxide radical to form peroxinitrite. However, this requires that equal amounts of NO and superoxide anions are produced simultaneously. Under such conditions, NO can prevent the toxic effects of the superoxide anion; which not only damages the cell membrane via iron-catalyzed lipid oxidation, but also damages the DNA. Conversely, an imbalance in the ratio of NO to superoxide anions causes an inhibition of peroxinitrite, consequently and reciprocally heightening the damaging consequences of prooxidative stress (Mies 1996). Peroxinitrite can redirect the initial phase of programmed cell death(triggered by the radicals NO and O_2^-), as long as enough reduced glutathione is available to compensate for the prooxidative/nitrosative stress (Brüne 1998).

In contrast to NO, peroxinitrite can stimulate, and even increase, the specific release of Ca^{2+} from mitochondria with an intact membrane potential. This happens when certain mitochondrial thiols, different than glutathione, are oxidized by peroxinitrite. This enables hydrolysis (splitting by water absorption) of the oxidized co-enzyme NAD^+. The products of the division of NAD^+—nicotinic acid amide and ADP ribose—regulate specific Ca^{2+} cycling in mitochondria with intact membrane potential (Schweizer 1996). Understanding this process is crucial because peroxinitrite is ineffective for Ca^{2+} cycling in mitochondria with intact membranes when co-enzyme remains reduced as NADH. The inhibition of NADH oxidation plays an important role at the onset of cancer.

Peroxinitrite is a double-edged molecule. When it is synthesized in the presence of free iron, it triggers the formation of ROS hydroxyl radicals (OH^-) which cause mutations in mitochondrial and nuclear DNA. This is the case when the antioxidative thiol pool becomes exhausted through high levels of NO and superoxide radicals. As DNA damage can also lead to programmed cell death or necrosis (Brüne 1996), extreme concentrations of gaseous peroxinitrite can do considerable damage to cells and tissue. Whether this happens depends on a multitude of counterregulations. One such counterregulation is the collective antioxidative capacity, which includes the thiol pool (glutathione, cysteine, and other thiols); antioxidative enzymes (SOD, catalase, glutathione peroxidase, glutathione reductase, transhydrogenase); the co-enzymes NADH, NADPH, FAD and FMN; vitamins C and E; and the polyphenols. When the fluctuating concentrations of the gaseous mixture of NO, O_2^-, peroxinitrite, and other ROS radicals increase in response to prooxidative/nitrosative stress, the redox milieu shifts to an oxidized state (proton deficit). If the antioxidative system can no longer mitigate this redox imbalance which poses a threat to the cell symbiosis, then the proton deficit leads to stimulation of transcription factors that activate the biosynthesis of special protective proteins. To this group belong, among others, the so-called heat shock proteins—ferritin, Bcl-2, and the enzymes hemoxygenase-1 and cyclooxygenase-2 (Kim 1995, Brüne 1998).

Counterregulation of the cellular symbiosis following stress from NO and oxygen radicals

The heat shock proteins primarily protect DNA from mutations, whereas ferritin binds iron and stores it in a non-redox form. This release of iron is important in preventing the formation of hydroxyl radicals (Miles 1996).

The inducible enzyme hemoxygenase-1 releases another type of gaseous monoxide: carbon monoxide (CO). The role of CO is still little researched, but there appear to be inverse interactions between NO and CO in various cell systems (Suematsu 1996, Rivier 1998).

Considerably more well-researched are the enzyme cyclooxygenase-2 and the protein Bcl-2, both of which play a crucial role in the toggle switch between the OXPHOS system of the mitochondria and aerobic glycolysis in the cytoplasm.

The enzyme cyclooxygenase converts arachidonic acid into the regulatory substances, prostaglandin and thromboxane (collectively termed "prostanoids").

Decisive in this context, are the prostaglandins (from the Greek: *prostatein* = protrude + *glandula* = gland). Though it was initially discovered in the male prostate gland, prostaglandin has a diversity of physiological and pathophysiological functions in all cell systems. Arachidonic acid is an unsaturated fatty acid, and is released by special phospholipid enzymes in the cell membrane. Under pathological stimulation, a heightened and long-term release of arachidonic acid is provoked by the enzyme phospholipase. Arachidonic acid is quickly converted, by the enzyme cyclooxygenase (COX) via intermediary products, into prostaglandin and thromboxane. There are two variations of the COX enzymes: COX-1 is widespread in a multitude of cell types and physiologically regulates the prostanoid levels; the second variation, COX-2, is induced by growth factors, cytokines and molecules that appear in inflammations. The decisive feature is that COX-2 synthesis is stimulated by the exact same factors as the inducible NOS enzyme (which synthesizes cytotoxic NO gas): microbial endotoxin lipopolysaccharide (LPS), type 1 cytokines, and platelet-activating factor (PAF).

High levels of prostaglandins are not only formed in acutely or chronically infected cells, but also in activated T-helper immune cells. All of these factors stimulate the activation of inducible NO synthase, but also interact with a series of receptors releasing a flood of communication signals, activating transcription factors and increasing the genetic expression for the biosynthesis of COX enzyme proteins (Goppelt-Struebe 1995, Appleton 1996, Herschman 1996, Minghetti 1998).

The connection between the common stimulation of the enzyme for cytotoxic NO production and the COX-2 enzyme for prostaglandins is key, as the prostaglandins are involved with the redisposition of T-helper cells from a type 1 (Th1 cells) to a type 2 (Th2 cells) cytokine profile (Betz 1991, Gold 1994, Hilkins 1995, Katamura 1995, Lucey 1996).

The activation of prostaglandin synthesis serves to protect the cellular symbiosis, and is evolutionarily conserved

In fact, the genes for the isoforms of NOS, at least for mammals and humans (Knowles 1994, Nathan 1994, Lincoln 1997), and the isoforms for COX-2 enzyme synthesis in various animals and humans (Fletcher 1992, Kosaka 1994, Bauer 1997, Minghetti 1998), are evolutionarily conserved and show a high degree of homology. Large increases in prostaglandin levels in activated T-helper immune cells suppress type 1 cytokine synthesis but not type 2 cytokine synthesis. A synergy takes place between the type 2 cytokines and high levels of prostaglandins, suppressing the synthesis of cytotoxic NO, as well as tumor necrosis factors which activate the superoxide anions (Milano 1995, overview Minghetti 1998). The depletion of the oxidative/nitrosative gases NO and O_2^- further inhibits peroxinitrite formation, thereby preventing the danger of programmed cell death or necrosis as a result of loss to the mitochondrial membrane potential. The upregulation of COX-2 enzymes and prostaglandins by acute and chronic pathological stimulation (microbial and non-microbial toxins, microbial and non-microbial antigens and alloantigens, immunotoxic pharmaceutical substances and drugs, etc.) serves to protect the cell symbiosis and is evolutionarily programmed.

Prostaglandins (PG E2) intervene in a further protective manner in the restriction of NO synthesis. PG E2 operates in the same way as a regulating factor related to type 2 cytokines (Abbas 1996): the transforming growth factor TGF-β (Vodovotz 1997, Minghetti 1998). TGF is a versatile cytokine that among other things increases the synthesis of prostaglandin and in conjunction with PG E2 suppresses large amounts of the cytotoxic NO production. PG E2 and TGF also activate in stimulated cells the genetic expression for the biosynthesis of the enzyme arginase. This converts arginine to ornithine in the first phase of the metabolic pathway of the synthesis of polyamines. The latter likewise inhibit the enzyme for the synthesis of cytotoxic NO (Szabó 1994). Since both NO synthase and arginase compete for the same amino acid, arginine, in the case of the simultaneous biosynthesis of both enzymes in stimulated cells, the amount of arginine available for NO synthesis diminishes (Modolell 1995). Additionally, there is the important fact that polyamines promote the proliferation and repair of various cell types; PG E2 and TGF-β thus lower the cytotoxic effects of NO, encourage the repair processes for damaged cells, and stimulate the formation of new cells. However, this also means an increase in aerobic glycolysis. It is striking that both cancer cells and parasitic cells show high concentrations of polyamines. This factor serves as a measure of success in chemotherapeutic treatment in oncology (Papadopulos-Eleopulos 1992b).

The Bcl-2 protein locks down the mitochondrial membranes and prevents the return from aerobic glycolysis (Warburg Phenomenon) to the OXPHOS phase of cellular symbiosis

Also impeding programmed cell death, is the simultaneous counterregulatory synthesis of Bcl-2 during excessive prooxidative stress (by NO and its derivatives, as well as ROS). Bcl-2 prevents disruption to the cellular Ca^{2+} equilibrium and thus inhibits ROS production. It is presumed that Bcl-2 shifts the ratio of oxidized NAD^+ to reduced NADH in favor of the latter. Thereby the release of Ca^{2+} from the endoplasmic reticulum (membrane structures in the cytoplasm) is inhibited. This release requires the hydrolysis of oxidized NAD^+ (Richter 1996). Bcl-2 is, furthermore, located in the membrane of the nucleus and in the outer mitochondrial membrane. It is here that Bcl-2 performs its crucial function: it is, so to say, the gatekeeper of the mitochondrial import/export lock-gates. Bcl-2 stabilizes the mitochondrial membrane potential, preventing energy loss, thereby modulating the flow of Ca^{2+} into and out of the mitochondria. The effect is controlled by interaction with protein complexes that keep the mitochondrial membrane permeable to Ca^{2+}ions and protein molecules. In the first phase of programmed cell death, which could ensue as a result of prooxidative stressors, the Bcl-2 proteins close the lock-gates thus preventing the "infection" of the host cell by the mitochondrial endosymbionts.

Bcl-2 belongs to a wide-ranging family of proteins that continue to be discovered. This assembly of proteins includes some that prevent programmed cell death (apoptosis, from the Greek: *apo* = from + *ptosis* = falling) as well as some that promote apoptosis. An imbalance in the genetic expression of these protein products has been established in roughly half of all human cancer forms (overview Zamzami 1997). Therefore it can be assumed that Bcl proteins also play an important role in the toggle switching of ATP production between the OXPHOS system of the mitochondria and aerobic glycolysis (Warburg Phenomenon), for the prevention or mitigation of NO and ROS stress in the closing mechanisms of the mitochondrial membrane. On one hand, this assumption is related to the transitory physiological barrier against the interaction between the cell symbionts and the maturing cells, during the embryonic development phase, during the S-phase of cell division, and in the transitional phases of heightened stress loads. On the other hand, under the substantial and long-term influence of pathological factors and their combinations, a hyperexpression of Bcl-2 proteins can be enforced which in synergy with other counterregulations blocks the switch from Warburg Phenomenon back to the mitochondrial OXPHOS system—at least for as long as it takes the redox milieu to re-establish self-organizing homeostasis. Dependent on cell type, the cells "re-fetalize" and, trapped in the cell division cycle, uncoordinatedly found a new cell colony as a tumor. Other cell types, which are no longer active in division, such as mature muscle and nerve cells, degenerate in specific ways to a state of cell dyssymbiosis (myopathy, encephalopathy, neurodegeneration) (Johns 1996, Wallace 1999).

The redox control of cell symbiosis, via interaction between NO and its metabolites and the sulfurous non-protein and protein thiols

Yet NO can also produce other important molecular bonds. Besides the binding with metalloenzymes (such as the ferrous enzyme guanylyl cyclase, which catalyzes the production of cyclic guanosine monophosphate, a secondary messenger which initiates growth processes and a multitude of biosyntheses), the redox status of many other enzymes can be altered by NO, thereby modulating the information profile in the cells. Such procedures control, for instance, the relaxation of blood vessels, the transfer or inhibition of impulses in the central and peripheral nervous system, intestinal peristalsis, and so on. For the understanding of cell-mediated immune deficiency and carcinogenesis, however, the tendency of NO in various redox states (NO°, NO^-, NO^+) to bond with sulfurous molecules is very important. These molecular bonds are termed S-nitrosothiols (RSNO), and when the RSNO bond is made with a thiol-containing protein, the term is S-nitrosylation. Many of the reactions associated with NO synthesis, of which NO alone is incapable, are stimulated by nitrosation or S-nitrosylation. Stimulation of T-cells, for instance, is triggered by S-nitrosylation of the protein molecule p21ras (Lander 1995). Also the efficiency of cytotoxic NO gases (and other NO derived molecular species) against microbes depends on the S-nitrosylation of microbial proteins (Stamler 1992, 1995, De Groote 1995). The nitrosothiols are produced in high concentrations in infectious and inflammatory conditions. Under normal physiological conditions, the S-nitrosylation of proteins serves as a reciprocal functional regulator in a variety of cellular control mechanisms, including: ion channels in both the cell and organelle membranes, signal-transmitting proteins (e.g. proteins that transfer or split phosphorus), various enzymatic proteins (e.g. controlling the glucose breakup for glycolysis and the OXPHOS system, for prostaglandin synthesis, and for the glutathione system), and many others (Han 1995, overview Stamler 1994, 1995).

Nitrosation and S-nitrosylation also intervene in the activation of transcription proteins that activate the transcription of certain genes to messenger RNA for the biosynthesis of enzyme proteins of the antioxidative counterregulation. Stamler's research group in the USA introduced the term "nitrosative stress" to describe the interaction of S-nitrosothiols (Hausladen 1996). Nitrosative stress, parallel to oxidative stress situations, depletes the intracellular thiol pool in the cytoplasm as well as in mitochondria and activates certain transcription factors. The redox-dependent expression for the biosynthesis of antioxidative and antinitrosative genes is increased via the altered redox-dependent transcription. This gene activity leads to an increased biosynthesis of thiols and enzymes which neutralize and metabolize the reactive O_2 species (ROS) and S-nitrosothiols (RSNO) (see illustration: Compensated/ decompensated oxidative and nitrosative cell stress (see table VI)).

But if the antinitrosative thiol capacity is exhausted, the S-nitrosothiols search for other thiol-containing target molecules. One such target is an important enzyme that ferries hydrogen ions from the co-enzyme NADH+H+ into the mitochondria. ADP ribosylation follows that irreversibly inhibits enzyme activities. The result is a disruption of the electron transfer in the respiratory chain of the mitochondria. At the same time, NO radicals can attack the iron-sulfur centers in the enzymes of the respiratory chain (oxidoreductase, cytochrome oxidase), enzymes of the carbon metabolic pathway from the breakup of glucose (cis-aconitase), enzymes from DNA synthesis (ribonucleotidase), and others. ATP production in the OXPHOS system begins to wane and the mitochondrial membrane is energetically destabilized (Brüne 1994, Richter 1996). Ca^{2+} cycling between the mitochondria and the cytoplasm gets out of control. If the loss of energy happens rapidly, then the cell dies through necrosis. Intracellular protein, DNA, and other molecules pass into the extracellular space and increasing numbers of autoantibodies are formed. If the energy loss is at a slower pace, so that there is still enough ATP for an energy-dependent dismantling of the nucleus and the remaining cell contents via programmed cell death when the cell membrane is still intact, then apoptosis takes place; without alloantigenic stimulation, no autoantibodies will form. If the cell switches on the "emergency power unit" (glycolytic ATP production in the cytoplasm) in time, and reacts to this state of cell dyssymbiosis with a coordinated counterregulation (the type 2 cytokine profile shuts down cytotoxic NO synthesis, dampening the calcium-dependent NO synthesis, upregulation of heat shock proteins, ferritin proteins, COX-2 enzymes, prostaglandin, Bcl protein family, etc.) then the cell symbiosis can be restored and the cell will survive. If the thiol pool and antioxidative/antinitrosative capacity remains depleted over the long-term (or intermittently, given that the causes continue to afflict, become more serious, or cannot be neutralized), then the cells—could simultaneously or successively suffer from cell dyssymbiosis, the outcome of which varies depending on cell, tissue and organ type.

The cytoplasm can accomplish its functions only in a highly reductive state. Under extensive oxidative and nitrosative stress, whether acute or chronic, the endosymbiotic eukaryote cells have a strategic dilemma: the cells must either seal the import/export lock-gates of the mitochondrial membrane (to calcium, proteins and other molecules), or keep them open. In the latter case, the cells are sacrificed to necrosis—or if it is still possible, to apoptosis. In the case of lock-down, the cells remain in the counterregulated state of cellular dyssymbiosis, at the expense of the number and vitality of the mitochondria. Cells that are no longer able to divide will degenerate, and those that are still capable of division may transform to cancer cells.

Programmed cell death is an evolutionarily conserved program that has already been proven in unicellular eukaryotes such as the trypanosomes. This is a sign that apoptosis is triggered by cell symbionts in these archaic eukaryotes, as well as in multicellular animals, and probably in fungi as well (Kroemer 1997).

The proliferation of tumor cells, within which the mitochondrial population is extremely reduced and inactive, apoptosis by NO and its derivatives cannot be easily induced experimentally but merely a cell inhibition (cytostasis) is attained; this fact supports the assumption that programmed cell death is dependent on the destabilization of the mitochondrial membrane (Hibbs 1987, Nussler 1993, MacMicking 1995, Wei 1995, Lincoln 1997).

Apoptosis is an important component of immune defense against intracellular agents, including viruses, as the dispersal of microbes within cells and to a certain extent in extracellular areas can be prevented by sacrificing the affected cells. A well placed fully-dosed gas cloud from NO and oxygen radicals of the Th1 immune cells, macrophages, microglia cells, natural killer cells, neutrophilic leukocytes, and many other immune and non-immune cells, is for all multicellular organisms, including humans, the most effective weapon of choice. The most primal of cell types of the nonspecific gas defense—the macrophages—are classified as the most evolutionarily ancient cells of natural immunity and stress defense. They synthesize a common pool of peptides (derived from proopiomelanocortin, which is also synthesized in brain cells), cytokines, biogenic amines (dopamine, adrenaline, noradrenalin [USA: epinephrine, norepinephrine]), glucocorticoids, as well as NO and its derivatives, and reactive oxygen species. Macrophages are deemed to be the evolutionary progenitors of both the immune network and the neuroendocrine systems (Ottaviani 1998). Like T-cells, macrophages can trigger apoptosis or necrosis by producing oxidative and nitrosative stress in microbial or bodily cells, but can for the same reasons also die by apoptosis or necrosis.

The immune cell network is a redox-sensitive early warning system for the cellular symbiosis

It is, however a gross oversimplification of the given physiological facts to attribute the immune cell network solely to the defense against foreign protein. Rather, the immune cell network is comprised of particularly redox-sensitive cells, whose diverse function it is to ensure a balance in the energy flows. If this can no longer be maintained on a cellular or intracellular level (i.e. too many immune cells and non-immune cells become apoptotic or necrotic), then in compliance with the rules of cell protection, the immune cells switch from intracellular home defense of the bioenergetic balance (based on redox equilibrium) to an extracellular shield; this is done mainly by increasing antibody production as an emergency measure. The active strategy is determined by the health of the cell symbiosis. *The immune cell network is thus an early warning system for the organism as a whole.* The immune cells are feelers and executors, sensors and effectors, that continuously measure and modulate the redox milieu as control variables for the continual perfusion of energy and substance flows.

The regulators of this process, however, are the gas-driven cell symbionts. An intensive exchange takes place between the immune cell network and the neuroendocrine system, as both cell systems synthesize, to all intents and purposes, the same signaling molecules (neurotransmitters)—biogenic amines, cytokines, NO, CO, prostaglandin hormones, etc. (Ader 1980, Spector 1985, 1988, Rivier 1998, McCann 1998a, 1998b). In this respect, the immune cells process all stress factors found in the blood or lymph pathways, in the extracellular liquids, or those mediated by cell-to-cell contact. *It makes no difference to the cell symbionts of the helper lymph cells whether, for instance, the disruption is caused by microbial antigens or alloantigens, psychic traumata and pain, protein deficiency syndrome or antioxidant impairment as a result of faulty nutrition, nitrites and nitrosamines, bacterial toxins or pharmatoxic substances, serious injuries or burns, operations or organ transplants, radiation damage or environment toxins, drug abuse or doping agents, contaminated coagulating proteins or multi-transfusions, vaccines or antibiotics, congenital or acquired factors.* The T-helper immune cells and other cell systems will always react, modulate, and adapt, following the same evolutionary biological laws.

The gas-controlled micro-Gaian environment of the cellular symbiosis allows room for the thermodynamic range of oscillation between solid and fluid phases

Cellular life happens from the outset almost four billion years ago, quantum dynamically speaking, in the marginal phase between solids (macromolecules) and fluids (liquids and gases), between order and chaos (Langton 1990). Macromolecules (proteins, nucleic acids) alone are not living materials. They require quantum dynamic oscillation by fluid molecules. An over-rigorous order is just as hostile as overstepping the boundaries to chaos. A fortnight before death, the heartbeat is completely regular. On the other hand, gaseous molecules have the highest degree of freedom for quantum dynamic fluctuations, and can quickly construct, alter, and destroy information patterns and energy flows. However, they must be constantly counterregulated in order to maintain the bio-energetic self-organization of the cellular "island of order in the middle of thermodynamic chaos" (Schrödinger 1967). In accord with the standard model of the development of life, the first storage of photonic energy from sunlight took place in the "thioester-iron world" (De Duve 1991). When the first macromolecules which could store information organized energy flows and metabolism in a membrane, away from thermodynamic equilibrium, the sulfur-iron centers in the substrates were already existent as were NO and its derivatives as terminal electron receivers instead of molecular oxygen. Anaerobic prokaryotes to this day use nitrite and NO for respiration and cell growth (Kucera 1983, Satoh 1983, Barton 1983, Papadopulos-Eleopulos 1988). So life began with nitrosative stress and still overcomes it with the help of reduced sulfur and selenium. Both elements, together with oxygen, belong in the same column of the periodic table and can exchange electrons with one another (Hässig 1999, Kremer 1999).

The global gas exchange of the prokaryotes in the autopoietic biosphere of the Gaian world (Lovelock 1974) was to become the driving force for the evolutionary quantum leap of cell symbioses (Margulis 1997). The micro-Gaian environment (endosymbiotic, gas-controlled hybrid cells) enabled a deeper thermodynamic oscillation to occur in the marginal zone between the solid and fluid matter phases, which allowed the evolution of the ever-increasing complexity of the human mind, intellect, and spirituality.

The list of the systemic and chronic diseases caused by functional and structural disturbances of the mitochondria grows even longer

It has taken modern medicine 150 years to understand the meaning and function of the laws of the most successful fusion in the history of evolution. The mitochondrial genome holds only 37 informational and operative genes all of which are indispensable. In all sexually-reproducing eukaryotes, humans included, the cell symbionts are exclusively passed down by maternal inheritance (Wallace 1999). There are huge amounts of mitochondria found in the ovarian cells. Within the last 30 years, an ever-increasing number of systemic diseases, serious myopathies and encephalopathies, Alzheimer's-like and Parkinson's-like diseases, diabetes and cardiac defects, multiple sclerosis and cancer as well as geriatric diseases have been recognized as resulting from maternally inherited mutations of the mitochondrial DNA, or as a result of oxidative/nitrosative stress of the OXPHOS system and an inability to repair the mitochondrial genome. The list is growing and already includes 200 defined diseases. It is remarkable that such mitochondrial diseases are not known in mammals living in the wild, and can only be found after being provoked by experimental tests in clinical studies (Wallace 1999). The clinical picture becomes complex and puzzling in congenital mitochondrial diseases through mutation of individual genes (genotypes) which cause a plethora of different disease symptoms (phenotype) and vice versa several mutations (genotype) causing a single symptom (phenotype). This phenomenon is deemed to be puzzling, despite the manageably small number of remaining genomes, as the interplay between the two genomes—the nuclear genome with roughly 25,000 genes and more than 3 billion base pairs and the mitochondrial genome with 37 genes and more than 16,000 base pairs, make the multitude of combination possibilities of both genomes difficult to determine.

These complicated interactions make a "gene therapy" on the mitochondrial genome of maternal ovarian cells at present utopian, although such "repairs" may become possible in the future (Johns 1996). Then again, acquired non-inherited mutations in Alzheimer's-like and Parkinson's-like diseases, primarily caused by oxidative free radicals, glutamates and NO, has been discussed (Johns 1969).

Somatic, non-inherited mutations have been identified in various tumors and tumor cell lines: "In principle, these mutations could contribute to neoplastic transformation by changing cellular energy capacities, increasing mitochondrial oxidative stress, and/or modulating apoptosis" (Wallace 1999).

AIDS and cancer are not puzzling phenomena, but overdriven counterregulations of the micro-Gaian milieu

To modern humans, the evolutionary-biologically programmed protection of cellular symbioses becomes a disadvantage, in that the immune and non-immune cells answer to every form of prooxidative (oxidative and/or nitrosative) stress with counterregulations, and have the potential for overreaction in today's toxic industrialized world. To counter the enormous quantity and diversity of synthetic and physically generated oxidative and/or nitrosative sources of stress, evolution could predispose no other strategy for achieving its aims than the capacity for social intelligence. The opportunity to exercise this, however, is left to the free will of individuals. Even the simplest bacteria have intelligence, in the spiritual sense of perception to environmental dangers and autopoietic adaptive response (Maturana 1987). As a rule, microbes are outgunned by the higher reduction powers of cellular symbioses in the human organism, as long as the micro-Gaian milieu is functional. The genetic make-up of human mitochondria has been under threat since the introduction of sulfonamide chemotherapy in 1935, and the ensuing prevalence of antibiotic therapy; as these pharmaceutical substances not only attack intracellular microbes, but also the cell symbionts in human cells. As the mitochondria are former bacteria, they are just as vulnerable to targeted attacks as actual bacteria.

To this day, nobody knows whether ever-increasing inherited mitochondrial DNA mutations and the associated degenerative and tumorous diseases (Johns 1996, Wallace1999) are caused by such pharmatoxic damage to the genetic make-up of human cell symbionts. For obvious reasons, up to now these problems have not been well investigated, although it has to be assumed that antimicrobial substances which can penetrate the cell membrane, also damage the cell symbionts. This has already been demonstrated with chloramphenicol, tetracycline and some macrolides like erythromycin and carbomycin: "The treatment of animals or man with antibacterial drugs can have harmful effects on mitochondrial function, especially in tissues that have a high proliferation rate" (Tyler 1992). As health diseases, ageing, and death of humans are dependent on the vitality of the micro-Gaian milieu, more precedence should be given to the study of *acquired energy dyssymbiosis syndrome* (AEDS) (Kremer 1998 b) for understanding AIDS and specific cancer diseases, than to the "*Invent[ed] . . . AIDS virus*" (Duesberg 1996).

The precious legacy of the human symbionts should have long ago been declared a protected species. In all primitive societies, cancer was practically unknown (with a few exceptions like Kaposi's sarcoma) before they came into contact with civilization (Goldsmith 1998). Recently, the WHO prognosticated that in 50 years, every second person will die of cancer; 100 years ago the figure was one in ten. In no way does this affect only the elderly, as cancer in children is increasing annually by 1% (Epstein 1998, White 1998). The growth of systemic human illnesses still reflects the strategic dilemma of the cell-symbiotic fusion of an archaeum and a protobacterium, some two billion years ago. Chronic systemic diseases are the answer in an energetic/spiritual sense to the cumulative burden of excessive stressors in an extremely different inner and outer environment which has not been previously experienced in the course of evolution (Kremer 1997 a).

The evolutionary-biologically programmed limits on how far the human cell symbioses can be stretched from equilibrium, within the border zones between solid and fluid matter phases (Langdon 1990) has, however, remained unchanged. 50 years ago, a doctor's practice would treat nine out of ten patients for acute complaints; today, nine out of ten patients need treatment for chronic illnesses. Taken as a whole, the spectrum of diseases reflects a clear shift towards cell dyssymbiosis. *AIDS and cancer are in no way puzzling phenomena, but simply overcompensated Type-II counterregulations of the micro-Gaian milieu* (see illustration: cell symbiosis and cell dyssymbiosis in dependence on NO and ROS production (plate VII) and illustration: Clinical examples of cell dyssymbioses resulting from Type-I overregulation or Type-II counterregulation (table VIII)).

Fig. 24) The development of organisms up to human beings. The O2 atmosphere after the appearance of the first nucleic eukaryote organisms.

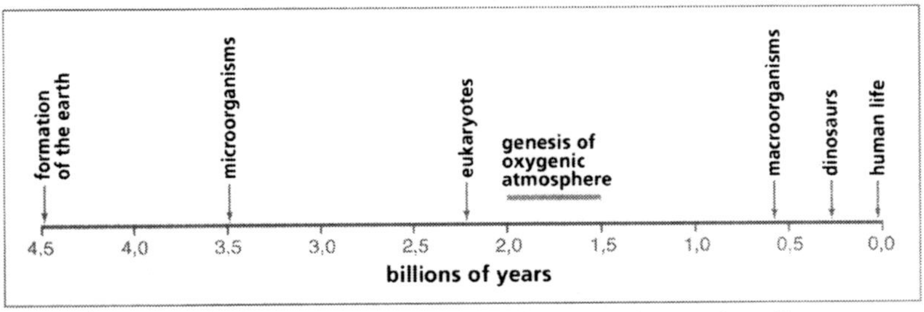
formation of the earth
microorganisms
eukaryotes
genesis of oxygenic atmosphere
macroorganisms
dinosaurs
human life
4,5
4,0
3,5
3,0
2,5
2,0
1,5
1,0
0,5
0,0
billions of years

Fig. 25) Diagram of the three domains of life. All eukaryotic cells, including human ones, derive from the symbiosis between proteobacteria and archaea that produce methane.

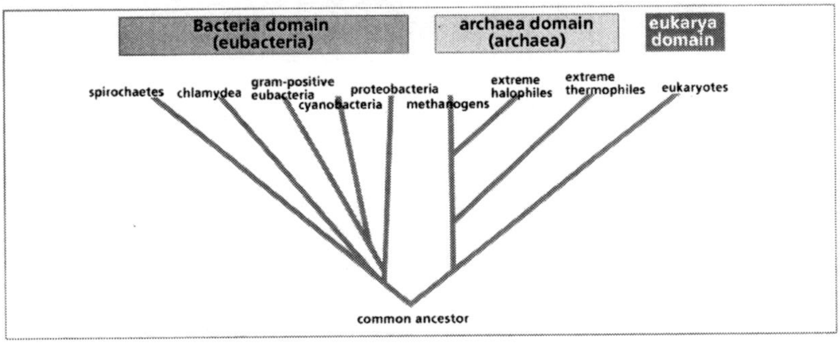
Bacteria domain (eubacteria)
archaea domain (archaea)
eukarya domain
spirochaetes
chlamydea
gram-positive eubacteria
cyanobacteria
proteobacteria
methanogens
extreme halophiles
extreme thermophiles
eukaryotes
common ancestor

Fig. 26) Diagram of present classification of life's kingdoms or domains. The section of the genome of archaeal origin predominates, tumor cells acquire the characteristics of the protists.

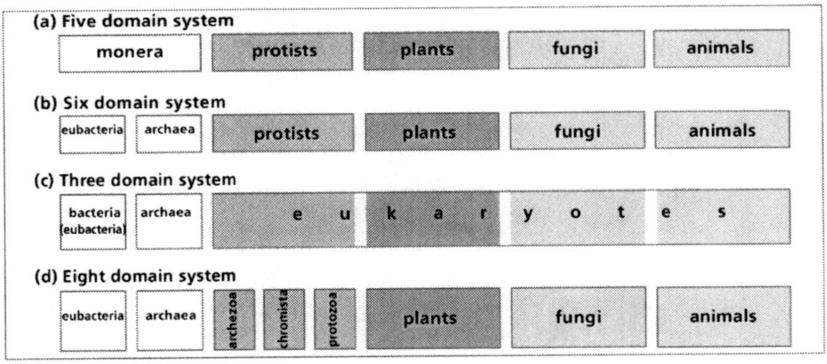
(a) Five domain system
monera
protists
plants
fungi
animals
(b) Six domain system
eubacteria
archaea
protists
plants
fungi
animals
(c) Three domain system
bacteria (eubacteria)
archaea
e u k a r y o t e s
(d) Eight domain system
eubacteria
archaea
archezoa
chromista
protozoa
plants
fungi
animals

Fig. 27) Diagram of the anaerobic synthesis of ATP in eukaryotes up to the predominant aerobic synthesis of ATP in humans. Tumor cells mainly revert to anaerobic synthesis of ATP.

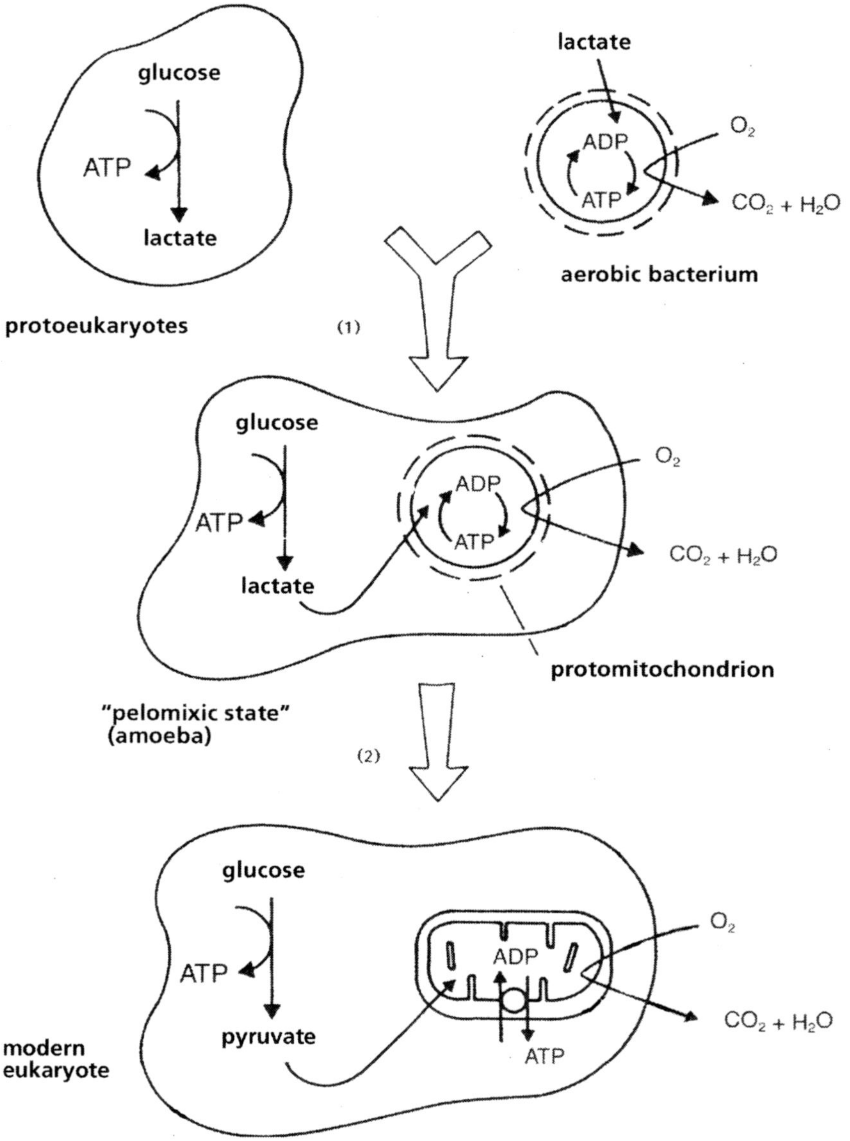

glucose
ATP
lactate
protoeukaryotes
lactate
ADP
ATP
O_2
$CO_2 + H_2O$
aerobic bacterium
(1)
glucose
ATP
lactate
ADP
ATP
O_2
$CO_2 + H_2O$
protomitochondrion
"pelomixic state"
(amoeba)
(2)
glucose
ATP
pyruvate
modern
eukaryote
ADP
ATP
O_2
$CO_2 + H_2O$

Fig. 28) Diagram of the main features of mitochondrial ultrastructure.

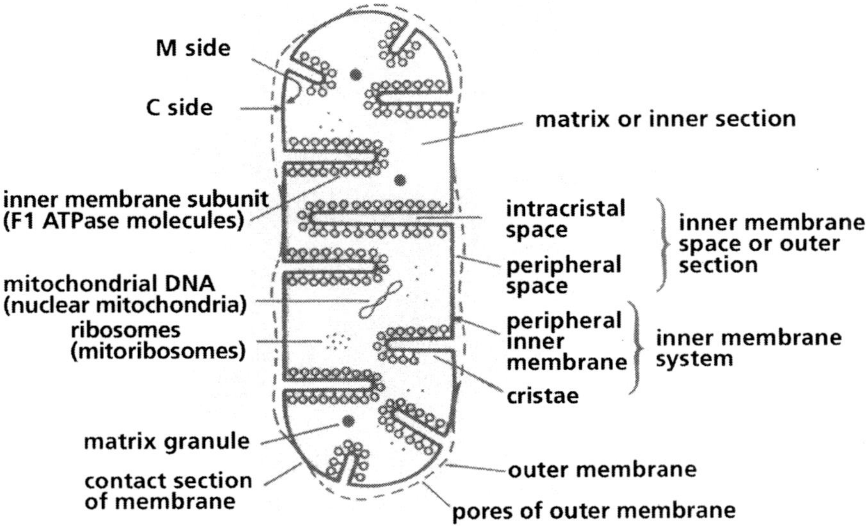
M side
C side
matrix or inner section
inner membrane subunit
(F1 ATPase molecules)
intracristal
space
peripheral
space
inner membrane
space or outer
section
mitochondrial DNA
(nuclear mitochondria)
ribosomes
(mitoribosomes)
peripheral
inner
membrane
cristae
inner membrane
system
matrix granule
contact section
of membrane
outer membrane
pores of outer membrane

Fig. 29) Electron microscopic photo of a mitochondrion. The inner membrane is always folded and includes several thousand respiratory chains in every mitochondrion.

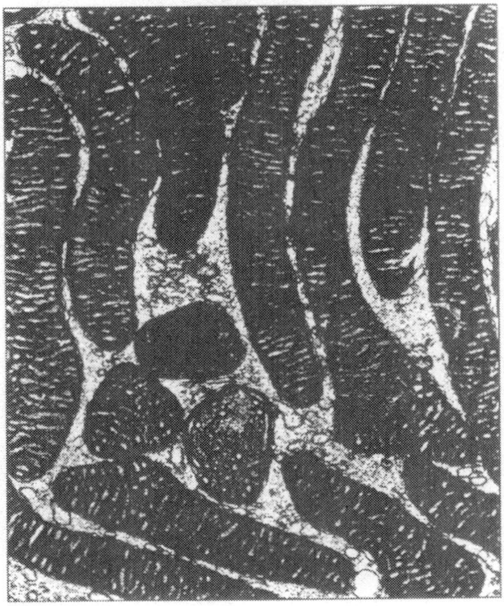

Fig. 30) Enlargement of Fig. 29.

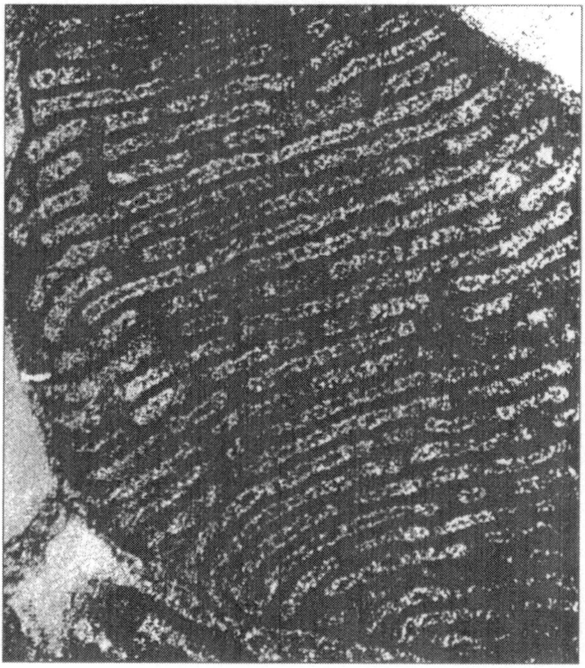

Fig. 31) Diagram of the inner and outer mitochondrial membranes. The mitochondrial locks (b) are often referenced in the book.

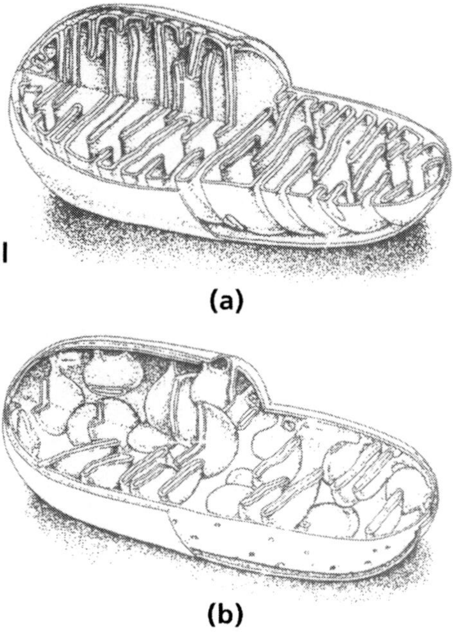

(a)

(b)

Fig. 32) Diagram of a typical animal/human cell and a vegetable cell. Each cell contains about 1,500 mitochondria.

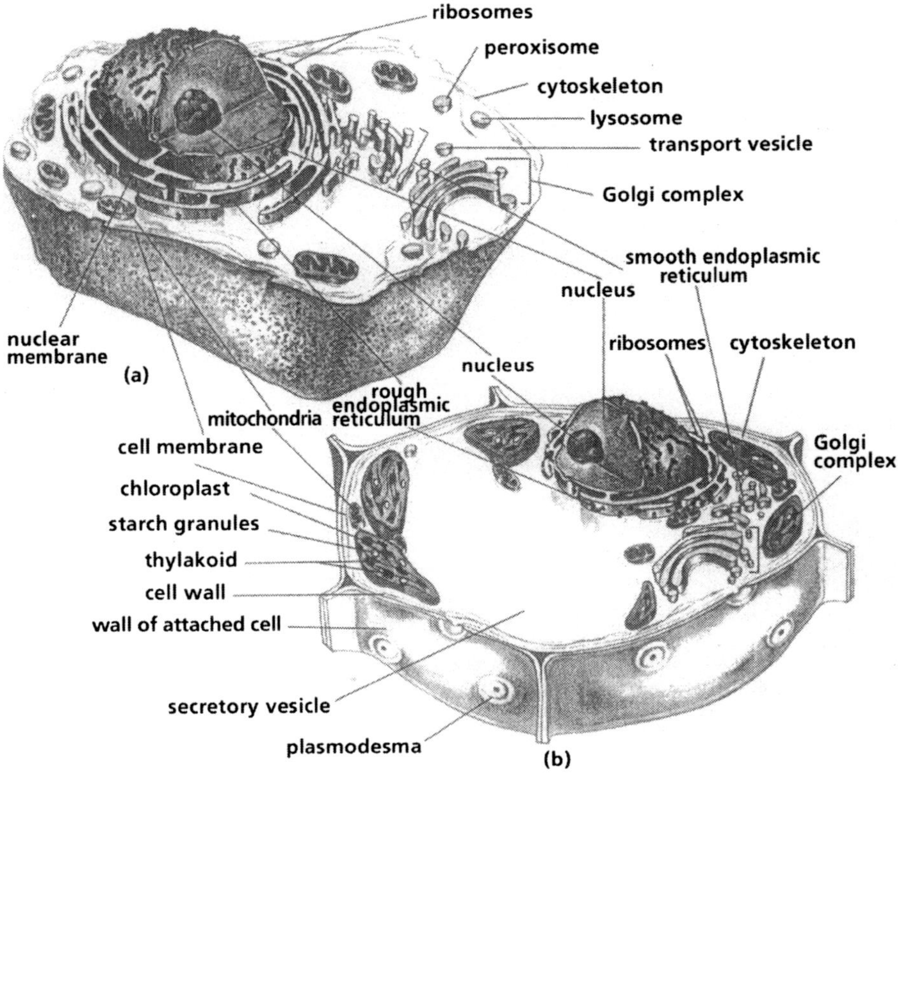
ribosomes
peroxisome
cytoskeleton
lysosome
transport vesicle
Golgi complex
smooth endoplasmic reticulum
nucleus
nuclear membrane
(a)
ribosomes
cytoskeleton
nucleus
rough endoplasmic reticulum
mitochondria
Golgi complex
cell membrane
chloroplast
starch granules
thylakoid
cell wall
wall of attached cell
secretory vesicle
plasmodesma
(b)

Fig. 33) Human mitochondrial genomes. The synthesis of the enzymatic complexes of the mitochondrial respiratory chain requires interaction between nuclear and mitochondrial DNA. This correlation is disturbed in tumor cells.

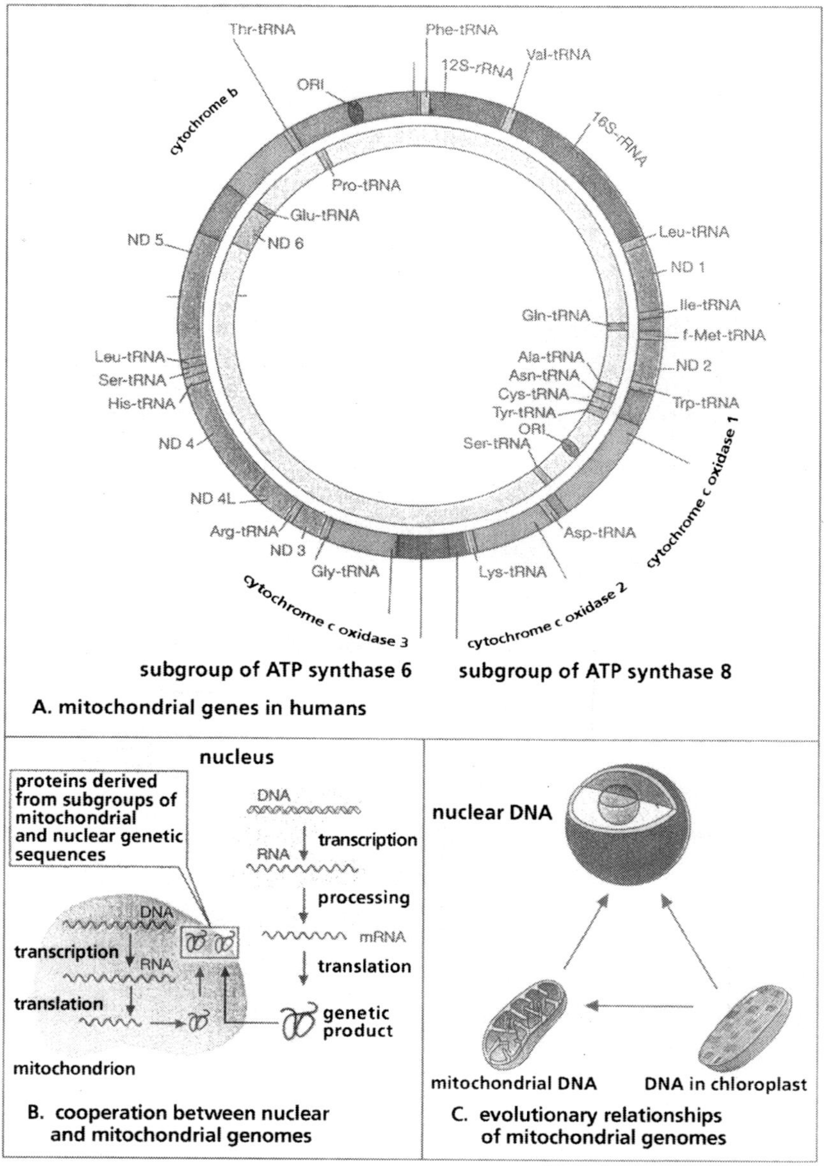

Thr-tRNA
Phe-tRNA
12S-rRNA
Val-tRNA
ORI
cytochrome b
16S-rRNA
Pro-tRNA
Glu-tRNA
ND 5
ND 6
Leu-tRNA
ND 1
Ile-tRNA
Gln-tRNA
f-Met-tRNA
Leu-tRNA
Ser-tRNA
His-tRNA
Ala-tRNA
Asn-tRNA
ND 2
Cys-tRNA
Trp-tRNA
Tyr-tRNA
ORI
Ser-tRNA
ND 4
cytochrome c oxidase 1
ND 4L
Arg-tRNA
Asp-tRNA
ND 3
Gly-tRNA
Lys-tRNA
cytochrome c oxidase 3
cytochrome c oxidase 2
subgroup of ATP synthase 6
subgroup of ATP synthase 8
A. mitochondrial genes in humans
nucleus
proteins derived from subgroups of mitochondrial and nuclear genetic sequences
DNA
transcription
RNA
processing
mRNA
translation
genetic product
DNA
transcription
RNA
translation
mitochondrion
B. cooperation between nuclear and mitochondrial genomes
nuclear DNA
mitochondrial DNA
DNA in chloroplast
C. evolutionary relationships of mitochondrial genomes

Fig. 34) Diagram of a cell and an electron microscopic photo. Mitochondria cooperate with all organelles and all structures of cells with the exception of the nucleus.

A. Diagram of an epithelial cell

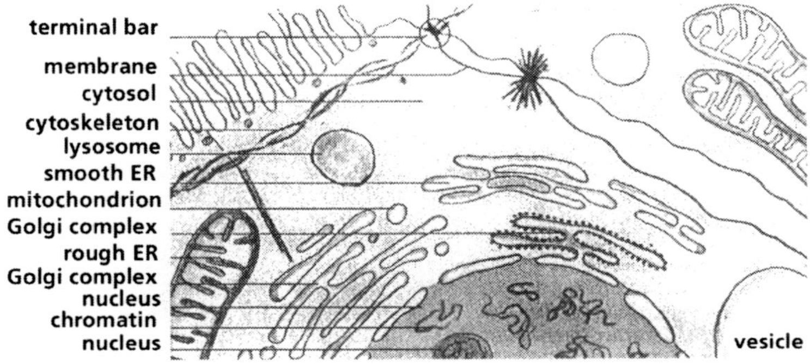
terminal bar
membrane
cytosol
cytoskeleton
lysosome
smooth ER
mitochondrion
Golgi complex
rough ER
Golgi complex
nucleus
chromatin
nucleus
vesicle

B. Structure of epithelial cell under electron microscope.

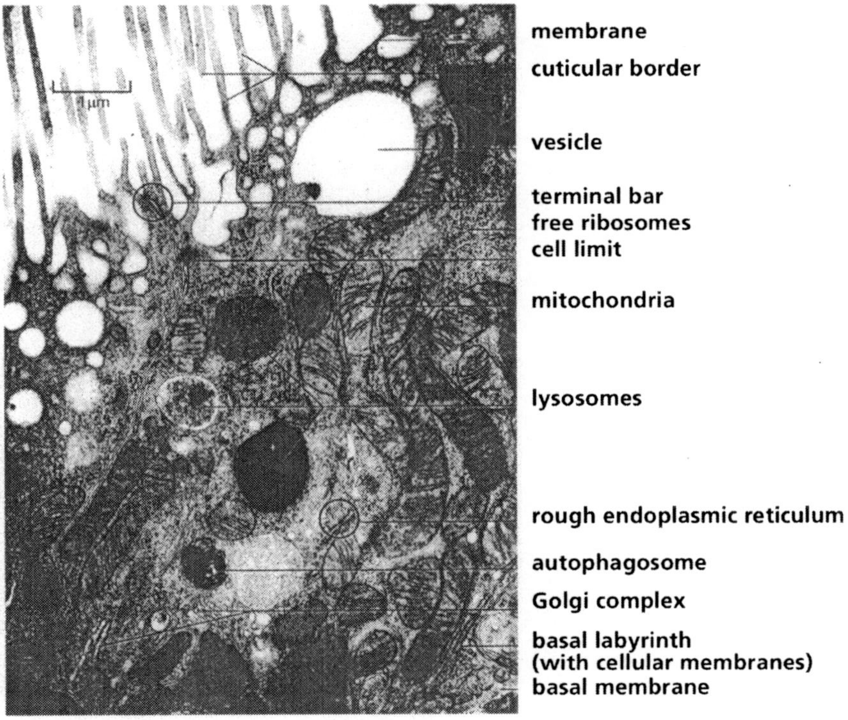
1 μm
membrane
cuticular border
vesicle
terminal bar
free ribosomes
cell limit
mitochondria
lysosomes
rough endoplasmic reticulum
autophagosome
Golgi complex
basal labyrinth
(with cellular membranes)
basal membrane

Fig. 35) Catabolism of food (proteins, fatty acids and carbohydrates) in the cytoplasm (top) and in mitochondrion (bottom) during the three stages of cellular respiration.

Phase 1: Oxidation of fatty acids, glucose and some amino acids produces acetyl CoA.

Phase 2: Oxidation of acetyl groups in the citric cycle includes four stages of electron splitting.

Phase 3: The electrons transmitted by NADH and FADH2 feed a chain of mitochondrial vectors of electrons (in bacteria they bond to the cellular membrane) / the respiratory chain reduces O_2 to H_2O. This electron flow feeds ATP production.

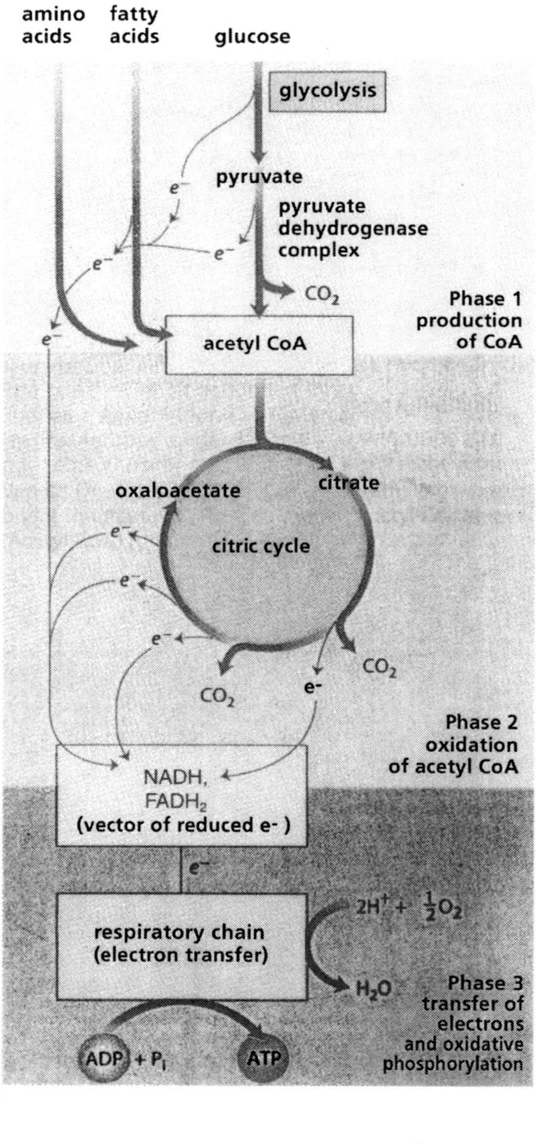
amino acids
fatty acids
glucose
glycolysis
pyruvate
pyruvate dehydrogenase complex
CO2
acetyl CoA
Phase 1 production of CoA
oxaloacetate
citrate
citric cycle
CO2
CO2
e-
Phase 2 oxidation of acetyl CoA
NADH, FADH2 (vector of reduced e-)
respiratory chain (electron transfer)
2H+ + ½O2
H2O
Phase 3 transfer of electrons and oxidative phosphorylation
ADP + Pi
ATP

Fig. 36) The visually similar structures of adenosine triphosphate (ATP) and the main molecules for the transfer of electrons and hydrogen ions (NADH, FAD and coenzyme A). The adenine group is shaded light grey, the ribose group black and the diphosphate group white.

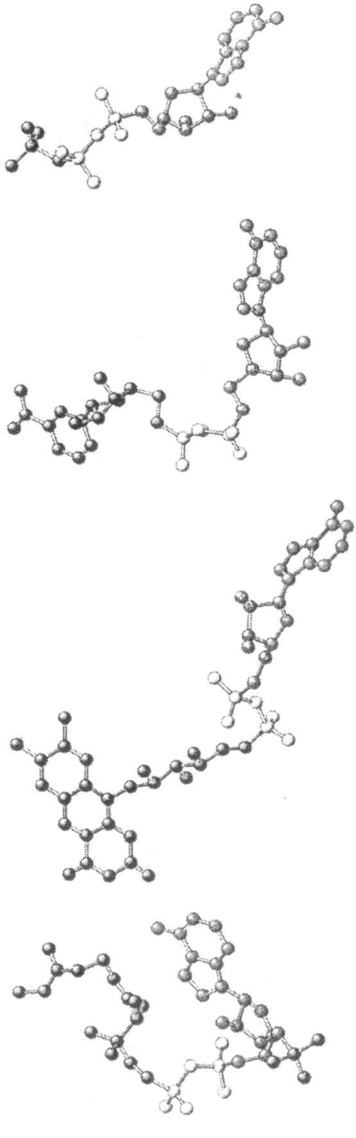
ATP
NADH
FAD
coenzyme

Fig. 37) The catabolism of glucose and the transfer of glucose hydrogen ions to NADH and enzymatic ATPase. In tumor cells the ATP, instead of being synthesized in the mitochondria, is synthesized enzymatically and hydrogen is transferred to lactate (strongly acidic in tissues).

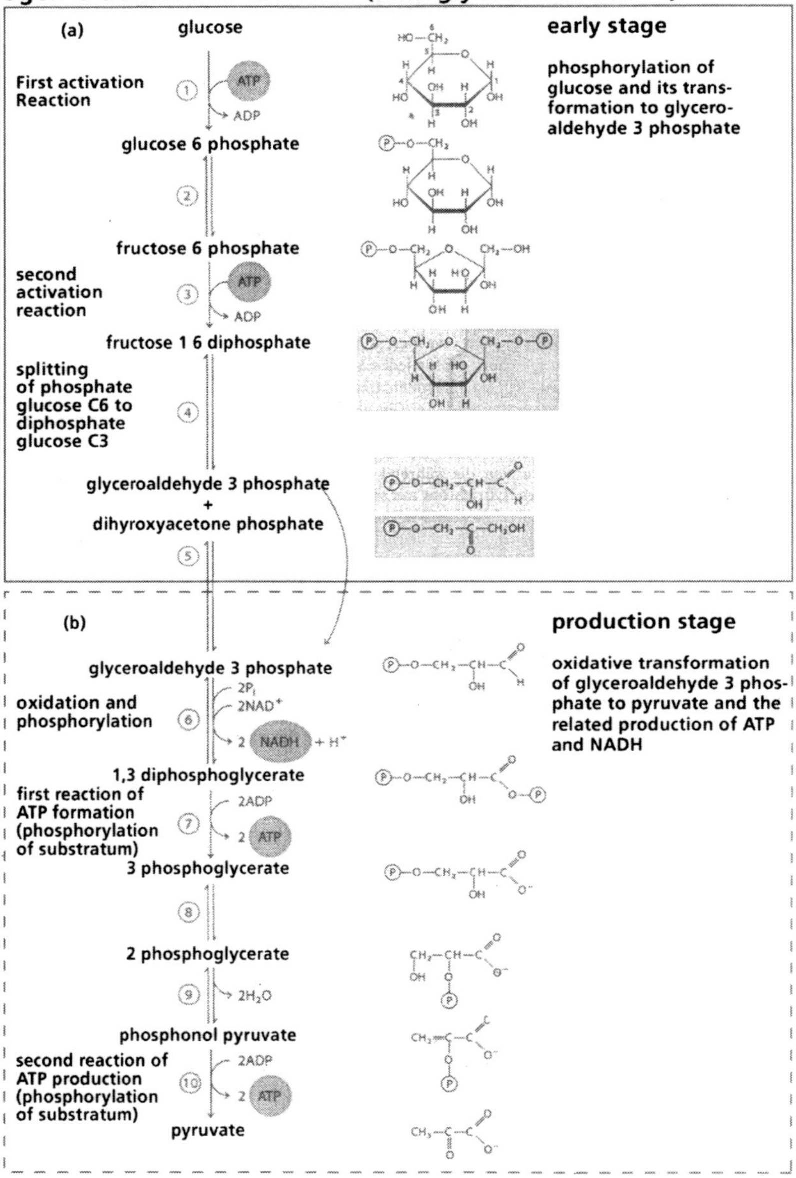
(a)
glucose
early stage
First activation Reaction
ATP
ADP
phosphorylation of glucose and its transformation to glyceroaldehyde 3 phosphate
glucose 6 phosphate
fructose 6 phosphate
second activation reaction
ATP
ADP
fructose 1 6 diphosphate
splitting of phosphate glucose C6 to diphosphate glucose C3
glyceroaldehyde 3 phosphate
+
dihyroxyacetone phosphate
(b)
production stage
glyceroaldehyde 3 phosphate
oxidative transformation of glyceroaldehyde 3 phosphate to pyruvate and the related production of ATP and NADH
oxidation and phosphorylation
2Pi
2NAD+
2 NADH + H+
1,3 diphosphoglycerate
first reaction of ATP formation (phosphorylation of substratum)
2ADP
2 ATP
3 phosphoglycerate
2 phosphoglycerate
2H2O
phosphonol pyruvate
second reaction of ATP production (phosphorylation of substratum)
2ADP
2 ATP
pyruvate

Fig. 38) Transfer of hydrogen ions to NADH and FADH2 in the citric cycle of the mitochondrial respiratory chain and the simultaneous production of CO_2.

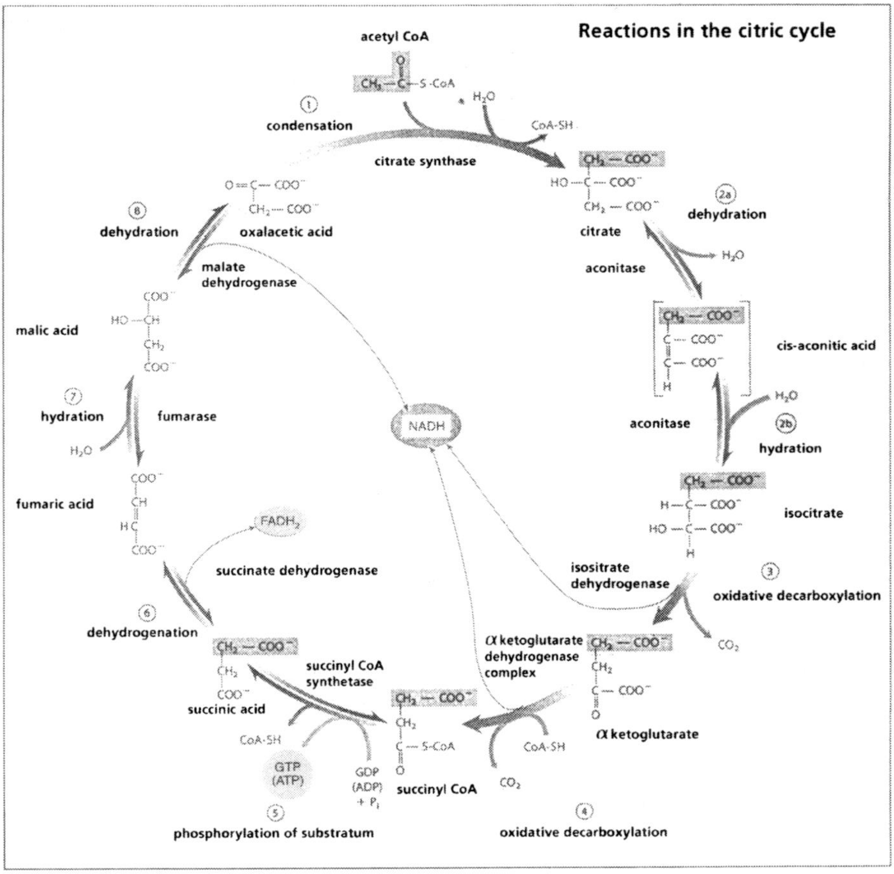

Reactions in the citric cycle
acetyl CoA
condensation
citrate synthase
citrate
dehydration
aconitase
cis-aconitic acid
hydration
isocitrate
isositrate dehydrogenase
oxidative decarboxylation
α ketoglutarate dehydrogenase complex
α ketoglutarate
oxidative decarboxylation
succinyl CoA
succinyl CoA synthetase
phosphorylation of substratum
GTP (ATP)
GDP (ADP) + Pi
succinic acid
succinate dehydrogenase
dehydrogenation
FADH2
fumaric acid
fumarase
hydration
malic acid
malate dehydrogenase
dehydration
oxalacetic acid
NADH
CoA-SH
H2O
CO2

Fig. 39) Fluorescent dyeing of the mitochondria of a fibroblast.

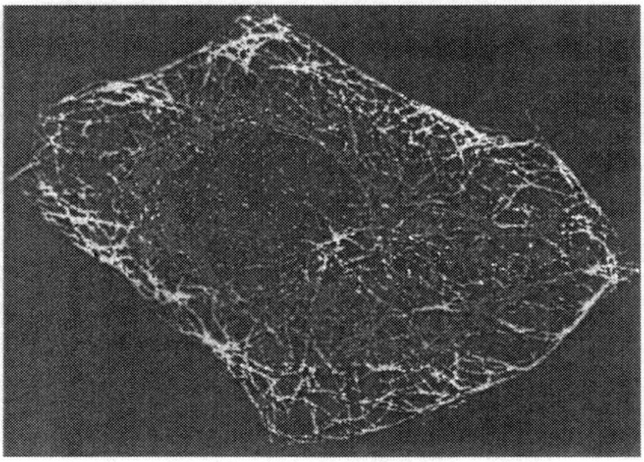

Fig. 40) Diagram of the complexes of the respiratory chain in the inner mitochondrial membrane. The electrons released by reducing food are transferred via the complexes to molecular oxygen, which is reduced to water, thus feeding the "proton battery" for ATPase. In tumor cells this process is severely inhibited.

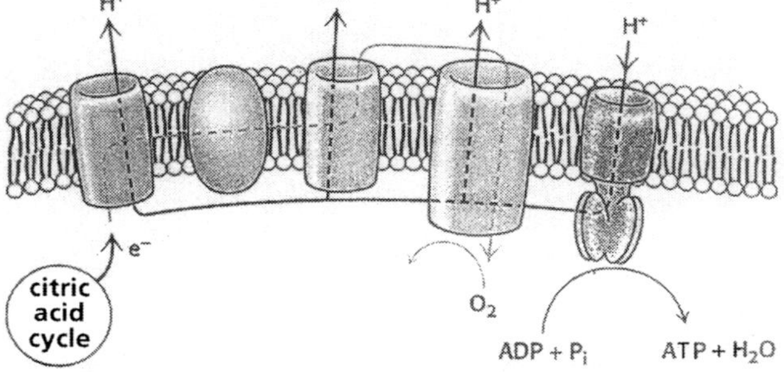
H+
H+
H+
H+
e−
citric acid cycle
O2
ADP + Pi
ATP + H2O

Fig. 41) The direction of the synthesis of the protein sub-groups of the enzymatic complexes of the respiratory chain are codified in the DNA of the nucleus and in the mitochondrial nucleus. The available proteins always have to be reassembled. Changes in this cooperation is decisive for transformation into tumor cells.

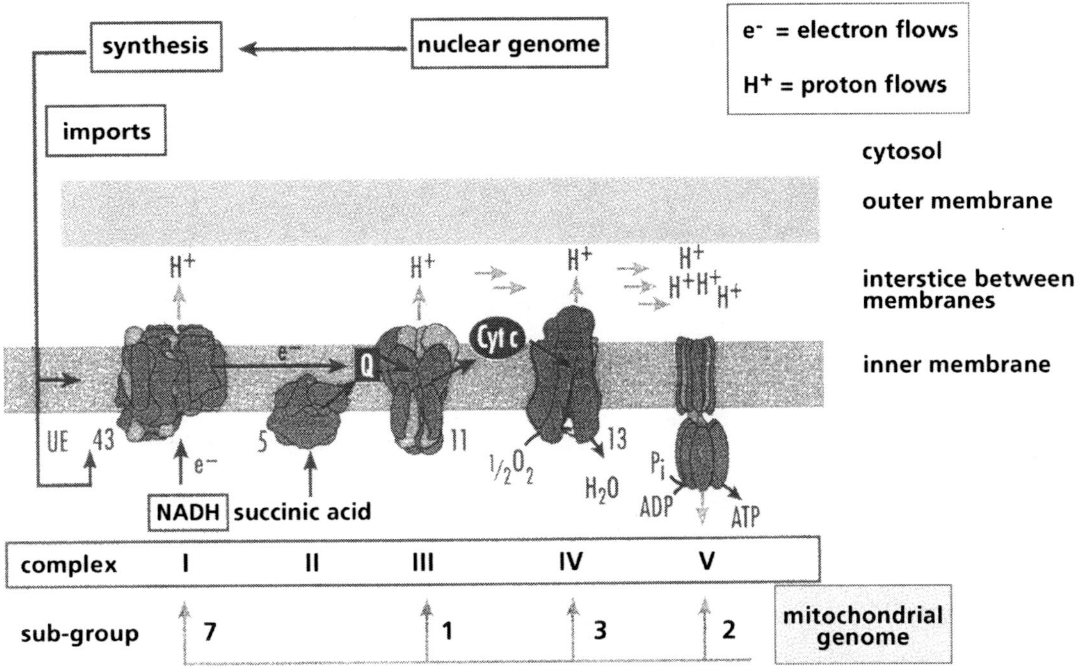
synthesis
nuclear genome
e⁻ = electron flows
H+ = proton flows
imports
cytosol
outer membrane
interstice between membranes
inner membrane
H+
e−
Q
Cyt c
UE
43
5
11
13
1/2 O2
H2O
Pi
ADP
ATP
NADH
succinic acid
complex
I
II
III
IV
V
sub-group
7
1
3
2
mitochondrial genome

Structure of the respiratory chain of the mitochondrial membrane.

Fig. 42) The electrochemical potential between the outer and inner mitochondrial membrane for feeding ATPase. This process guarantees up to 90% of the total requirements of cellular ATP. In tumor cells this synthesis capacity is severely curtailed and in order to survive cells are compelled to turn either to enzymatic ATPase in the cytoplasm or to oxidize other substrata.

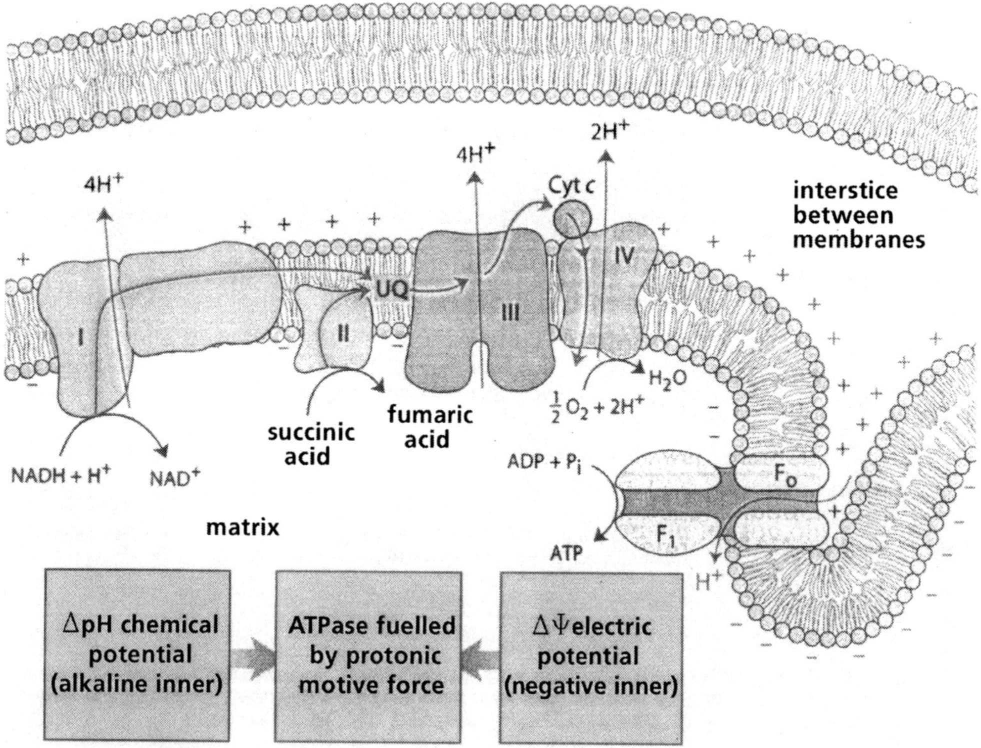
4H+
4H+
2H+
Cyt c
interstice
between
membranes
UQ
I
II
III
IV
H2O
1/2 O2 + 2H+
succinic
acid
fumaric
acid
NADH + H+
NAD+
ADP + Pi
Fo
F1
ATP
H+
matrix
ΔpH chemical
potential
(alkaline inner)
ATPase fuelled
by protonic
motive force
ΔΨ electric
potential
(negative inner)

Chapter VII

Collective Tunnel Vision

Why "HIV characteristics" are the outcome of evolutionary-biological programming, and are not specific causes of acute and/or chronic immune stress—what the "HIV test" really measures

The Nobel Prize winner for Chemistry in 1993, American research scientist Kary Mullis, gave an account of his experiences while searching for scientific references for the disease theory that "HIV is the probable cause of AIDS". His account is a astonishing document of contemporary history, and highlights the mass psychological staging of "the most devastating epidemic of the 20th Century" (Gallo 1991).

"In 1988 I was working as a consultant at Specialty Labs in Santa Monica, setting up analytic routines for the Human Immunodeficiency Virus (HIV). I knew a lot about setting up analytic routines for anything with nucleic acids in it because I had invented the Polymerase Chain Reaction. That's why they had hired me."

The Polymerase Chain Reaction (PCR) is a laboratory process in which the tiniest DNA fragments can be amplified. The prerequisite is that the DNA sequences that flank both ends of a given region of interest are known, and that a short fragment of the corresponding start sequence is available to bootstrap the amplification process. Today, PCR is one of the most important methods in every medical and molecular biological laboratory (Wirthmüller 1997). In his 1993 Nobel Prize acceptance speech, Mullis addressed the problem of lacking evidence for the hypothetical retrovirus HIV as the supposed cause of AIDS. *In over 100 years of the Nobel Prize, his speech is the only one that was not published.*

The futile search of the Nobel Prize winner Mullis for the original publication showing "HIV is the probable cause of AIDS"

> "Acquired Immune Deficiency Syndrome (AIDS), on the other hand, was something I did not know a lot about. Thus, when I found myself writing a report on our progress and goals for the project, sponsored by the National Institutes of Health, I recognized that I did not know the scientific reference to support a statement I had just written: "HIV is the probable cause of AIDS". So I turned to the virologist at the next desk, a reliable and competent fellow, and asked him for the reference. He said I didn't need one. I disagreed. While it's true that certain scientific discoveries or techniques are so well established that their sources are no longer referenced in the contemporary literature, that didn't seem to be the case with the HIV/AIDS connection. It was totally remarkable to me that the individual who had discovered the cause of a deadly and as-yet-uncured disease would not be continually referenced in the scientific papers until that disease was cured and forgotten. But as I would soon learn, the name of that individual—who would surely be Nobel material—was on the tip of no one's tongue. Of course, this simple reference had to be out there somewhere. Otherwise tens of thousands of public servants and esteemed scientists of many callings, trying to solve the tragic deaths of a large number of homosexual and/or intravenous (IV) drug-using men between the ages of twenty-five and forty, would not have allowed their research to settle into one narrow channel of investigation. Everyone wouldn't fish in the same pond unless it was well established that all the other ponds were empty. There had to be a published paper, or perhaps several of them, which taken together indicated that HIV was the probable cause of AIDS. There just had to be. I did computer searches, but came up with nothing. Of course, you can miss something important in computer searches by not putting in just the right key words. To be certain about a scientific issue, it's best to ask other scientists directly. That's one thing that scientific conferences in faraway places with nice beaches are for. I was going to a lot of meetings and conferences as part of my job. I got in the habit of approaching anyone who gave a talk about AIDS and asking him or her what reference I should quote for that increasingly problematic statement, "HIV is the probable cause of AIDS". After ten or fifteen meetings over a couple years, I was getting pretty upset when no one could cite the reference. I didn't like the ugly conclusion that was forming in my mind: The entire campaign against a disease increasingly regarded as a twentieth century Black Plague was based on a hypothesis whose origins no one could recall. That defied both scientific and common sense.

Finally, I had an opportunity to question one of the giants in HIV and AIDS research, Dr Luc Montagnier of the Pasteur Institute, when he gave a talk in San Diego. It would be the last time I would be able to ask my little question without showing anger, and I figured Montagnier would know the answer. So I asked him. With a look of condescending puzzlement, Montagnier said, "Why don't you quote the report from the Centers for Disease Control?" I replied, "It doesn't really address the issue of whether or not HIV is the probable cause of AIDS, does it?" "No," he admitted, no doubt wondering when I would just go away. He looked for support to the little circle of people around him, but they were all awaiting a more definitive response, like I was. "Why don't you quote the work on SIV [Simian Immunodeficiency Virus]?" the good doctor offered.

"I read that too, Dr Montagnier," I responded. "What happened to those monkeys didn't remind me of AIDS. Besides, that paper was just published only a couple of months ago. I'm looking for the original paper where somebody showed that HIV caused AIDS". This time, Dr Montagnier's response was to walk quickly away to greet an acquaintance across the room" (Mullis 1996).

The astonishing confession from the "HIV" discoverer Montagnier, that the self-defined standards for genuine retrovirus isolation were ignored

Beside Dr Gallo, the former director of the Laboratory for Tumor Biology of the National Cancer Institutes in the USA, Dr Montagnier is a worldwide authority on HIV. Since 1983 he is considered to be the discoverer of the "retrovirus HIV". Together with Gallo he is the patent holder for the "HIV test" and earns a certain share on every "HIV test". Montagnier has led the research team for viral cancer research at the world-famous Pasteur Institute in Paris since 1972 and has been the leader of the AIDS and retroviral department at the same institute since 1991. Dr Montagnier has also been President of the World Foundation for Aids Research and Prevention since 1993.

In 1997 Dr Montagnier gave a detailed scientific interview in which in answer to the final question about his belief in the existence of "HIV" he stated: "Oh, it is clear. I have seen it and I have encountered it". In the same interview Montagnier explains why the electron microscopic photographs of the supposed "new agent" produced and publicized by his research team were made only from cells in the cell culture and not, in accordance with the standard rules of virology, after the purification of the supposed virus particle from the remaining cell debris: "There was so little production of virus it was impossible to see what might be in a concentrate of virus from a gradient" (density gradient: the separation of the tested material in a sucrose solution after ultracentrifugation of the cell fluids of the stimulated cell culture. This process is one of the standard rules of isolation of a retrovirus).

"There was not enough virus to do that. Of course one looked for it, one looked for it in the tissues at the start, likewise in the biopsy. We saw some particles but they did not have the morphology typical of retroviruses. They were very different. Relatively different. So with the culture it took many hours to find the first pictures. It was a Roman effort! It's easy to criticise after the event. What we did not have, and I have always recognized it, was that it was truly the cause of AIDS" (Tahi 1997).

Montagnier was referring in his interview in 1997 to findings in cell cultures of T-helper immune cells. These experiments were carried out by Montagnier's viral cancer research group at the Pasteur Institute in 1982/1983 and publicized in the leading scientific journal *Science* in March 1983, the same month as the historic conference in New York postulated a "new agent" as the cause of AIDS. The findings of the Montagnier team were not presented at the historic conference, but only the discovery by the Gallo team of a supposed retrovirus HTLV-1 in T-cells of two American AIDS patients. The T-cells analyzed by the Montagnier team originated from the blood serum of patients who had shown clinical and immunological signs of a Th1-Th2 switch. The cells were treated in a culture with a growth factor (type 1 cytokine interleukin-2) and heavily oxidized substances like PHA as mitogens. After a few days physical and biochemical analyses were carried out both on the surface of some of these cells and in the cell fluids. These resulted in unspecific findings. In 1972 researchers at a symposium at the Pasteur Institute—Montagnier has led the research team for viral cancer there since 1972—established the standard practice for the isolation of retroviruses from cell cultures, which were supposed to exclude the possibility that unspecific findings from cell cultures and cell fluids of human cells could be confused with specific characteristics of retroviruses (Sinoussi 1973, Toplin 1973, Bader 1975, Papadopulos-Eleopulos 1993a). In the publication of the Montagnier team in *Science* of March 1983, which later was deemed to be the first publication about the discovery of the "human immune deficiency virus HIV", the authors emphatically refer to the standard rules of isolation of retroviruses in human cell cultures from 1972, as proof for the isolation of a "new retrovirus" in human T-helper immune cells (Barré-Sinoussi 1983, Montagnier 1985).

The most important standard rule for isolation of a retrovirus in human cell cultures is the separation of the cell material gained in the cell culture from all cell debris other than the cell particles thought to be retroviral, which after stimulation of the cell culture have budded out of the cell membrane. The cell particles that are considered retroviral particles have to be separated from the cell culture fluids by ultracentrifugation and absorbed in a sucrose solution. From experimental analysis it is known that during this process retroviruses band at a certain level known as the density gradient. 1.16 gm/ml is the accepted level. Molecules, cell debris, virus particles and non-virus particles from the centrifuged cell fluids of different cell cultures all band at this density gradient as the components separate not according to molecular weight but according to the density of the components in the sucrose solution. In order to be sure that, as far as possible, only the supposed virus particles have banded at the 1.16 gm/ml density gradient, purification and concentration procedures have to be carried out, as only the particles at the density gradient may be tested as to whether they correspond in diameter and volume to the supposed retroviral particles that were ascertained by studying electron-microscopic (EM) photographs during maturation from the cell membrane. As there are many non-viral particles in stimulated cell cultures whose shape, structure and appearance cannot with absolute certainty be distinguished from actual retroviruses, the contents of the particles have to be biochemically processed after isolation by purification. The proteins of the particle's membrane together with proteins from the inner particle membrane, including the characteristic enzyme proteins of retroviruses and nucleic acids, have to be exactly identified by a routine molecular biological process.

Only if structurally completely identical proteins and nucleic acids are present in the isolated and purified particles, and only if the nucleic acids in these particles form RNA instead of DNA molecules, can it be assumed as a probability that they are retrovirus particles. The findings can only be considered to be sure proof of the existence of a retrovirus in human cells when the RNA molecules in these particles construct genes which present the coded instruction for the biosynthesis of proteins within this particle and if these proteins can actually be identically synthesized. Once these findings have been verified it is still not possible to say whether these retroviral particles are exogenous, transmittable and infectious retroviruses as they could be endogenous retroviruses that have often been identified in the center of the genotype of many human cell types and are not infectious. In order to enable a differentiation between exogenous and endogenous retroviruses in human cells the properly isolated and biochemically characterized retroviruses would have to be transferred to human cell cultures, mature out of the cell again, it has to be separated again from any cell material by means of proper isolation and purification, successful isolation would have to be confirmed by EM photographs, the biochemical identity of the proteins and nucleic acids have to be substantiated and the RNA of the particle as coded genotype for the specific protein synthesis of the retrovirus particle would have to be verified.

In an interview in 1997 Montagnier admitted that he and his colleagues did not carry out purification of the cell particle. “I repeat, we did not purify” (Tahi 1997). Montagnier also conceded that only an “assemblage of properties” of the cell particle was detected by his team on the cell membrane and only components were found in the density gradient. No EM photographs were published to show which cell material had banded at the density gradients. Nevertheless, non-identified proteins from the density gradients were used as substrate for the “HIV test” patented by Montagnier in 1983 with the claim that they were retrovirus proteins of the “newly isolated HIV”.

The financial battle between the Pasteur Institute in Paris and the National Cancer Institute of the USA, litigation over the patent rights to the “HIV test”

The Pasteur Institute receives half its finance from the state and the other half through the production of vaccines, test diagnostics etc. The Pasteur Institute, in competition with the Gallo team from the National Cancer Institute in the US, very definitely had commercial interests in capturing the worldwide market for test substrates against the “new AIDS agent”. What in fact happened was that in 1983, three months after the first publication of the Montagnier team’s “isolation” of a new retrovirus in T-helper cells from the blood serum of risk-group AIDS patients, the license for the Pasteur Institute’s vaccine against hepatitis B was cancelled, for example, in Germany and Switzerland. Instead the use of hepatitis B vaccines from the US was recommended. This hepatitis B vaccine was approved in the US in October 1981 and in Germany and Switzerland in October 1982. The justification for the international ban on the Pasteur Institute’s substrate was, according to a confidential official memo: “suspicion of AIDS contamination of the French vaccine”. Although the American and French vaccines were extracted from comparable human cell cultures the National Health Authority’s suspicion of “AIDS contamination” only fell on the Pasteur vaccine. In the same issue of *Science* in which the Montagnier team reported about the “isolation” of a “new human retrovirus”, the Gallo team published about the “isolated retrovirus HTLV” in T-helper cells of homosexual patients, allegedly carried out in 1980 (Marx 1983, Barré-Sinoussi 1983). By mid-1983 the irrational notion of a "lethal AIDS/sex plague" was psychologically programmed on the basis of a few hundred cases of "infection" among anal receptive homosexuals with a long-standing abuse of nitrite inhalants and antibiotics. By mid-1983 an interaction between retroviral and cancer laboratory specialists, national health authorities and the mass media had long established that AIDS diseases were the consequence of a "new agent" and a "lethal new plague of sex and blood". It was only a question of who would control the "invisible hand of the market" for the marketing of the worldwide test substances. The Gallo team evidently needed to win time to come up with the decisive laboratory trick of how to isolate enough "HIV" in order to produce enough "HIV proteins" for mass testing. "HIV production" in a test tube was not sufficient for this purpose. In September 1983, Gallo announced that the Montagnier team could not have discovered a "new retrovirus" as they could not provide evidence of continuous "HIV production". In an interview in 1997 Montagnier stated: "For example Gallo said: "They have not isolated the virus . . . . and we (Gallo et al.), we have made it emerge in abundance in an immortal cell line." But before making it emerge in immortal cell lines, we made it emerge in cultures of normal lymphocytes from a blood donor. That is the principal criterion" (Tahi 1997).

Gallo and Montagnier's statements are both objectively misleading and are based on deliberate acts of deception.

But in the economic war between the French and the Americans the Americans initially retained the upper hand. The denunciation of the Pasteur Institute's hepatitis B vaccine as "AIDS contaminated" had its effect. Montagnier's patent application for an "anti-HIV antibody test" was rejected in the USA, the patent application of the National Cancer Institute for Gallo's "anti-HIV antibody test" was authorized in record time even before Gallo had published one line in scientific journals about the "isolation of HIV" and the development of an "anti-HIV antibody test" on the basis of proteins from his "isolated HIV". Only after year-long litigation between the USA and France were the patent charges for the "anti-HIV antibody test" awarded equally to Gallo and Montagnier at a conference between President Reagan and the then Mayor of Paris, Chirac and then given in an apparently noble gesture to the World Foundation for AIDS whose president Montagnier was to become. In reality this absurd dispute over the patent rights served as a distraction from the real problem—namely the fact that neither Gallo nor Montagnier had "isolated" a human retrovirus and that the source of the proteins for "HIV tests" had by no means been established as having a retroviral origin. The worldwide public was led to believe that when two specialists from such renowned research institutes like the Pasteur Institute and the National Cancer Institute quarrel about the honor of discovery, then "Public Enemy No.1" (President Reagan 1984) must really exist and be the cause of the "most devastating epidemic of the 20th Century" (Gallo 1991), and also that the "AIDS test" would protect the world population from this "deadly mass plague".

The ramifications of the psychological mass suggestion of a "new plague of sex and blood"

Nobel Prize winner Mullis' "little question" as to the original references that demonstrated that "HIV is the probable cause of AIDS", which neither Montagnier nor any other specialists would or could answer, answered itself by virtue of scientific historical facts. Fear of plagues is deeply anchored in the archaic subconscious of mankind as a legacy of evolutionary experience. It is very easy to trigger especially in association with sex and blood. When non-stop images are shown on television and in other mass media of condemned, relatively young people in connection with a "puzzling plague" and it is suggested that this "deadly incurable mass plague from the malicious depths of Nature" affects homosexuals today and tomorrow every man, woman and child, then people are scared. Then the question of whether the causes of the disease are correct will already have been answered, before a rational analysis could even be initiated. The all-or-nothing approach is adopted when confronted with archaic fears. You are either frightened of not. Reason confirms with hindsight what apparently the emotions already had known. With the continuous barrage of horrific images in the media and the statements of medical authorities, apparently in the know, terms like "HIV" and "AIDS" become provisory triggers whose objective truths can no longer be queried. The majority of people surrender helplessly to suggestive manipulation. There are plenty of object lessons in the history of the 20th Century in totalitarian systems and also in the world of modern media. Psychologists name this process "operant conditioning". When a non-specific, diffuse prospect of fear is associated contemporaneously with enough concrete stimuli or projections, the appearance of the stimulus without a concrete reason for fear is sufficient in the future, to search for and find a collective consensual protective mechanism for fear. There is no need to seek out original scientific references to prove whether the statements associated with these fears are justified. They are secure as they have been collectively internalized as a "healthy strategy". The people who are considered dangerous are those who reject the apparent dangers through rational analysis. The standard answer, since the "outbreak of AIDS epidemic" among uninformed doctors remains to this day "Do you want send millions of people to a certain death?" or "You should be happy that the young are frightened of something during sex and are more careful". When reasons are given as to why the false disease theory "HIV causes AIDS" is a danger to millions of people and that making the sex life of young people neurotic by means of HIV/AIDS propaganda detracts from the real dangers, you get at most a look of "condescending puzzlement" just as Nobel Prize winner Mullis did from Dr Montagnier in reply to his "little question" (Mullis 1998). After verifying that there were no scientific references to show that "HIV is the probable cause of AIDS", Mullis publicly described this fact as one of the greatest scientific scandals of the 20th Century (Mullis 1998).

The self-delusions and other mistakes of the "HIV discoverers" and the "disastrous results"

In the first publication about the "isolation of a human retrovirus" in the T-helper immune cells of AID and AIDS patients in 1983 the Montagnier team claimed to have followed all the procedural steps according to the standard rules of isolation of a retrovirus with the exception of electron-microscopic photographs of the density gradients. Such photographs are, however, of crucial importance to verify which proteins are present in the band of the density gradient. An arbitrary choice of these proteins may not be used as antigen substrate for the "HIV test". If decay proteins from the stimulated human cells in the cell culture have banded in the density gradient, then "HIV positive" will register as increased quantities of antibodies are found in the blood serum of test subjects which formed naturally against decay proteins inside the organism, against alloantigens (e.g. foreign semen after anal intercourse) or against microbial antigens. These antibodies in "HIV positive tests" then also react against decay proteins from the foreign human cells of the cell culture. This means, however, that millions of patients have received the medical death sentence of a "lethal retroviral infection" as a consequence of a natural antibody reaction and in countless cases the patients have been treated with highly toxic drug cocktails which have been proven to trigger AIDS and cancer. The electron-microscopic control of the protein components at the density gradient in the "isolation of HIV" and the construction of the "HIV test" is of immense importance to a large number of people and their dependents.

Yet, between 1983 and 1997, the EM photographs of the protein components of the density gradient were not published either by Montagnier, Gallo, or any other retro-virologist. The very first EM photographs of the density gradient of "HIV isolation" were published in March 1997 by two research groups, fourteen years after the first apparent "HIV isolation" by Montagnier and Gallo. These EM images showed "disastrous results", as judged by Professor De Harven, one of the pioneers of the use of electron-microscopy for the control of the isolation of retroviruses in mammalian cells (De Harven 1998 a). The first EM photographs, as truth test for the cell material of the density gradient after "HIV isolation" from human cells showed "practically only cell material" from human cells of the cell culture (Papadopulos-Eleopulos 1998 a). So, fourteen years after the alleged "first isolation of HIV" and thirteen years after the introduction of "HIV tests" it transpired that the retrovirus cancer researchers Montagnier and Gallo feigned the "isolation of HIV" and that the cell proteins for the protein antigens of the "HIV test" were nothing more than decay proteins from human cell cultures. The test result "HIV positive" meant the reaction of natural, if increased, antibody levels in the blood serum of test subjects.

Whatever else the retrovirus cancer researchers fabricated by laboratory trickery, the omission of EM photographs of the test proteins for the "HIV test" objectively amounted to grievous bodily harm, in uncounted cases leading to death, as patients as a rule were treated with highly toxic pharmaceutics, which could trigger AIDS and cancer. The explanation of Montagnier in an interview in 1997 is significant in understanding the grave charge that is based on firm scientific documents. Montagnier suddenly denies that he and his research team adopted the standard rules of isolation of retroviruses during the "first isolation of HIV". This statement is a direct contradiction to the claims in several publications by Montagnier and his colleagues in which it is explicitly reported, with reference to the rules determined by the Pasteur Institute in 1972, that these procedures were carried out for the "isolation of HIV", excluding the crucial EM cell material images at the density gradient after centrifuging the cell fluids of the suspected retrovirus cell culture of lymph cells from the AID and AIDS patient's blood serum (Barré-Sinoussi 1983, Brun-Vezinet 1984, Vilmar1984, Rey 1984, Klatzmann 1984, Montagnier 1985). As to the question of whether the standard rules for the isolation of retroviruses (Sinoussi 1973), defined at a symposium at the Pasteur Institute in 1972 and which he and his colleagues referred to in the initial publication of the "Isolation of HIV" were respected—namely:

- "culture [the suspected T-cells], purification of the material by ultracentrifugation, Electron Microscopic (EM) photographs of the material which bands at the retrovirus density, characterisation of these particles, proof of the infectivity of the particles"

Montagnier answered unequivocally in an interview in 1997: "No, that is not isolation" (Tahi 1997).

There are only two possible explanations for this response from one of the leading HIV specialists in the world:

- Either Montagnier and his team, contrary to the claims in their publications, did not follow the standard rules of retrovirus isolation during the "isolation of HIV", in which case these publications are scientific falsifications
- Or they did follow standard procedures and realized that the required results—the existence of human retroviruses in the T-immune cells of AID and AIDS patients—were not to be proven, in which case we are dealing again with a serious case of scientific falsification.

The fact that Gallo and his team published the same procedure as the Montagnier team for "HIV isolation" and that the Pasteur team sent the cell fluids from its cell cultures to the Gallo laboratories in 1983, speaks against the first possibility (Popovic 1984). In an interview in 1997 Montagnier admits that in 1983 he had seen only unspecific factors for the existence of retroviruses, but that through an assemblage of unspecific factors his mind's eye perceived the retrovirus "HIV" and this speaks for the latter possibility: "It is not one property but the assemblage of the properties which made us say it was a retrovirus of the family of lentiviruses. Taken in isolation, each of the properties isn't truly specific. It is the assemblage of them. So we had: the density, RT, pictures of budding and the analogy with the visna virus. Those are the four characteristics" (Tahi 1997).

All four characteristics are absolutely unspecific, they are found in many human cells, normal cells and cancer cells in cell cultures (overview Papadopulos-Eleopulos 1998 a). For fifteen years (1982-1997), both Montagnier and Gallo and all other retrovirologists dispensed with the only specific characteristic, a highly specific characteristic, namely the EM control of the density gradient after purification by ultracentrifugation, in order to be able to determine whether human cell proteins or retrovirus proteins were to be found in the density gradient for the "HIV test" construction. This is a routine matter in laboratories. "Dangerously enough, EM was progressively dismissed in retrovirus research after 1970. Molecular biologists started to rely exclusively on various "markers", and what was sedimenting in sucrose gradient at density 1.16 gm/ml was regarded as "pure virus". It is only in 1997, after fifteen years of intensive HIV research, that elementary EM controls were performed, with the disastrous results recently reviewed in *Continuum*. How many wasted efforts, how many billions of research dollars gone in smoke . . . . Horrible. Errare humanum est sed diabolicum perseverare . . . . [To err is human. To repeat error is of the Devil]" (De Harven 1998 a).

So Montagnier and Gallo must have blindly fished out of their "cell soup" protein antigens for the test substrate of the "HIV test", a test which in positive cases meant horrific suffering and death for millions of people, for the healthy and ill "HIV positives", for those with symptoms and those without. "How sad it is to think that a simple EM control of such "bands" (which takes about two days, and costs a few hundred dollars, but has never been done before 1997) could have prevented these highly misleading interpretations of "markers" (De Harven 1998 a).

It is, however, very difficult to imagine that of the thousands of highly specialized laboratory scientists in countless retrovirus research laboratories all of which have an electron-microscope on hand, with a budget of over 200 billion dollars in research funds, nobody in 15 years thought of running an EM control of the sucrose gradient in the "cell culture soup". The acceptance of such a syndrome, in light of the alleged threat to mankind of a "deadly mass HIV plague", required a devout deference to authority. Gallo, Montagnier and a few of their colleagues were proclaimed as "HIV discoverers", consultants in chief and lords of the greatest capital investment in modern medical history. The majority of retrovirologists profited knowingly and silently from the funding. "It was like having a money-printing machine in the basement, when you based a funding application on HIV, irrespective of what you wanted to research, the funds flowed. Without HIV every funding application was a lottery" (anonymous laboratory researcher about research practices in the AIDS era).

The most absurd thing about the statements from Montagnier and his co-workers is the fact that every interpretation of the observed phenomena in the cell cultures, the cell fluids, the density gradients and the interaction of cell cultures had to be objectively false. In the 1980s there was still a lack of knowledge among laboratory researchers and clinicians about the fundamental processes in human cell systems. The less they definitely knew, the more dictatorial the assertions that the research findings had been properly rendered (Epstein 1996, Lang 1996).

"The emergence of acquired immunodeficiency syndromes (AIDS) in 1981 gave the retrovirus establishment an opportunity to transform what could have been only an academic flop into a public health tragedy"

The first trailblazing insights of NO research, cytokine research, mitochondrial research and many other research fields have heralded a radical change in the understanding of many apparently puzzling phenomena. For the first time it is possible to recognize all phenomena in the context of "HIV isolation", "HIV test construction" and "HIV test findings" as being within the bounds of evolutionary biological laws. The insights suggest a more than strong suspicion that Montagnier, Gallo and their colleagues had not only examined the four unspecific standard characteristics for the isolation of retroviruses in human cells, named by Montagnier in an interview in 1997, but had also made up the standard characteristic—the EM control of the material in the sucrose solution in the density gradient. The logical reason for this assumption is the fact that the Montagnier and Gallo teams had made publications of EM photos of budding particles from the cell membrane of human cell cultures that they had stimulated with strong oxidizing substances. Why, then, would they not be interested in checking these EM findings with a control of the purified materials in the density gradient. Both teams have, to this day, sold these unspecific EM photos of budding from the cell membrane as evidence for the existence of "HIV". The budding of particles from stimulated cells is not specific evidence for retrovirus particles, not even if this particle arouses unspecific initial suspicions that it could be a retrovirus particle. Presenting the unsuspecting public with budding EM photos as evidence of the "existence and isolation of HIV" is a premeditated act of deception and a deliberate scientific falsification. Noted virologists have clearly proven that: "budding virus-like particles from the cell membrane can be ascertained in numerous non-infected normal cell lines and transformed cell lines, in T-cell lines, in transformed B-cell lines; and in cultures of primary human lymphoid cells from cord blood, which were either PHA stimulated or not and grown with or without serum and in cord lymphocytes directly after Ficoll separation". (Dourmashkin 1991, overview Papadopulos-Eleopulos 1993 a, 1993 b, 1996, 1998 a, 1998 b). Such budding particles have been demonstrated in the cell membranes of cells in enlarged lymph nodes in 90% of cases of "HIV associated" AID and AIDS patients as well as in the cell membranes of cells in enlarged lymph nodes in 87% of cases of non-"HIV associated" AID and AIDS patients (O'Hara 1988). In the same way as the embryonic umbilical cells and the transformed cells, all cases were concerned with cells after a Th1-Th2 switch and a type 2 cytokine dominance. Montagnier and Gallo knew nothing at the beginning of the 1980s about the existence of the two T-helper lymph cell populations, Th1 and Th2. They also did not know that these cells synthesize different cytokine profiles and that this was the reason why they showed differing patterns in the regulation of cellular symbiosis. They also did not know that T-helper cells produce or do not produce NO depending on the redox status. They also did not know that, depending on the redox status and the stimulation by oxidizing substances, T-helper cells activate counterregulations that either accelerate or inhibit apoptosis/necrosis and activate glycolitic energy production from outside the mitochondria.

The latter, however, meant an increase in lactate formation and the export of cell debris, accrued by proteolytic enzymes activated by the lactate. The budding of virus-like particles from the cell membrane is the garbage collection of the type 2 cytokine cells. The proof is the findings in typical Th2 cells: transformed T- and B-cell lines, embryonic lymphoid cells in umbilical tissue, productive lymph nodes independent from antibody levels obtained in the "HIV test" (Dourmashkin 1991, O'Hara 1988).

But Montagnier and Gallo definitely had a dire need to confirm, by means of EM photos of the materials in the sucrose solution, their initial suspicion, on the basis of the budding EM photos, of being on the trail of a "new retrovirus". If, after ultracentrifugation, there was a banding at the density gradient of predominantly retrovirus-like particles, then it could be possible by biochemical identification of the proteins and amino acids of this particle to prove that it was a new retrovirus. The disappointment must have been immense when, exactly like the first EM photos from 1997, practically only cell debris from the human cells of the stimulated cell culture was represented (Bess 1997, Gluschankof 1997). Such EM photos were the counter-evidence of the "isolation of a new agent". Proteins from human cell debris are not suitable to be sold as protein antigens for a worldwide antibody test. So Montagnier and Gallo declared the four unspecific characteristics for "HIV" for specific by a generous interpretation of the set theory—four times minus equals plus (Montagnier in interview 1997, Tahi 1997). They expounded the unspecific budding EM photos as specific evidence of a "new agent HIV". The specific EM photos of the sucrose gradient were not published; the unspecific budding EM photos were sufficient to quench the thirst of the mass media craving for images of the plague. Photofit images of "HIV" were later supplied together with computer designed monster-like excrescences, so-called knobs and spikes, to stimulate the collective plague fantasies, how the "new agent of the deadly mass plague" enters the immune cells and how it goes about its deadly deeds (see illustration: HIV photofit [table IX]). In reality the best-known electron microscopist for "HIV" EM photos had published that the "HIV particle" on average only exhibited 0.5 knobs per particle. These protein complexes on the cell membrane of the "HIV particle" are supposed to be decisive for the infectiousness of "HIV". This protein with a molecular weight of gp120 is one of the proteins—the alleged "HIV protein" in the "HIV test"—that reacted to the antibodies in the human serum and can produce positive results in the test. The EM researchers established that knob-like structures could be observed, even when gp 120 proteins were not present, the EM results could then be falsely positive (Layne 1992). But how is "HIV" without the gp 120 configuration supposed to dock onto the immune cells, if, according to the unanimous view of the "HIV" researchers it could not possibly be infectious without it? The act of deception with the budding EM photos and the gp 120 protein complex for the "HIV test" is of crucial importance to the virus hunters for the optical staging of the trick series. As the human sensory organs receive some 11 million bits per second, of which roughly 10 million are optical bits, pictorial presentation is the best means to generate fear or fancy. From a mass psychological viewpoint it is not to be assumed that Montagnier and Gallo had forgone the opportunity to produce considerably more specific EM photos of the sucrose gradient as there were very convincing EM photos of retrovirus particles in the sucrose gradient after purification by ultracentrifugation even in the 1960s. Such EM photos were published by, among others, the Pasteur Institute under Montagnier and by the National Institute of Cancer in the USA under Gallo. These EM photos were taken of cell cultures of mice suffering from leukaemia. EM photos of particles from human cancer cells and other cell types after purification could, however, never be demonstrated. The scientific contemporary witness, De Harven, who as one of the pioneers of retrovirus research had already shown in the 1950s convincing EM photos of purified retrovirus particles from animal cancer cells at the most famous American cancer research center—the Sloan-Kettering Institute in New York—stated: "In the 1950s and 1960s many EM cancer research centers [in the USA and Europe], were spending a considerable amount of time in attempts to demonstrate virus particles associated with human cancer cells. "Virus-like particles" were occasionally reported but convinced nobody. Typical viruses were never conclusively demonstrated. This was in sharp contrast with the highly reproducible demonstration, by EM, of viruses in a variety of murine and avian leukemias and tumors. Very few papers were published to report on these negative findings in human cancers and leukemias. However, Haguenau, in 1959, reported on the difficulty of identifying any typical virus particles in a large series of human mammary carcinomas. Bernhard and Leplus, in 1964 in an EM survey of cases of Hodgkin's disease, lymphosarcomes, lymphoid leukemias and metastatic diseases failed to recognize virus particles associated with these malignant conditions. At Sloan Kettering in New York, I decided, in 1965, to stop surveying cases of leukemias and lymphomas by EM for the presence of viruses in view of our entirely negative results. This was reported at a conference on Methodological Approaches to the Study of Leukemias held at the Wistar Institute, in 1965 (Haguenau 1959, Bernhard 1964, De Harven 1965). Publication of these negative findings failed to discourage fanatical virus hunters! An explanation for these negative results had to be found somewhere! Perhaps the technique of EM by the thin section method was not the best approach? (although it worked perfectly for mice!). Preparing thin sections was time-consuming and skill-demanding! Who had time for that, when research funding was getting difficult, and when major pharmaceutical corporations were starting to finance "crash programs" for speedy answers? . . . . It became acceptable to postulate that when viruses cannot be seen by EM in cancer cells, biochemical or immunological methods supposedly identifying viral "markers" were enough to demonstrate viral infection of the cells under scrutiny. Such markers can be an enzyme (RT), an antigen, various proteins, or some RNA sequences. "Never seeing the viral particles was conveniently explained by the integration of the viral genome into the chromosomes of the alleged infected cells. To accommodate such interpretations implied complete oblivion of all we knew from previous research on cancer of experimental animals . . ." (De Harven 1998 b).

The fact that the leading lights of "HIV isolation" and the patentees of the "HIV antibody test", Montagnier and Gallo, were not in the position to produce a specific EM photo of purified cell debris and instead of this were able to feign for 17 years the unspecific budding EM photos as the official "wanted" poster for "HIV" just goes to show that counter controls no longer work in medical research: "As far as scientific policy is concerned, research on potentially oncogenic viruses was dominated by the retrovirus hypothesis. Federal funding took the same direction, amplified by the incredibly naive idea that success was primarily a matter of money! Unusually large levels of federal support resulted in the creation of a retrovirus research establishment. Large numbers of research jobs were created in this venture. The intellectual freedom to think along other avenues of cancer research was rapidly dwindling, especially when major pharmaceutical companies started to offer tantalizing contracts to support polarized retrovirus research . . . . The top priority was to demonstrate, at any cost, that retroviruses had something to do with human cancer, a hypothesis, however, which didn't receive the slightest support throughout the 1970s. Such a misdirected research effort would have been relatively inconsequential as long as public health was not involved. Unfortunately, the emergence of acquired immunodeficiency syndromes (AIDS) in 1981 gave the retrovirus establishment an opportunity to transform what could have been only an academic flop into a public health tragedy" (De Harven 1998 b).

Using the concept of cell dyssymbiosis, specific "HIV Characteristics" can be consistently accounted for as a legitimate evolutionary biological product after prooxidative stress

The remaining unspecific characteristics can also be explained by the concept of cell dyssymbiosis. The Montagnier team and the Gallo team specified as second characteristic, besides the budding of cell particles from the stimulated human T-helper cells, evidence of the repair enzyme reverse transcriptase (Barré—Sinoussi 1963, Popovic 1984). Such enzymes transcribe the RNA sequences to DNA sequences. From an evolutionary-biological viewpoint, information storage began in living cells, with less stable RNA codings, as "RNA world" (overview De Duve 1991). DNA coding is, however, more stable and in all living cells the carrier of information for protein synthesis in the cytoplasm. Mobile messenger RNA, after redox dependent activation, is transcribed to the DNA form. Up until 1970 the biological dogma was that flows of genetic information always ran from DNA to RNA. As Temin and Baltimore discovered in 1970 that there is also a counter-flow of information from the RNA form to DNA form, they termed the enzyme involved reverse transcriptase (RT). At first it was thought that this enzyme was present exclusively in animal cell identified RNA tumor viruses (retroviruses). This assumption was soon recognized as a mistake. RT is active in all eukaryotic cells and in bacterial cells (Temin 1972, 1974, 1985, Baltimore 1985, Varmus 1987, 1988).

The claim by Montagnier and Gallo that RT was fished out of the density gradient 1.16 gm/ml, which was shown to contain Montagnier's impure cell debris from the cell fluid (Tahi 1997), and that this find is exclusive proof of the presence of "HIV" and so the proteins from the same density gradient are exclusively "HIV proteins" is a grave scientific deceit. As Montagnier and Gallo did not purify the material from the banding by ultracentrifugation and also did not wish to verify the presence of retrovirus particles with EM photos, in order to disguise the absence of retrovirus particles (!) the whole process becomes a dreadful game with concealed cards. Montagnier said in an interview in 1997, after the 1997 EM photos (Bess 1997, Gluschankof 1997) had exposed the non-existence of the retrovirus particle in the sucrose gradient which had been intimated since 1983: "I repeat, we did not purify . . . Gallo? . . . I don't know if he really purified. I don't believe so" (Tahi 1997).

The safest and clearest procedures for the isolation of retroviruses from stimulated human cells was not employed and substituted by the objectively false statement that evidence of RT is exclusive proof of the "isolation of HIV".

As the discoverer of RT, the Nobel Prize winners Temin and Baltimore and Nobel Prize winner Varmus (Temin and Baltimore 1972, Varmus 1987,1988) had unequivocally shown that RT features in all cells, the presence of RT in the cell debris of cell fluid from human cell cultures, which were stimulated with strong oxidizing substances, was to be expected.

Montagnier and Gallo as well as all the other HIV researchers were only able to demonstrate "HIV characteristics" in stimulated cells (Klatzmann 1986, Papadopulos-Eleopulos 1993, 1998 a). The stimulation of the cell cultures took place as a result of the addition of strong oxidizing mitogens (PHA, Con A etc.) and type 1 cytokine interleukin-2 (IL-2). IL-2 activates, however, Type 1 cytokine interferon-γ (IFN-γ). IFN-γ stimulates cytotoxic NO production. As the Montagnier team and the Gallo team stimulated T-helper cells (TH cells) from homosexual AID and AIDS patients and it has been demonstrated that such patients show a TH-2 dominance (overview Lucey 1996), these cells have mostly been counterregulated, this means on activation of NO synthesis by interferon-γ these cells either die by apoptosis or necrosis, as IL-2 also stimulates tumor necrosis factors and as a consequence increasingly ROS. Or the cells increase the counterregulation to protect against apoptosis/necrosis which means that by activating the type 2 cytokine profile (IL-4, IL-5, IL-10 etc.) the formation of the enzyme COX-2, prostaglandin (PGE) and the repair enzyme, transforming growth factor (TGF) is increased. PGE and TGF suppress the NO synthesis and activate from arginine the metabolic path for the synthesis of polyamines that stimulate the proliferation and repair mechanisms. The synthesis of reverse transcriptase, the enzyme for the neosynthesis of DNA from RNA, also belongs to the repair sequence.

"HIV positive" tested people have a conspicuously low thiol pool in T-helper cells. Both the cysteine levels in the blood plasma are lower as well as the intracellular glutathione levels in the T-helper cells that are on average 30% lower (Dröge 1988, Eck 1989, Buhl 1989, Gmünder 1991, Roederer 1991 a, 1991 b, Harakeh 1991, Kinscherf 1994, Dröge 1997 a, 1997 b, Herzenberg 1997). Thiol depletion is to be expected in long-term stress in which a number of factors are involved and is a specific expression of a profound cell dyssymbiosis in AID and AIDS patients. The antioxidative and antinitrosative emergency status of the T-helper immune cells can only be remedied by massive counterregulation or apoptosis/necrosis. The stimulation by IL-2 and heavily oxidized mitogens and antigens of these thiol depleted immune cells in the cell culture triggers oxidative and nitrosative stress. Considerable cell damage can be expected through this provocation of the synthesis of cytotoxic

NO gases, which in the cell culture also diffuse to the neighboring cells. The net effect is that the RT levels also increase in counterregulated cells.

In plain language the procedures of the virus hunters meant that they placed the immune cells that were already dyssymbiotic under artificial prooxidative/nitrosative stress, inevitably provoking apoptosis/necrosis and /or increased counterregulation. Finally the released cell products, including RT and other cell specific proteins, RNA and DNA molecules as well as the export particles of the stressed cells (budding) are interpreted by chicanery as unspecific, but then again apparently *in toto* specific, characteristics of a "new retrovirus". The "HIV test" is assembled using disintegrating proteins with the full awareness that people with an increased antibody count (Th2 status with increased antibody production) and/or cross-reacting antibodies and autoantibodies according to the natural laws could show an antigen antibody reaction on contact with human foreign protein. The selection of the "HIV positive" stigmatized is governed by an arbitrary specification of the measuring threshold of the test, this means at which point of sensitivity the antigen antibody reaction counts as "positive". With this technique of measuring a targeted haul can be made within the population as a whole as it is already known which particular subgroups will be stigmatized. Subsequently the necessity was suggested to those who had been scared to death at being stigmatized, for a long-term therapy with highly toxic pharmaceutical combinations to combat the phantom retrovirus that a few thousand laboratory specialists with a simple EM photo costing "a few hundred dollars" were apparently unable to conceive for 17 years. Then again the extremely expensive pharmaceutical cocktails, the unfailing implementation of the "planned experiments on human beings" promoted at the historic conference of the *manqué* retrovirus cancer researchers in March 1983, have been shown to cause prooxidative/nitrosative stress and compound cell dyssymbiosis. The circle closes, the pharmatoxic consequences, to the point of fatal organ failure, are interpreted as "specific characteristics" of the "lethal HIV infection".

The "HIV" test measures an antibody reaction against what is put into the test substrate: indeterminate proteins excreted by repeatedly stressed human immune cells

Countless experimental studies with all kinds of cell types have proven that the "four HIV-specific characteristics" (Montagnier) observed in cell cultures can equally arise in "HIV negative" cell cultures under stimulation stress. When HIV researchers say that they have infected previously "non-infected cell cultures" with "HIV" it always means that they have stimulated oxidative/nitrosative stress (without stimulation stress there are no "HIV characteristics"!) and that these cells, dependent on cell type or the state of cell symbiosis, have reacted with counterregulations. The subsequent diagnosis of "HIV positive" in the cell culture is reached in that budding was observed, a portion of RNA (or DNA!) was re-modelled to DNA in an artificial initial sample, and that this is regarded as evidence for the presence of the enzyme RT, that the one or the other protein is proven by molecular weight, as occurs in every cell, but that this one is defined as an "HIV protein" in advance and that possibly these proteins will react to antibodies in animal or human blood serum. In the last case it is claimed, from a scientific viewpoint incorrectly, that these antibody reactions are specific and exclusively a reaction to "HIV proteins".

In reality there are no "specific" antibodies. Rather there are special protein molecules that are formed by the million each day by B-cells in every human being. They are positively charged whereas T-cells are negatively charged. Antibodies have varying charging centers on the molecular surface. When they come into contact with an antigen, mostly proteins but also other molecules, then one or more of the positively charged centers on the antibody react to one or more negatively charged centers on the antigen. The antibodies are, so to say, the molecules with the positive plug that fit into the antigens' negative socket. If you have a negatively charged antigen many different antibodies with roughly the same positive "plug" can fit the negative "socket" of the same antigen. Conversely many different antigens with the same negatively charged "sockets" can couple with positive "plugs" of the same type of antibody. This process is called cross-reaction. The logic is that the more different antibodies a person has formed in the blood serum in increasing amounts, the higher the statistical probability is that they will react on contact with antigens. It is not known, however, whether these antibodies were originally produced "specifically" against these particular antigens or against other antigens. As antibodies remain a long time in blood serum, sometimes lifelong, it cannot be stated for certain whether the antibody activating incidents are backdated or persist from the time of the test (Guilbert 1985,1986, Pontes de Carvalho 1986, Chassagne 1986, Termynck 1986, Matsiota 1987, Parravicini 1988, Gonzalez-Quintial 1990, Berzofsky 1993, Fauci 1994, Owen 1996, Papadopulos-Eleopulos 1998 a).

The claim of the retrovirologists that a positive "HIV test" signifies a "specific" antibody reaction against "HIV proteins" is thus consciously misleading. As Montagnier admitted in an interview in 1997, originally he and Gallo brought the "unpurified" protein mixture from their "real cell culture soup", as Montagnier described it in the same interview (Tahi 1997), into contact with the serum from AID and AIDS patients. If there was shown to be an antigen antibody reaction in the serum, which was by no means the case in all the serums, then the reaction as such would be published as evidence that "HIV" must exist and that the patients must be suffering from AID and AIDS because they had become infected with "HIV". This meant that T-helper immune cells extracted from the serum of immune-stressed AID and AIDS patients were exposed to a further immune stress through oxidizing substances in a cell culture. The highly oxidized proteins, released by the overstrained immune cells by cell disintegration or cell particle export were ultracentrifuged and then banded in a sugar solution, but not purified and identified. Finally a sample was taken from the material that had banded at a particular density (a level at which according to procedures in earlier experiments with animal cancer cells, retrovirus particles, among other things, had concentrated)—blindly and without identification of the material. Taking the protein as antigen from the sample it was allowed to react with antibodies from the blood serum of likewise immune-stressed AID and AIDS patients. Nobody, not even the most imaginative retrovirologist, could even with the remotest semblance of certainty say which proteins from the cell culture had reacted to which antibodies from the serum of AID and AIDS patients. It could only be said that if the proteins from the immune cells of immune-stressed patients were treated prooxidatively/nitrosatively in a laboratory and the released proteins were made to react with antibodies from the serum of equally immune-stressed AID and AIDS patients, then an antigen antibody reaction can be seen. This arcane process and the alleged evidence that unspecific repair enzyme RT is released in immune-stressed immune cells after immune stress in a cell culture is up until now the only evidence for the "existence and isolation of HIV" as well as for the "infection with the immune cell killing HIV".

The first "HIV test" process was called the ELISA test. It was said later that the ELISA test was wrongly positive in 90% of the positive results. In reality all ELISA tests are wrongly positive as without proper isolation of a retrovirus no test can be constructed that can display the antibody formation against a retrovirus. Later the proteins from the blind sample from the cell culture soup were run through an electric field and defined as "HIV proteins" a handful of proteins that stood out distinctively according to particular molecular weights. In laboratory jargon this process is called Western Blot. The ELISA test becomes the screening test and Western Blot the confirmatory test. If the ELISA test is positive twice then a subsequent Western Blot test is carried out. If this is also positive then the patient is considered to be "HIV positive".

In reality the Western Blot test also does not measure antibody formation against a "retrovirus HIV". It measures an antibody reaction against what was put into the test substrate: undefined proteins, released by repeatedly stressed human immune cells.

The screening test also cannot find what it is looking for, namely the human antibodies against a "retrovirus HIV" that Dr Gallo and Dr Montagnier also failed to find. The confirmatory test also cannot confirm the antibody formation against "retrovirus HIV", as Dr Gallo and Dr Montagnier only saw "unspecific characteristics" and for the only specific characteristic that could confirm the existence of a "retrovirus HIV", namely EM control after purification of the cell fluids, they evidently did not want to expend "two days time and a few hundred dollars" (De Harven 1998 b).

Nevertheless, can the "HIV test" give information about the condition of a human's immune system? As the test substrate contains human proteins it can only indicate the degree of sensitivity that a test subject reacts to human proteins. From this alone it cannot be deduced why a proband reacted to a particular protein with antibodies of a particular intensity. There might be, for instance, a cross-reaction between antibodies against tubercular bacteria, leprosy bacteria, pneumocystis carinii fungi, candida fungi and the proteins of the "HIV test". There are many other cross-reactions that have still been little researched (Mathews 1998, Calabrese 1989, Müller 1990, 1991, Ezekowitz 1991, Tumijama 1991, Kion 1991, Kashala 1994, O'Riordan 1995, Fraziano 1996, Papadopulos-Eleopulos 1997 c). The test cannot provide information about the concrete significance of an antibody reaction against the proteins of the "HIV test" for the past, present or future of test subjects. At the very most a test can indicate that the proband could have Th2 dominance with an increased antibody production. The "HIV test" has no more informational value than the simple DTH test that measures the reaction of the skin lymphocytes to antigen stimulation. As was demonstrated with surgical patients (Christou 1986) the DTH skin reaction could give significant indications about which patients could develop sepsis after severe traumata, burns and operative intrusions. In this respect the DTH skin reaction is superior to the "HIV test" as it indicates the readiness of stimulation of the Th1 immune cells. As the "HIV test" merely shows an increased antibody sensitivity, which can have a lot of different or evident causes in excessive immune stress, and as antibodies are not decisive for the development of opportunistic infections and certain cancer forms but for the elimination capability of Th1 immune cells for an intracellular agent and the antioxidative capacity for the efficiency of cell symbiosis, the "HIV test" is unsuited as an aid to diagnosis and prognosis. But as the construction of the "HIV test" is based on sham particles this test should be banned internationally as quickly as possible and the groundbreaking work of NO research, cytokine research, mitochondria research and other seminal research fields should be implemented into medical practice.

The experimental findings of the Montagnier team as counter-evidence against the disease theory "HIV is the cause of AID and AIDS"

From the numerous experiments with different cell cultures, two experiments from Gallo and Montagnier should demonstrate how they themselves have shaken their "HIV causes AIDS" theory (Zagury 1986, Laurent-Crawford 1991). At the time of the cell experiments the fact of the existence in humans of different cytokine profiles (type 1 and type 2) of the T-helper cells, Th1 cells and Th2 cells, were not yet published. Likewise the fact that during excessive or long-term immune stress of the redox milieu a re-programming of the cytokine profile of the T-cells can take place. These facts were finally verified in 1991 (Romagnani 1991). The additional fact that Th1 cells and Th2 cells can be differentiated as Th1 cells produce cytotoxic NO gas after stimulation with interleukin-2, while Th2 cells suppress the formation of cytotoxic NO gas was only demonstrated in 1995 (Barnes 1995). In this respect the consequence of a Th1-Th2 switch to Th2 dominance was also not known then, namely the fact that after severe immune stress Th2 dominance impairs or totally prevents the elimination of intracellular agents. The further consequence that with a Th2 dominance massive counterregulations are triggered resulting in a cell dyssymbiosis in mitochondria and that these cells export highly oxidized proteins by transporting particles from the cells as well as producing an increase in repair enzymes instead of NO gas production was also at that time not understood.

The Montagnier team (Laurent-Crawford 1991) provoked by mitogen and cytokine stimulation (PHA, interleukin-2) in three human cell lines the appearance of "unspecific characteristics".

The experiments of the Montagnier team (Laurent-Crawford 1991) show that the four "HIV characteristics" cited by Montagnier as evidence supply the counter-evidence; that we are dealing with cell products under prooxidative and nitrosative stress (see illustration: Experimental findings of the Montagnier team as counter-evidence against the disease theory "HIV is the cause of AID and AIDS" (see table X)).

The results demonstrate the following findings:

1. In T-helper immune cells and other human blood cells that have been acutely stimulated in cell cultures with highly oxidized mitogens (PHA) and the type 1 cytokine interleukin-2 (IL-2) cell disintegration always occurs (cell culture A, C, D).
2. Those cells in the cell culture showing no signs of cell disintegration are those that have reacted with counterregulations to stress provocation by PHA and IL-2 or those that were already counterregulated (cell cultures A, B, C). The counterregulations lead to a shutting down of cytotoxic NO production and to the choking of ROS production in the OXPHOS system of the mitochondria (cell dyssymbiosis).
3. The maximum cell disintegration appears a few days before the maximum appearance of "HIV characteristics" (cell culture A).
4. Cell disintegration occurs after stimulation by PHA and IL-2 even when there are no cells in the cell culture that had previously been provoked for the formation of "HIV characteristics" by stimulation with PHA and IL-2 (cell culture D).

Explanation: In case A, the cell culture was stimulated with mitogens and IL-2 for as long as it took some cells from the cell culture to show signs of "HIV characteristics" (in a cell culture it is always only individual cells that are "HIV positive"). This cell culture is then declared as "HIV infected". After further stimulation the cells that are not counterregulated (or have not been counterregulated through the additional stimulation) die (apoptosis/necrosis). These are mainly the Th1 cells. If these Th1 cells are thiol-depleted, as has been proven in numerous studies on AID and AIDS patients (Herzenberg 1997 et al.), they die even more quickly as the provoked NO gas and the ROS in the Th1 cells can no longer be neutralized quickly enough. Thiol-depleted Th2 cells have a better chance of survival as with a type 2 cytokine profile they can shut down the enzyme for cytotoxic NO synthesis and slow down calcium-dependent NO synthesis in the cytoplasm. In doing this the level of the powering gases for the mitochondrial channels in the mitochondrial membrane sinks. The import and export facilities of the mitochondria are reduced, the mitochondrial membrane relatively or totally closed, the Ca^{2+} level in the cytoplasm is lowered, apoptosis or necrosis (depending on the diminished ATP level) is prevented. In the cell culture there remain, in essence, the cells that already before stimulation ("HIV characteristics") or during stimulation ("HIV characteristics") were no longer capable of apoptosis or necrosis (cases A and

B). The cell culture is "chronically HIV infected" and shows no apoptosis /necrosis. Logically the maximum apoptosis/necrosis has to precede the maximum "HIV production" as is the case in cell culture A. The length of time for maximum apoptosis/necrosis after prooxidative/nitrosative stimulation (case A) is well known: an attack of flu in immune healthy people lasts a week, with or without treatment. The Th1 cells react to the intracellular agents. For people with a Th2 dominance, for instance the elderly, a flu infection can be lethal because hitherto compensated cell dyssymbiosis can decompensate which could lead to organ failures ending in death. The same critical period of time was also apparent in the surgical sepsis patients. If the anergic DTH skin reaction as expression of Th2 dominance failed to improve after seven days a significant sepsis developed (Christou 1986). In cases C and D apoptosis/necrosis occurred in Montagnier's experiment, independent of whether the T-helper cells for the provocation of "HIV characteristics" had been placed under immune stress. In case D without previous "HIV stimulation" apoptosis/necrosis occurred somewhat later than in case C. That is easily explained by the thiol usage of the preceding prooxidative/nitrosative stimulated cells of cell culture C some of which, although not the majority, had developed "HIV characteristics". Subsequently through further stimulation with PHA/IL-2 even more cells died even more quickly. As can be seen in all four cases it is the stimulation by PHA/IL-2 that is decisive in cell disintegration and not the formation of "HIV characteristics". These are in fact the results of counterregulation and not the cause of cell disintegration (see especially cases A and B).

As the "HIV researchers" measured the cell effects after stress stimulation only as a net effect of the total amount of cells in the cell culture, the differentiated reaction and regulation (or as the case may be the counterregulation of individual cells) remained concealed. Up until now there have been no publications from the "HIV researchers" about NO-induced effects on an individual cell level. Mitochondria researchers, however, have carried out such studies with the fluorescence-activate cell sorter. In human myelomonocytes from bone marrow after a direct dose of an NO-donating substance at 2mM some 30% of the cells showed necrosis and 30% apoptosis depending on time and dose. The loss of the electric membrane potential of the cell symbionts (mitochondria) preceeded in each case cell disintegration (Richter 1996).

The experimental findings of the Gallo team as counter-evidence against the disease theory "HIV is the cause of AID and AIDS"

The findings of the experimental studies of Gallo and his assistants confirmed, in principle, the results of the Montagnier team (see illustration: Experimental findings of the Gallo team as counterevidence of the disease theory "HIV causes AID and AIDS", table XI).

The Gallo team stimulated three T-lymph cell cultures with oxidizing mitogens (PHA) and type 1 cytokine IL-2. Previously cell culture A showed signs of "HIV characteristics" in some cells after stimulation with PHA and IL-2 but the majority of the cells in cell culture A showed no "HIV characteristics". Cell cultures B and C were not previously stimulated with PHA and IL-2 and had no signs of "HIV characteristics. The Gallo team then exposed the two cell cultures, the "HIV infected" cell culture and one of the two "HIV negative" cell cultures, to the same amounts of immune-stress-triggering PHA and IL-2. The third "HIV negative" lymph cell culture was not stimulated as a control. All three T-lymph cell cultures had a 34% proportion of T-helper cells (Zagury 1986). The AEDS concept (acquired energetic cell dyssymbiosis syndrome = acquired cell dyssymbiosis) now predicts that:

1. Cell cultures A and B will feature a cell loss of T-helper cells after stimulation with PHA and I-2,
2. Cell culture C will show no loss of T-helper cells,
3. Cell culture A will show a greater loss of T-helper cells than cell culture B as the cells from cell culture A were previously treated with oxidizing substances (PHA, IL-2) and some cells had shown signs of "HIV characteristics".

The latter is a sign of a relative thiol deficiency. These cells will respond to stress stimulation with a stronger apoptosis/necrosis as the previously damaged cell symbioses will react more sensitively to the induction of cytotoxic NO gas and oxygen radicals with cell disintegration (as they had not previously responded with counterregulation). Their cell receptors alter in such a way that they respond to PHA and IL-2 in a reduced way. This would mean that a proportion of the Th1 cells do not die but can no longer be measured as Th1 cells due to monoclonal antibodies. The results must have been as follows:

- T-helper cell loss in cell culture A > cell culture B > cell culture C
- T-helper cell loss in cell culture C = 0

The data of the Gallo team were unequivocal (Zagury 1986). The findings confirmed the later results of the Montagnier team that apoptosis/necrosis in T-helper immune cells is dependent on stress stimulation. The strength and duration of the reaction of the T-helper immune cells, either as a type 1 reaction (apoptosis, necrosis) or a type 2 reaction (counterregulation with loss of Th1 characteristics) is dependent, among other things, on the thiol pool. In the Gallo team's experiment there were probably among the 3% of T-helper cells, those that could be traced a few days after cultivation through stress stimulation, cells that featured signs of "HIV characteristics" (the publications, however, do not mention this). These cells on further cultivation will "continuously produce HIV" (Laurent-Crawford 1991) as in case B of the Montagnier team's T-lymph cell cultures, and show no signs of apoptosis or necrosis. This process of counterregulation has been demonstrated by NO researchers. When liver cells were pretreated with low, tolerable amounts of NO gas (NO-donating substances) then a resistance to apoptosis/necrosis was subsequently induced by the addition of higher amounts of NO gas. This resistance was linked to an increased counterregulation through the synthesis of heat shock proteins, the enzyme hemoxygenase and ferritin proteins that can store iron in a non-redox active form (Kim 1995).

The system of genetic and supragenetic counterregulation against nitrosative and oxidative stress is proven in all animals

As already documented the system of genetic and supragenetic counterregulations is much more comprehensive and complex. A crucial point is that a part of the counterregulation for the stabilization of the redox milieu is the export of highly oxidized proteins by "retrovirus-like" particles and an increased synthesis of the repair enzyme RT. Montagnier identified both of these factors as being "unspecific HIV characteristics" (Tahi 1997). They actually occur in AID and AIDS patients not as causes, but on the contrary as consequences of a severe or long-term immune stress status and have nothing to do with an "HIV infection". This evolutionary-biological switching from a Type I reaction to a Type II reaction in states of highly acute or long-term immune stress has been demonstrated in all animals from microbes to human beings. As the cell symbionts in human cells were former bacteria they are also confronted, under severe and/or long-term stress, with the strategic dichotomy, literally, of "gas pedal" or "brakes". The net result of the counterregulation of the gas-driven micro-Gaian milieu are subject to intricately networked, non-linear adherence to the rules that have only recently, at least in principal, been recognized. The knowledge that all plant cells also react to stress stimuli by producing NO as a protective gas is helpful here. What is remarkable is the fact that plant cells using the unique messenger substance NO and its capacity to diffuse, can relay alarm signals to distant plant cells within its cell system. These primarily unaffected plant cells become subsequently and in increasing numbers resistant to the same initial stress stimulus, as the warning signal triggered an adequate counterregulation in good time. Plants have also developed a dual strategy although they do not have a specific immune cell network. They react by closing down NO production and the formation of ROS (superoxide anion, hydrogen peroxide) when confronted with microbial toxins that trigger a physical/chemical reaction, with a too strong UV irradiation or with heat stress. The affected plant cells respond to acute stress attacks with a hypersensitive Type I reaction and programmed cell death or necrosis. Simultaneously a series of transcription factors are stimulated via a highly networked alternating cooperation between NO and ROS that activate, on a genetic level, a multitude of expressions for the biosynthesis of enzymes. These effect a Type II protective reaction that inhibits NO/ROS/ONOO production and lowers the increased calcium level (Delledonne 1998, Dangl 1998, Hachtel 1998). The ratio of cyclic guanosine monophosphate (cGMP) to cyclic adenosine monophosphate (cAMP) plays an important role in this process. The cGMP, activated by NO, participates in many productive metabolic processes, while the cAMP, as opponent, brakes overreactions. The ratio of cGMP to cAMP is regulated in human cells by corticosteroid hormones (glucocortico steroids) from adrenal glands in favor of cAMP. Practically all stress influences provoke in T-cells as net effect a strong increase of cAMP. The result is a loss of function and the dwindling of T-helper cells (AID) (Fauci 1974, 1975, Hadden 1977, Haynes 1978, Cupps 1982, Coffey 1985, Calvano 1986). Glucocorticoids infiltrate the T-helper cells, bond with transcription factors and inhibit via a chain reaction the synthesis of all cytokines, type 1 cytokines and type 2 cytokines. The only exception is the synthesis of certain repair phase cytokines, like transforming growth factor (TGF) and platelet derived growth factor (PDGF) (Brattsand 1996). Every doctor knows this fact, including the laboratory specialists Gallo and Montagnier.

Polyamines are synthesized by TGF and prostaglandin PGE2 from arginine in competition with the NO synthesis via the enzyme arginase. These inhibit the production of cytotoxic NO and activate repair mechanisms. Included in this process is an increased production of the repair enzyme reverse transcriptase (RT) (overview Lincoln 1997).

Gallo left a lead as evidence for his ploy. In 1984 the Gallo team had used T-helper cells from homosexual AID and AIDS patients "as evidence of the isolation and continuous production of cytopathic retroviruses" as well as for the production of the "anti-HIV antibody test" (Popovic 1984, Gallo 1984, Schüpbach 1984, Sarngadharan 1984). External colleagues participated in the laboratory work. Two of these assistants worked for Litton Bionetics,

Kensington, MD, USA. In 1987 they reported on the way the Gallo team had treated the T-helper cells of the AID and AIDS patients. Among other things they disclosed: "Stimulation in vitro [in cell cultures] could be provided by mitogen or added cells (allogenic antigens) . . . . Certain manipulations of culture conditions were found to improve the outcome, e.g., cocultivation of patient cells with mitogen stimulated peripheral blood leukocytes from uninfected donors. Isolation of virus from cultured cells also was substantially facilitated by inclusion of hydrocortisone in the culture media" (Sarngadharan 1987). The statement by scientists participating in the "HIV isolation" in Gallo's laboratory confirmed the simulated "HIV isolation" and the use of released proteins from human cells from the cell culture as protein antigens for the "anti-HIV antibody test" (Kremer 1998 a, 1998 c):

1. Hydrocortisone is a glucocorticoid.
2. Glucocorticoids inhibit the increase and proliferation of human T-helper cells. They effect in all physiological, psychological and pathophysiological states of stress an effective immune suppression (Gabrielsen 1967, Machinodan 1970).
3. Real existing retroviruses in human T-helper cells can only proliferate when the enzymes for the duplication and division of the DNA strand of the T-helper cells—the DNA polymerases—are present and active (Levine 1991).
4. Glucocorticoids inhibit the synthesis and activities of the DNA polymerases of the T-helper cells (Gillis 1979 a, 1979 b).
5. Glucocorticoids inhibit the genetic expression of the enzyme NO synthase for the production of cytotoxic NO on the genetic transcription level and at the translation stage of RNA transcripts in the biosynthesis of proteins (Kunz 1996).
6. Glucocorticoids promote the synthesis of repair enzymes and the repair processes in T-helper cells (Brattsand 1996, Lincoln 1997).
7. The indispensable prerequisites for the production of "HIV" in T-helper cells are stimulation by the type 1 cytokine IL-2 (Gallo 1984, Montagnier 1985) and mitogens. Glucocorticoids block the effects of IL-2 and mitogens (Gillis 1979 a, 1979 b).
8. The production of type 1 cytokines in the human organism is subject to a day/night rhythm. When the glucocorticoid (cortisol) level in the blood serum is at its lowest during the night and in the early morning, the production of inflammatory type 1 cytokines is at its peak (Petrovsky 1998).
9. Glucocorticoids are employed clinically for the treatment of type 1 cytokine overreactions in countless inflammatory and autoimmune

> diseases, leukaemia, and tumors as well as for organ transplant patients to prevent rejection of the transplant (Cupps 1982).

The statement: "Isolation of virus from cultured cells also was substantially facilitated by inclusion of hydrocortisone in the culture media" (Sarngadharan 1987) is objectively misleading. All specialists are agreed that the indispensable prerequisite for the cultivation of retroviruses from human T-helper cells is blocked by the glucocortico steroid hydrocortisone. In order to be scientifically correct the quoted passage should read: "The production of the repair enzyme reverse transcriptase (RT) in human cells, which were cultivated by stimulation with mitogens and type 1 cytokine IL-2, was substantially facilitated by the inclusion of hydrocortisone in the culture media".

In his original publication in 1984 Gallo kept quiet about the manipulation of the cell culture of T-helper cells of AID and AIDS patients with hydrocortisone for "isolation of HIV" (Gallo 1984). After publication of these facts (Kremer 1998 a, 1998 c) Gallo was asked at an international press conference at the World AIDS Congress in Geneva in 1998 whether it was the case that: 1. He and his assistants had added hydrocortisone to the culture media "for proof of isolation and the continuous production of HIV" in T-helper lymph cell cultures of homosexual AID and AIDS patients. 2. Whether the "HIV isolation" from cells that had been previously activated by stress stimulation with mitogens and interleukin-2 had been substantially facilitated by the addition of hydrocortisone.

Gallo countered with the question: "What are you implying?" After persistent questioning by journalists Gallo admitted that it was correct and that during the first experiments for "isolation of HIV", hydrocortisone was added to the "HIV infected" culture media. All other comments as to how the "retrovirus isolation" had been substantially facilitated when he and is team had blocked the proliferation of "retroviruses" with hydrocortisone, were declined by Gallo. The questions to Gallo, Montagnier and their colleagues, posed by representatives of the German Research Group for Investigative Medicine and Journalism (regimed) have remained unanswered to this day. A few weeks after the World AIDS Congress it was prematurely announced in the press that Gallo was to be awarded the most prestigious medical research prize in Germany. The HIV/AIDS establishment was alarmed, the award ceremony was planned for a number of months later in 1999. A statement from the president of the Paul-Ehrlich-Stiftung, which awards this research prize, declared: "This prize is not being awarded for the discovery of HIV"

(Paul-Ehrlich-Stiftung 1998). An absurd statement as bar the "isolation of HTLV-I, HTLV-II and HTLV-III (HIV)" by Gallo there is no "discovery of human exogenous retroviruses" (the reason for the prize). HTLV-I and HTLV-II were produced by Gallo with the same laboratory techniques as the "retrovirus characteristics" in leukaemia cell cultures and in contrast to "HIV" play no role clinically. "HIV", however, was supposed to be threatening all of mankind, why then should the most prestigious German research prize be awarded to Gallo "for not discovering HIV"? In his acceptance speech for this special honour Gallo does not mention a single word explaining whether "HIV isolation" had been substantially facilitated by hydrocortisone. He also did not waste a single word about concrete isolation techniques for "retroviruses", the "discovery" of which, under his auspices, he described in detail. In the listing of "retroviruses" that he had discovered, Gallo remained silent about the "very first human retrovirus", HL23V, propagated by Gallo in 1976. This oversight is interesting because for the "isolation" of that particular "human retrovirus" Gallo was still using the standard rules that he ignored for the "isolation of HIV".

The absurdity of this "first human retrovirus" is, however, that this particle of "HL23V" did not constitute a "retrovirus" and also that Gallo no longer tried to maintain this assertion (Papadopulos-Eleopulos 1996, 1998 a).

Also, it has also to be said that it is an irresolvable logical contradiction to claim that retroviruses find it considerably easier to propagate in human T-helper cells with the addition of hydrocortisone.

The assumption that evidence of the repair enzyme RT under the influence of hydrocortisone, is the result of the activation of TGF and prostaglandins as a Type II counterregulation of cell dyssymbiosis against oxidative and nitrosative stress stimulation, has been supported by an overwhelming amount of clinical and experimental research data. The fact that Gallo remained quiet about the inclusion of hydrocortisone and to this day is not prepared to give an explanation proves that he has systematically suppressed all evidence that contradicts this claim of "HIV isolation" and all evidence that the protein antigens used for the "HIV test" could be exposed as human cell proteins. The only possible explanation is that Gallo had sold the products of evolutionary-biological counterregulation of human T-helper cells under oxidative and nitrosative stimulation stress as "retrovirus HIV" and as "anti-HIV antibody test" to the scientific community and the population of the world as a whole.

But how could Gallo "cultivate the virus en masse" (Montagnier in an interview 1997, Tahi 1997) in order to gain enough "HIV proteins" as protein antigens for the "HIV test"?

The laboratory trickery behind the mass production of "HIV Proteins" needed for the assembly of the "HIV test"

T-helper cells only have a limited lifespan. As Gallo had made his "retrovirus HTLV-I and HTLV-II" appear in leukemic lymph cell lines, it seemed appropriate to establish the mass production of "HIV proteins" by having the "HIV particles" mature out of unlimitedly cultivatable, transformed leukaemia cancer cells via prooxidative and nitrosative stress stimulation. For this purpose Gallo chose cell line H9 (HUT78) that came from patients with T-helper cell leukaemia. Gallo cultivated this H9 cell line together with T-helper cells from AID and AIDS patients and claimed that the observed "unspecific characteristics" were proof that "HIV" had relocated from the T-helper cells to the T-helper cells leukaemia cells (Gallo 1984). This process is called co-cultivation. As the cancer cells are highly counterregulated cells in a state of decompensated cell dyssymbiosis we can say according to the AEDS concept that these leukaemia cells in a co-cultivated cell culture will respond to the NO gas production in the T-helper immune cells by increasing counterregulation. The NO gas produced after oxidative and nitrosative stress stimulation also diffuses between the two cell types. The "immortal" T-leukaemia cells that as a consequence of the decompensated cell dyssymbiosis (heavily reduced vitality and number of mitochondria) no longer show signs of programmed cell death, behave in the mixed stimulated cell culture similarly, but even more distinctly, to cell culture B in the Montagnier team's experiment in 1991. The leukaemia cells increase the already running counterregulations and display chronic "HIV characteristics" (increased RT production, increased budding of export particles for oxidized cell proteins). And exactly that was the case. Cancer cells respond to NO exposure, depending on the dosage, with cell inhibition (cytostasis), subsequently with a heightened counterregulation (Brüne 1996, Lincoln 1997). Up until now nobody has been able to demonstrate actual "HIV production" in the H9 leukaemia cells, as was also the case of the T-helper cells of AIDS patients. Also the H9 cells were by no means destroyed by "HIV" as they should have been according to the "HIV/AIDS theory". Again in these limitlessly cultivatable leukaemia cells unspecific "HIV characteristics" remained, nobody has demonstrated the actual presence of "HIV retroviruses" in these cells. Though in this way any old cell debris from the cell fluid from this "immortal" cell culture can be centrifuged out and some of these scrap proteins can be used as antigens to assemble the "HIV test" (Sarngadharan 1984). In "HIV tests" these proteins from the special refuse of co-cultivation (foreign proteins from human cells) could react with increased amounts of antibodies in the blood serum of probands. An absurd vicious circle with tragic consequences.

The "invisible hand of the market"

Unspecific pseudo evidence was published for the "isolation of HIV" and the "existence of HIV"—unspecific "HIV characteristics" and unspecific "molecular markers"—but never challenged in scientific discourse. The scientific contemporary witness, Professor De Harven, after decades of laboratory experience and as an internationally renowned expert in the field of detection and isolation of retroviruses categorically stated:

"When around 1980, R. Gallo and his followers attempted to demonstrate that certain retroviruses can be suspected of representing; human pathogens, to the best of my bibliographical recollection, electron microscopy was never used to demonstrate directly viremia in the studied patients. Why? Most probably, EM results were negative and swiftly ignored! But over-enthusiastic retrovirologists continued to rely on the identification of "viral markers", attempting to salvage their hypothesis. When retrovirus particles are legion, the study of molecular markers can be useful, and provide an approach to quantification probably better than direct particle counting under the EM (which I always found very difficult). But when, using EM, retrovirus particles are absent relying exclusively on 'markers' is a methodological nonsense. 'Markers' of what? . . . In conclusion, and after extensive reviewing of the current AIDS research literature, the following statement appears inescapable: neither electron microscopy nor molecular markers have so far permitted a scientifically sound demonstration of retrovirus isolation directly from AIDS patients" (De Harven 1998 c).

The "invisible hand of the market" that had produced the conditions for heavy and long-term immune stress (AID) (nitrite gases, the raw materials of recreational drugs, pharmaceutical substances for antibiotic, chemotherapeutic and analgesic abuse, highly contaminated coagulating protein preparations and blood products etc. etc., conditions for poverty), then arranged the patented marketing of "unspecific HIV characteristics"—the subsequent symptoms not the causes of acquired immune stress syndrome: "anti-HIV antibody tests", "anti-retroviral" substances for "anti-HIV prevention" and "HIV synthesis inhibition".

The agencies of the "invisible hand of the market" (Centers for Disease Control, CDC, National institutes for Health, NIH, Food and Drug Administration, FDA) had already issued warnings about the "human immunodeficiency virus" (CDC and NIH 1982, CDC, FDA, and NIH 1983) before the desired product design was developed and marketable (Popovic 1984, Gallo 1984, Sarngadharan 1984, Schüpbach 1984).

"Unfortunately, the emergence of acquired immunodeficiency syndromes (AIDS) in 1981 gave the retrovirus establishment an opportunity to transform what could have been only an academic flop into a public health tragedy . . . Soon after the first cases of "Gay related immune deficiency" were described by Gottlieb it was obvious for all observers that Gallo and his associates were going to jump on the new syndrome as a Godsent opportunity to attempt to justify the lavish federal budgets they had consumed on retroviruses over the past 10 years. In 1980, the scientific community was getting more and more concerned about the absence of results in "The War against Cancer" based on retrovirus hunting. The minor episode of HTLV 1 was not enough, by far, to calm the fears of grossly misdirected federal research funds. The fact that the syndrome, soon tactically renamed "AIDS", had nothing to do with cancer was apparently of little embarrassment for Gallo. Frequent association with Kaposi sarcoma helped to blur the difference in the eyes of the public. Dominated by the media, by special pressure groups and by the interests of several pharmaceutical companies, the AIDS establishment in his efforts to control the disease lost contact with open-minded, peer-reviewed medical science since the unproven HIV/AIDS hypothesis received 100% of the research funds while all other hypotheses were ignored. The general public and the medical community were made to believe that the presence of circulating antibodies is diagnostic of this disease . . . And to ensure that the AIDS establishment could profitably continue to flourish, research on any dissenting (i.e. non-HIV) hypothesis was carefully prevented by tight control of research funding and by the extreme difficulty of publishing anywhere any dissenting views . . . . In the late 1980s, I was considering adding to my research program in Toronto more EM observations on samples from AIDS patients. Unfortunately, by that time the media and the CDC had so perfectly orchestrated the panic of a plague-like epidemic that I was quickly made to understand that my assistants would all transfer out of the lab if I had insisted to activate such a program . . . . The HIV seropositivity test was still at that time regarded as providing reliable diagnostic data. Since then, Papadopulos and the Australian team have demonstrated that this is very far from the truth" (De Harven 1998 b, Papadopulos-Eleopulos 1993 a).

In comprehensive scientific analyses the internationally renowned research group of Eleni Papadopulos-Eleopulos and her colleagues at the Royal Perth Hospital and the University of Western Australia have published numerous critical publications about the "isolation of HIV", the construction of the "anti-HIV antibody test", AIDS-indicating diseases, their causes and proliferation as well as about HIV/AIDS therapy (Papadopulos-Eleopulos 1988, 1992 a, 1992 b, 1993 a, 1993b, 1995 a, 1995 b, 1995 c, 1996, 1997 a, 1997 b, 1997 c, 1998 a, 1998 b, 1999, 2000 a, 2000 b, Turner 1998).

In German-speaking countries the most important critical studies on the same questions about "HIV isolation", "HIV test", AIDS diseases, AIDS therapy and AIDS politics have been published by the study group Ernährung und Immunität (Nutrition and Immunity) in Bern and the research group regimed (Research Group for Investigative Medicine and Journalism) in Stuttgart as well as the Zentrum zur Dokumentation für Naturheilverfahren (ZDN) (Center for the Documentation of Natural Healing Processes) in Essen (Hässig 1993,1994 a, 1994 b, 1996 a, 1996 b, 1997 a, 1997 b, 1998 a 1998 b, Kremer 1990, 1994, 1996 a, 1996 b, 1998 a, 1998 b, 1998 c, 2000 b, 2000 c, Lanka 1994, 1995, 1997, ZDN 1995, 1998).

Chapter VIII

The Solution to the Cancer Puzzle

Why normal cells become cancerous—degeneration of the cancer cells into an embryonic state is programmed by evolutionary biology, and is the result of mitochondrial inactivation

Three quarters of a century ago the German biochemist Otto Warburg made a crucial discovery: He had recognized that unlike normal differentiated cells, cancer cells could produce the universal energy-bearing molecule adenosine triphosphate (ATP) mostly without the assistance of molecular oxygen from the cell symbionts—the mitochondria. Warburg was the first to demonstrate "Atmungsferment" in mitochondria. This German term for one of the indispensable enzymes of the mitochondrial respiratory chain has remained in use to this day in English scientific terminology. The astonishing thing about Warburg's discovery was that the cancer cells that he studied synthesized ATP, to a large extent outside of the mitochondria in the cytoplasm, from the degradation products of glucose with the aid of enzymes, even when oxygen was available (Warburg 1924). This finding contradicted the Pasteur effect of the 19th Century French chemist and discoverer of microbes, Louis Pasteur, who stated that enzymatic glucose degradation is inhibited by microbes in the presence of oxygen (Pasteur 1876).

As the ATP production of the cancer cells occurred directly from the degradation products of glucose in the metabolic chain up to pyruvate, before entry of pyruvate in the mitochondria, Warburg called this process aerobic glycolysis (in the presence of oxygen, while the fermentative glucose degradation observed by Pasteur in the absence of oxygen is termed anaerobic glycolysis).

The controversy on the Warburg Phenomenon and on RNA-tumor viruses

Warburg and his colleagues at the Kaiser Wilhelm Institute in Berlin deduced from the anomaly in the Pasteur effect in cancer cells that the oxygen in the respiratory chain could no longer be used due to a defect of the Atmungsferment (Warburg 1949, 1956). This original substantiation of the "Warburg phenomenon" prompted controversy and bitter scientific feuds for decades with no satisfactory explanation for cancer metabolism. Some years before his death there was a final historic confrontation at the annual meeting of Nobelists at Lindau on Lake Constance. Warburg was awarded the Nobel Prize in 1931 for his discovery of Atmungsferment as well as for the evidence of aerobic glycolysis in cancer metabolism, and a second Nobel Prize in 1944, but was prevented from receiving the award. Warburg gave a lecture at Lindau in 1966 on "The Prime Cause and Prevention of Cancer" that triggered fierce criticism among his colleagues:

"Oxygen gas, the donor of energy in plants and animals, is dethroned in the cancer cells and replaced by an energy yielding reaction of the lowest living forms, namely, a fermentation of glucose . . . . Nobody today can say that one does not know what cancer is or what the prime cause of cancer is. On the contrary, there is no disease whose prime cause is better known, so that today ignorance is no longer an excuse that one cannot do more about prevention. That prevention of cancer will come there is no doubt, for man wishes to survive. But how long prevention will be avoided depends on how long the prophets of agnosticism will succeed in inhibiting the application of scientific knowledge in the field of cancer research. In the meantime, millions of men must die of cancer unnecessarily" (Warburg 1967, Werner 1996).

There are a number of objective objections to the assumption that the "Warburg phenomenon" is caused by a primary structural defect in the respiratory chain of mitochondrial cell symbionts. But in 1966 due to the research techniques at that time Warburg's hypothesis on the structural blockade of the OXPHOS system could neither be definitively refuted nor confirmed. Instead, Warburg was confronted with criticism that he had not made sufficient allowances for the tumorigenic role of the retroviruses that in those days were still termed RNA tumor viruses (Racker 1981).

The postulate of RNA retroviruses originated in 1911. The cancer researcher Peyton Rous filtered a cell-free extract from a muscle tumor though gauze with extremely fine pores (diameter under 120 nanometers). He injected the filtrate into chickens and was able to induce malignant sarcomas (cancer of the connective tissues). From then on it was referred to as Rous sarcoma virus (from the Latin: *virus* = poison). Rous himself had misgivings in viewing his filtrate as infectious cells: "The first tendency will be to regard the self-perpetuating agent active in this sarcoma of the fowl as a minute parasitic organism. Analogy with several infectious diseases of man and the lower animals, caused by ultramicroscopic organisms, gives support to this view of the findings, and at present work is being directed to its experimental verification. But an agency of another sort is not out of the question. It is conceivable that a chemical stimulant, elaborated by neoplastic cells, might cause the tumor in another host and bring about in consequence a further production of the same stimulant" (Rous 1911).

Rous' discovery was confirmed in countless experiments on birds and mice. In the ensuing development of electron microscopes in the 1930s the possibility of making such virus particles visible played an important role. As Claude, after the WWII demonstrated via electron microscopic photographs of the Rous sarcoma virus particles in chickens, "the direct observation of virus particles in these experimental tumors gave an enormous [today, we would perhaps say excessive!] impetus to virus research in oncology" (Claude 1947, De Harven 1998 b 1998 c). But intensive and elaborate experiments to demonstrate virus particles in human cancer cells met a complete lack of success:

"Virus-like particles were occasionally reported but convinced nobody. Typical viruses were never conclusively demonstrated. This was in sharp contrast with the highly reproducible demonstration, by EM, of viruses in a variety of murine and avian leukemias and tumors" (De Harven 1998 b, De Harven 1965).

Evidence of retroviruses in human cancer cells has never been demonstrated

And while Warburg was confronted by colleagues with the notion that RNA tumor viruses were the probable cause of human cancer cells, the retrovirus cancer research scene had decisively changed:

"Publication of these negative findings [about the lack of EM evidence of retroviruses in human tumor cells] failed to discourage fanatical virus hunters! . . . Unfortunately many cell debris and vesicular fragments, when air-dried for negative staining, form similar 'tailed' structures. Interpreting 'tailed' particles as RNA tumor viruses was therefore a bonanza for virus hunters! Still, we had demonstrated that 'tailed' virions were preparation artifacts which can be avoided by proper control of the osmolarity and by osmium fixation prior to negative staining, or by critical-point drying. The chaos created by reports on 'tailed' particles damaged the credibility of EM in the search for cancer related viruses. Cow's milk and human milk were being screened for 'tailed' particles and Sol Spiegelman (then a well-known retrovirus researcher) was eloquent on the possible risks of breast feeding . . ." (De Harven 1998 b).

From this point in time onwards the combined electron microscopic and biochemical identification of retroviruses, precisely following the predetermined standard rules, became gradually displaced to be replaced by "molecular markers" (De Harven 1998 c) for "proof, isolation and identification" (Popovic 1984) of retroviruses in human tumor, leukaemia and, finally, lymph cells. According to the latest figures from the German Krebsforschungszentrum (Cancer Research Center) of "viruses responsible for tumors" in humans there are about 220 different viruses that "promote the growth of human cells" (Kohlstädt 2000), almost double the number of human cancer types. Decisive insights for understanding the cancer puzzle were gained, roughly thirty years after the introduction of "molecular markers" as a substitute for proper retrovirus isolation, through the groundbreaking findings of NO and cell symbiosis research which were able to integrate research data from many other fields of research into a unified understanding.

The Warburg Phenomenon and the transformation of cancer cells are not primarily dependent on structural defects in DNA in the nucleus or in mitochondria

Warburg's hypothesis that the primary cause of the transformation of differentiated cancer cells to undifferentiated cancer cells is brought about by a primary structural defect in the complexes of the oxidative respiratory chain of mitochondria was logical as the cancer cells, despite the normal oxygen tension in the cells, use it only in greatly reduced amounts for the production of ATP. Warburg's assumption, however, turned out to be incorrect:

"In contradiction to the assumption of Warburg those cell lines that are defective in respiration are less tumorigenic than cell lines with active respiration" (Mazurek 1997).

This statement is of fundamental importance, as the earlier research findings confirmed that human cells without traceable structural defects of the mitochondrial DNA (overview Cuezva 1997) or rather without structural defects of the DNA in the nucleus (Lijinsky 1973, 1992), transform to cancer cells. These findings, however, shake the doctrine prevailing to this day—that the transformation to cancer cells is triggered by structural defects of the DNA sequences in the nucleus (chance mutations, viral infections, toxic DNA damage, radiation injury etc.).

Warburg's original discovery in the 1920s that cancer cells gain their operational energy mostly from glucose degradation in the cytoplasm without using the available oxygen, thus through aerobic glycolysis, was time and again confirmed in many experiments on cancer cell cultures and in animal experiments (Warburg 1929, Crabtree 1929, Burk 1967, Krebs 1972, Racker 1976, Weinhouse 1976, Eigenbrodt 1980, Racker 1981, Argiles 1990, Bagetto 1992, Mathupala 1997, Mazurek 1997, Bannasch 1997, Brand 1997 a, Capuano 1997).

Aerobic glycolysis as a source of energy for transformed cells, however, is not the only energy source. In cases of glucose deficiency cancer cells also use other nourishing substrates, for instance by oxidizing glutamine or degrading galactose (McKeehan 1982, Mazurek 1997). However, the seperation and migration of tumor cells as metastases requires aerobic glycolysis as a driving force and for biosyntheses (Mazurek 1997).

The considerably increased rate of aerobic glucose degradation, around 18- to 38-fold, up to the pyruvate and lactate stage in the citric acid cycle of mitochondria (Golshani-Hebroni 1997, Brand 1997 a 1997 b) balances out the low energy yield of aerobic glycolysis, a mere 5% of the energy available in glucose (Mazurek 1997). The increased glucose turnover and the resulting 19-fold lactate production compared to normal cells in a quiescent state was considered from the time of Warburg's discovery until a few years ago a "metabolic enigma" (Mathupala 1997, Brand 1997 a).

Crucial to the solution of the cancer puzzle is the fact that in liver cancer cells, as well as in other tumor cells, exactly the opposite of the differentiation and proliferation of mitochondria could be demonstrated. The number of mitochondria and activity of the mitochondria in liver cancer cells drastically declines. An apparent paradox appeared (exactly as in the case of the fetal cells shortly before birth) in that the transcripts of RNA messages for the syntheses of the protein complexes of the respiratory chain and for complex V for ATP production (OXPHOS) in comparison to adult liver cells were synthesized in increasing numbers without being converted to protein synthesis. This finding equally applied to the RNA messages of the corresponding nuclear genes and the RNA transcripts of the mitochondrial genes.

By contrast the synthesis of the enzymes for glycolytic ATP production in the cytoplasm is considerably higher in comparison to the adult liver cells. These enzymes are, however, identical in cancer cells to isoforms of the fetal enzymes for glycolysis (above all hexokinase II, whose genetic expression increases 5-fold). As is the case in fetal cells, the synthesis of nucleic acids, enzymes and co-enzymes together with other molecules for enforced DNA synthesis for an increase of cell division is considerably boosted. These molecules are synthesized from components of glucose degradation via a special metabolic pathway (pentose phosphate pathway). Inversely, the influx of glucose degradation products for oxidation in the citric acid cycle of the mitochondria remained moderate, analogous to the fetal cells in liver cancer cells. Also similar to the fetal cells, the transport of hydrogen ions for the mitochondrial OXPHOS system by means of molecular ferries (glycerol 3-phosphate shuttle and malate aspartate shuttle) is restricted or blocked. The hydrogen in normal differentiated cells with an active OXPHOS system is transferred onto shuttles by $NADH^+H^+$ formed in the glycolytic metabolic chain, and then is ferried into the mitochondria.

The similarity between fetal and cancer cells on the genetic, metabolic and bioenergetic level

On a genetic level an equally astonishing similarity occurs between fetal and cancer cells. In both cell types redox-dependent altered transcription factors are stimulated. These switch on promoters (promoters define which gene sequences are expressed for the biosynthesis of proteins and enzyme proteins) and gene sequences that are sensitive to glucose, hypoxia, pseudohypoxia, insulin and glucagon in differentiated adult cells. As a result of the amount of genetic, metabolic and bioenergetic harmony between fetal and cancer cells, "re-fetalization" of tumor cells was coined as the appropriate terminology (overview Cuezva 1997, Capuano 1997, Brand 1997 b, Mathupala 1997, Mazurek 1997, Bagetto 1997, Bannasch 1997, Dorwand 1997, Dang 1997, Golshani-Hebroni 1997).

The bioenergetic cooperation of mitochondrial symbionts with the fetal cells (Cuezva 1997), the replicating cells in the late S-phase of division (Brand 1997 b), the regenerating cells during the wound healing process (Capuano 1997), and tumor cells with varyingly quick rates of reproduction (Cuezva 1997) evidently obey the same rules. The elementary difference between the activity states of the cell types arises from the fact that the fetal cells and the cell symbionts up until birth have not yet been regulated by the OXPHOS system, the replicating cells in the S-phase of division and cells in the early regeneration stage of healing have temporarily not been regulated and the tumor cells are no longer regulated.

The fundamental supposition of the evolutionary biological program of Type-II counterregulation, for the understanding of fetalization and the Warburg Phenomenon

To understand re-fetalization and the Warburg Phenomenon, the following assumptions must be established:

- Like all eukaryotic cells, the human genome developed from the integration of two genome cultures—the archaeal genome and proteobacterial genome. The informational genes originate mostly from archaeal genes, while the operational genes are primarily from proteobacterial genes (Gray 1999).
- The energy-gaining system of the archaeal stem cells in archaic cell symbiosis is glycolysis for enzymatic ATP production. The reduction product is lactate. The genetic equipment for the glycolytic enzymes is evolutionarily conserved. The original energy gain system of the proteobacteria, the precursor cells of the mitochondria (before installation of the respiratory chain) is the energy provision of hydrogen as the reduced end product (by means of hydrogenosomes). In addition, oxidation from glutamine (glutaminolysis) in the citric acid cycle of proteobacteria, that metabolically and evolutionarily is pre-switched to the respiratory chain and the OXPHOS system, could be used as energy source. The oxidation product is glutamate.
- The glycolytic replication system (cell division) is dominated by the archaeal genome portion, the biogenesis of the mitochondria, probably, is dominated by the proteobacterial genome portion (in an interplay between archaeal and proteobacterial genes in the nucleus and the proteobacterial genes in the mitochondria). During the activity phase of cell division (S-phase in physiological cell division, early wound healing phase, fetal cell division, tumor cell division) an effectual production of glycolytic enzymes and phosphometabolites is provided for cell division. The primary stimulation for glycolytic enzymes (hexokinase II etc.) is hydrogen ion diffusion through the mitochondrial membrane. The "quantum dynamic depth" of photon oscillation is less than during the active OXPHOS phase of respiratory cell symbiosis. These reduced quantum dynamic states in tumor cells are interpreted as "dedifferentiated."
- The quantum dynamic states are not, however, linear on/off switches but are subject in their marginal phases to non-linear quasi-deterministic rules that are modulated by complex cellular and cell-spanning influencing variables (Waliszewski 1998).

- The increased "quantum dynamic depths" of the activated cell symbioses enable a greater fluidity via the production of increased amounts of liquid oxides (nitrogen oxide, superoxide, peroxides). Peroxinitrite as product of equal amounts of NO and superoxide anion (O_2^-) seems to play a vital role in the maintenance and variability of the bioenergetic potential of the mitochondrial membrane. The latter serves as a checkpoint for Ca^{2+} cycling. Too high amounts of oxides lead to a sinking of the membrane potential and to an increased membranal permeability (as trigger for apoptosis and necrosis), too small amounts of oxides lead to a stabilization of the membrane potential and a reduced permeability of the membrane (as trigger for degeneration and transformation). As information-bearing genes, the archaeal components of the genome are more sensitive to increased oxide production than the proteobacterial components. In oxidative and nitrosative stress on a genetic level the expression for the biosynthesis of counterregulators is activated via redox-dependent transcription factors. Part of the system of counterregulation is the biosynthesis of type 2 cytokine proteins that inhibit the synthesis of NO as well as the superoxide anion and peroxides and trigger a further cascade of counterregulations (here compactly termed Type-II counterregulations of cell dyssymbiosis).
- The Type-II counterregulation that is modulated beforehand via steroid hormones, insulin hormone, thyroid hormone and other hormones, restricts the OXPHOS activities, increases the membrane potential and diminishes the mitochondrial membrane's permeability as well as weakening the sensitivity of immune and non-immune cells to external stress stimuli. This redox-dependent switch to Type-II status is among other things determined by the strength, duration and type of external and internal stress stimulation, as well as by the cell type, the previous damage to cell symbiosis and the depletion of the antioxidative thiol pool and other enzymatic and non-enzymatic antioxidants.
- Phases of excessive nitrosative stress as a consequence of the bonding of NO and its derivatives to non-protein thiols (nitrosation of glutathione (GHS) to GSNO, cysteine to SNO-Cys etc) lead to the formation of nitrosothiols. After depletion of the thiol pool, NO and its derivatives bond on thiol-containing proteins (nitrosylation of R-SH to RSNO). As a result, the function-regulating characteristics of the cellular control of membrane receptor proteins and ion channels, signal-carrying protein substances, transcription proteins, and enzyme proteins are altered (overview Stamler 1995).

Dissociation of the interaction between different sections of the cellular and mitochondrial genomes

Considering the well-founded conclusion that there are varying thresholds of sensitivity in the archaeal and proteobacterial genome elements against states of nitrosative stress, a dissociation of the interplay between the differently structured genome elements is to be expected. On the one hand under these conditions a massive Type-II counterregulation is triggered by archaeal gene activities to minimize nitrosative stress. On the other hand the proteobacterial gene activities continue synthesizing transcripts for the biosynthesis of the protein complex of the respiratory chain and the OXPHOS system. Because of the continuing blockade of the mitochondrial membrane channels to proteins and ions (especially calcium ions) as a result of the increased membrane potential (Golshani-Hebroni 1997), the proteins for the complexes of the respiratory chain and the OXPHOS system can no longer be optimally supplied.

This networked function model explains the apparent paradox of the provision of transcripts for mitochondrial proteins without a sufficient conversion to protein synthesis, as well as the dwindling number and activities of mitochondria in the transitional activity phases of cell division (fetal cells, late phase of physiological cell division, early wound healing phase) and the permanent cell division phases of tumor cells.

Cancer cells are no longer able to perish (apoptosis or necrosis) from prooxidative stress, since the mitochondrial membranes remain closed after mitosis, due to long-term counterregulation against oxidative and nitrosative stress

Regarding the tumor cells, they are prevented from executing programmed cell death (apoptosis) or sudden cell death (necrosis) as they require a lowering of the mitochondrial membrane potential and the opening of the mitochondrial channels. Instead of this there is a forced aerobic glycolysis for enzymatic ATP production in the cytoplasm. The driving element is hydrogen diffused from the mitochondria. The glucose degradation products of glycolysis are invested in nucleic acid and DNA syntheses for cell division via the pentose phosphate metabolic path. An increased number of phosphorus metabolites from the pentose phosphate metabolic path keep mitosis running. The glycolytic cells transform to tumor cells and remain trapped in the cell division cycle.

The cancerous cells as permanent regression of cellular symbiosis into the early evolutionary-biological stage of protista

So the tumor cell is a permanent regression of oxidative cellular symbiosis to the early evolutionary stage of cell symbiosis between archaea and proteobacteria, the phase of the first eukaryotes that are termed protista (Kremer 1997 b, 1998 d, 1999). In this symbiotic stage (proto-cell symbiosis of the protista) the eukaryotes profited from the hydrogen diffusion of the proteobacteria (overview Gray 1999). Only the later development of a respiratory chain, as electron transport pathway for the electromotive powering of the hydrogen ion compression pumps, enabled the reversion of the hydrogen driving of hydrogenosomes for the oxidative phosphor coupling (OXPHOS) to increase ATP synthesis in mitochondria drastically.

Under pathophysiological conditions, the fluctuating bioenergetic rhythm of cellular symbiosis can be over—or underdriven in two directions (Type-I overregulation or a respective Type-II counterregulation)

Under pathophysiological conditions the “hybrid impulse” of cell symbiosis can be overdriven or underdriven: on the one hand, under the influence of versatile acute stressors the production of oxidative/nitrogen oxides, superoxides and peroxides can be too strongly increased and lead to a breakdown in the counterregulation of the thiol pool and other antioxidative systems. The consequence is a too high fluidity and “acute infection” by the cell symbionts. The membrane potential of the mitochondria sinks below a critical threshold, the permeability of the lock-gates of the mitochondrial membrane, the permeabiity transition (PT), increases leading to too many Ca^{2+} ions and induced proteins being released from the cell symbionts, the cell nuclear DNA and other cell structures are degraded by a cascade of protein-splitting enzymes. Programmed cell death or necrosis occurs dependent on the speed of the decline of oxidative ATP production (overview Richter 1996, Kroemer 1997, Zamzami 1997). The mitochondrially triggered apoptosis and necrosis are the expression of a decompensated dysregulation of cell symbiosis that is dependent on a dominance of the type 1 cytokine profile. That is why this form of reaction of cell symbiosis will be termed here as a Type-I overregulation of cell dyssymbiosis (Type-I AEDS). Clinical manifestations are acute infections, inflammatory processes and, after necrotic cell death, autoimmune reactions and autoimmune illnesses (overview Mosmann 1996, Abbas 1996, Lucey 1996).

On the other hand, under the influence of versatile chronic stressors a too-high nitrosation of non-protein thiols and secondary nitrosylation of thiol proteins can severely inhibit the production of nitrogen oxides, superoxides and peroxides. The consequence is too little fluidity and "chronic infection" by the cell symbionts: The PT channels are severely restricted, and the impaired Ca^{2+} cycling leads to inhibition of the biogenesis of the number and activities of the mitochondria. The bioenergetic "hybrid impulse" reverses, the supply of hydrogen ions by the glycerol 3-phosphate and malate aspartate shuttling from the cytoplasm to the mitochondria is disturbed, and the compression of hydrogen ions by electron transfer in the respiratory chain for the OXPHOS system of the mitochondria is impeded. The cell symbionts produce smaller amounts of ATP for their own needs. Surplus hydrogen ions diffuse into the cytoplasm and increase the "antioxidative stress" of transforming cells resulting from the critical shifting of the phase of the negative redox potential. The consequence is the continued genetic expression of the fetal isoform of the glycolytic enzyme hexokinase II, which switches on the metabolic chain for a predominant ATP production through aerobic glycolysis.

Why, without compensation of the thiol pools, chemotherapeutic agents selectively strengthen the Type-II counterregulation of cancer cells, favoring the formation of resistant metastases

The degradation products of sugar metabolism are invested in forced cell division via the pentose phosphate metabolic pathway. The cells are re-fetalized, the alternate switch of the previously intact cell symbiosis no longer functions, and the transformed cells remain trapped in the division cycle (overview Cuezva 1997, Capuano 1997, Brand 1997 b). Without the compensation of the thiol pools and the phase reversal to an adequate negative redox potential aerobic glycolysis can no longer be switched off. The primary preventative and therapeutic consequence can only be the biological compensation therapy of the thiol pool.

According to this model of an overdriven Type-II cell dyssymbiosis (identical to the archaic cell symbiosis of the hydrogen-donating proto-mitochondria) it is to be expected that highly glycolytic tumor cells are most strongly counterregulated and feature only minor NO synthesis. For this reason NO-insensitive daughter cells of highly glycolytic tumor cells should have the best chances of survival on their metastatic wanderings as, due to their high lactate production, they secrete increased proteolytic (protein-splitting) enzymes, metalloproteinases and other proteinases which pave the way through the extracellular matrix, and they gain access to the capillary blood vessels. On the other hand chemotherapeutics, which activate the synthesis of cytotoxic NO gas, for instance cisplatin (Kröncke 1995, Son 1995) or taxol (Jun 1995), increase the risk of selectively further increasing a Type-II counterregulation and favoring the formation of resistant metastases.

From the very beginning a constant fine tuning is required via the thiol pool and other enzymatic and non-enzymatic antioxidants, in order to be sure of the best gas mixture from NO, ROS, and peroxinitrite for the micro-Gaian milieu of an intact cell symbiosis. Under these conditions peroxinitrite subsequently oxidizes neighboring sulfhydryl groups (SH groups) in proteins in the inner mitochondrial membrane and short-circuits the SH groups. In this way the opening of the mitochondrial membrane is facilitated without loss of the membrane potential. Analogously peroxinitrite oxidizes SH groups from mitochondrial proteins and enables the enzymatic division of oxidized NAD^+ by hydrolysis. The split product of NAD^+, ADP ribose, activates the specific release of Ca^{2+} from the mitochondria into the cytoplasm. The enzyme Cyclophilin (peptidyl-prolyl cis/trans isomerase) participates in the hydrolysis of NAD^+ (in ADP ribose and nicotine acid amid) that also opens the PT channels for the Ca^{2+} metabolic pathway (Richter 1996, Zamzami 1997, Kroemer 1997).

The treatment of organ transplant patients with Cyclosporin A, an immunosuppressive and carcinogenic mycotoxin, as model of the provocation of cancer cell transformation via closing of the mitochondrial membranes

The blockade of Cyclophilin enzymes through long-term medication with Cyclosporine A is an illuminating model for the onset of cancer resulting from the reversal of the bioenergetic and metabolic differentiation and maturation of the cell symbionts and the related re-fetalization of tumor cells (Type-II counterregulation of cell dyssymbiosis). This substance isolated from fungi (an undecapeptide) has been used since 1983 on organ transplant patients to inhibit rejection reactions, but is also employed on patients with autoimmune illnesses. This drug has induced the development of lymphomas (cancer of the B-cells) and other lymphoproliferative disorders, as well as carcinomas and opportunistic infections in a not inconsiderable proportion of transplant patients (Penn 1991). This clinical manifestation equates in a fatal way to the appearance of Kaposi's sarcomas, lymphomas, carcinomas and opportunistic infections since the 1960s in organ transplant patients (Krikorian 1978, Penn 1979, 1981).

Cyclosporin A forms a complex with Cyclophilin that is termed immunophilin in immune cells. This complex bonds to calcineurin (serine-threonine phosphatase) and inhibits its activities. Calcineurin is activated in type 1 T-helper cells when they react with their receptors to the signal of a suitable antigen MHC complex of antigen-presenting cells. In this case the calcium level in the Th1 immune cells is raised and calcineurin splits a phosphoric ester off a particular transcription factor in the cytoplasm. This then moves into the nucleus and triggers the transcription for the biosynthesis of type 1 cytokines, interleukin-2 (IL-2). IL-2 induces the synthesis of interferon-γ, which in turn triggers the synthesis of cytotoxic NO gas as antigen defense.

The bonding of CSA Cyclophilin complexes to calcineurin does not make the latter active and the synthesis of IL-2 does not take place (Clipstone 1992, Schreiber 1992, Bierer 1993). The deficient production of cytotoxic NO in organ transplant patients treated with CSA, provoked by IL-2 inhibition, explains the acquired immune deficiency (i.e. transplantation AIDS) of these patients against intracellular opportunistic agents (fungi, parasites, and mycobacteria).

The operating mechanism of CSA attacks on two different levels:

- The first CSA effect is the inhibited synthesis of type 1 cytokine profiles that favor a Th1-Th2 switch. Subsequently CSA promotes the counterregulation of Type-II cell dyssymbiosis. Increased numbers of type 2 cytokines become effective when the mutual balance between type 1 and type 2 cytokines is disrupted (overview Del Prete 1998, London 1998, D'Elios 1998. O'Gara 1998, Murphy 1998, Carter 1998, Morel 1998, Muraille 1998, Viola 1999, Coffman 1999). Type 2 cytokine stimulates the formation of prostaglandin (PGE 2) that in turn inhibits NO synthesis and causes the peroxinitrite level to sink (overview Lincoln 1997). The peroxinitrite function for the opening of the PT channels is impeded. The result is a limitation of the central function of the mitochondria as balancing pool for the modulation and maintenance of cellular Ca^{2+} homeostasis (overview Richter 1996). The surplus calcium ions are bonded to membranes of cell structures by the over-expression of proteins from the Bcl-2 family. This takes place on the outermost membrane of the mitochondria, the effect being an increased impermeability of the mitochondrial membrane. Bcl-2 acts in this way to impede apoptosis/necrosis in the presence of too large amounts of oxides. The over-expression of Bcl-2 proteins has also been demonstrated in many tumor cells (Mazurek 1997). The expression of the Bcl-2 genes as oncogenes has been traced back to a mutation effect but their biological function can only be grasped once the evolutionary history of cell symbiosis has been sufficiently understood. The increased formation of TGF and PGE triggers simultaneously the production of polyamines that are present in tumor cells in increasing numbers. Polyamines force cell division processes and repair mechanisms of DNA (overview Lincoln 19979.

- The second CSA effect takes place within the mitochondria and combines with the first CSA effect. Cyclophilin D is found in the mitochondrial matrix. It activates a protein complex in the inner mitochondrial membrane (adenosine nucleotide translocator, = ANT) that facilitates the opening of the PT channels. If CSA bonds with Cyclophilin D, ANT is not activated. At the same time CSA blocks the hydrolysis of oxidized NAD^+ so that the specific Ca^{2+} cycling between the mitochondria and the cytoplasm is disrupted. In combination with the depleted peroxinitrite level resulting from the CSA effect in the cytoplasm the CSA effect in the mitochondria builds up. The PT channels of the mitochondria open inadequately or not at all. As the energy potential of the mitochondria can be maintained or even increased programmed cell death or necrosis can no longer be triggered (overview Richter 1996, Kroemer 1997, Zamzami 1997). (See table XII: Model of the mitochondrial channels—open with Cyclophilin and peroxinitrite—close with CSA and peroxinitrite deficiency and Table XIII: The channel rhythm in mitochondrion).

The CSA effects are in no way only selectively operative in T-helper immune cells but also in other immune cells and non-immune cells. Besides the toxic damage to the kidneys and other organs, the appearance of tumors in CSA-treated transplant patients could also be explained by the provocation of a Type-II cell dyssymbiosis (proto-cell symbiosis).

The striking similarities between the cellular symbiosis behavior of immune and cancer cells in organ transplant and AIDS patients

The fact is that there are striking similarities in the immune cells and tumor cells of organ transplant patients (Kaposi's sarcoma, lymphoma, carcinoma) and AIDS patients (Kaposi's sarcoma, lymphoma):

- Type 1 to type 2 cytokine switch
- Inhibition of cytotoxic and calcium-dependent NO synthesis as well as the formation of peroxinitrite by the type 2 cytokine profile

- Closing of the PT pores of the mitochondria due to the absence of oxidation by peroxinitrite of the sulfhydryl groups of the ANT protein complexes (or other protein complexes) in the inner membrane of the mitochondria
- Deficient NDA+ hydrolysis in the mitochondria because of too little peroxinitrite formation, resulting in no release of Ca^{2+} with maintenance of the energy potential of the mitochondrial membrane
- Inadequate permeability of the mitochondrial membrane for calcium ions and for the proteins coded in the nuclear DNA for the complexes of the respiratory chain and the OXPHOS complexes
- Increased readiness of the RNA transcripts for the biosynthesis of proteins of respiratory chain complexes and the OXPHOS complexes (inhibition of the conversion of fetal cells up until the first breath and in tumor cells a permanent inhibition)
- Missing balancing pool of the mitochondria for the calcium ions of the cytoplasm due to increased impermeability of the mitochondrial pores
- Inhibition of apoptosis/necrosis in the mitochondria normally triggered by increased amounts of NO°, ROS, and peroxinitrites, simultaneous maintenance or increase in the energy potential of the mitochondrial membrane
- Inhibition of the biogenesis of mitochondria, strong reduction in numbers and activities, loss of differentiation and maturation of cell symbionts
- Hydrogen ion diffusion from the mitochondria into the cytoplasm
- Forced aerobic glycolysis for enzymatic ATP production, stimulated by the expression of the fetal isoenzyme, hexokinase II, located on the outermost mitochondrial membrane, in tumor cells always the expression of hexokinase II, irrespective of the hexokinase type of the differentiated original cells (hexokinase type I to IV)
- Enzymatic ATP synthesis mainly by aerobic glycolysis and investment of the glucose metabolic products, via the pentose phosphate metabolic pathway, in an increased rate of division
- Production of higher amounts of lactate and higher amounts of fetal metalloproteinases and other proteinases

The network of energy and information flow is a program that is self-organized by the variable "semi-conductor function" of macromolecular protein complexes

Cuezva and his colleagues have demonstrated the processes of re-fetalization of tumor cells at the transcription level (transcription of the DNA sequences in the nucleus and in the mitochondrial genome resulting from the signals by transcription factors into messenger RNA) and at the translation level (the translation of messenger RNA in protein synthesis for the biogenesis of mitochondria). As a consequence of the striking similarities between the genetic processes in the fetal cells shortly before birth and in tumor cells they conclude: "The million dollar question here is who orchestrates this cellular response?"

And after debating the role of genetic factors for the expression of tumor cells they summarize: "We are still far from reaching the expected answer that could explain the altered energetic metabolism of tumor cells, a challenge of the scientific community set out more than 60 years ago" (Cuezva 1997).

In the article by Cuezva and his co-workers there is no mention of the studies of NO research. The question about the orchestrator of the transformation processes of tumor genesis, on a genetic or non-genetic level, was wrongly posed. The answer is:

There are no orchestrators. The popular dogma that genes have stored and can retrieve the program of life is a biological myth. The network of energy flows is the program and it is self-organizing. The information pattern of living cells and cell systems is modulated and dependent on fluidity and "quantum dynamic depths." The macromolecular components (genes, proteins, transcription factors, enzyme proteins and many others) perform a "semiconductor" function for the upping and downing of regulations of the complex supragenetic network of cellular symbiosis. Physically the electron flows do not alter in proportion to the voltage as with metals but in "tailback stages." The electrons have to physically overcome the energy gaps in order to be able to move from the valance band to the conduction band in which they can move freely. Biophysically the macromolecules feature a relatively large energy gap of several millivolts that enable a corresponding modulation range.

During cancerous transformation, the macromolecular semiconductor function of the mitochondrial membranes is invariably inhibited, via forced restriction of the fluidic micro-Gaian gas mixture

The macromolecular protein complex of the PT lock-gates of the mitochondrial pores is one such "tailback stage." There are variable physiological and pathophysiological states of the opening and closing of the PT lock-gates. These determine the fate of cell symbiosis and are governed by the proportions of fluid NO and superoxide anions (O_2^-), respectively, and the diffusion product of both oxides—fluid peroxinitrite (micro-Gaian milieu). Extreme, intolerable amounts of the components of the oxide mixture (overoxidation) lead to programmed or unprogrammed cell death (apoptosis/necrosis) (Richter 1996) via an energy loss of the membrane potential of the cell symbionts. The result is an uncontrollable opening of the PT lock-gates and an outflux and influx (Ca^{2+} cycling) of large amounts of calcium ions inducing a cascade of energetic and metabolic chain reactions ending in cell death. *Too small amounts of the diffusion product peroxinitrite can trigger a transformation to tumor cells (permanent regression to the state of proto-cell symbiosis before the development of the respiratory chain in mitochondria) in cells that are actively dividing.* Analogous degradation states are provoked in cells that are no longer actively dividing (mature nerve and muscle cells and the retina). The synthesis and regulatory tasks of the fluid oxides are interlaced in a highly complex manner with all energetic, metabolic and informational procedures of the complete cell and the organism as a whole.

Since isomerase enzymes modulate the semiconductor properties of the macromolecules, the manipulation of the isomerase enzyme Cyclophilin with Cyclosporin A in organ transplant patients leads to cancer cell transformation

In cellular terms it is more important that Cyclophilins are isomerases. They are enzymes that catalyze the isomery (from the Greek: *isos* = same + *meron* = part) of the molecules. Isomery is the phenomenon that molecular substances with the same configurations with diverse atoms (sum formula) can assume a different structural composition of the atoms. For instance, lactic acid has the same sum formula as glycerine aldehyde and dihydroxy acetone but a different structural formula. In addition the spacial composition of the same molecules with the same sum and structural formula can be different. The biochemical and biophysical characteristics, including the semiconductor functions of the macromolecule, can considerably change through isomery. Isomerase enzymes such as Cyclophilin can influence the energy flows and informational patterns dramatically by activating or inhibiting. The evident interaction of Cyclophilin isomerases with calcium cycling, NO synthesis, oxide synthesis, peroxinitrite formation as well as NAD^+ hydrolysis for the regulation of intact cell symbiosis and the pathologic inhibition of these regulating processes by CSA manipulation of Cyclophilin isomerases demonstrate the basic model of tumor genesis.

The successful evolutionary-biological solution—uncoupling the genomic sections of the cell nucleus and the mitochondria upon low fluid levels during the physiological cell division phase—becomes permanently fixed during cancer cell transformation at the expense of the mitochondrial activity

The explanation of Brand's research group of the archaic regression of energetic and metabolic processes during fetal development, the late phase of the cell division cycle and the early wound healing phase and the necessity of protection from oxidative stress at the expense of energy exploitation is not alone convincing as the mitochondrial genes have, as a general rule, survived without defects for around 2 billion years in an oxidative milieu without the presence of protective proteins. In contrast, during fetal development and also in tumor cells they are particularly inactive despite having their own energy supplies through glutaminolysis and oxidative remnant ATP production. It is more likely that during the increasing cell division phases the cooperation of the archaeal and proteobacterial genome elements in the nucleus is altered and the symbiotic competition-free cooperation with the proteobacterial genes in the mitochondria in this phase is not assured. In these cell division phases, a regulated function of the archaeal genomes is only possible on low fluid levels with a simultaneous choking of the synthesis of nitrogen and oxidative oxides at the expense of mitochondrial activity.

This assumption is also supported by the fact that the cell division apparatus had to have functioned after symbiotic fusion, before the OXPHOS system was installed in mitochondria, and later could not be accommodated to the OXPHOS system. Instead of this the toggle switch between aerobic glycolysis in the late division phase and the OXPHOS system in the active operational phase was the successful solution. This splitting of responsibility has, after all, been able to function for about 2 billion years.

Medications with mitochondrial toxicity lead to an inability to utilize oxygen (pseudohypoxia)

In the case of the transplantation of a foreign organ the massive provocation by alloantigens is answered by excessive nitrosative and oxidative stress. This is suppressed medicamentally by the complex formation of Cyclosporin A with Cyclophilin isomerase. The effect is the inhibition of the synthesis of type 1 cytokines and the compensatory increase in type 2 cytokine profiles. These trigger a cascade of Type-II counterregulations. The result is a choking of NO synthesis, the synthesis of ROS as well as the formation of peroxinitrite, the inhibition of calcium cycling, a strong reduction of mitochondrial activity and the closing of the mitochondrial membrane with a maintained or increased energy potential. Dependent on dosage and duration of the medication and the disposition of the patient, the redox milieu concerning particularly sensitive cells is manipulated according to the physiologically based functional phases of the increased cell division cycle. In the end the same bioenergetic state is signalled in the supragenetic network that also precedes the active cell division cycle. The state corresponds to a pseudohypoxia (an apparent oxygen deficiency from failure to exploit oxygen) and can be termed as such because the OXPHOS machinery of the mitochondria merely performs as if it were dormant (Brand 1997 b) despite sufficient quantities of oxygen being available—almost as if the cell symbionts were suffering from a real oxygen shortage.

The pseudohypoxic state reactivates the evolutionarily conserved biological programs for survival without oxygen

If it is assumed from the well-founded supposition that the original archaea were facultative anaerobes with a capacity for non-oxidative energy extraction and that the respiratory chain with oxidative phosphorus bonding for ATP production was composed at a later stage, after the act of symbiosis (Gray 1999), then it is to be expected that in a state of pseudohypoxia the evolutionary-biologically conserved programs for survival could be reactivated without oxygen.

The findings of genetic expression studies with pseudohypoxia are in fundamental contrast to the prevailing theories of carcinogenesis by random mutation

Pedersen's research group was able to demonstrate that the promoter for hexokinase II genes in tumor cells is regulated by various signal transmission pathways including, among others, glucose, insulin and glucagon. Although insulin and glucagon are hormones that have opposite actions, surprisingly they stimulate the same genes. The response element of the promoters for the hexokinase II gene in tumor cells overlaps the element that corresponds to hypoxia. Pseudohypoxia in diabetes with a simultaneous NO inhibition (overview Lincoln 1997) can be associated with a higher incidence of cancer in those suffering from diabetes (overview Bannasch 1997). The hexokinase II enzyme, located on the outer mitochondrial membrane, catalyzes glucose degradation to the first phosphorus metabolic product and in fast growing tumor cells there is a 5-fold amplification compared to normal differentiated cells. Furthermore genetic studies showed that the promoter for the hexokinase II gene in tumor cells resembles the promoter of hexokinase II genes in normal differentiated cells by up to 99%. From this and other findings the researchers concluded that the hexokinase gene normally remains mute and is not activated by mutation but by the type of combination of transcription factors on a different level: "Therefore, altered DNA sequences within respective promoters cannot be involved in the changes observed during reporter gene expression studies" (Mathupala 1997).

This statement fundamentally opposes the prevailing theories of carcinogenesis by random mutation. The findings support the concept stated here that cancer originated from a primary comprehensive switch in the micro-Gaian milieu to a level of early proto-cell symbiosis (Type-II cell dyssymbiosis) and followed by the activation of evolution-biologically conserved gene programs. Pedersen and his colleagues confirm indirectly this pathogenesis model of tumors by finally stating about the genetic findings:

"The studies indicate a strategy used by highly malignant tumors to survive as well as thrive within a host using a remarkable set of coordinated molecular mechanisms. These mechanisms, which are very similar to those utilized by some highly successful parasites, indicate a "sophisticated strategy devised by tumors to survive even the most inhospitable microenvironments within the host" (Mathupala 1997).

In other words: "Highly successful parasites" (protozoa and fungal microbes) are those which under permanent conditions of hypoxia/pseudohypoxia, analogous to re-fetalized cancer cells, can switch to a Type-II counterregulation of cell dyssymbiosis (regression to the early protista stage, Kremer 1999). That is how they can survive the body's own immune defense (inhibition of cytotoxic NO gas synthesis in the neighboring immune and non-immune cells by type 2 cytokine associated cancer cells similar to parasitic cells) in "the most inhospitable microenvironments within the host" almost as if they were counterregulated cancer parasites with an increased proliferation rate and even survive targeted chemotherapeutic attacks as "resistant agents" (similar to fungal and parasitic microbes in full-blown AIDS).

The survival of metastatic and non-metastatic cancer cells does not depend on coincidence but upon non-linear bioenergetic conditions

The term strategy is misleading, as all eukaryotic cells have the evolutionary-biological capacity to switch back to archaic proto-cell symbiosis as the physiological reproduction phases demonstrate. The micro-Gaian milieu conditions both within cells and, in multicellular organisms, between the cells—with respect to the organism as a whole and its environment—which promote or inhibit assimilations in the self-organized network, are highly complex. We should rather speak of an evolutionary-biological option as the bioenergetic processes are nonlinear and can only be realized with a high degree of selection. This does not mean that every individual parasite or cancer cell can choose arbitrarily a "sophisticated strategy" to "survive even the most inhospitable microenvironments within the host" (Mathupala 1997). From colonized daughter cells of a primary tumor, for instance, roughly one in 10,000 survive in the bloodstream with the potential to colonize another organ (metastatic cells, from the Greek: *meta* = other + *histanai* = place). As most cancer patients do not die from their primary tumor, but of cachexy and metastatic formation, this fact is of great importance. However, cancer cells do not survive or die by accident. Metastatic cells are clone cells, meaning that they originate from a single cancer cell that has formed a tumor cell cluster. These contain heterogenic subpopulations of cells. In order to discover where the difference lies between metastatic and non-metastatic daughter cells, the capacity for stimulation of the enzymes for the synthesis of cytotoxic NO (iNOS) was studied in these cancer cells (Xie 1996).

Experimental evidence that programmed cell death in non-metastatic cancer cells depends on the activity of the iNOS enzyme for the production of cytotoxic NO gas and can also be activated in metastatic cancer cells via strong and repeated iNOS stimulation

Metastatic melanoma cancer cells from mice that had lung metastases were treated with different type 1 cytokines and bacterial lipopolysaccharides (LPS) for the stimulation of iNOS. There were no signs of iNOS activity and no cytotoxic NO production. The same procedure with non-metastatic cells from the same tumor, however, activated a high iNOS level and high amounts of cytotoxic NO. In the cell culture it was shown that after stimulation, cytotoxic NO-producing cancer cells died by apoptosis.

This experiment demonstrates that cancer cells differ energetically and metabolically from normal differentiated cells by a limited production of NO and O_2^-, or rather the product of both—peroxinitrite. This deficiency led to the closing of the PT pores of the mitochondria and impeded the normal toggle switch between aerobic glycolysis and OXPHOS, thereby blocking programmed cell death. In contrast stimulation of the non-metastatic cancer cells with type 1 cytokines, or as the case may be, LPS, stimulated iNOS synthesis and O_2- synthesis and in doing this also peroxinitrite formation. The sudden opening of the PT channels starts Ca^{2+} cycling and triggers apoptosis. In order to discover why the metastatic cancer cells did not react to the stimulation with iNOS, the same research group manipulated metastatic melanomas by genetic transfection in three ways:

The first cell group was equipped with functioning iNOS genes, the second with non-functioning iNOS genes, the third with neomycin resistance genes. A fourth non-manipulated metastatic cell group served as control.

All cell groups remained highly metastatic, except the first group with the functioning iNOS genes. After implanting the four cell groups in nude mice, which are especially sensitive to tumor cells, the first cell group developed slow growing tumors under the skin and the metastatic cell groups fast growing tumors.

In a further experiment the researchers demonstrated with sarcoma cancer cells in the lungs of other strains of mice that after a repeated injection of synthetic lipopeptides (similar to stimulation with bacterial lipopolysaccharides) the genetic expression of the enzyme proteins of iNOS was switched on in the metastatic cells and cytotoxic NO was produced. The metastases completely regressed. The scientists concluded: "These data demonstrate that the expression of iNOS in tumor cells is associated with apoptosis, suppression of tumorigenicity, abrogation of metastasis, and regression of established metastases" (Xie 1996).

(See illustration: Programmed cell death in metastatic cancer cells after transfer of a functioning iNOS gene (see table XIV) and after repeated injection of synthetic lipopeptides (see table XV))

In cancer cells the delicate balance of calcium-dependent NO gases plays a role in the complex Type-II counterregulation and "resistance" after chemotherapy

The fact that initially metastatic cells on repeated and strong stimulation display iNOS activities and die off, indicates that in metastatic cells the sensitivity of the transcription barrier of the expression of the iNOS genes is altered. Such changes in the behavior of transcription of the iNOS genes in tumor cells can appear selectively because of the nonlinearity (Waliszewski 1998) of the highly complex Type-II counterregulations. They can also be selectively triggered by chemotherapy and are then termed as "resistance" of tumor cells. Of the counterregulations the increased expression of type 2 cytokine transforming growth factor (TFG-β) for the control of NO production in tumor cells (Vodovotz 1997) as well as for the spreading of metastatic cancer cells via proteinases (Zvibel 1993) seems to have gained a special importance. The role of NO gases in tumor cells in relation to the inhibition of the tumor's growth and the new formation of capillaries through the deployment of NO-donating and

NO-inhibiting substances has been examined in many experimental and clinical studies. The results are contradictory. The findings showed that tumor cells require a low calcium-dependent NO synthesis for the sprouting of new capillaries and a higher NO synthesis that inhibits tumor growth (Chinje 1997). In the systemic treatment of cancer patients with interleukin-2, leaks in the capillary vessels occurred that were traced back to an increased cytotoxic NO stimulation and that could be retarded by the simultaneous dosage of NO inhibitors. On the other hand, NO-blocking substances alone could reduce tumor growth and metastatic formation so that it can be assumed that cancer cells require a fine balance of low calcium-dependent NO levels (Orucevic 1998) that are no longer sufficient to maintain an intact cell symbiosis. Then again this assumption corresponds to the very low lipid peroxidation in cancer cells (Horrobin 1990).

The causal relationship between chronic fungal and parasitic infections and the development of cancer, after the exhaustion of the thiol pool and inhibition of the synthesis of cytotoxic NO

The explanation of the old clinical observation that fungal and parasitic infections often precede a cancer disease can be found in the fact that chronic infections lead to an increase in cytotoxic production, which in turn leads to the inhibition of the type 1 cytokine profile, while the type 2 cytokine profile is more vigorously synthesized. The cross-regulation between type 1 cytokines and cytotoxic NO evidently impedes overreactions of Th1 immune cells and inflammatory processes (overview Lincoln 1997). On the other hand chronic overproduction of NO after the exhaustion of the thiol pool and S-nitrosylation (NO formation on sulfhydryl groups in function proteins and enzyme proteins (overview Stamler 1995) leads to considerable counterregulations (Type II cell dyssymbiosis).

Chronic parasite infections (and probably fungal infections) can trigger secretion of substances on the part of the agents (e.g. glyco-inositol phospholipids), which can inhibit NO synthesis (Liew 1994). This effect is comparable to the effect of the fungal extract Cyclosporin A on the Cyclophilin isomerases and the thereby triggered inhibition of interleukin-2 resulting in inhibition of cytotoxic NO synthesis as well as the blockade of NAD^+ hydrolysis and the closing of the mitochondrial lock-gates.

For many decades, nitrosamine researchers sought the primary cause of cancer in the wrong place: in the genome of the cell nucleus

The causal link between chronic infections and chronic inflammatory processes has been proven in many studies and been associated with the nitrosamine formation from endogenous NO (overview Tannenbaum 1994, Oshima 1994, Kerwin 1995). Nitrosamine research, furthermore, has shown with absolute certainty, in wide-ranging experimental and clinical analyses, an immense number of exogenous sources, e.g. in nutrition, in drinking water, in tobacco, at industrial places of work, but also through antibiotics, chemotherapeutics, analgesics, cosmetics etc. A large number of N-nitroso compounds as well as similarly operating alkyl hydrazine, alkyl azoxy, alkyl triazine, compounds have been demonstrated as being highly carcinogenic substances in a large variety of animals including apes. Carcinogenic nitroso compounds are formed by N-nitrosation reactions between different secondary and tertiary amines and nitrites and other substances capable of nitrosation. These reactions can take place in the environment and within an organism (overview Lijinsky 1992, Loeppky 1994 a).

The "fingerprints" of these chemicals in DNA are discussed as evidence of the carcinogenic effect of nitrosamines and related substances in humans. It concerns changes in the bases, the building blocks of DNA, which have been established in the DNA in the formation of tumors by UV light on the skin and by the fungal toxin, aflatoxin in liver and other tumors. They are changes to the tumor suppressor gene p53, that expresses a protein that promotes programmed cell death and is considered to be the opposite number of oncogene Bcl-2, whose protein product bonds Ca^{2+} ion to membranes forcing the closure of the PT lock-gates of mitochondria (Vogelstein 1992, Oshima 1994). The American pharmacologist Magee, a pioneer of nitrosamine research of the Thomas Jefferson University Cancer Research Institute in Philadelphia, after 40 years of research into the links between nitrosamines and cancer observed:

"N-nitroso compounds (NNOC) are toxic in human beings, causing acute and subacute pathological changes that are closely similar to those found in experimental animals. There is convincing epidemiological evidence that the cancer chemotherapeutic drug semustine, an N-nitrosourea derivative, is a human carcinogen. On the plausible assumption that all the NNOCs, including N-nitrosamines, act as carcinogens through the formation of the same active intermediates, probably alkyldiazionum ions, it seems reasonable to conclude that all the carcinogenic nitroso compounds are human carcinogens. Whether the compounds play any significant part in the causation of human cancers remains problematical. The proposal is attractive because of their ubiquitous occurrence in the environment, albeit in very small amounts, and the potential for their formation within the body from amine precursors and nitrite or other nitrosating agents. Definitive evidence might be obtained by the demonstration of mutations in oncogens specific for nitroso carcinogens, as has been shown with aflatoxins and UV light. So far this has not been achieved and further research in this area could be rewarding. Even though conclusive proof has not been obtained that the NNOCs are important causes of human cancer, it is clearly desirable that their occurrence in the environment and their formation in the body are reduced to the lowest practicable levels" (Magee 1996).

The ambivalence conveyed by these words after 40 years of nitrosamine research underlines the bewilderment of a whole generation of cancer researchers, who in countless experiments with more than 300 nitrosamine links in a wide range of animals and in all kinds of human cell cultures time and again observed the transformation to tumor cells. The researchers, consistent with the prevailing school of thought in cancer research as a whole, had manifestly sought the primary cause of cancer in the wrong place. The fixation with gene mutations, based on the dogma that the nuclear genome was the command center of the living cell, had clouded their judgement that the bioenergetic network is a self-organizing (autopoietic) program. The cancer researchers could not have realized without the fundamental knowledge from NO research, cytokine research and cell symbiosis research the possibility that cancer cells could represent a permanent regression to an archaic status of protosymbiosis, as executed for a limited time span in fetal cells and in certain cell division phases.

Now these findings have been available for over 10 years and the observations of respected nitrosamine researchers even for 30 years are again highly topical. *Gene mutations are neither sufficient nor necessary to trigger transformation of cancer cells as cancer also develops without traceable gene changes* (Lijinsky 1973, 1992). Mitochondria researchers, too, for a long time have confirmed that cancer, if anything, is more likely to develop with intact mitochondrial DNA than after gene toxic mutations (overview Mazurek 1997).

The assumed "fingerprint" of the nitrosamine effect, the altered p53 gene in tumor cells (Vogelstein 1992), on the basis of the concept of Type-II dyssymbiosis—a long-term or overly strong activation of NO and its derivatives that force a continual counterregulation to evolutionary-biologically programmed protosymbiosis (state of pseudohypoxia = seemingly deficient oxygen state)—can be explained in another way, without "altered

DNA sequences within the respective promoters" (Mathupala 1997) having to be involved:

"Recent studies have shown another interesting observation for the Type II hexokinase promoter within tumor cells, where functional p53 elements were identified within the same promoter region that harbors the glucose and hypoxia responsive elements. This correlated with the presence of a p53 protein with an enhanced half-life expressed in the same tumor. Co-expression of this protein with the Type II hexokinase promoter during reporter gene analysis resulted in enhanced transcription. The proximity of the p53 elements to the hypoxia and glucose response elements, as well as the recent observation that tumors within hypoxic regions promote p53 mutations at a high rate, implicate an important relationship between hexokinase expression, the expression of mutated p53, hypoxia, enhanced glucose catabolism, and cell-cycle progression or proliferative capacity of highly glycolytic, rapidly growing tumors" (Mathupala 1997).

The concept of Type 2 counterregulation of cell dyssymbiosis as an alternative explanation of the primary causes of cancer

In other words the altered gene expressions are not the cause but the response to the loss of fluidity and the "quantum dynamic depths" resulting from the forced choking of the synthesis of nitric and oxygenic oxides (NO, O_2^-, peroxinitrite) and the closing of the PT lock-gates of the mitochondria.

The Bcl-2 gene, the p53 gene and their protein products are components of an ever increasing ensemble of genes and proteins that are involved in the opening and closing of the PT lock-gates of the mitochondria (Richter 1996, Zamzami 1997). Protein patterns are synthesized dependent on the sensitivity of the expression of genes that inversely either force the opening or the closing of the PT lock-gates. The kind and variability of the gene expression and the following synthesis of the protein pattern is dependent on the fluidity of the redox milieu. In this way the semiconductor characteristics of the macromolecular DNA, namely the thresholds of the electron flows which define the transcription profile, can be variably modulated. Redox-dependent modulation of the genes thus govern whether and which RNA messages for the biosynthesis of function, structural, signal and enzyme proteins are mediated. So the genes do not have to be altered by mutations in the sense of a biochemical structural defect.

The "Warburg Phenomenon" of aerobic glycolysis, not understood for more than 80 years, is switched on as a strategy for survival in states of pseudohypoxia based on the scenario of archaic protosymbiosis. The pseudohypoxia is based on a secondary NO/peroxinitrite deficiency that leads to a Type-II cell dyssymbiosis.

"These mechanisms, which are very similar to those utilized by some highly successful parasites"(Mathupala 1997) are not only very similar, but the tumor cells are actually trapped in the division cycle by facultative anaerobic parasites (protista) and after every cell division cycle try in vain to offer their atrophying cell symbionts (mitochondria) the transcripts for proteins for the respiratory chain and the OXPHOS system (Cuezva 1997) in order to re-animate mitochondrial respiration.

As the unaltered p53 protein is involved in the opening of the mitochondrial lock-gates, the altered p53 gene through co-expression in the hypoxic region, which can be assigned to the archaeal genome part, is jointly responsible for the blockade of the switch back to the OXPHOS system. On the other hand, the transcripts for the synthesis of proteins for the respiratory chain and the OXPHOS complex could be coded on the proteobacterial portion of the nuclear genome. This assumption would explain the paradox that these transcripts continue to be supplied. In contrast the behavior of the transcripts makes sense in fetal cells because immediately after the first breath the necessary proteins for the respiratory chain and OXPHOS system can be implemented. The variable for this evolutionary-biologically programmed switch of the bioenergetic and metabolic network is the thiol pool (glutathione, cysteine etc.) and the nitrosylation of vital enzymes and signal proteins (overview Stamler 1995).

This alternative concept explains the primary cause of cancer and the relative inefficacy of conventional cancer therapy substantially more plausibly than any theories of mutation or fictitious retrovirus hypotheses

This causal link explains the fact of tumorigenesis through nitrosamines and other nitroso compound considerably more plausibly than any mutation theories and fictitious retrovirus theories. But it also explains the relative lack of success in the elimination of tumor cells by operations, radiation and chemotherapy. Without a balance to the excessive nitrosation and nitrosylation, enforced Type-II dyssymbiosis counterregulations will intensify, in the long run in even more cell systems, and as a result of the increased nitrosative and oxidative stress, selective subpopulations of metastatic tumor cells will proliferate. The epidemiological result is that the life expectancy of conventionally treated cancer patients is considerably shorter than that of untreated patients (Abel 1990), which reflects the short-sightedness in prevailing tumor research and cancer treatment.

Certainly the excessive stress of nitrogen compounds only demonstrates one section of the wide-ranging causal spectrum of cancer origins as, theoretically, longer-term disruptions can occur at every junction in the self-organizing bioenergetic network in the grey areas between solid and fluid phase. In general, however, the response to extreme stress will follow the same archaic evolutionary-biological rules. In this respect, the development of Kaposi's sarcoma as Type-II dyssymbiosis (regression to protosymbiosis) resulting from a primary NO overload and secondary NO^-/O_2^-/peroxinitrite choking, is a plausible model for understanding tumorigenesis.

The drastic decline of infections and inflammatory processes as major causes of death and disease in industrialized nations well before the introduction of vaccines, chemotherapeutic agents and antibiotics

During the long process of evolution the human organism was primarily confronted with biological sources to stress with nitrogen oxides. The main factor probably was endogenous NO stimulation by microbial toxins and antigens (acute and chronic infectious and inflammatory processes). Additionally, nitrite-bonding bacteria in contaminated drinking water and nitrite-contaminated foodstuffs (in later cultural history through preserved meat and sausage products) could play a role. The increased bonding of sulfur-containing thiols and thiol proteins through the formation of nitrosothiols could, however, be dramatically intensified by famine and malnutrition. These involve an accelerated utilization of the thiol pool and antioxidative capacities through a depletion of thiol-containing amino acids (cysteine, methionine), folic acid deficiency, deficits in antioxidative vitamins, essential fatty acids, polyphenols, polyanions, minerals and trace elements.

In industrialized countries acute and chronic infectious and inflammatory processes were continuously minimized as causes of disease and death from the middle of the 19th to the middle of the 20th Century by improved nutrition, hygiene, living conditions, drinking water purification, sewage, pest management, education as well as progress in modern medicine and the natural sciences (Sagan 1987, 1992). This drastic decline in the rates of infection and mortality was reached before the introduction of vaccines, chemotherapeutics and antibiotics (see illustration: Examples of the continuous decline of disease and mortality rates by infectious illnesses from the mid 19th Century to the mid 20th Century [see table XVI]).

The dramatically modified nitrosative and oxidative load created in industrialized nations can be answered by the archaic cellular symbiosis no differently than in the pre-industrial evolution phase and is the cause for cancer and other chronic degenerative illnesses

In the poorer countries malnutrition and deficient nutrition, in combination with higher exposure to microbes, favored by contaminated drinking water, hygiene problems, unfavorable living conditions, marginal education, lack of medical infrastructure etc., continue to be the dominating factors for the origins of acute and chronic infectious and inflammatory processes including opportunistic diseases (nutritional AIDS, Beisel 1992, 1996). In the industrial countries, however, completely new load profiles of insidious chronic nitrosative and oxidative states of stress are developing as a result of the products of civilization. This chronic nitrosative and oxidative load, unique in this combination in the history of evolution, can be answered by the archaic cellular symbiosis no differently than by using the same counterregulations used for chronic nitrosative and oxidative stimulation from parasites and worms. The result is a type 2 dominance and under the described conditions a fixed switching to Type-II dyssymbiosis. This evolutionary, biologically programmed, unchangeable option to the disruption of the micro-Gaian milieu as a result of chronic nitrosation, which in extreme cases can only be answered by the choking of the cells' own synthesis of nitrogen and oxygen oxides, is the cause of the reversion of ratios of acute to chronic diseases in the last fifty years, manifested by degenerative and cancer illnesses as the major cause of deaths. This view is supported by the evidence of many research groups, which shows that malign tumors are associated with type 2 cytokine dominance (Clerici 1998).

After 20 years of Kaposi's sarcoma research all relevant scientific data confirms excessive nitrosative stress and the exhaustion of the thiol pool as the primary cause of the exclusive incidence of Kaposi's sarcoma in homosexual men

Unique in history of mankind, however, is the sum-total prooxidative burden of a minority of promiscuous homosexual men, engaging in unprotected anally-receptive intercourse, combined with long-term sex doping through inhalation of nitrite gases ("poppers"); excessive abuse of nitrosative antibiotics, antiparasitics, antimycotics, virustatics, numerous "recreational drugs," etc.;

chronic multiinfections; and massive exposure to oxidative/nitrosative alloantigens via intake of foreign semen (overview Root-Bernstein 1993).

In 1985, animal experiments demonstrated that the simultaneous administration of nitrites and antibiotics provoked the formation of tumors (Brambilla 1985). The American pharmacologist Ignarro, who at the same time as his American research colleague Furchgott first proved the existence of gaseous NO molecules and their physiological functions in human cell systems, had demonstrated that NO is formed from nitrite in the endothelial cells of blood vessel walls. NO gas molecules that do not directly bond to iron in the enzyme guanylate cyclase for regulating blood pressure are stored as nitrosothiols via nitrosation from molecules from the thiol pool, and via nitrosylation as nitrosoproteins in special cell organelles—the lysosomes (Ignarro 1992).

If the thiol pool is exhausted by exogenous nitrite supply, the same regulations will be triggered by the thiol sensor as those by sustained and strong NO synthesis by stimulation through microbial toxins, microbial antigen loads or non-microbial alloantigen loads. The thiol pool becomes even more quickly depleted when NO from exogenous nitrite and other NO syntheses (through microbial stimulation, alloantigen load and the degradation of nitrosative drugs) have to be metabolized synchronously. Under such conditions, the cells' own NO^-/O_2^-/peroxinitrite production is choked, the altered redox milieu effects a switch from a type 1 to type 2 cytokine profile, and the OXPHOS system of the cell symbionts switches off in favor of aerobic glycolysis. The sensitivity of the signal-transferring proteins, transcription factors, and transcription genes become altered. If the bioenergetic and metabolic network remains decompensated and cannot regain an equilibrium on a non-genetic and genetic level, then the endothelial cells transform into Kaposi's sarcoma (Type-II counterregulation of cell dyssymbiosis).

Numerous studies have confirmed that "HIV positive" patients in the earliest stage of seroconversion display a drastic depletion of the thiol pool. Both the cysteine and glutathione levels are severely diminished in the blood plasma and within the cells (overview Herzenberg 1997, Dröge 1997 a).

Also clearly demonstrated in many studies is the switch of the intracellular cytokine pattern from a type 1 to a type 2 profile in the earliest stage of seroconversion in "HIV positive" patients as well as an immune status identical to worm infections, chronic parasitic and fungal infections and chronic mycobacterial and spirochete infections (overview Lucey 1996).

In Western countries, the appearance of Kaposi's sarcoma is clinically diagnosed almost exclusively in anal receptive homosexuals with a history of nitrite inhalation. *Since the decline in nitrite consumption among homosexuals, a decline in the incidence of Kaposi's sarcoma has also been observed, in contrast to the increased incidence predicted by the HIV/AIDS theory* (overview Levine 1982, Marmor 1982, Lauritsen 1986, Haverkos 1988, 1990, Papadopulos-Eleopulos 1992 b, Duesberg 1996, Kremer 1998 a, 1998 c).

Clinical HIV/AIDS research also published disparate cases of Kaposi's sarcoma: patients were diagnosed as KS cases who did not register "HIV positive" and whose immune status was not characteristically altered. This observation corresponds to the fact that endothelial cells, in isolated cases, can transform after counterregulation against nitrite abuse without the frequently synchronous Th1-to-Th2 switch. As a result of this and other clinical and laboratory data, orthodox HIV/AIDS researchers have come to the conclusion that HIV is not the cause of Kaposi's sarcoma and that KS cannot be the result of a sexually transmitted retroviral infection (Beral 1990).

On the whole, the clinical, anamnestic, epidemiological and laboratory data confirm, after 20 years of KS research, the bioenergetic, metabolic and genetic concept of tumorigenesis as a result of the decompensated regression of cell symbiosis to the archaic stage of proto-cell symbiosis due to excessive nitrosation and exhaustion of the thiol pool.

In contrast to the "Retrovirus AIDS/Cancer" theory, the concept of Type-II cell dyssymbiosis can integrate all decisive research data on the origins of cancer without contradiction

The prediction made at the historic conference of retrovirus researchers in March 1983—that by researching the "intriguing puzzle" (Friedman-Kein 1984 a) of Kaposi's sarcoma, useful information could be gained for the study of cancer in general (Thomas 1984)—has proven to be correct. However, the concepts of retrovirus-AIDS and retrovirus-cancer research have led to a dead end, even though the dogma of the disease theory "HIV causes AIDS" is stoutly defended with all available means, and kept alive by massive research grants and the ubiquitous media dictatorship. The crucial knowledge, which nobody had during the propagation of the HIV/AIDS theory in 1983/84, was gathered from outside of retrovirus-AIDS and—cancer research by, most notably, bioenergetic cell symbiosis research.

The evolutionary-medical concept of the Type-II cell dyssymbiosis of tumorigenesis based on bioenergetic investigation of the micro-Gaian milieu can integrate, without any contradiction, all pivotal research data gained since the quiet revolution in fundamental medical research in the 1980s.

Two statements from two of the most prominent, internationally acclaimed retrovirus cancer researchers promptly throws the spotlight on how they evaluate their theory—that retroviruses are the cause of cancer—as a contribution for the solution of the cancer puzzle.

Baltimore, who together with Temin in 1970 discovered the reverse transcription of RNA in DNA, a discovery which gave the crucial impulse for the retrovirus/cancer research within the framework of President Nixon's 1971 "War on Cancer," and who was awarded the Nobel Prize in 1975 for retrovirus/cancer research, stated in 1988 as president of the Rockefeller University in New York:

"I have no idea when we'll know enough to develop anything [for oncology] that's clinically applicable, and I don't know who's going to do it . . . It's not a high priority in my thinking" (Angier 1988).

Varmus, 1989 Nobel prize winner for retrovirus/cancer research, and director of the National Institutes of Health in the USA, the most prestigious research authority for all the US health authorities, including the National Cancer Research Institute stated, in 1988: "You can't do experiments to see what causes cancer. It's not the sort of thing scientists can afford to do" (Angier 1988).

In actual fact the retrovirus/cancer researchers, mutating to retrovirus/AIDS researchers at the historic conference in March 1983 in New York, had suggested just such experiments on AIDS patients with immune weaknesses, some of whom had developed Kaposi's sarcoma. The ensuing million-fold treatments on AIDS patients stigmatized as "HIV positive" with immunotoxic and cytotoxic antibiotics and chemotherapeutics could not finally solve the "cancer puzzle." However, the clarification of fatal mistakes and deceitful practices have contributed to a profound change in opinion about the nature of cancer cells and accordingly the effective therapy and prevention.

Warburg was basically right: The unplanned and planned pharmatoxic experiments on humans had proven that cancer is caused by a primary functional and secondary structural inactivation of mitochondrial symbionts. The functional blockade of cell respiration activates, in the case of prevented cell death, the evolutionary-biologically programmed survival competition of the archaeal genome and inactivates the cooperation with the proteobacterial genome elements inside the nucleus and in mitochondria. The result is a permanent Type-II counterregulation of cell dyssymbiosis.

Fig. 43) Types of tumors frequently found in humans. Before being approved new anti-tumor drugs have to pass strict testing in three phases: I (security, risks), II (dosage/efficacy), III (efficacy). [figures from Germany, *N.d.T.*]

1) Brain Tumors
- 6,400 new cases annually
- genetic therapy, phase III

2) Mouth, Neck and Head Tumors
- 13,800 new cases annually
- genetic therapy, phase II
- chemotherapy and overheating therapy, phase III

3) Lymph Node Tumors
- 9,800 new cases annually
- mabthera antibodies tried since 02/06/98
- antibodies with radioactive markers, phase II

4) Lung Tumors
- 38,000 new cases annually
- cytotoxic active principle called hycamtin administered, also for brain metastases
- chemotherapy and genetic therapy with p53 genes, phase II

5) Large Intestine tumors
- 33,000 new cases annually
- cytotoxic active principle called camptosar administered

6) Uterus tumors
- 18,000 new cases annually
- new form of antitumor vaccination, phase I
- overheating, phase III

7) Skin Tumors
- 6,400 new cases annually
- chemotherapy and genetic therapy, phase III
- chemotherapy and overheating therapy, phase III

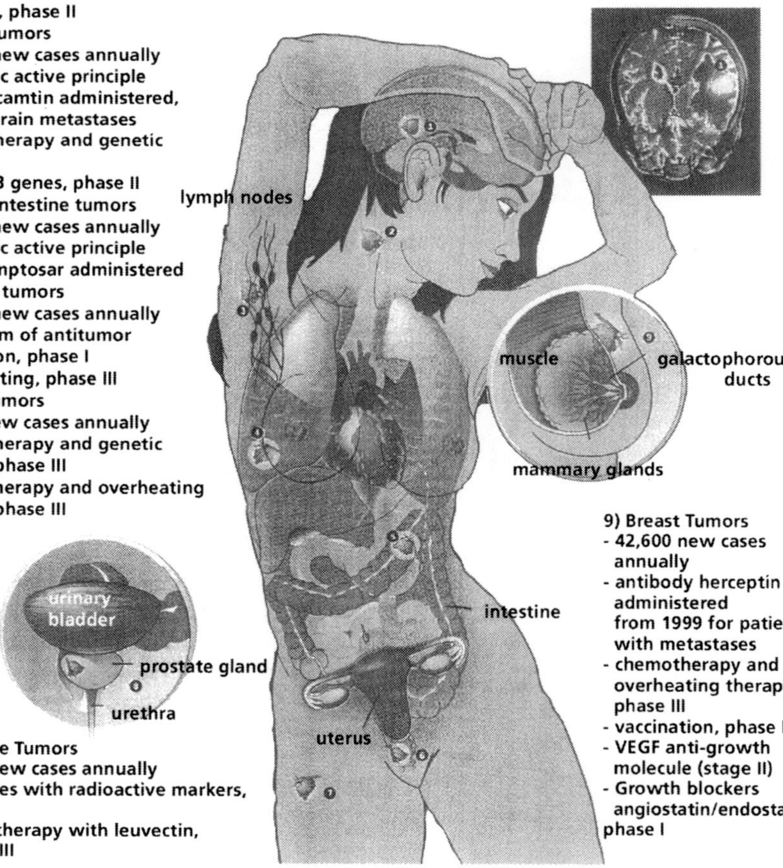
lymph nodes
muscle
galactophorous ducts
mammary glands
intestine
urinary bladder
prostate gland
urethra
uterus

8) Prostate Tumors
- 22,000 new cases annually
- antibodies with radioactive markers, phase II
- genetic therapy with leuvectin, phase II/III

9) Breast Tumors
- 42,600 new cases annually
- antibody herceptin administered from 1999 for patients with metastases
- chemotherapy and overheating therapy, phase III
- vaccination, phase I/III
- VEGF anti-growth molecule (stage II)
- Growth blockers angiostatin/endostatin, phase I

Fig. 44) The stages of development of a carcinoma

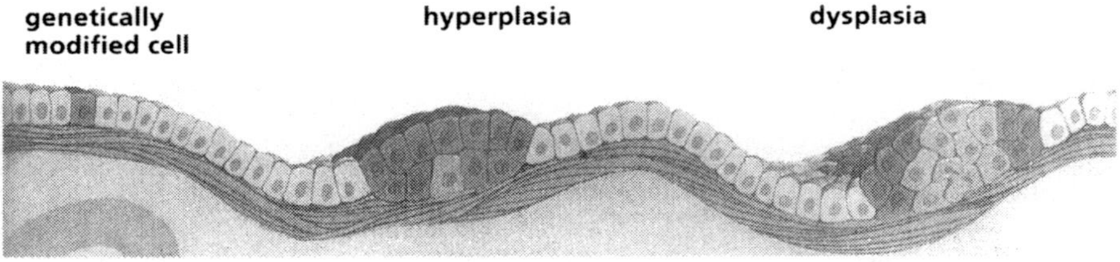
genetically
modified cell
hyperplasia
dysplasia

1. The developmentof a tumor begins with a genetic mutation: an ordinary cell that is part of the normal population undergoes a mutation, thus increasing its tendency to divide even when this should not happen

2. The modified cell and its newborn cells continue to be normal externally but proliferate excessively. Tissue displays hyperplasia and after some years one in a million of these cells could undergo a second mutation loosening the mechanisms of growth control at a later stage

3. The newborn cells from the highly proliferating cells now have a different appearance. Their shape and mutual orientation are abnormal. Sometimes a rarer third mutation occurs changing the behavior of the cell at a later stage.

Fig. 45) Stages of development of a carcinoma (cont.)

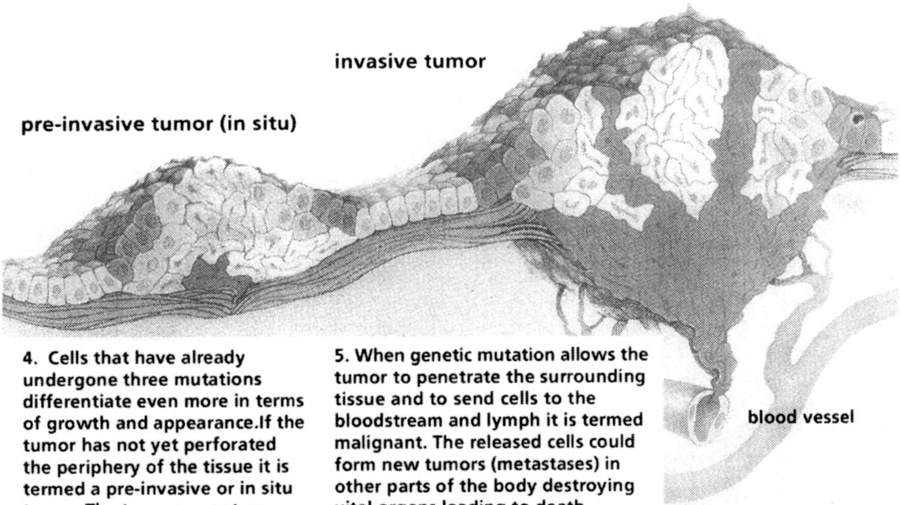
invasive tumor
pre-invasive tumor (in situ)
blood vessel

4. Cells that have already undergone three mutations differentiate even more in terms of growth and appearance.If the tumor has not yet perforated the periphery of the tissue it is termed a pre-invasive or in situ tumor. The tumor cannot go beyond the confines of the tissue but after a period of time a second mutation could occur.

5. When genetic mutation allows the tumor to penetrate the surrounding tissue and to send cells to the bloodstream and lymph it is termed malignant. The released cells could form new tumors (metastases) in other parts of the body destroying vital organs leading to death.

Fig. 46) Formation of a metastasis

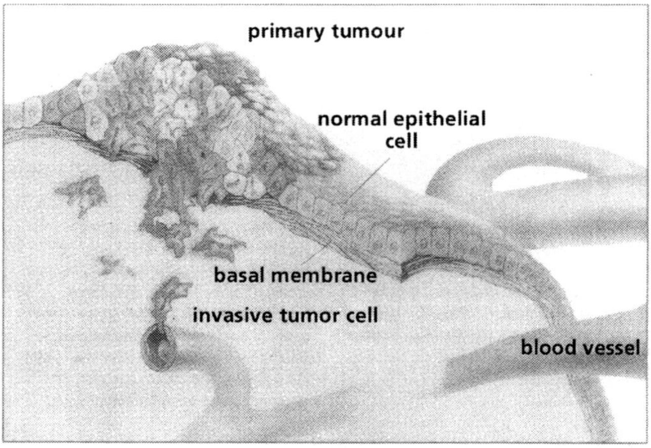
primary tumour
normal epithelial cell
basal membrane
invasive tumor cell
blood vessel

Tumor cells penetrating other tissues and the formation of metastases are responsible for the fatal spread of the tumor in the body. In the first stage, cells separate from the primary tumour (that comes often from the epithelial tissue) and break through the basal membrane that separates the epithelium from other tissues. Some of these cells also penetrate the basal membrane of the surrounding vessels and the endothelium of the vascular wall. They can then circulate freely throughout the body most of them will be destroyed but a few cells still remain in capillaries. If this type of cell manages to stick to the endothelium and to penetrate the vascular wall, it will be able to form a secondary tumor in the surrounding tissue. One in 10.000 cells released from the original tumour succeeds in founding a colony in another area.

Fig. 47) Formation of a metastasis (cont.)

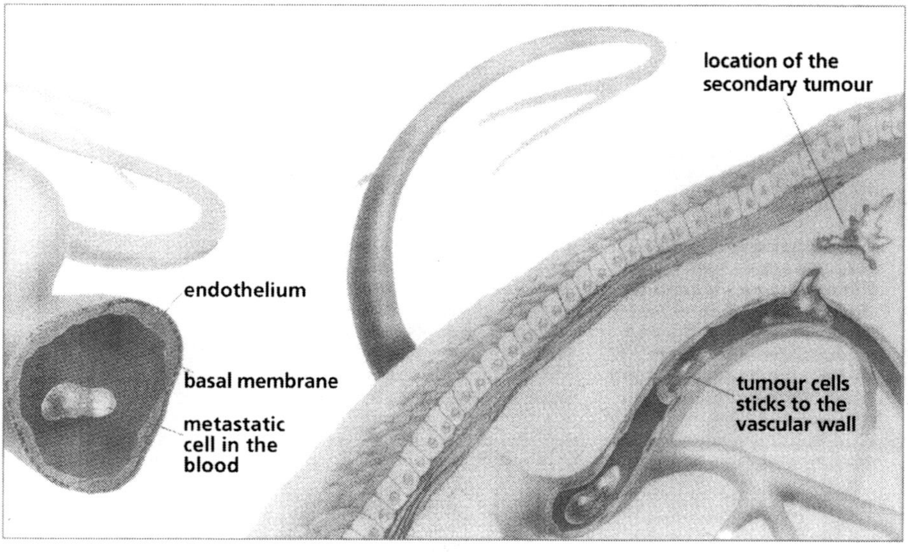
location of the secondary tumour
endothelium
basal membrane
metastatic cell in the blood
tumour cells sticks to the vascular wall

Fig. 48) Diagram of the spreading of a metastasis through the extracellular matrix (ECM) and into the bloodstream.

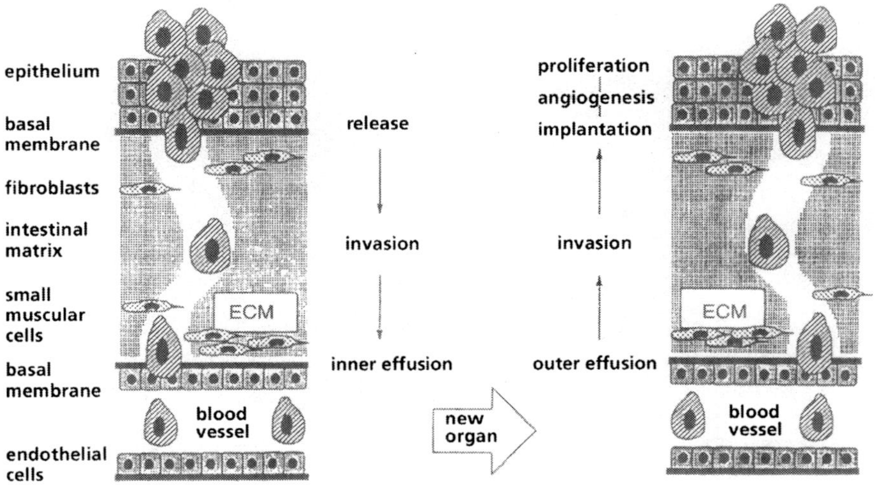
Primary Tumor
Metastasis
epithelium
basal membrane
fibroblasts
intestinal matrix
small muscular cells
basal membrane
endothelial cells
ECM
blood vessel
release
invasion
inner effusion
new organ
proliferation
angiogenesis
implantation
invasion
outer effusion
ECM
blood vessel

Fig. 49) Diagram of the cell division cycle.

G2 Phase

No DNA synthesis. The synthesis of RNA and proteins continues.

M Phase

Due to the mitosis (division of the nucleus) and the cytokinesis (division of the cells) two newborn cells are formed.

G0 Phase

The differentiated cells leave the temporary cycle.

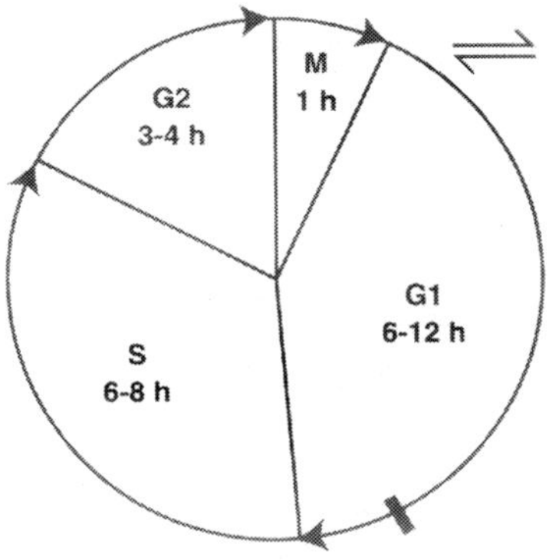
M
1 h
G2
3-4 h
S
6-8 h
G1
6-12 h

Re-entry point

A cell coming from G0 returns to the cycle in the early G1 phase.

G1 Phase

RNA and protein synthesis. No DNA synthesis.

S Phase

When the synthesis of DNA takesplace, the amount of DNA in the cell doubles. RNA and proteins are also formed

Restriction point

When a cell goes beyond this point it must go on to the S phase.

Fig. 50) During mitosis the chromosomes become visible

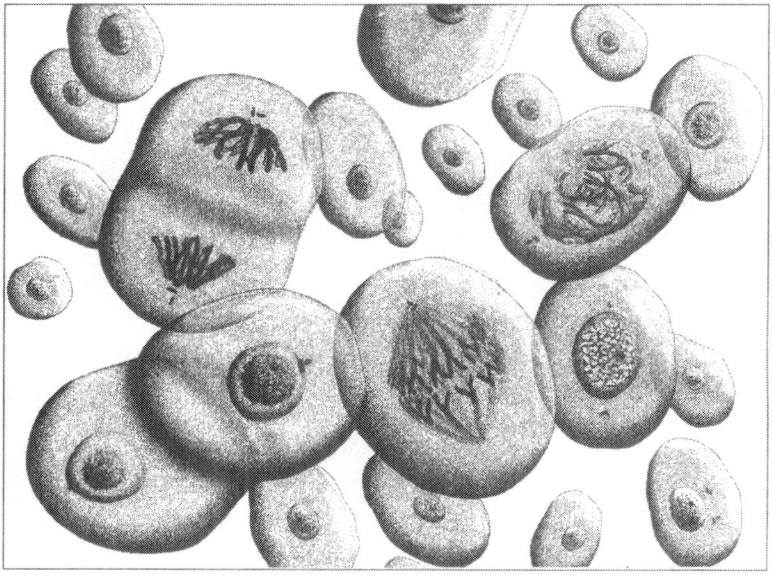

Fig. 51) Diagram of the effects of cytostatics on the phases of the cell division cycle.

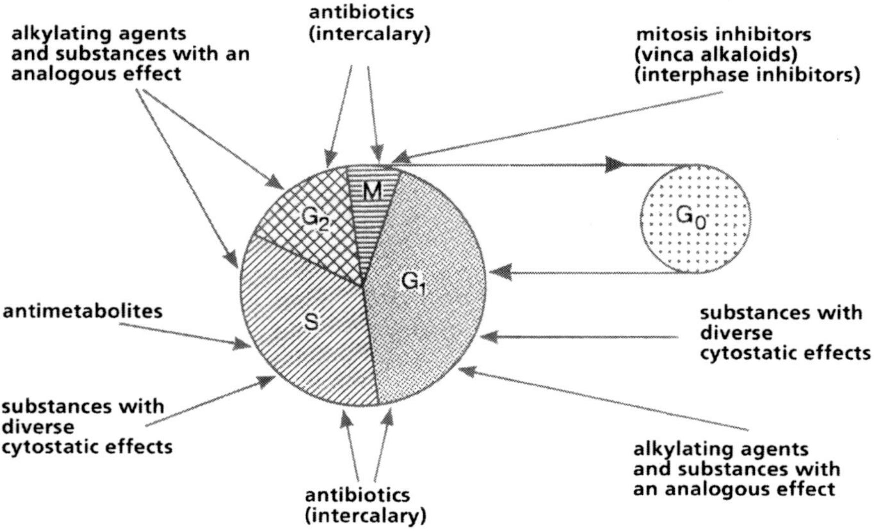

antibiotics (intercalary)
alkylating agents and substances with an analogous effect
mitosis inhibitors (vinca alkaloids) (interphase inhibitors)
M
G2
G0
G1
S
antimetabolites
substances with diverse cytostatic effects
substances with diverse cytostatic effects
alkylating agents and substances with an analogous effect
antibiotics (intercalary)

Fig. 52) Diagram of the mitosis phases during the cell division cycle

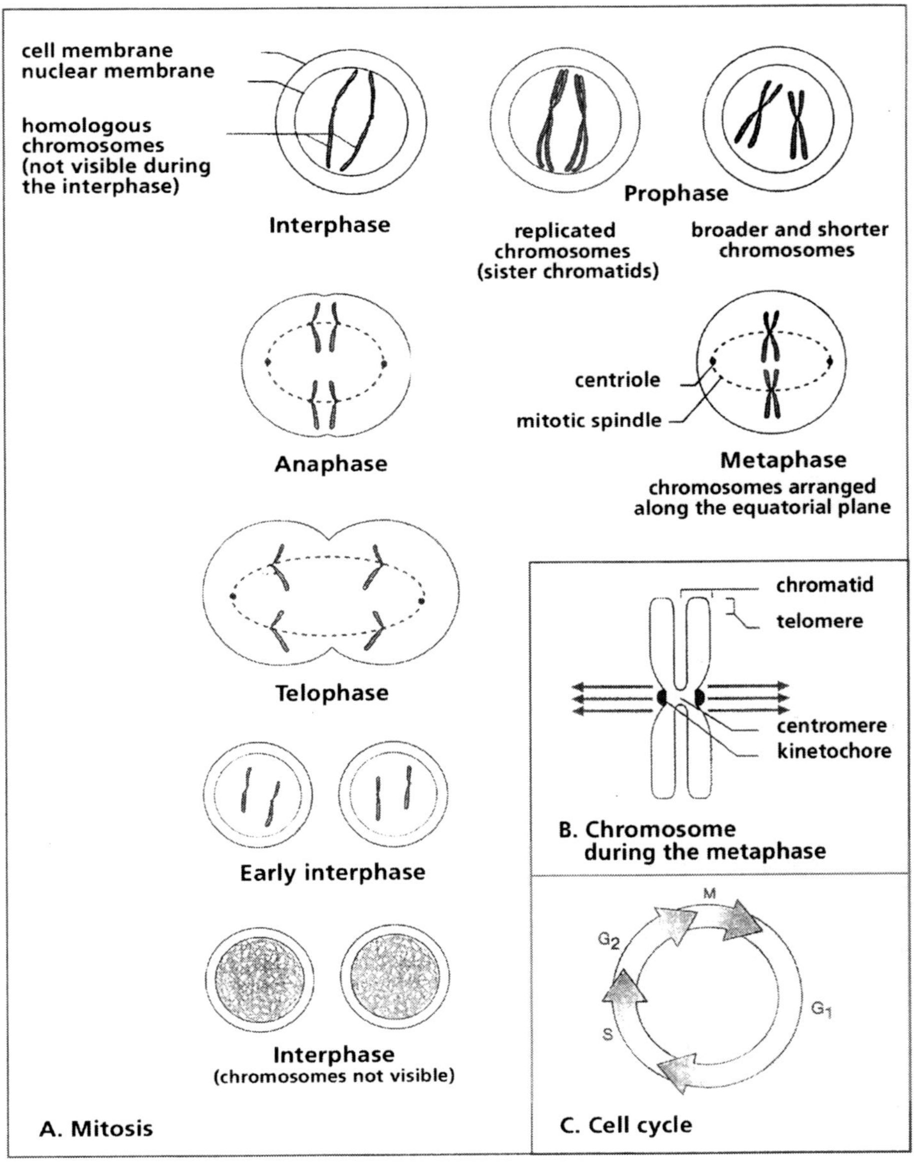
cell membrane
nuclear membrane
homologous chromosomes (not visible during the interphase)
Interphase
Prophase
replicated chromosomes (sister chromatids)
broader and shorter chromosomes
Anaphase
centriole
mitotic spindle
Metaphase
chromosomes arranged along the equatorial plane
Telophase
chromatid
telomere
centromere
kinetochore
Early interphase
B. Chromosome during the metaphase
M
G2
G1
S
Interphase
(chromosomes not visible)
A. Mitosis
C. Cell cycle

Fig. 53) Electron microscope photos. The process of transformation into a tumour is illustrated with an unusual distinctness.

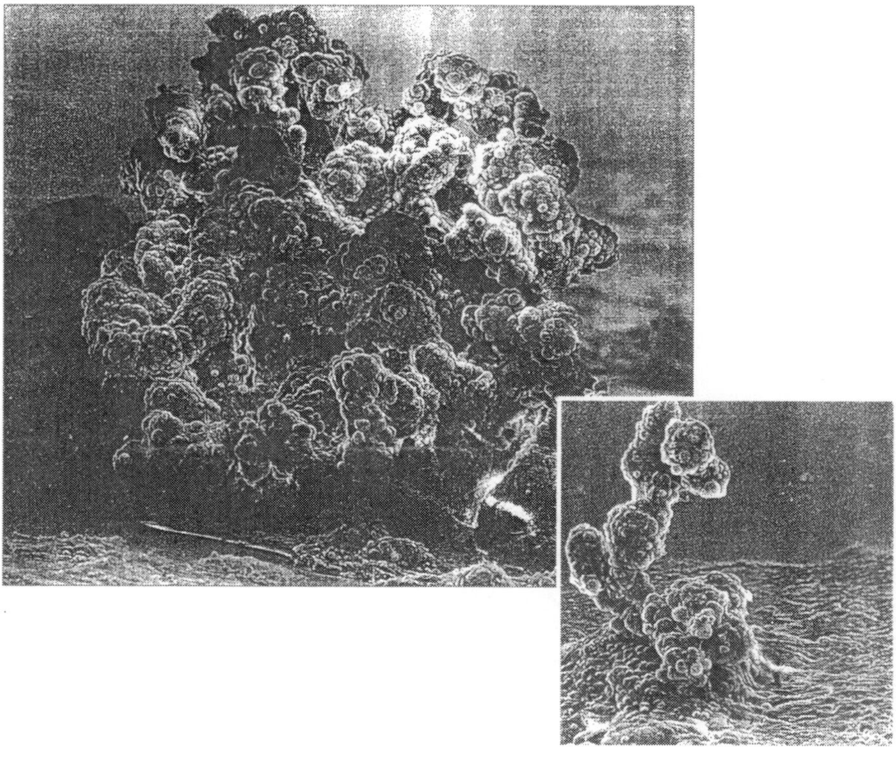

Fig. 54) The effects of chemotherapeutic agents on the synthesis of DNA, RNA and proteins.

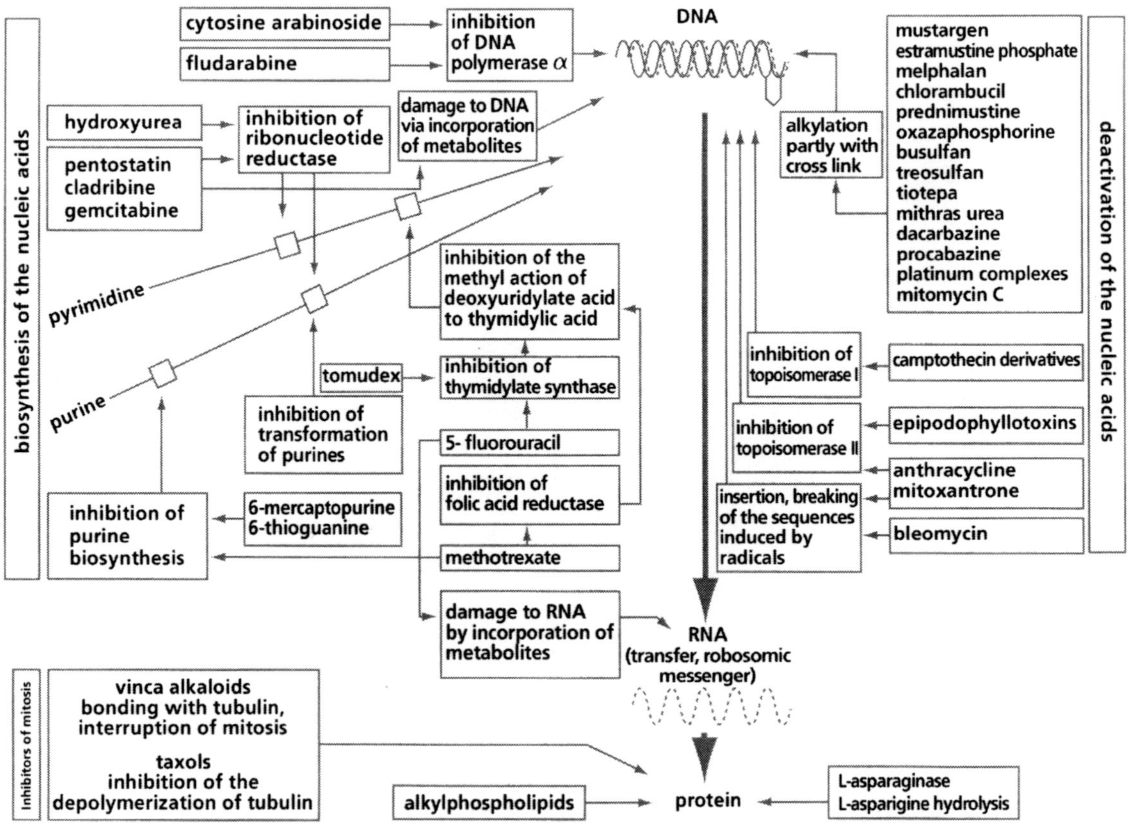
biosynthesis of the nucleic acids
cytosine arabinoside
fludarabine
inhibition of DNA polymerase α
DNA
hydroxyurea
pentostatin
cladribine
gemcitabine
inhibition of ribonucleotide reductase
damage to DNA via incorporation of metabolites
pyrimidine
purine
inhibition of the methyl action of deoxyuridylate acid to thymidylic acid
tomudex
inhibition of thymidylate synthase
inhibition of transformation of purines
5- fluorouracil
inhibition of folic acid reductase
inhibition of purine biosynthesis
6-mercaptopurine
6-thioguanine
methotrexate
damage to RNA by incorporation of metabolites
RNA
(transfer, robosomic messenger)
alkylation partly with cross link
mustargen
estramustine phosphate
melphalan
chlorambucil
prednimustine
oxazaphosphorine
busulfan
treosulfan
tiotepa
mithras urea
dacarbazine
procabazine
platinum complexes
mitomycin C
deactivation of the nucleic acids
inhibition of topoisomerase I
camptothecin derivatives
inhibition of topoisomerase II
epipodophyllotoxins
anthracycline
mitoxantrone
insertion, breaking of the sequences induced by radicals
bleomycin
Inhibitors of mitosis
vinca alkaloids
bonding with tubulin, interruption of mitosis
taxols
inhibition of the depolymerization of tubulin
alkylphospholipids
protein
L-asparaginase
L-asparigine hydrolysis

Fig. 55) Effects of some chemotherapeutic agents.

Antimetabolites

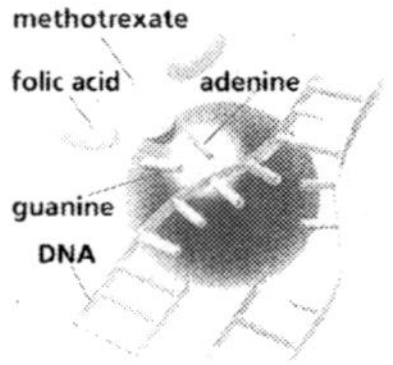
methotrexate
folic acid
adenine
guanine
DNA

Examples: methotrexate, fluorouracil, gemcitabine.

Some antitumor drugs act by sabotaging biochemical reactions in living cells. The most important example is methotrexate, a chemical analog of the vitamin folic acid. It binds to an enzyme that usually contributes to the transformation of folic acid to two components of DNA, adenine and guanine. In this way it prevents the cells from replicating: the cells lose their ability to generate new sequences of DNA for replication.

Topoisomerase inhibitors

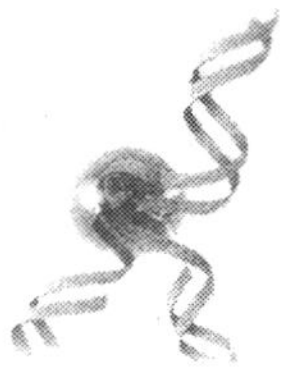

Examples: doxorubicin, CPT-11.

For the replication of the genomes of a cell a medium is needed to subdivide the double helix of the DNA into two sequences. As a rule this role is carried out by a special topoisomerase enzyme which temporarily shears the sequence, it allows the second sequence to pass through the opening and afterwards it reseals the ends. Some drugs inhibit the ability of topoisomerase to reseal the free ends, thus provoking a rupture in the DNA sequences at the replication stage leading to the cell's death.

Alkylating substances

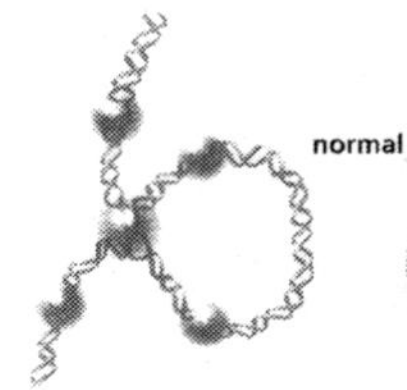

Examples: cyclophosphamide, chlorambucil.

Some chemical products bind to certain components of DNA provoking defects in the structure of the double helix, e.g. ruptures or mismatched links between (or within) sequences. When the cell is not able to counter the damage by means of one of its DNA repair mechanisms, programmed cell-death is provoked.

Vegetal alkaloids

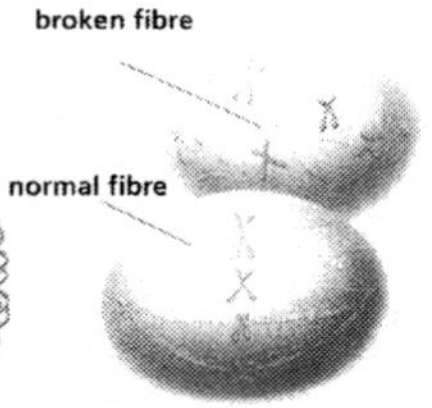
broken fibre
normal fibre

Examples: vinblastine, vinorelbine, paclitaxel, docetaxel.

Some active principles of vegetal origin stop cell division, binding themselves to tubulin protein, that is responsible, as the name suggests, for the generation of microtubules that are essential for cell division. These fibres separate the doubled chromosomes and after division arrange for each newborn cell to receive a complete genome. The drugs that interfere with the construction or the elimination of the tubulin fibres stop cell division.

Fig.) 56 Oncogenes and tumor suppressive genes.

Oncogenes

Growth factor genes and their receptors

PDGF — Codifies platelet-derived growth factor; contribute to some brain tumors (gliomas).

erbB — Codifies for the receptor of epidermic growth factor (EGF); contributes to some brain tumors (glioblastoma) and breast tumors.

erb-B2 — Also called her/2 or neu; codifies a growth factor receptor; contributes to breast, salivary gland and ovary tumors.

RET — Codifies a growth factor receptor; contributes to thyroid tumors.

Genes for relaying cytoplasmic proteins in stimulatory signals.

Ki-ras — Involved in lung, ovary, large intestine and pancreatic tumors.

N-ras — Involved in leukemias.

Transcription factors genes that activate genes that promote growth

c-myc — Involved in leukemias as well as to breast, stomach and lung tumors.

N-myc — Involved in neuroblastoma (a tumor of the nerve cells) and glioblastoma.

L-myc — Involved in lung tumors.

Other protein genes

Bcl-2 — Codifies a protein that stops programmed cell death (apoptosis); involved in follicular lymphoma of B cells.

Bcl-1 — Also called PRAD 1; codifies cyclin D 1, a component that stimulates the mechanism of the cellular cycle; involved in brain, head, and neck tumors.

MDM-2 — Codifies an opponent of tumor suppression protein p53; involved in connective tissue tumors (sarcomas) and other tumors.

Tumor suppressive genes

Cytoplasmic protein genes

APC — Involved in large intestine and stomach tumors.

DPC-4 — Codifies a messenger protein in the signalling system that stops cell division; involved in pancreatic tumors.

NF-1 — Codifies a protein that inhibits a stimulation protein (Ras); involved in neurofibromas, peripheral nervous system tumors (pheochromocytoma) and myeloid leukemia.

NF-2 — Involved in some brain tumors (meningioma and ependymoma) and schwannoma.

Nuclear protein genes

MTS 1 — Codifies the p16 protein, which is a restraining component of the mechanism of the cellular cycle; involved to a wide range of tumors.

RB — Codifies pRB, which is an essential suppressor of the cell cycle. Involved in retina tumors (retinoblastoma), bone, breast and bladder tumors and in pulmonary carcinoma.

p53 — Capable of stopping cell division and inducing programmed cell death in abnormal cells. Involved in a wide range of tumors.

WT-1 — Involved in renal tumors (Wilms tumor).

Genes for the proteins whose location in the cell has not yet been explained

BRCA1 — Involved in breast and ovary tumors.

BRCA2 — Involved in breast tumors.

VHL — Involved in kidney cell tumors.

Fig. 57) Comparisons between fetal, tumor and adult cells in relation to enzymatic and oxidative ATPase, the amount and the activity of mitochondria and the formation of lactate.

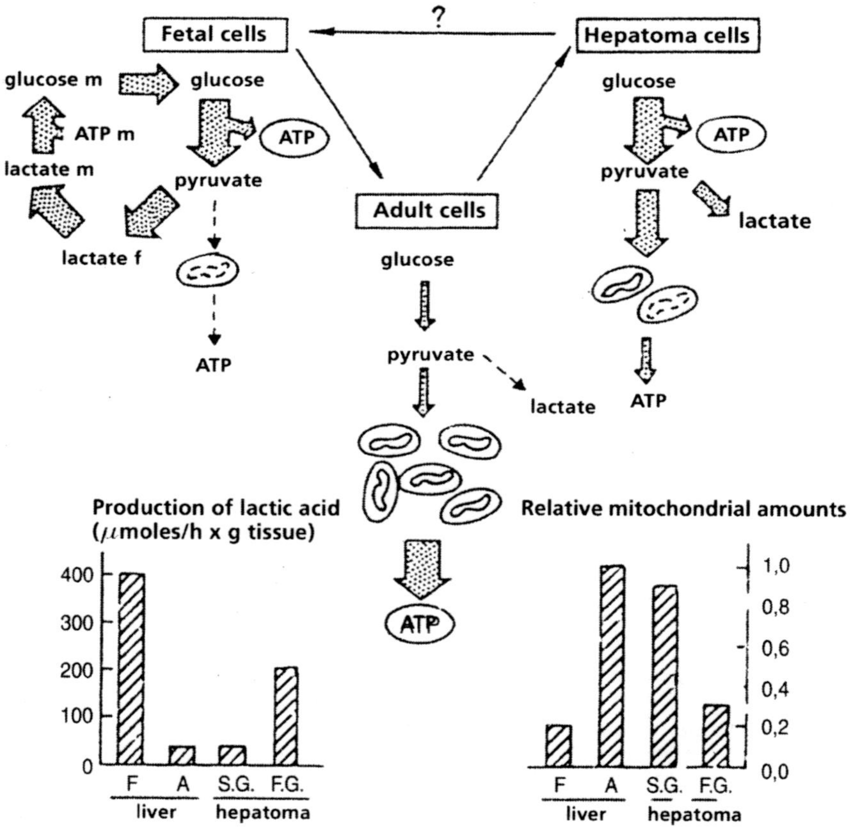
?
Fetal cells
Hepatoma cells
Adult cells
glucose m
glucose
ATP m
ATP
lactate m
pyruvate
lactate f
ATP
glucose
ATP
pyruvate
lactate
glucose
pyruvate
lactate
ATP
ATP
Production of lactic acid
(μmoles/h x g tissue)
400
300
200
100
0
F
A
S.G.
F.G.
liver
hepatoma
Relative mitochondrial amounts
1,0
0,8
0,6
0,4
0,2
0,0
F
A
S.G.
F.G.
liver
hepatoma

Fig. 58)
Diagram of programmed cell death due to release of cytochrome c by mitochondria after highly prooxidative stress. This reaction is blocked in tumor cells. The proteins of cytochrome contain heme molecules from the tight bond that contains iron, whose splitting in tumor cells is forced by enzymes. The consequence is the inhibition of cell respiration and apoptosis, as well as an increase in the production of carbon monoxide (CO) and cyanide (CN). This reaction explains phenomena that have been puzzling up until now, i.e. the transformation to tumor cells and the failure of chemotherapy and radiotherapy.

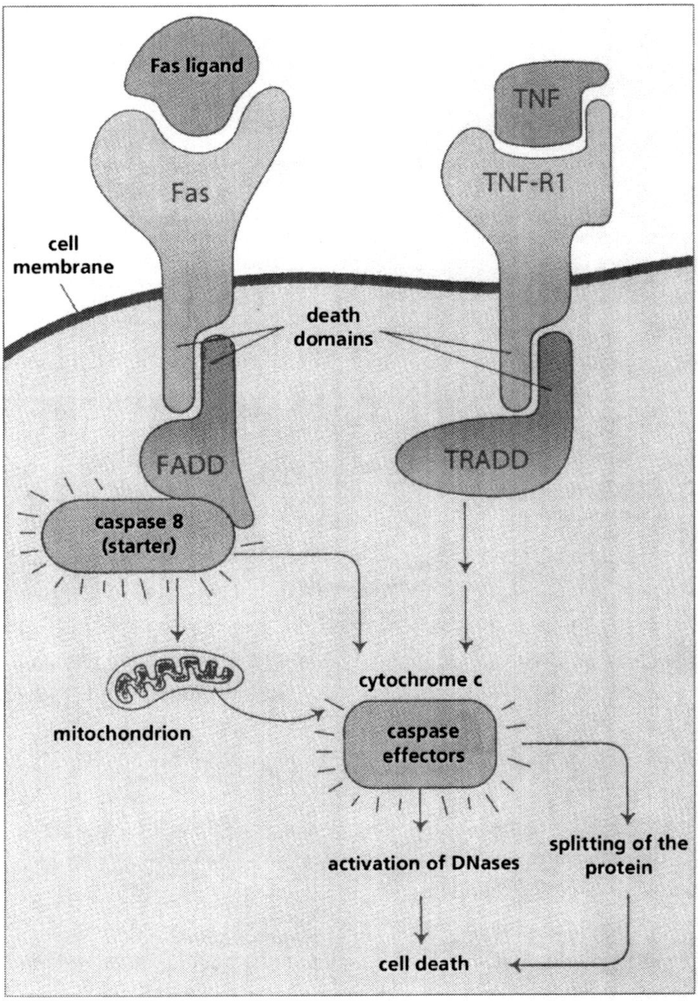
Fas ligand
TNF
Fas
TNF-R1
cell membrane
death domains
FADD
TRADD
caspase 8 (starter)
cytochrome c
mitochondrion
caspase effectors
splitting of the protein
activation of DNases
cell death

Fig. 59) First and last stages of mitochondrial synthesis.

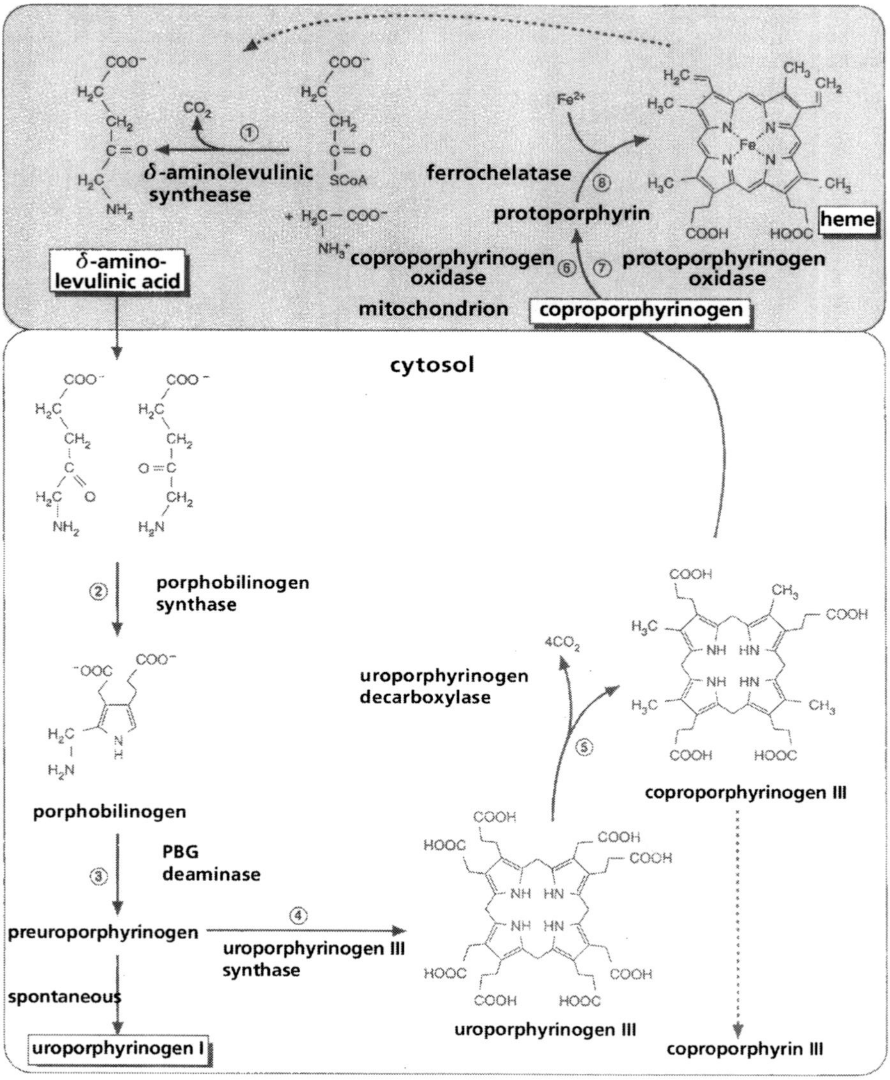
δ-aminolevulinic
synthease
ferrochelatase
protoporphyrin
heme
δ-amino-
levulinic acid
coproporphyrinogen
oxidase
protoporphyrinogen
oxidase
mitochondrion
coproporphyrinogen
cytosol
porphobilinogen
synthase
porphobilinogen
uroporphyrinogen
decarboxylase
coproporphyrinogen III
PBG
deaminase
preuroporphyrinogen
uroporphyrinogen III
synthase
spontaneous
uroporphyrinogen I
uroporphyrinogen III
coproporphyrin III

Fig. 60) The forced splitting of the heme molecules causes the formation of CO and catabolic products (biliverdin/bilirubin) with a high absorption of photons. These processes promote the transformation to tumor cells

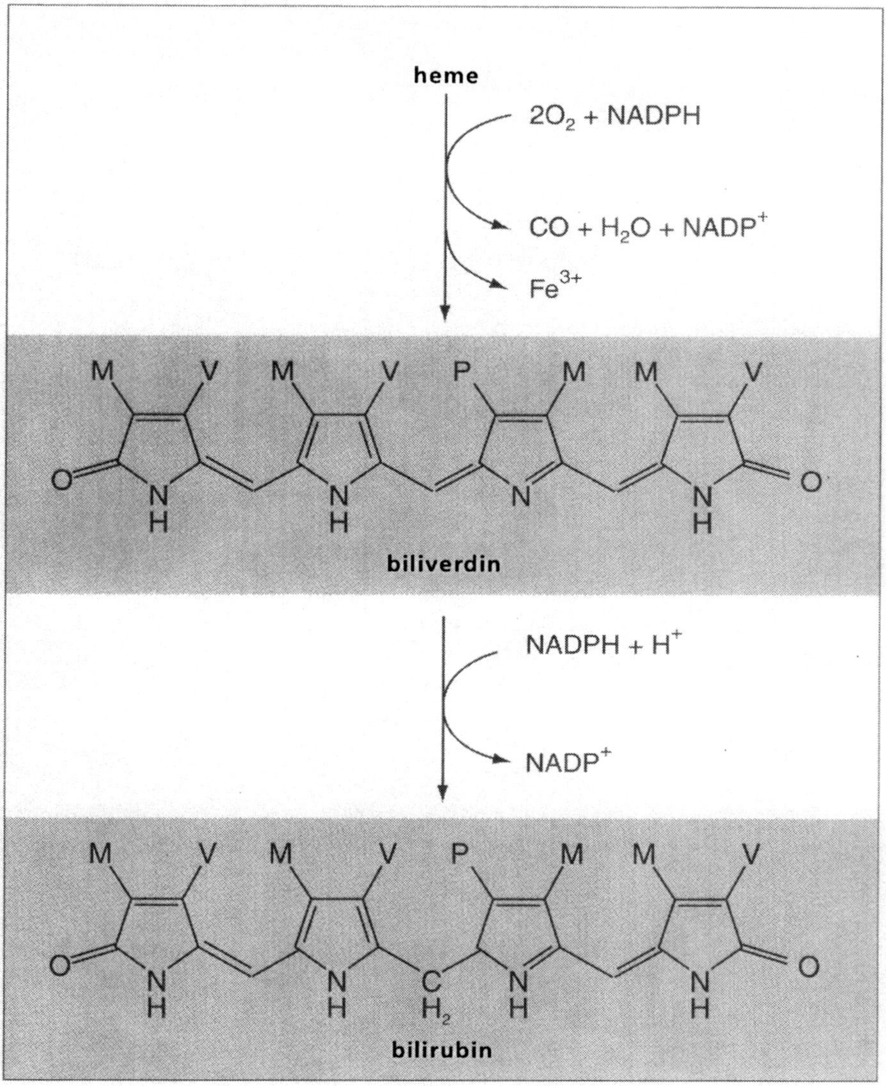
heme
2O2 + NADPH
CO + H2O + NADP+
Fe3+
M V M V P M M V
O N H N H N N H O
biliverdin
NADPH + H+
NADP+
M V M V P M M V
O N H N H C H2 N H N H O
bilirubin

Fig. 61) Blockade of the electron transport chain in complex IV of cellular respiration in the mitochondrion by means of CN, CO and the nitrogen group N^{---}.
The CN and the CO blockade similar to the N^{---} blockade (for instance the immunosuppressor Azathioprine (AZT), the "anti HIV" drug, and chemotherapeutic agent Bactrim could lead to the transformation to a tumour cell.

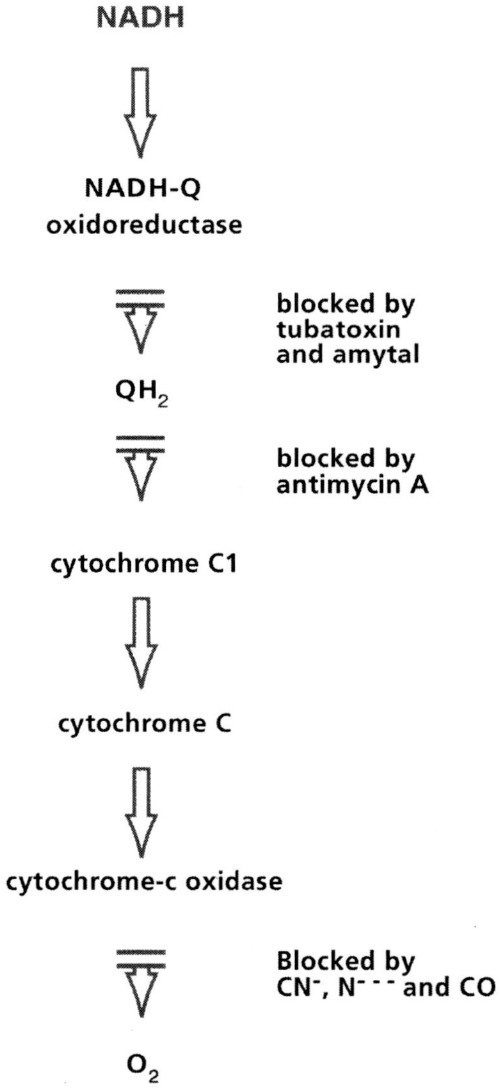
NADH
NADH-Q
oxidoreductase
blocked by
tubatoxin
and amytal
QH_2
blocked by
antimycin A
cytochrome C1
cytochrome C
cytochrome-c oxidase
Blocked by
CN^-, N^{---} and CO
O_2

Fig. 62) The attack on inner vascular wall cells following the inhalation of nitrate gases ('poppers', a sexual stimulator for anal intercourse) leads to an increase in the amount of NO gas and in certain doses and depending on the length of consumption provokes Kaposi's Sarcoma.

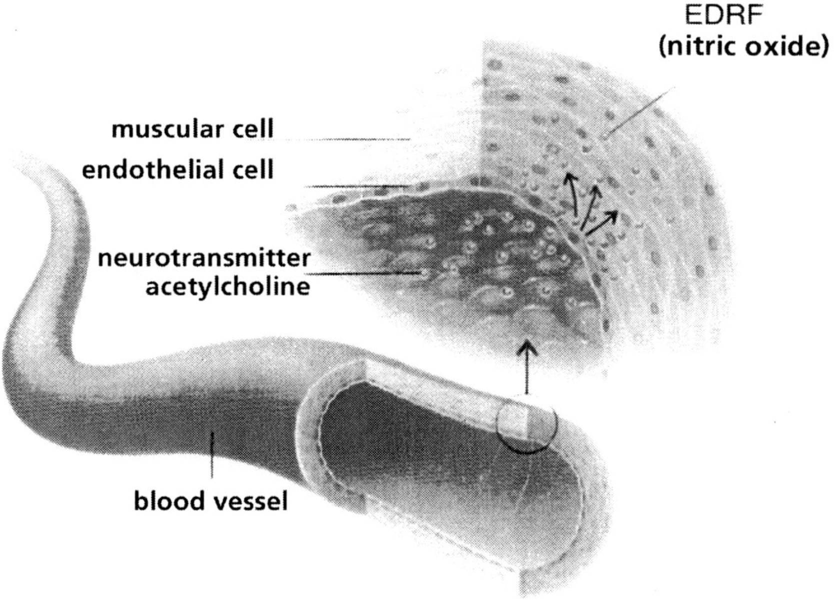

EDRF
(nitric oxide)
muscular cell
endothelial cell
neurotransmitter
acetylcholine
blood vessel

Chapter IX

HIV/AIDS Medicine Run Amok

Why AIDS drugs cause cancer, degenerative changes in muscular and nervous cells, and even AIDS itself-the explanation of how AZT, Bactrim/Septra, and their ilk actually work.

The three "most successful" immunosuppressive (Azathioprine), antimicrobial (Trimethoprim) and "antiretroviral" (AZT) drugs originate from the same laboratory: all three substances have immunotoxic, mitochondriotoxic and carcinogenic (primary and secondary AIDS indicator diseases) effects.

The products of laboratory research initiated more than 50 years ago whose target was to plant analog transformed bases in the biosynthesis of the building blocks of nucleic acid of the DNA—the purine bases, adenine and guanosine as well as the pyrimidine bases thymine and cytosine—were supposed to inhibit the biosynthesis in microbe, immune and cancer cells. Hitchings' laboratory team from Burroughs Wellcome synthesized three substance groups, which in their molecular composition contain nitro structure groups as a common characteristic. These substances produce both antimicrobial effects in microbe cells and immune suppressive and carcinogenic effects in immune and non-immune human cells on top of degenerative DNA damage.

- The first substance was Azathioprine, adopted as an immune suppressive drug for organ transplant patients since the 1960s (Chen 1987). Azathioprine triggered clinically opportunistic infections, Kaposi's sarcoma and lymphomas (transplantation AIDS) (overview Penn 1979, 1981).
- The second substance was Azidothymidine (AZT), from 1986 until today the most frequently prescribed drug for the prophylaxis of AIDS. AZT is supposed to inhibit the proliferation of the hypothetical "HIV retrovirus" in "HIV positive" and AIDS patients. AZT is highly toxic has

antimicrobial, immune suppressive and carcinogenic effects and causes degenerative DNA damage in numerous human cell systems (overview Duesberg 1996, Giraldo 1999, Brink 2000).

- The third substance was Trimethoprim (TMP). TMP as a combination preparation with sulfamethoxazole, a sulfonamide derivative, was authorized as co-trimoxazole in 1969 in the USA and Europe as an antimicrobial drug (DTB 1969). Trimethoprim as sole medication or in combination with sulfamethoxazole (co-trimoxazole) produced in addition to its antimicrobial mechanisms, immunosuppressive and carcinogenic effects and degenerative DNA damage in numerous human cell systems.

All three substances, Azathioprine, Azidothymidine (AZT) and Trimethoprim respectively co-trimoxazole (T+S) possess the chemical attributes to realize the clinical research program postulated by the retrovirus cancer researchers at the historic conference in New York in March 1983 in "a series of human experiments, planned and executed in order to answer the sort of question which automatically raises itself: what would happen if you were to remove the putative defense mechanism of cellular immunity in human beings? Would this affect either the incidence or clinical course of cancer?" (Thomas 1984).

Background and manipulations behind the introduction of AZT for planned human experiments

The assumption that T-helper immune cells are destroyed by a hypothetical retrovirus was extremely helpful in leading to proof of whether the loss of the function of T-helper immune cells could cause the development of tumor cells. This hypothesis allowed for the deployment of a substance group that was known to have immunosuppressive effects and to cause the formation of tumor cells. Using the excuse of retrovirus inhibition in order allegedly to prolong the life of, according to medical opinion, the inevitably moribund AIDS patients it was possible to prescribe such experimental substances without ethical scruples to willing patients.

There was one such substance. It was first isolated in 1961 from herring sperm cells and in 1964 was synthesized as 3'-azido-3'-deoxythymidine by Horwitz from the Michigan Cancer Foundation (Horwitz 1964). Animal experiment trials in mice and rats with leukaemia showed the development of lymphomas (Yarchoan 1987, Adams 1989). As a result of its tumor-causing effects and the lack of inhibition of leukaemia cells this substance was not authorized for clinical human trials (Duesberg 1996). In 1985, shortly after the worldwide introduction on the market of the "anti HIV antibody tests," developed according to the patented production procedures of Gallo at the National Cancer Institute in the USA, publications appeared from the same institute in which it was reported that Azidothymidine (AZT), a chemotherapeutic from nucleoside analog substances, inhibited the proliferation of "retrovirus HIV" in cell cultures (Mitsuya 1985).

Since 1984 it had been acknowledged that nucleoside analog substances not only cause lymphomas but also exercise massive immunosuppressive effects on the T-helper immune cells and provoke opportunistic infections.

"Each of the nucleoside analogs is associated with a profound lymphocytopenia [loss of T-helper immune cells], with a reversal of the CD4/CD8 [the ratio of T-helper immune cells to T8 lymph cells] and opportunistic infections" (Cheson 1997).

So nucleoside analog substances cause AIDS and cancer. AZT is consequently the suitable propagated substance for the "removal of cellular immunity" (Thomas 1984) and tumorigenesis.

After only a 17-week trial in a multi-center study in a number of US clinics in 1986/87 AZT was authorized in record time as a medication for AIDS patients. Clinical trials of a new medicament in the USA usually take on average 8 to 10 years. Burroughs Wellcome, the same US pharmaceutical firm that produced Azathioprine, undertook the marketing of AZT. The global British/American pharmaceutical giant Burroughs Wellcome, which in the 1990s merged to become the largest pharmaceutical company in the world—Glaxo Wellcome (now GlaxoSmithKline)—had an unusual historical company policy: a large portion of the profits were directed to research foundations and donated to biochemical research institutes and clinical studies. As a result of this financial flow a close financial dependency developed between the researchers in laboratories and university clinics and the national health authorities and pharmaceutical companies. Burroughs Wellcome financed many experimental and clinical studies on chemotherapeutic treatment. The head of research there, Barry, had previously worked as a virologist for the American authority responsible for the admission and surveillance of food and drugs—the FDA. He was, conveniently, the right man at the right place at the right time to organize the mass human experiments of the cancer therapeutic, AZT on AIDS patients, and to use the right channels of cooperation for the very rapid approval of AZT by the FDA. The National Cancer Institute had transferred the data and technology for the synthesis of AZT to Burroughs Wellcome. In July 1985 Burroughs Wellcome was accorded "orphan drug status" for AZT by the FDA, even before the first scientific publications from researchers of the National Cancer Institutes on the "anti HIV effect" of AZT in October 1985.

"Orphan drugs" are medications that are required by fewer than 200,000 patients annually in the USA, so production by pharmaceutical companies is not financially lucrative. The respective US law provides for seven years of exclusive marketing rights and tax relief for the production of such "orphan drugs." In the case of AZT, which is extremely expensive, the FDA did not assign a price limit for Burroughs Wellcome. In February 1986 Burroughs Wellcome transformed from a non-commercial organization into a corporation. In November 1986 Barry, together with his colleagues from the National Cancer Institute, published research data on "anti HIV inhibition" in T-helper immune cells of AIDS patients after AZT treatment. This caused a furor. Burroughs Wellcome stock almost quadrupled within a year (Adams 1989). The "invisible hand of the market" had ensured, as in the case of the patenting of Gallo's "anti-HIV test" before the first publication of data that could be analyzed, that strategic decisions for the global marketing of "planned human experiments" for the "removal of cellular immunity" by medication with immunosuppressive and carcinogenic chemotherapeutic AZT had already taken place before the research data of the first experimental study (October 1985) as well as the second experimental and first clinical study (November 1986) were published.

At the time of publication of the latter, clinical tests were already under way in a multi-center study in the USA. AZT was authorized by the FDA and was already being deployed for all AIDS patients in the early summer of 1987. Barry's co-workers were the then leader of the research and development department and later director of the National Cancer Institute (1989-95), Broder, and the clinical retrovirologist Bolognesi from Duke University in North Carolina (Duesberg 1996). As authors they were responsible for the key publication in the proceedings of the National Academy of Science in 1986, in which it was claimed that AZT was 100 times more effective at inhibiting DNA synthesis in "HIV infected" cells than in "non-HIV infected" cells in cell cultures. The same non-specific "molecular markers" were cited as proof of the presence of the "retrovirus HIV" that Gallo and Montagnier had deliberately misinterpreted as "evidence of the isolation and continuous production of cytopathic retroviruses" by virus-like particles (Popovic 1984). At the same time the allied experimental scientists from the pharmaceutical company Burroughs Wellcome, The National Cancer Institute and Duke University, claimed after intake of AZT in the first clinical studies on AIDS patients that the substance was 2,000 to 20,000 times more effective at inhibiting the replication of "HIV DNA" (measured by means of unspecific markers) than the nuclear DNA of "HIV infected" T-helper immune cells (Furman 1986).

These claims have since been refuted in numerous experiments of orthodox HIV/AIDS researchers who had followed the same assumptions about the existence of "retrovirus HIV" on the basis of molecular markers and the workings of AZT (overview Chui 1995). The supposition of a higher affinity for the integration of AZT in "retroviral DNA" in comparison to nuclear DNA of human cells has to this day not been corrected by the researchers of the producers, Burroughs Wellcome (now GlaxoSmithKline), the National Cancer Institute or Duke University. On the basis of this false assumption and these false claims countless doctors all over the world have prescribed AZT to AIDS patients since 1987. They have also prescribed the proven dangerous drug to healthy, asymptomatic "HIV positive" patients since 1990 (Volberding 1990).

Before the global marketing of AZT for "life-prolonging treatment of AIDS patients through inhibition of retroviral replication" in 1987 and the "preventative inhibition of HIV replication in T-helper immune cells of asymptomatic HIV patients" neither the researchers from the company producing AZT, nor the researchers from the NCI or any other researchers had tested the actual functioning mechanisms of AZT. Without exception all researchers and prescribing physicians, independent of the respective assumptions about the affinity of AZT to "retroviral DNA" or to nuclear DNA, took for granted, without checking, that AZT as a transformed molecular building block is integrated into the DNA chain in place of the natural building block, thymidine, either by the "HIV enzyme RT" or by the natural nuclear enzymes of the DNA polymerases.

In the long drawn-out chain of about 25,000 human genes, spread out on 23 paired chromosomes, several billion building blocks are strung together. These nucleotides (from the Greek: *nucleos* = core) are molecular, composed from a sugar, a base and three phosphate group atoms. Nucleotides contain one of four bases (adenosine, cytosine, guanosine or thymidine). These bases have an OH molecule group to which the respective proximate nucleotide is attached. The sequence of the bases in each case with three bonded sets of paired nucleotides form the coding pattern for the building instructions for the synthesis of proteins from amino acids in the cytoplasm. This DNA coding profile is transcribed, after redox-dependent stimulation by transcription factors, to a messenger RNA and translated into the biosynthesis of proteins. This process is called expression and one talks of genes being expressed.

According to the dogmatic doctrine of HIV/AIDS medicine it is this process that the transformed building block AZT affects. In the thymidine base of this molecule the OH group is replaced by an azido group. Should the false building block AZT be integrated into a DNA copy of the "HIV RNA" via the RT enzyme of the supposed "retrovirus HIV," then on this location of the short DNA string of "HIV" (termed provirus) no further nucleotides could align as the integrated AZT has the wrong pairing. The provirus genome of "HIV" would remain incomplete and could no longer be reproduced, with the aid of the cell division apparatus of the host cell, as new infectious "retrovirus HIV."

That is the theory anyway by which the "invisible hand of the market"-manipulated HIV/AIDS doctors suggest, to this day, to their asymptomatic "HIV-positive" patients and AIDS patients, that the intake of AZT for life, alone or in combination with other substances, will prolong their lives through the inhibition of the sooner or later "deadly retrovirus infection with HIV." This doctrine is spread by an immense propaganda input throughout all countries in the world. Unfortunately it has nothing to do with the biological realities and those responsible know this full well.

Clarification about the real working mechanisms of AZT

AZT is a synthetic nucleotide, the precursor of a nucleoside triphophate that merely docks one phosphate atom. In order to be integrated into DNA, regardless of whether it is "HIV provirus DNA" or nuclear DNA, the nucleoside monophosphate AZT in the nucleus must have three phosphate atoms and could only then be incorporated at the growing end of the DNA as a nucleotide by an "HIV RT" or the nuclear enzyme DNA polymerase. In this case the synthetic nucleoside monophosphate AZT would become the DNA nucleotide Azidothymidine triphosphate (AZT TP) that is capable of integration. Countless studies over the last decade, however, have clearly shown that only about 1% of AZT is transformed to AZT TP—thus, at prescribed AZT doses of between 500 and 1,500 mg per day, much too little to be able to cause any kind of inhibition of "HIV provirus DNA" or nuclear DNA as a "DNA terminator" as the claimed effects of AZT state (overview Papadopulos-Eleopulos 1999).

When in 1961 Azidothymidine was isolated from the sperm cells of herrings and subsequently synthetically produced in 1964 (Adams 1989) the obvious question that nobody asked should have been: What was the natural function of Azidothymidine in the sperm cells of vertebrates? Two reasons are conceivable: the fertilization of the ova and the development of the embryo. Firstly, all eukaryotic organisms that propagate sexually, inherit their mitochondria only through the maternal hereditary line (Wallace 1999). The mitochondria of the sperm cells thus have to be somehow inactivated before penetration of the egg cell, yet nobody has subsequently studied how this happens. Secondly, the sperm cells must not introduce intracellular agents to the egg cells as the embryonal cells, as a result of their type 2 cytokine dominance, are not able to adequately eliminate intracellular agents (Coffman 1986, Mosmann 1996). Azidothymidine, as a nitrosative substance, serves both purposes. The azido groups of Azidothymidine inhibit the mitochondrial enzyme cytochrome oxidase (Tyler 1992). The biological logic is that the inhibition of cytochrome oxidase in sperm cells takes place shortly before they penetrate the egg cell, and the sperm cell mitochondria are inactivated by azidothymidine. Azidothymidine is thought to have the same effect on cytochrome oxidase in microbes.

After the worldwide licensing of AZT as an AIDS drug for the supposed blockade of the "retrovirus HIV," a number of research groups reported that the administration of AZT caused damage to DNA and mitochondria (overview Lewis 1995). These findings did not concur with the claims of the HIV/AIDS researchers that AZT is exclusively incorporated into "HIV proviral DNA," as a selective DNA chain terminator.

In order to test the causes of AZT damage to mitochondria and to study whether the observed DNA damage was responsible for the subsequent growth inhibition of the cells after AZT treatment, researchers from the State University in New York carried out experiments of the effect of AZT on mitochondria. They allowed mitochondria to grow in a medium for five days with a pharmacotherapeutic AZT dose (5 micromoles for five days). As soon as three hours after the addition of AZT, the mitochondria showed signs of characteristic changes: reduced number of mitochondria, a reduction in the intake of oxygen, reduced ATP synthesis and an increased lactate synthesis. As the new formation of DNA takes considerably longer than three hours, the change in mitochondrial quantity and energy production, and the glycolytic formation of lactates, could not be based primarily on the inhibition of mitochondrial DNA (Hobbs 1995).

Research teams from a number of French research institutes studied the effects of AZT and two other AIDS drugs (the nucleoside analogs ddI and ddC) in human muscle cells. All three substances cause a dose-dependent reduction in the proliferation and differentiation of cells, a reduction in enzyme activity in the mitochondrial respiratory chain (cytochrome c-oxidase in complex IV and succinate dehydrogenase in complex II of mitochondria as well as an increase in glycolytic lactate synthesis). The researchers concluded that AZT, ddI and ddC exercise a cytotoxic effect on human muscle cells and cause functional changes through the blockade of mitochondrial respiratory enzymes.

A number of fundamental consequences arose from the research findings that were not explicitly discussed by researchers:

Warburg discovered the "Atmungsferment" cytochrome in the 1920s. This molecule transports electrons in the respiratory chain from complex III to complex IV, where the electrons are transferred to molecular oxygen O_2 by the enzyme cytochrome c oxidase. Through the reaction O_2 is reduced to water. 90% of oxygen used worldwide, in algae, plants, fungi, parasites, animals and humans is converted by this reaction. The transferred electron energy in the mitochondrial respiratory chain compresses the hydrogen ions in the mitochondria, the hydrogen generator activates the synthesis of the energy-carrying molecule ATP, and the whole cell is then provided with energy for biosyntheses. Azidothymidine inhibits the enzyme cytochrome c oxidase and thus interrupts the ATP synthesis. This effect is easy to follow: The azido group of azidothymidine is made up of N_3. This triple nitrogen atom configuration is just as reactive as nitrosative molecules, such as NO and its derivatives. The azido group analogous to NO and its derivatives, can oxidize metal ions such as those found in cytochrome oxidase; and likewise oxidizes sulfhydryl groups in thiols (glutathione, cysteine) and thiol proteins (R-SH).

In fact, this characteristic of azide (N_3) has long been used by mitochondria researchers to inhibit the electron transfer from complex IV to molecular O_2 in the respiratory chain of the mitochondria (overview Tyler 1992).

This is why it is incomprehensible why the HIV/AIDS researchers did not want to know about this function of azidothymidine, and instead claim to this day that AZT is incorporated in "HIV provirus DNA" as a selective DNA chain terminator, although AZT is only marginally transformed into AZT triphosphate.

The blockade of cell respiration in mitochondria can be short and it can be reversible. Depending on the dosage AZT can cause, however, with a sudden reduction of ATP through the blockade of cytochrome c oxidase, programmed cell death due to the loss of tension of the electric mitochondrial membrane potential and massive Ca^{2+} cycling. Adenosine triphosphate (ATP) is formed in mitochondria from adenosine diphosphate (ADP) and inorganic phosphate (P_i). If the ratio of ADP to ATP sinks below the critical level of 0.2, necrosis begins (Richter 1996).

However, a multitude of Type-II counterregulations can be triggered by longer-term exposure to AZT. These are dependent on the depletion of the thiol pool through nitrosative stress. The type 1-type 2 balance shifts to a type 2 cytokine dominance (overview Lucey 1996). The type 2 cytokine profile effects an increased expression of the cyclooxygenase-2 enzyme (COX 2) and transforming growth factor (TGF-β). COX 2 controls the increased formation of prostaglandine E2 (PEG2) from arachidon acid, which is formed from essential fatty acids (overview Minghetti 1998). TGF-β and PEG2 suppress the inducible enzyme of cytotoxic NO synthesis and activate the enzyme arginase, which transforms arginine to ornithine. The diminished concentration of arginine in the cytoplasm leads to a diminished production of NO and peroxinitrite, that contributes to a closing of the mitochondrial membrane. The resulting Type-II cell dyssymbiosis (proto symbiosis) triggers an increased expression of heat shock proteins, Bcl-2 proteins (calcium bonding on membranes) and transformed p53 proteins, ferritin protein (bonding on free irons) and the enzyme protein hemoxygenase (overview Lincoln 1997).

The latter leads to the excessive formation of carbon monoxide (CO), which as well as NO regulates many processes (Suematsu 1996, Rivier 1998). CO can likewise block the enzyme cytochrome c oxidase of the mitochondrial respiratory chain. Under the influence of CO increased polyamines are formed from ornithine via the decarboxylase reaction. Polyamines activate repair processes and increase the cell division cycles (McCann 1987, Bachrach 1989, Lincoln 1997). The ornithine decarboxylase reaction induces simultaneously via the putrescine product, enzymes for ATP synthesis via aerobic glycolysis (Brand 1997 b). So the result is the "Warburg Phenomenon", a puzzle for more than seventy years, as a consequence of a nitrosative and/or oxidative provoked pseudohypoxia (an apparent oxygen deficiency). The genetic and non-genetic programmes in response to pseudohypoxia are evolutionary biologically conserved and are regulated by the autopoietic micro-Gaian milieu.

So the effects of azidothymidine inactivate mitochondria by blocking the enzyme cytochrome oxidase, which contains iron and copper ions, inhibit ATP synthesis and depending on the dosage and the duration of administration, together with the disposition of the antioxidative capacity of the cells, trigger a Type-I cell dyssymbiosis (apoptosis /necrosis) or a Type-II cell dyssymbiosis (immune deficiency, degradation or the formation of tumors). Clinically all forms of compensated and decompensated cell dyssymbiosis have been more than abundantly documented (overview Giraldo 1999, Brink 2000).

The therapeutic pseudo-benefit of AZT administration

The observed changes of mitochondrial DNA by nitrosative or oxidative effects analogous to the DNA transformations by NO, peroxinitrite, nitrosamine and ROS are viewed as secondary effects (overview Lijinsky 1994, Loeppky 1994, Lincoln 1997, Wallace 1999).

By inactivating cell respiration enzymes, azidothymidine not only has immunosuppressive and carcinogenic effects, but also antimicrobial ones. The enzyme cytochrome c oxidase and other enzymes able to be oxidized by AZT, are also present in bacteria, fungi and protozoa. The clinically apparently beneficial effects of AZT, which for the stated reasons can by no means be traced back to the inhibition of any “HIV provirus DNA”, are based on a different absorption of the substance both in the body’s cells and in microbial cells. This effect of AZT can lessen microbial stress over a limited period of time if as a consequence of the type 2 cytokine dominance the T-helper immune cells of the patient no longer produce cytotoxic NO and can no longer eliminate intracellular microbes. At the same time, however, the cell dyssymbiosis of immune and non-immune cells of the patient deteriorate depending on the remaining thiol pool. As surviving microbes can also respond to nitrosative stress from AZT with a Type-II counterregulation, the question is who will win the competition for the best possible assimilation to the targeted attack by AZT and a whole battery of other cytotoxins, man or microbe. On the one hand counterregulated intracellular microbes find in counterregulated human cells a favorable environment as they can no longer be eliminated due to the lack of cytotoxic NO gas. On the other hand AZT can only inhibit fungi and parasites that have not been counterregulated.

When confronted with AZT drugs, microbes capable of survival switch to glycolysis and glutaminolysis and can profit even better in cell systems whose defense is weakened by the lack of cytotoxic NO gas as the formation of lactate enables the acidification of the neighboring tissue as well as the penetration of the blood vessels and the possibility of movement through cell areas with an undersupply of oxygen by means of the activation of proteinase enzymes like heparanase (Liew 1994, Brand 1997 b). The fact that highly malignant tumors behave in a very similar manner to some highly successful parasites (Mathupala 1997) proves that the cell types are conforming to the same archaic evolutionary-biological rules.

The important question of whether male sperm cells contain immunotoxic and carcinogenic azidothymidine (AZT)

Whether azidothymidine or similar substances are formed in human sperm cells and other cells has not been studied, but there are indications that this could be the case. Human sperm cells, like highly malignant cancer cells or quickly proliferating microbes, contain high amounts of polyamines that are formed by the ornithine cycle. Lethal protozoa infections as well as the fungal agents of *Pneumocystis carinii* pneumonia (PCP), the most frequently diagnosed AIDS-indicating disease, can be effectively treated by ornithine decarboxylase inhibitors (alpha difluoromethylornithine) (Sjoerdsma 1984). This form of treatment for analog cancer cells has not been tested as apparently it was not taken into consideration that:

- The inactivation of the mitochondrial respiratory chain through nitrosative and/or oxidative nucleosides (for instance through the change in reaction of nucleosides in nitrosamines)
- The counteractivation of CO synthesis through hemoxygenase I

In 1991 a Japanese research team stated: "Oxidative damage of mtDNA can be accumulated during even short period of AZT administration .... For AIDS patients, it is urgently necessary to develop a remedy substituting this toxic substance, AZT" (Hayakawa 1991).

This appeal did not particularly impress the retrovirus cancer hunters or their hunting companions on the HIV/AIDS front. AZT is still the most frequently prescribed AIDS drug (Papadopulos-Eleopulos 1999).

The suppression of toxicological evidence on the carcinogenic properties of AZT by the FDA (the US approval authority), and the worldwide clinical aftermath of AIDS and cancer caused by AZT medication

Before the approval of AZT by the FDA in spring 1987 their toxicologist had internally issued an urgent warning about AZT as a possible carcinogenic rat poison. The study of AZT using the toxicological standard method of "cell transformation assay" and other processes produced the following results:

"This behavior is characteristic of tumor cells and suggests that AZT may be a potential carcinogen. It appears to be at least as active as the positive control material, methylcholanthrene [an extremely potent carcinogen] ... Dose-related chromosome damage was observed in an *in vitro* cytogenetic assay using human lymphocytes ... Although the dose varied, anemia [maturation inhibition of red blood cells] was noted in all species (including man) in which the drug was tested" (Chernov 1986, overview Lauritsen 1987, 1988 a. 1988 b, 1990 b, Young 1988).

The FDA on the licensing of AZT ignored this unequivocal toxicological report by one of their own staff, violating their own guidelines. The producers Burroughs Wellcome (now GlaxoSmithKline) falsified toxicological findings with the directions on the information leaflet for AZT stating: "The significance of these *in vitro* results is not known."

The FDA's toxicologist criticized this claim and unmistakably stated:

"The sentence: 'The significance of these *in vitro* results is not known.' is not accurate. A test chemical which induces a positive response in the cell transformation assay is presumed to be a potential carcinogen" (Chernov 1986).

In the USA the therapeutic use of potential carcinogens on humans is forbidden by law (Nussbaum 1990). The FDA's internal toxicological reports about the AIDS and cancer-causing effects of AZT first became public knowledge when the FDA was forced to release them under the US "Freedom of Information Act" (Lauritsen 1987, 1990 a). Nevertheless, the majority of doctors and media expressed no doubts about its use for symptom-free "HIV positive" and AIDS patients. The toxicological test results before the authorization of AZT were very quickly confirmed in the clinical use of AZT on AIDS patients both regarding its AIDS-causing and carcinogenic effects.

After a more or less short phase of prooxidative mobilization of the reserve capacities of the immune cells, depending on dosage, AIDS patients developed a massive inactivation of mitochondria and DNA effects, profound damage to the immune cell functions and the maturation of red blood cells as well as tumorigenesis, degeneration of nerve and muscle cells, liver failure and wasting syndrome and other toxic syndromes (Richman 1987,1990, Pizzo 1988, Lauritsen 1988 a, 1989, 1990, 1990 b, 1990 c, Young 1988, Ostrom 1989, Bach 1989, Marx 1989, Cherfas 1989, Pluda 1990, Dalakas 1990).

In 1989, on the recommendation of the National Institute of Allergies and Infectious Diseases, under the directorship of the most senior assessor of research funding for HIV/AIDS medicine in the USA, Dr Fauci, the FDA's approval of azidothymidine (AZT—biochemically termed zidovudine, trade name Retrovir) for the unlimited treatment of symptom-free "HIV positives" was forced through under massive political pressure (Farber 1989, Larhoven 1990, Lauritsen 1989 a, 1989 b, 1990 a, 1990 b, 1990 c, 1990 d, 1993, Cotton 1990, Friedland 1990, Volberding 1990, Fischl 1990, Duesberg 1996, Lang 1998). From 1990, all the health authorities in Western countries, as already was the case in 1987 in accepting the FDA's decision to approve AZT for the treatment of manifest AIDS patients, sanctioned AZT for unlimited treatment of symptom-free "HIV positives," newly born babies, children, adolescents, pregnant and non-pregnant women, and men with and without recognizable risks.

As might have been expected with the chemical characteristics of such a substance, clinical studies in numerous human immune and non-immune cells revealed toxic damage through AZT medication that were not in accordance with the preservation of life. Not even the crushing abundance of scientific evidence published on the state-sanctioned poisoning excess through administration of AZT to pregnant women, newly born babies and children could end this medically irrational and therapeutically useless worldwide mass poisoning (Gill 1987, Richman 1987, Bessen 1988, Gorard 1988, Helbert 1988, Yarchoan 1989, 1991, Pluda 1990, Till 1990, Dalakas 1990, Smothers 1991, McLeod 1992, Bacellar 1994, Parker 1994, Kumar 1994, Rosenthal 1994, Chiu 1995, Zaretsky 1995, Moye 1996, Giraldo 1999 b, Brink 2000).

The manufacturer of AZT admits that the toxic consequences of AZT administration cannot be differentiated from the theoretical "HIV symptoms"

Even the manufacturers, the pharmaceutical company Glaxo Wellcome (now GlaxoSmithKline), who marketed AZT under the chemical name of Zidovudine and the trade name Retrovir, felt compelled to state, as a legal safeguard against the right of recourse:

> "Retrovir (Zidovudine [= AZT]) may be associated with severe hematologic toxicity including granulocytopenia and severe anemia particularly in patients with advanced HIV disease . . . Prolonged use of Retrovir has also been associated with symptomatic myopathy similar to that produced by human immunodeficiency virus" (Glaxo Wellcome 1998).

Nothing can more clearly demonstrate the callous loss of medical ethics than the admission of a global pharmaceutical concern, that a substance, which on the basis of numerous indubitable experimental findings cannot objectively accomplish its claimed effect, namely the integration of AZT allegedly selectively in the DNA chain of a "provirus DNA of retrovirus DNA," but instead causes severe toxic damage to blood and muscle cells. This statement by the manufacturer justifies the criminal charge of grievous bodily harm with fatal consequences. Nobody had in actual fact isolated a "provirus DNA of retrovirus DNA" (Papadopulos-Eleopulos 1993 a, 1998 a) and nobody had been able to prove the pathogenetic mechanism of the "provirus DNA of retrovirus DNA," despite the largest capital investment and the most intensive research efforts in medical history (Balter 1997).

On the contrary, severe maturation disruptions of immune and non-immune cells were diagnosed with absolute regularity in the million-fold AZT prescriptions all over the world. The statement by Glaxo Wellcome that the associated severe cell damage in quick maturing white blood cells "particularly in patients with advanced HIV" appear after AZT medication means no more than AZT aggravates the shift to type 2 cytokine dominance, as shown in numerous studies of the earliest stages of "HIV positive" (overview Lucey 1996), resulting from the chemical characteristics of the substance. "Advanced HIV disease" means that the detoxication capacity of the immune and non-immune cells fails due to a permanent nitrosative and/or oxidative stress status. To administer a highly nitrosative and oxidative substance to a patient in this diagnostic situation, instead of improving the detoxicative performance of the cell systems, is in a legal sense wilful poisoning that sooner or later must result in death for already poisoned patients. The admission by Glaxo Wellcome that "symptomatic myopathy similar to that produced by human immunodeficiency virus" (Glaxo Wellcome 1998) proves that the symptoms of the "HIV disease" cannot be differentiated, diagnostically or pathologically, from a medicamentous intoxication by AZT. AZT causes an "HIV disease" in exactly the same way as an "AZT disease" is caused by excessive and permanent nitrosative and oxidative stress.

The working-mechanism of Bactrim/Septra (Trimethoprim + Sulfamethoxazole)

The fact that the "antiviral" AIDS drugs (nucleoside analog and non-nucleoside analog substances as well as protease inhibitors for the supposed inhibition of the replication of "HI viruses") due to the given biochemical attributes could not inhibit the reproduction of "HI viruses," whatever the immunotoxic, carcinogenic and degenerative effect they had on immune and non-immune cells, raises a further decisive question, and that is to what degree the antimicrobial substances that are deployed for the prophylaxis and therapy of opportunistic infections in "HIV positives," AIDS patients and other groups of patients can also provoke immunotoxic, carcinogenic and degenerative effects.

The first AIDS patients were, from 1980, routinely treated with Trimethoprim/Sulfamethoxazole (co-trimoxazole, T+S, trade name Bactrim, Septra, Eusaprim, Cotrim Forte etc) against the agent of *Pneumocystis carinii* pneumonia (PCP), which is still the most frequent AIDS-indicating disease in Western countries (CDC 1981 a, Gottlieb 1981, Masur 1981). When T+S failed the medication was changed to drugs with pentamidine, an antiparasitic substance in use since 1939, Pyrimethamine, Dapsone and others as well as combinations of these substances. The exact working mechanisms of most of these substances were not known but were employed on a trial-and-error basis both as long-term prophylaxis and in acute treatment as chemotherapeutic inhibitors of fungi and parasites.

Trimethoprim bonds to an enzyme whose function is indispensable in all cell systems from microbe to man. The enzyme converts essential folic acid to the biologically active form tetrahydrofolate (THF). The enzyme is named dihydrofolate reductase (DHFR). THF supplies, among other things, carbon building blocks for the construction of the purine bases, the building blocks for nucleic acid for the synthesis of DNA and the co-enzymes NAD(P)H, FAD, and FMN. THF also participates in the synthesis of the pyrimidine base thymine, which as the phosphate-coupled DNA molecule thymidine triphosphate (TTP) is supposedly suppressed by azidothymidine (AZT). The blockade of THF through inhibition of the enzyme DHFR leads to major disruptions to DNA synthesis, co-enzyme synthesis and the metabolism of certain amino acids. That is why the effects of this disruption affect a multitude of central biosyntheses. At the end of the 1940s, Methotrexate was developed as one of the substances acting as a DHFR inhibitor. This substance effectively bonds to the human DHFR enzyme and is deployed as a blocker of the biologically active forms of folic acid in leukaemia cells and carcinogenic cells. Methotrexate bonds relatively solidly to the DHFR enzyme in cancer cells and healthy cells; nevertheless folic acid turnover, dependent on cell type, is also inhibited in the latter. The results are the side effects of this chemotherapy, which dependent on cell type and the redox conditions proceed both as biochemical target effects and as the target effects against cancer cells.

Soon further DHFR blockers were developed and it was recognized that the DHFR enzymes in bacterial, parasitic, fungal and mammalian cells, including humans, feature minor structural differences. This fact was used to synthesize DHFR enzyme blockers that could selectively bond to the respective microbe enzymes more solidly than to the human DHFR enzymes. This expectation proved to be a dangerous illusion in clinical practice.

One of these substances is Trimethoprim (TMP) whose selective bonding to DHFR enzymes was recognized in 1965. Selective always means merely a relatively strong bond to the enzyme of microbe species as they are dependent on the presence of the co-enzyme NAD and a multitude of bioenergetic conditions. Depending on the preferred bonding to the DHFR enzyme it was possible for the DHFR inhibitors to inhibit folic acid metabolism in bacteria with Trimetoprim, in parasites like the malaria agent with Pyrimethamine, and in tumor cells with Methotrexate and other substances. Trials on Trimethoprim for the inhibition of bacterial growth gave the researchers the idea of combining TMP with other chemotherapeutics containing folic acid inhibiting sulfonamides introduced since 1935. The active principal of sulfonamides was based on the fact that most bacteria, many parasites but also fungi like *Pneumocystis carinii* (the PCP agent) cannot transport available folic acid through the cell membrane but must assemble it from three molecules within the cells. The middle molecule is para amino benzoic acid whose integration to folic acid is regulated by an enzyme that is inhibited by sulfonamide so that insufficient amounts of active folic acid can be synthesized.

Decisive was the consideration that bacterial inhibiting effects of the individual substances could strengthen TMP and sulfonamides in such a way that the combination of substances had a bacteria-killing effect. At the same time it was hoped that through this combination preparation the unpleasant "resistance capacity" of the microbes against the individual substances might be prevented (Bushby 1968). This double folic acid blocker, appearing on the market in the USA and Europe in 1969 (DTB 1969), was going to have an exemplary career as "one of the most successful agents ever developed" (Then 1993). In 1972 Trimethoprim was introduced as a single substance and since then TMP as a stand-alone preparation is annually prescribed to between four and five percent of the population (Steen 1985). The amounts of T+S prescribed in Western countries is considerably higher:

"Co-trimoxazole, Bactrim etc., the fixed combination of sulfamethoxazole and Trimethoprim, constituted until recently the best option for many mundane infections in outpatient practices" (Gysling 1995).

The dangerous illusion of safeguard from infection by continual prophylaxis with Bactrim among promiscuous homosexuals during the 70's

The introduction on the market of T+S as the then unique chemotherapeutic strategy of inhibiting the colonization of human organisms by bacteria, parasites and fungi through the simultaneous inhibition of two essential enzymes of folic acid metabolism in microbes, occurred at the same point in time as the beginning of the decade of sexual liberation for homosexuals. The minority of multi-infectious promiscuous homosexuals and the doctors in the cities specializing in this clientele had the illusory feeling that there was in Bactrim etc. a prophylactic and therapeutic safeguard from infection. The list of infections with agents from all kinds of species, above all in homosexuals with a preference for unprotected anal receptive intercourse, is long and without precedent (Jaffe 1983, Callen 1990, Root-Bernstein 1993).

"Gay men were aware of their disease susceptibility long before AIDS emerged as a problem .... They made chronic use of antibiotics, some prophylactically and some to treat recurrent venereal and other infections. I have been told by a number of gay men that it was not uncommon to take a few antibiotics and sniff an ampule or two of amyl nitrite on the way to the baths or bars for a round of anonymous sex .... Over 40% of the men surveyed responded that they 'routinely' treated themselves with prescription antibiotics. Chronic and high-dose antibiotic abuse can lead to significant immune suppression" (Pifer 1987; Root-Bernstein 1993).

After a series of Bactrim-related deaths, it was recommended that its use be restricted, except for the treatment of already immune-damaged "HIV positives" and AIDS patients

One of the chemoantibiotics most frequently consumed by homosexuals in Western countries, whether prescribed or not, was T+S (co-trimoxazole). However, there was a lack of studies about long-term consumption of T+S both in AIDS risk groups and in the population as a whole. One of the few studies, which at least covered a time span of 45 days after the beginning of the administration, came from the General Practice Research Database. The data were gathered from 420 general practitioners in Great Britain after prescription of T+S and other chemoantibiotics between 1988 and 1993. A treatment time of 45 days is insufficient for an assessment of the long-term consequences as folic acid can be stored in human cell systems for roughly 45 days. Serious long-term damage through lack of folic acid became manifest after months-long T+S medication, for instance in urinary passage infections or in unlimited prophylaxis in "HIV positives" and AIDS patients usually up to six weeks after the beginning of treatment, and was not at that time associated with a folic acid deficiency. Unwanted acute effects were relatively unusual in the studies of the British general practitioners, but dependent on the disposition of the patients they could be serious. Already in 1985 cases of mortalities after T+S medication were published. After a series of deaths heavy restrictions on the indications for T+S were issued in Great Britain (Jick 1995, Committee on the Safety of Medicines 1985, 1995). Also in the USA indications for T+S were stringently revoked and a maximum medication time of no longer than one week recommended.

The remaining European countries have up until now drawn no consequences from the resulting data (overview Lacey 1985, DTB 1995). However, it is rationally incomprehensible that in the terms of the pseudo-logic of the state doctrine that "HIV causes AIDS" T+S medication for unlimited long-term prophylaxis of PCP in "HIV positives" was excluded from this restrictive administration as the only exception, even in Anglo-Saxon countries. The admission of the unlimited indication for T+S medication for immune cell-damaged HIV-stigmatized patients is a blatant contradiction as the restrictions were recommended principally because of serious damage to the blood formation systems resulting from T+S medication (overview Gysling 1995, DTB 1995). This recommendation to prescribe co-trimoxazole, above all in patients who had been diagnosed as being in danger of opportunistic infections as a result of a functional disruption of cells in the immune cell network, for an unlimited long-term prophylaxis, defies all medical logic. "They must have been out of their minds," was the stunned diagnosis of one pharmaceutically independent therapist. However, there was method in the madness.

A crucial problem arose from these findings: A decade before the "sudden" appearance of opportunistic fungal infections as AIDS-indicating diseases in homosexual men, it was already recognized that long-term medication with folic acid inhibitors could provoke neutropenia and systemic fungal infections. At the same time it was known that long-term inhalation of nitrite gases had an intoxicating effect, which also favored fungal infections. It was known that homosexual men with opportunistic fungal infections (AIDS) were habitual T+S abusers and chronic nitrite gas consumers (CDC 1981 a, Gottlieb 1981, Masur 1981). What was the rationale that found the appearance of opportunistic fungal infections in homosexuals puzzling and declared that long-term prophylaxis with T+S was the chosen therapy method for these patients, if indeed they had survived acute treatment with T+S (Gottlieb 1981, Masur 1981)? How could the medical logic be rationally understood when it had been emphatically stated that in the same homosexual patients with fungal infections (AIDS) "Aggressive chemotherapy . . . contributes to the final degree of immunologic incompetence" (De Wys 1982)? Why instead did they seek recourse in the "new agent" (Haverkos 1982) which was eventually created as a fictitious "retrovirus HIV" in test tubes in the Pasteur Institute in Paris and in the National Cancer Institute in the USA?

There is only one rational explanation for the most calamitous failure of modern medicine: The collective repression of the fact that the would-be "miracle weapons" of the 1970s like co-trimoxazole (Bactrim, Septra, Eusaprim etc.) had led to a disaster. The admission of these facts, namely that microbial enemies and malign cancer cells had to be eliminated by aggressive chemotherapy, had so shaken the leading minds and business interests of modern medicine at such a time that the fundamental knowledge of the fluidity principle of the micro-Gaian milieu as archaic laws of the co-evolution of man and microbe had yet to be gained. As a result of this there was a collective stampede and much trumpeting on the virus hunt and new chemo-cocktails that were inevitably to make the disaster even worse. 20 years after the first diagnosis of opportunistic fungal infections in homosexual patients, the dreadful consequence of this obsession is to this day blindly being executed using all the instruments of power as the events before and during the World AIDS Congress in South Africa in July of 2000 demonstrated.

Evidence from animal experiments on the immunosuppressive effects of Azathioprine and Trimethoprim (Bactrim)

In 1970, shortly before the launch of Bactrim, Septra etc. a research team at St. Mary's Medical School in London carried out a revealing study on animals. The clinical researchers were interested in whether the Trimethoprim analog to Azathioprine caused immunotoxic effects. The study was based on three facts:

- The substances Azathioprine and Trimethoprim have similar biochemical structural characteristics and attack the nucleic acid synthesis of DNA as well as the synthesis of nucleotides of the co-enzymes NAD^+, FAD and FMN.
- Azathioprine had suppressed as an immunosuppressive substance the cellular immunity in organ transplant patients and other patients with systemic illnesses and caused opportunistic infections, Kaposi sarcomas, lymphomas and degenerative cell transformations.
- Azathioprine had, like Trimethoprim, inhibited the proliferation of microbial cells.

From these facts the researchers produced the hypothesis that the immunosuppressive substance Azathioprine (producer Burroughs Wellcome) via the same functional mechanism caused antimicrobial effects and vice versa the antimicrobial substance Trimethoprim (producer Burroughs Wellcome) via the same functional mechanism caused immunosuppressive effects.

The researchers transplanted from a strain of brown mice a same-sized piece of skin to four groups of white mice from the same strain. The first group were injected with Trimethoprim, the second group with Azathioprine, the third group with Trimethoprim + Tetrahydrofolate (THF). The fourth group, not injected, served as control.

During the experiment the concentration of hemoglobin, hematocrit, white blood cells and their differential number, the weight of the mice and other readings were measured. The dosage of the substances was so chosen as to be the equivalent of that used in oral therapy in humans (on the basis of comparative weight). The weight of the mice in all groups was comparable for the duration of the experiment, and there were no signs of either suppression of bone marrow cells or a general toxicity. In order to differentiate the non-specific toxic effects from the immunosuppressive effects, the blood concentration of Trimethoprim was measured in the mice blood. Up to the end of the experiment it did not overshoot the relative concentration in humans after oral Trimethoprim medication.

The findings were clear:

The immunosuppressive inhibition of rejection of the transplanted skin in the mice treated with Trimethoprim took exactly as long as the mice treated with immunosuppressive Azathioprine.

The rejection of the skin transplant in mice treated with Trimethoprim + Tetrahydrofolate (THF) took place just as quickly as the non-immonusuppressed control group (Ghilchick 1970).

According to today's knowledge Trimethoprim, just like Azathioprine and later azidothymidine (AZT) (producer Burroughs Wellcome, today GlaxoSmithKline), suppressed the function of NO gas-producing Th1 immune cells and caused, after a few days, a Th1-Th2 switch of cellular immunity. In the third group of mice the immunosuppressive effects of the folic acid blockade by Trimethoprim were compensated for by the simultaneous dose of THF. So the assumption was justified that a medicamentous folic acid blockade with long-term medication with Trimethoprim could, similarly to Azathioprine, induce opportunistic infections, Kaposi's sarcomas, lymphomas, carcinomas and degeneration of muscle and nerve cells (AIDS). Kaposi's sarcomas appeared in organ transplant patients treated with Azathioprine within a few weeks or up to 12 years later and on average after 36 months (Penn 1979).

The London research team subsequently stated:

"The site of the immunosuppressive action of Trimethoprim is the same as that of its antibacterial action—at the conversion of folates to folinates" (Ghilchick 1970).

The study was funded by Burroughs Wellcome, the findings of the study failed to prompt the producers of the T+S preparation to issue a warning about long-term immunotoxic effects of Trimethoprim (Bactrim, Septra, Eusaprim etc) or about even a warning to people with an immunosuppressive disposition about the short-term effects.

The medical establishment denies the toxic consequences of its chemotherapeutic "miracle weapons" in order to preserve the status quo

To understand rationally why a whole generation of doctors since the 1970s is unwilling to give up the antimicrobial "miracle weapons" and to consciously realize their immunotoxic manifestations in "HIV positive" and AIDS patients as substance-induced effects one has to look at why the fact that immunotoxicity of "one of the most successful antimicrobial agents ever developed" (according to the Research Department of the Bactrim, Septra producer Hoffmann-LaRoche, in 1993) is still being denied. The blinkered adoption of the fictitious HIV/AIDS theory had system supporting advantages and stabilized the complex network of give and take between the offering pharmaceutical industry and a reluctant generation of doctors understandably averse to considering its own activities as a major contributor to systemic diseases. The advantage of this system is thus precisely substantiated, to view severe damage to immune cells and non-immune cells as the cause of an apparently unavoidable deadly "retrovirus infection," which requires a battery of chemotactic substances as "life-prolonging therapy"; the toxic consequences of its own activities are explained and exculpated from the outset as the destructive consequences of this "deadly retrovirus infection" (Glaxo Wellcome 1998).

The analogy to chemotherapy in oncology and other fields of clinical medicine is blatant. This system of thought and trade conceals the fact that the half-life of medical theory is becoming ever shorter, thus the practicing doctor unavoidably acts erroneously, a correction to medical malpractice is as a rule only possible once those responsible have lost their influence. The price of the constraints of the system is paid by those affected, for whom medicine is the last bastion of credibility in which they have to confide.

This tragedy, intrinsic to the system, more than clearly demonstrated by Dr. Montagnier, Dr. Gallo and their adherents before and during World AIDS Conferences, poses the question by which right they withheld the knowledge, for example from the people of the Third World, that folic acid deficiency due to undernutrition or malnutrition (nutritional AIDS, Beisel 1992, 1996) and/or chemotherapy against tuberculosis (Davis 1986) and/or Bactrim, Septra etc. and/or other antibiotics can cause exactly the same opportunistic infections and other AIDS-indicating diseases which have been, according to the disease theory "HIV causes AIDS," accredited exclusively to exactly these "HI viruses" that are detected by extremely questionable "HIV Tests."

Instead of offering the required discourse they gathered roughly 5,000 signatures of doctors and scientists in the leading scientific journal *Nature* to keep up appearances. A medical science that is no longer prepared to continue what it does or does not do on the basis of data and facts, which are available for all to verify, deserves no confidence and disqualifies itself as a guarantor of credibility. Scientifically based questions on production procedures of the "HIV tests" remained unanswered by the patent holders Dr. Gallo and Dr. Montagnier and those responsible from the national authorizing institute, stereotypically referring to the relevant secrecy clauses of the producing companies. The control processes demanded by law in all Western countries on the simple suspicion of damaging aftereffects of already authorized medications were not carried out on the "anti-HIV" and anti-AIDS drugs with the claim that it was a lethal infection to which there were no alternatives to the "life prolonging" substances. Referring to the dominant doctrine of HIV/AIDS medicine, the charges of failure to adhere to the control processes demanded by law were rejected. The impression that the established HIV/AIDS group operate above the law can only be counteracted by free discourse within established medical science without being dictated by business personalities like Dr. Montagnier and Dr. Gallo.

Explanation of the mitochondriotoxic working mechanisms of the components of Bactrim

The causal link between folic acid deficiency and chronic and/or opportunistic infections as well as the incidence of tumors has been demonstrated by numerous studies. It has been observed, for instance, that people with a sufficient supply of folic acid have a 35% decrease in the incidence of colon carcinomas compared to those with a smaller provision of folic acid. Comparable findings apply to other tumors (Tönz 1996). Equally, there is no doubt that "persistent infections" (De Wys 1982), for instance in "HIV positive" homosexuals, require an increased demand of folic acid (Davis 1982). Folic acid deficiency inhibits a diversity of biosyntheses and metabolic processes. The blocking effect of Trimethoprim is accordingly complex for the availability of biologically active folate. Trimethoprim disrupts the metabolism of amino acids, for instance the transformation of the amino acid serine to glycine, which supplies one of the three building blocks essential to the sulfurous antioxidant, glutathione. Glycine also participates in the recovery of the essential sulfurous amino acid methionine from homocysteine. The sulfurous amino acids homocysteine and cysteine, which are essential to the organism, can be synthesized from methionine. Homocysteine levels play a important role in all systemic diseases (De Groote 1996). Cysteine is the central building block for glutathione and vital for the detoxification processes of all cell systems. Active folic acid is in turn necessary for the enzyme that can equip methionine in such a way that it can act as indispensable donor for methyl groups in mammalian metabolism.

Activated folic acid is closely related to vitamin B12 and the degradation path of histidine. Additionally, activated folic acid plays an important role for enzymes that are involved in the synthesis and transformation of biogenic amines (dopamine, adrenaline, noradrenaline, serotonin, melatonin) (Lambie 1985). This incomplete list shows that it is misleading to restrict chemotherapeutic substances like Azathioprine, Trimethoprim or Azidothymine (AZT) to either their "immunosuppressive" or "antimicrobial" or even their "anti-retroviral" effects. Chemical substances with or without the decorative epithet "therapeutic" have to be judged on which biochemical compounds they can respond to on the basis of their structural attributes and which metabolic reactions they can indirectly disrupt on the basis of their bonding characteristics. Trimethoprim attacks in a diversity of ways the maturation, function and detoxification of immune cells but at the same time disrupts the synthesis of the co-enzymes which are indispensable for the synthesis of defensive NO gases in immune cells and non-immune cells. The impairment of the co-enzymes through the blocking of activated folic acid resulting from Trimethoprim medication applies, besides many other biosyntheses, also to the co-enzymes of the respiratory chain in cell symbionts, the mitochondria. There is an interaction, a cycling between enzymes and co-enzymes. Trimethoprim attacks this cycling in mitochondria in an incalculable way.

The question of how the doubled folic acid inhibitor in combination of Trimethoprim/Sulfamethoxazole (Bactrim, Septra, Eusaprim etc) is metabolized is of vital interest. The well-founded assumption is that the already synthesized folic acid, on account of its molecular size, is unable to penetrate the mitochondrial membrane. Mitochondria in all human cells originate from proteobacteria (Gray 1999). All bacteria, just as fungi and parasites, which in contrast to bacteria contain mitochondria, have to assemble folic acid from the three single building blocks within the cytoplasm or as the case may be in the mitochondria. The consequence is that T+S medication attacks a diversity of the functions of mitochondria leading to the following assumptions:

- Sulfamethoxazole blocks the synthesis of folic acid in human mitochondria as well as in microbes.
- Human mitochondria are just as vulnerable to Sulfamethoxazole as bacteria cells.
- Trimethoprim blocks the activation of folic acid in mitochondria as well as in intracellular microbes, the bonding affinity of Trimethoprim to the enzyme DHFR is an analog to the bonding affinity of the substance in bacteria cells.
- Human mitochondria are just as vulnerable to Trimethoprim as bacteria cells.
- The metabolic product of Sulfamethoxazole, above all the toxic hydroxylamine, has to be detoxified by glutathione. Toxic nitroso compounds form in cases of increased glutathione use an ensuing deficit of the forming glutathione. This leads through nitrosative and oxidative stress to inhibition of cytochrome oxidase in the respiratory chain, to a decreased ATP production, to DNA damage and disruption to protein synthesis, to increased cell disintegration (Type-I overregulation of cell

dyssymbiosis) or to cell transformation as glycolytic tumor cells (Type-II counterregulation of cell dyssymbiosis).

- The metabolic product of Trimethoprim, especially the nitro groups, caused nitrosative and oxidative stress effects in mitochondria analogous to those in bacteria cells, and the mitochondrial stress effects are analogous to the effects of NO radicals as well as the nitro groups of Azathioprine and azidothymidine (AZT).
- The bacterial stem cells of the human mitochondria can, during the course of a glutathione deficit (through increased use and disturbance of the new syntheses) and deficits of other antioxidants under prolonged medication with T+S, react more vulnerably than opportunistic agents that are able to switch facultatively and selectively to a Type-II counterregulation: T+S provokes T-helper immune cells (NO gas-producing Th1 cells) to die at a faster rate (Type-I overregulation) and/or newly maturing T-helper stem cells from the thymus to switch to a type 2 cytokine profile (Th2 cell dominance, Type-II counterregulation) and stimulate increased antibody production. Other T+S provoked immune cells can also die at a faster rate (neutrophile granulocytes, neutropenia, Type-I overregulation) or be increasingly activated (eosinophile granulocytes, eosinophilia, Type-II counterregulation). T+S-provoked non-immune cells can also die at a faster rate (apoptosis/necrosis, Type-I overregulation) or degenerate (myopathies and encephalopathies through a Type-II counterregulation in muscle and nerve cells no longer active in division).
- Trimethoprim respectively Trimethoprim/Sulfamethoxazole (and pentamidine, pyrimethamine, dapsone analogs) alone or synergetically with other immune stressors and immunotoxic/cytotoxic substances can provoke "HIV positive" test reactions, opportunistic infections (AIDS), cancer cell transformations and degeneration in muscle and nerve cells no longer active in division.
- Trimethoprim or as the case may be, Cotrimethazole induced damage of human mitochondrial DNA is passed on over generations from mother to child via the exclusive inheritance of the mitochondrial DNA of the egg cells and can trigger a diversity of systemic diseases like AIDS, cancer and degenerative muscle and nerve illnesses in progeny. These are dependent on the ratio of still intact to already defective mitochondria in the specific cell systems (heteroplasmy). In the course of the load from lifetime stressors the mitochondrial functions which have until that time been compensated could decompensate and congenital mitochondrial damage strengthened through acquired mitochondrial diseases which exponentiate to systemic deficits (Johns 1996, Wallace 1999).

Nobody knows how the mitochondria status in the population as a whole is obtained as the appropriate survey has not been carried out yet. It is to be feared that after 65 years of chemoantibiotic treatment (the introduction of sulfonamide was in 1935) lasting mitochondrial effects have accumulated and exponentiated both transmitted from mother to child and a brought on by an insidious disposition for Type-II cell dyssymbioses. This founded assumption also applies to AIDS and cancer dispositions by the corresponding exposure to prooxidative stress (Kremer 1997 a).

The pathogenetic causal link of mitochondrial damage through the combined inhibition of folic acid metabolism in human cell systems and the enforced appearance of acquired immunodeficiency syndrome (AIDS) dependent on dose and duration of medication and the disposition of the patients was first broached for discussion as a research concept for an experimental study in 1996 (Kremer 1996 c; 1996 a, 1996 b, 1997 a).

An inquiry about experimental and clinical studies of the effects of combined TMP/SMX (T+S, co-trimoxazole) on the functions of human mitochondrial cell symbionts at the pharmaceutical company Hoffmann LaRoche in Basel, producer of Bactrim and Septra with the highest global turnover, produced a clear disclosure from the "pre-clinical research" department:

"Over the years I have time and again been dealing with different aspects of the TMP/SMX combination, but with regret have to inform you that I know of no studies on the questions you addressed. Also my other colleagues involved with co-trimoxazole are unable to help . . . A colleague with extensive knowledge is on holiday at the moment. I will contact you again on his return should he have information on the themes addressed" (Then 1996).

The "colleague with extensive knowledge" was also unable to name one single publicized study on the effects on the ultrastructure and function of human mitochondria resulting from medication with Bactrim, Septra etc., "one of the most successful agents ever developed" (Then 1993). Additional questions to the research departments of the pharmaceutical companies Glaxo Wellcome (now GlaxoSmithKline) and Bayer confirmed the negative results: There were no experimental or clinical studies about the mitochondriotoxic effects of the single substance Trimethoprim or the combination substance co-trimoxazole. Extensive research in medical literature confirmed the statement from the producers of T+S. The discussion among specialists on, "Thoughts about an experimental study on the effects of folic acid inhibitors on the ultrastructure and function of mitochondria in human lymphocytes and in human microbial opportunists" (Kremer 1996 c) made the community aware of the deficit of experimental and clinical mitochondrial research and the rationally incomprehensible lack of knowledge of doctors, about whether and which effects chemoantibiotics like Trimethoprim and Sulfonamide or the combined chemoantibiotic co-trimoxazole and other antibiotics actually cause in mitochondrial immune and non-immune cells.

The strong suspicion of transferring irreparable mitochondrial damage from toxic chemoantibiotics and chemotherapeutic agents, over the maternal germline as an inherited disposition for AIDS, cancer and other chronic illnesses

The internationally respected mitochondria researcher Professor Richter from the Laboratory for Biochemistry at the Federal Technical University in Zürich stated in a proposal for the research project "Antibiotic-induced damage to mitochondria":

"The survival of mitochondria and thus the cell as a whole crucially depends both on an intact mitochondrial DNA and protein synthesis. Studies of diseases associated with mDNA, show that a large number of degenerative processes and cell death are caused by defects of mitochondrial oxidative phosphorylation [the supply of energy]. Antibiotics are compounds that are aimed against microorganisms that cause diseases. They operate by destroying the cell wall structure, changing the membrane permeability, transforming DNA, inhibiting protein syntheses or altering energy metabolisms. As former bacteria, mitochondria still possess many attributes that are otherwise only found in microorganisms. Thus it is possible that antibiotics also lead to changes in mitochondria . . . Up until now there have been no studies on antibiotic-induced mitochondrial damage in higher organisms. It seems urgently necessary to study the effects of antibiotics on the hereditary structure and functionality of mitochondria . . . In contrast to nuclear DNA, damage to mDNA, according to the present state of knowledge, is either not or only partially repaired . . . In the suggested study we expect to find evidence of medication-induced damage to the mitochondria. Of particular importance is the possibility, which has not been tested up until now, that antibiotics can provoke congenital mutations of mitochondrial DNA, which could be passed down via the germline from mother to the following generation. Evidence of antibiotic-induced damage to mitochondria obviously has far-reaching political, social and economic consequences" (Richter 1997).

Richter's intended research project failed to attract funding, the fact that the world's largest pharmaceutical concern, the Eusaprim producer Glaxo

Wellcome demanded to have a say in the research publication as a condition of funding throws a bad light on the practices in present-day medical research when concerned with controlling the research findings that have obvious "far-reaching political, social and economic consequences" (Richter 1997).

There are, however, a few studies on damage to mitochondria by chemoantibiotics. It was first demonstrated in 1973 that chloramphenicol inhibited protein synthesis in mitochondria. Protein synthesis was blocked in isolated mitochondria by lincomycin and antibiotics from the macrolide classes (erythromycin, oleandomycin, spiramycin, tylosin and carbomycin). Possible mitochondrial damage in human cells is dependent on whether the antibiotics can pass the cell membrane.

"The treatment of animals or man with antibacterial drugs can have harmful effects on mitochondrial function, especially in tissues that have a high proliferation rate, such as bone marrow, intestinal epithelium, and tumor cells. Chloramphenicol causes a dose-dependent depression of bone-marrow function during treatment, probably by inhibiting mitochondrial protein synthesis. It can also cause a lethal late-onset toxicity (aplastic anemia) long after treatment has ceased . . . . In the rat, inhibition of mitochondrial protein synthesis by prolonged tetracycline treatment causes a substantial decrease in the content of respiratory-chain-phosphorylation complexes in intestinal and in skeletal muscle. Fortunately, the apparent overcapacity in the catalytic activity of these complexes can provide protection against these effects, so that an 80% decrease in intestinal cytochromic *c* oxidase activity is tolerated without adverse effects" (Tyler 1992).

The research findings on the reduction of the oxygen respiration of mitochondria after prolonged administration of tetracycline were already published in 1981 (Busch 1981), but the consequences of the research data were not understood at that time. The fact that an 80% decline in the performance of the respiratory chain was still tolerated shows the necessity, according to the laws of nature, for all cell systems that are dependent on the supply of oxygen and its conversion, to still be able to tolerate a broad spectrum of fluctuations in performance.

But the research findings also demonstrate that at 20% remaining capacity of the complexes of the mitochondrial respiratory chain the critical threshold is reached beyond which the energy supply of ATP for the whole cell is endangered. This performance parameter corresponds very well to the stable levels of the alternate switch under physiological conditions from oxygen-dependent cell respiration for ATP production in cell symbionts to oxygen-free enzymatic ATP production in the cytoplasm.

The sudden loss of more than 80% of the cytochromic c oxidase activity of the respiratory chain can be caused by nitrosative stress through chemotherapeutics and antibiotics (for instance Azathioprine, azidothymidine (AZT), co-trimoxazole) and/or oxidative stress and/or structural damage of the DNA and protein syntheses after too high usage of antioxidants and/or too little absorption or neosynthesis of antioxidants (thiol pool, enzymatic and non-enzymatic antioxidative molecules). The result is a too weak transmission of electron flows to molecular oxygen (O_2) at the end of the respiratory chain, a quick degradation of mitochondrial ATP production, a sudden sinking in the membrane potential, increased Ca^{2+} cycling and increased formation of reactive oxygen species (ROS) and NO and its derivatives (Richter 1996, Kroemer 1997, Zamzami 1997).

The above-mentioned processes cause "infectious" cell death for the whole cell through the additional release of "apoptosis-inducing factors" from the mitochondria. The procedure here corresponds to a Type-I regulation of cell dyssymbiosis and can also be understood to be a hypercatabolic reaction.

The fundamental problem of aggravated Type-II counterregulation and cellular dyssymbiosis in AIDS and cancer patients, forced by chemoantibiotics and chemotherapeutic agents

Richter's statement follows the laws of nature:

"The survival of mitochondria and thus the cell as a whole is crucially dependent both on an intact mitochondrial DNA and protein synthesis" (Richter 1996), however, has to be amended on one decisive point:

Mitochondria and thus the cell as a whole can survive a more than 80% loss of the performance capacity of the respiratory chain, if the bioenergetic membrane potential of the mitochondria can be stabilized or overstabilized by a Type-II counterregulation and the energy supply for the whole cell can be safeguarded mostly independently of the OXPHOS system of the mitochondria (Type-II counterregulation of cell dyssymbiosis).

Under these conditions the number and activities of the mitochondrial cell symbionts are substantially reduced to a fifth of their norms (Mathupala 1997). The bioenergetic, metabolic and proliferative prolonged transformation of the cells active in division, which happens largely on the performance level of archaic protista (Kremer 1999) are termed undifferentiated tumor cells. However, it is misleading to view, as does mainstream oncology, the formation of tumor cells primarily as the result of degradative mutations of nuclear DNA. The prime cause of transformation to tumor cells is to be understood as a bioenergetic process which, under a strong and prolonged nitrosative and oxidative stress, triggers survival strategies in the cells active in division after persistent inhibition of the OXPHOS system.

DNA damage can be caused after depletion of the antioxidizing capacities synchronously or sequentially and in a vicious circle aggravating the stable switch of the supragenetic network to a quantitatively and qualitatively lower fluidity level.

Degradation mutations alone in nuclear DNA and mitochondrial DNA involve deficient cell performance and the corresponding clinical syndromes. The fact that tumor cells can also develop without DNA mutations in the nucleus and in mitochondria confirms this consequence of the concept of Type-II counterregulation of cell dyssymbiosis that is represented here. Awareness of this obviously has a far-reaching significance for prevention and therapy.

"Tumor cells divide more frequently than normal cells and often have a low reserve capacity for respiratory-chain phosphorylation. The deliberate inhibition of mitochondrial protein synthesis *in vivo* by antibiotic treatment could be used to block the growth of malignant tumor cells, and it might offer some clinical advantage when used in conjunction with other therapeutic methods" (Tyler 1992).

Chemotherapeutics and antibiotics can indeed block, under certain circumstances, tumor cells from the reserve capacity of the OXPHOS system, which not only often but regularly is lower than the critical thresholds (Mathupala 1997), but this is a cause and not a result of tumor formation (Kremer 1999). Chemotactic attacks, however, can eliminate cancer cells not only by blocking the reserve capacities of the cell symbionts but also selectively strengthen the Type-II counterregulation in cancer cells. This is demonstrated in cancer cells that are characterized by higher sensitivity thresholds of the genetic expression of calcium-dependent NO synthesis and very low NO gas productions; they grow and divide especially quickly (Chinje 1997). But there could be other cells in the critical areas of performance capacity of the mitochondrial respiratory chain that are forced to a Type-II counterregulation by chemotherapeutic and antibiotic treatment and then secondarily transform to cancer cells. Equally there is the danger that after chemotherapy and/or radiation treatment a few metastatic cells form selectively, as through forced counterregulation the sensitivity barriers for the genetic expression of inducible calcium-independent NO synthesis in these cancer cells is seriously increased. Metastatic cells are characterized by a very low capacity for the stimulation of inducible cytotoxic NO gas and can thus prevent the cytokine stimulation of the cytotoxic NO gas synthesis in the metastatic tumor cells that have been induced by immune cells and non-immune cells (Xie 1996). Apart from cachexy the majority of cancer patients die from metastases. The fact that in the Deutsches Krebsforschungszentrum (German Cancer Research Center) after evaluation of the results of chemotherapeutic treatment on cancer patients over many years it was observed that:

" . . . Even after decades of clinical use the cytostatics have proved to be a failure in broad areas of oncology" (Abel 1990). This reflects the effects of a Type-II counterregulation of cell dyssymbiosis and the forced switch through chemotherapeutics and antibiotics.

The same observations apply to nerve cells no longer active in division as well as heart and skeletal muscle cells, whose oxygen-dependent performance can degenerate as a result of chemotactic influences through a Type-I overregulation or a Type-II counterregulation.

However, in the age of chemotherapeutics and antibiotics the evolutionary-biological programmed counterregulation can be disastrous. As a rule, chemotactic acute treatment of intra- and extracellular agents in humans is successful if the patients still have sufficient thiol reserves and other protective antioxidizing molecules as well as a reasonably well functioning cytotoxic NO gas defense of T-helper immune cells, as the performance, antioxidizing capacity, and the reduction power of the complex human cell symbiosis is superior to the comparable capacity of single and multicellular microbes. If, however, the human immune and non-immune cells are exposed to a continuous pharmacotoxic bombardment and manifold immune stressors over a long period of time, then even in "previously healthy patients" (Gottlieb 1981) after the loss of critical reserve capacities the cell symbiosis in immune and non-immune cells responds to previously tolerable chemotherapeutics, antibiotics and immune stressors with "acquired immune deficiencies" in the form of clinically manifest opportunistic infections (AIDS) and/or specific tumors.

However, there is another factor in play. As a few especially successful opportunists, which just like successful cancer cells (Mathupala 1997) could survive chemotactic attacks in human organisms by counterregulating, these selected opportunistic agents could be relatively more tolerable to these chemotactic weapons than human immune and non-immune cells which have become dyssymbiotic.

The same process could take place when people with “acquired immune deficiencies” in symptom-free intervals are given long-term prophylaxis with immunotoxic antimicrobial substances such as co-trimoxazole, Trimethoprim, Sulfonamides, Trimetraxate, Pentamidine, Pyrimethamines, Dapsone and many other pharmacotoxins (antiparasitics, antifungals, antibacterial and antiviral substances), singularly or in combination, or with “antiretroviral” nucleoside analogs or non-nucleoside analogs or protease inhibitors, alone or combined. Or when various immunotoxic and cytotoxic preparations are temporarily allotted, combined and exchanged as “life prolonging cocktail or combitherapy” in a colourful mixture and sequence, on a trial and error basis, until a respective “incompatibility” is reached, as usual without an antioxidative compensation therapy.

The clinical diversity of short-term effects following Bactrim/Septra medication

That alone the doubled folic acid inhibitor co-trimoxazole achieved the basic condition of a toxic chemo-antibiotic, not only to penetrate the membrane barriers of single-celled and multi-celled microbes but also the cell membranes and mitochondrial membranes of human cells, is demonstrated by a choice from a long list of serious cell damage following short-term medication with Bactrim, Septra, Eusaprim, Cotrim Forte etc.:

- “Hematologic toxicity [toxic damage to blood formation]: Leukopenia/ Neutropenia, various forms of anemia, thrombocytopenia [deficiency of blood platelets], hypoprothrombinaemia [deficiency of coagulation factor II]
- Vascular changes: Vasculitis, periarteriitis nodosa (seldom)
- Central nervous system: Ataxy [inability to coordinate muscles], tremors, convulsions, aseptic meningitis, psychoses with hallucinations, depressions
- Metabolic problems: hypercalcemia [elevated calcium levels], hyponatremia [reduced sodium levels], hypoglycemia [reduced sugar levels],
- Stomach/intestinal problems: Vomiting, inappetence, diarrhea, pseudomembranous colitis [inflammation of the mucous membrane of the colon]

- Liver and pancreas: Transaminase elevation [increase in liver enzymes], hepatitis, intrahepatic cholestasis [biliary stasis], liver necrosis [liver cell degradation], pancreatitis
- Nephrotoxicity [toxic damage to the kidneys]: Creatinine increase, interstitial nephritis [kidney infection], crystalluria [excretion of crystals in urine], urolithiasis [kidney stones]
- Skin reactions: exanthema, exfoliative dermatitis, erythema multiforme, Stevens-Johnson Syndrome, toxic epidermal necrolysis [degradation of the skin cells], urticaria [nettle rash]
- Further allergic/toxic phenomena: Fever, angioedemas" (Gysling 1995).

Proof of the toxic effect of Bactrim/Septra on the DNA

Already in 1981 a research team published the proof by means of a micronucleus test that pathological transformations of nuclear DNA appeared in patients who had been treated to customary doses and durations of co-trimoxazole for urinary tract infections:

"The present study shows that trimethoprim-sulfamethoxazole [co-trimoxazole], like other folic antagonists [for instance, methotrexate for the treatment of leukaemia], damage the human genetic material" (Sørensen 1981).

This clear research finding was published in the same year that AIDS specialists were recommending unlimited medication with co-trimoxazole as a long-term prophylaxis for patients who had already been seriously immunotoxically and cytotoxically impaired (CDC 1981 a, Gottlieb 1981, Masur 1981, De Wys 1982).

The fact of DNA damage due to co-trimoxazole medication established the compelling logic that such DNA transformations would also be apparent in the mitochondrial DNA that was decoded for the first time in 1981(Tyler 1992). Nuclear DNA is protected by special histone proteins and repair mechanisms while mDNA can either not be repaired or only partially (Richter 1997) and the damage rate is ten times higher than nuclear DNA (Yakes 1997). The working mechanisms of the doubled folic acid inhibition of nucleic acid synthesis of nuclear and mitochondrial DNA as well as the inhibition of co-enzymes essential for all biosyntheses change in many ways, indirectly and directly, the redox milieu of human cell systems. These redox transformations in turn influence the whole pharmacokinetics and pharmacodynamics of folic acid inhibitors and their bonding to enzymes and co-enzymes, which via the biological activation of folic acid drive other enzymes that regulate the nucleic acid metabolism, the synthesis of amino acids and biogenetic amines (Mathews 1985, Stone 1986, Zimmermann 1987, Oefner 1988, Hitchings 1989, Gilli 1990, Margosiak 1993, Sasso 1994).

The excessive demand created by Bactrim/Septra on the detoxification performance of the glutathione system, and the incalculable interactions with other chemoantibiotics and chemotherapeutic agents

The toxic effects of medication with folic acid antagonists like co-trimoxazole become aggravated when various chemoantibiotics influence the bioenergetic and biochemical patterns of absorption, bioavailability, distribution of the metabolic reactions and detoxification. Even small changes to the distribution of substances in organisms (pharmacokinetics) and actions and interactions in organisms (pharmacodynamics) can induce severe unwanted and inestimable consequences (Van Meerten 1995).

The degradation products of Sulfamethoxazole, in particular, play an important role in the toxic short-term effects of co-trimoxazole on immune and non-immune cells. Sulfonamides are converted to highly reactive metabolic products in an enzyme-driven process. The first stage of this biological activation is the oxidative metabolism of sulfonamides to hydroxylamine. This degradation product can under physiological conditions be oxidized quickly and spontaneously to nitroso compounds. These are even more highly reactive and even more toxic than hydroxamines (Uetrecht 1985, Shear 1985, 1986, Rieder 1988, Spielberg 1989, Cribb 1990, 1992).

Nitroso compounds (initially N-nitrosodimethylamine, Magee 1956) have been recognized as carcinogenic substances in hundreds of variations since 1956 (Loeppky 1984 a). They have to be detoxified, particularly by sulfurous reduced glutathione, which in all cells and above all in mitochondrial cell symbionts as reduction equivalent breaks down oxidized metabolic products (Siliprandi 1978, Meister 1983, Beutler 1985). The toxic sulfonamide product, hydroxylamine from co-trimoxazole is reduced by glutathione and prevented from transforming to potential carcinogenic nitroso compounds (Shear 1985, Rieder 1988, Spielberg 1989).

Asymptomatic "HIV positives," however, already showed signs of a systemic glutathione deficit in immune and non-immune cells before and after the laboratory reaction "HIV positive" (Buhl 1989, overview Herzenberg 1997).

In addition to high glutathione usage through enforced detoxification actions in excessive chemoantibiotic medication and exposure to other immune stressors, glutathione deficiency was encouraged in promiscuous homosexuals for other reasons by the deficit of biologically active folic acid: As a result of chemoantibiotic abuse, frequently intermittent intestinal infections lead to resorption dysfunctions in the small intestine. This impedes the absorption of important nutrients including folic acid and the glutathione building blocks of the sulfurous amino acid cysteine or respectively sulfurous methionine which can be metabolized to cysteine in the liver (Lambie 1985, Davis 1986).

Methionine on the other hand requires methyl groups for the formation of cysteine, which is supplied by active folic acid (tetrahydrofolate, THF). Trimethoprim in turn intervenes in the formation of THF from folic acid and thus depletes the provision of cysteine from methionine as a building block for the neosynthesis of glutathione. A too high usage of glutathione and the inhibition of the neosynthesis of glutathione lead to a systemic glutathione deficit.

This in its turn then favors nitrosative and oxidative stress under specific risk loads, which in acute cases leads to an increased cell death (apoptosis/necrosis: Type-I overregulation of cell dyssymbiosis) in immune and non-immune cells and/or with a time lag to exhaustion of the long-term effects of the performance of cell respiration in immune and non-immune cells (asymptomatic acquired immune deficiencies with NO inhibition, Th2 cell domination and increased humoral immunity [AID], symptomatic acquired immune deficiencies with clinically manifest opportunistic infections [AIDS, and/or specific tumors in endothelial and lymph cells], cancerous disposition in the cells active in division / degeneration in the nerve, cardiac muscle and skeletal cells inactive in division) (Type-II counterregulation of cell dyssymbiosis).

The question of responsibility for the deadly consequences of "HIV/AIDS" medicine run amok

There is no need to possess a particularly medical imagination to picture what actually happened in the 1970s on the proclamation of "sexual liberation" in the homosexual scene in Western cities before the first Kaposi's sarcoma in 1978 and the first PCP fungal infection in 1980 were diagnosed in homosexual patients. How could these patients be termed "previously healthy" (Gottlieb 1981) although it had been ascertained that "Aggressive chemotherapy . . . contributes to the final degree of immunologic incompetence" (De Wys 1982)? How could it be stated that these diseases developed "without a clinically apparent underlying immunodeficiency" (CDC 1981 a) although it was recognized that the immunotoxic co-trimoxazole promoted systemic fungal diseases through neutropenia (Lehrer 1971 a, 1971 b) and chronic inhalation of organic nitrites (poppers) caused very serious damage to cellular immunity (overview Haverkos 1988) and 95% of the homosexuals from Washington, New York, San Francisco and Los Angeles examined in a study on nitrite usage by the US surveillance authority reported use of nitrites, often regularly (Jaffe 1983)? How was it possible to assume that "a speculative new virus" (Haverkos 1982) was the cause of the disease although the long list of infections with all kinds of agents, particularly in promiscuous homosexuals with a preference for unprotected anal receptive intercourse, was unprecedented (Jaffe 1983, Callen 1990, Root-Bernstein 1993)?

Doctors and patients knew full well the causes of AIDS-indicating diseases but still the specialists spoke in unison at the historic conference of March 1983 in New York (the first World AIDS Conference) of a "new agent" and the "intriguing puzzle" of Kaposi's sarcoma (Friedman-Kein 1984 a) although animal experiments had clearly demonstrated the carcinogenic effects of simultaneous administration of chemoantibiotics and organic nitrites (Bambilla 1985). How could the international medical fraternity tacitly and almost without objection accept in the light of the accumulated knowledge that patients who had already been severely immunotoxically and cytotoxically damaged or even immune healthy patients who through a more than obscure antibody reaction test had been stigmatized as death candidates, were treated with chemotherapeutics and antibiotics in open-ended "planned experiments" (Thomas 1984) "practically like guinea pigs in one of the largest and most expensive experiments of our time" as the *Wall Street Journal* reported in 1996? Every informed person in the medical profession has known for more than 30 years that these drugs trigger AIDS and cancer as well as nerve and muscle degradation and that patients on long-term medication with these substances die of internal poisoning of the cellular respiration in immune and non-immune cells. Who is responsible for the deadly consequences of HIV/AIDS medicine run amok? Was it incomprehensible incompetence, twisted obsession or indifferent professional routine, which allowed a host of international doctors to become accomplices, lackeys or bystanders in one of the most disastrous tragedies of modern medicine? There is only one explanation: The dictates of the "invisible hand of the market" has since the approval of patents of medical laboratory findings, techniques and products at the end of the 1970s, polluted modern medicine and used the unscrupulous international media and professional media reliant on sponsorship in order to create an atmosphere of plague panic and mortal fear and to exploit helpless victims in all corners of the world.

As a consequence of the rash chemotherapeutic free-for-all during the 1990s "HIV positives" increasingly fell ill to life-threatening bacterial infections not previously seen in these patients

At an international press conference at the World AIDS Conference in Geneva in 1998 Dr. Fauci, director of the National Institute for Allergy and Infectious Diseases in the USA, was asked by a specialized journalist:

"The American surveillance authority, the CDC, has explicitly excluded bacterial infections from the catalog of AIDS-indicating diseases (CDC 1993). Why do AIDS patients in Western countries develop almost exclusively systemic fungal infections?"

The immune specialist Dr. Fauci answered amicably:

"Oh yes, I have many AIDS patients with bacterial infections."

The journalist, in the presence of many colleagues, countered:

"Yes, and these HIV positives and AIDS patients were treated with AZT."

To the astonishment of the journalists instead of answering Dr. Fauci stormed out without uttering a word. Most of the journalists were unclear about why Dr. Fauci was in such a hurry. The journalist had exposed the pivotal question of HIV/AIDS medicine: Why were patients with an acquired immune deficiency being treated with a "cocktail therapy" of substances which trigger acquired immune deficiencies?

Dr. Fauci, a long-standing coordinator for HIV/AIDS research, had endorsed in 1989, as chief medical evaluator, the approval of AZT as the "retroviral" prophylaxis for the medication of asymptomatic HIV positives. For this endorsement AZT was approved by the FDA, the American authority for the licensing of drugs, without having to wait a number of years for the mandatory clinical studies on the effects and side effects of the substance. AZT suppressed the maturation of blood cells in the bone marrow and inhibited the formation of antibodies against bacterial agents (Rosenthal 1994). At the beginning of the 1990s suddenly an increase in massive bacterial pneumonias appeared in previously asymptomatic HIV positives who had been treated with AZT; until that point in time these pneumonias had not been diagnosed to this serious degree in HIV positives.

The pneumonias, more over, were often fatal: "Bacterial pneumonias account for up to 40-50% of hospital admissions for lower respiratory tract infections among people with HIV" (Arzuaga 1994, Marco 1998).

The sudden increase in the appearance of bacterial infections, which by a characteristic "HIV positive" Th1 immune cell deficiency is usually inhibited by a compensatory increase in antibody production and an increase in other cells of the immune cell network, was explicitly traced back to medication with AZT:

"Neutropenia [loss of neutrophile white blood cells which mature in the bone marrow] is becoming more common because of the use of myelotoxic [those which damage bone marrow cells] drugs such as AZT, ganciclovir and other bone marrow suppressive agents" (Wilder 1998).

Dr. Fauci, Dr. Montagnier and all their colleagues know precisely why they have to decline open discourse: They had tried to drive out the Devil "retrovirus HIV" with Beelzebub "AZT etc." and fear the cross-complaints of the victims and their family and friends, as HIV/AIDS therapy is not rationally sustainable. An Australian doctor sums up the swashbuckling virus hunt, the poisoning of the already poisoned by a blind dogmatic "cocktail therapy," which responds to one medically induced symptom with the induction of ever increasing symptoms by means of pseudo-rationally combined pharmacotoxins:

"It is therapeutic chaos. Doctors are prescribing what patients ask for, or they're guessing, adding different drugs when they feel like it. I've never seen anything in Medicine quite like it" (Christie 1997).

Every antimicrobial substance also attacks human cells, since our own cells bear the heritage of the archaic cellular symbiosis acquired from single-cellular microbes

The "HIV positive" patients, who through an unrestrained publicly staged campaign of hysteria were metaphorically scared to death, in turn believed that they could be saved from the phantom-like deadly virus by an almost masochistic belief in the promises of the pharmaceutical industry of the healing powers of a multitude of immunotoxic, mitochondriotoxic, glutathione-consuming mixture of substances—substances of which they should perhaps have been more scared. In this mutually delusional world the only real puzzle is why patients and doctors still believed in the fiction that AIDS drugs would solely target the microbes so that without progressive cell destruction by the "HI viruses" the diversity of toxic symptoms up to fatal organ failure would not be able to develop. This fiction was based on a fundamental error: Every toxic antimicrobial substance also attacks human cells, as all human cells are descended from archaic cells that have developed from the cellular symbiosis of single-celled microbes. Human cells differ from microbial cells, in principal, through a relatively better capacity for detoxification—as long as cell symbiosis is intact. But precisely this fundamental prerequisite has been endangered by the rapid change in external and internal toxic load patterns of the development of civilization over the last 150 years. AIDS and cancer diseases in Western countries are only a symptomatic reflection of overstepping the load limits. Modern medicine will have to find a more intelligent response to the challenge than a collective mobilization of deep-rooted fears of plague and uninformed "shotgun" virus hunting. Without the strict observance of the laws of co-evolution within human cells, between human cells and microbes as well as between human transformed and non-transformed cells the vital heritage of the micro-Gaian milieu will be irreparably squandered by a medicine governed by totalitarian commerce and ignoring evolutionary developments not only for the limited number of individuals of today's generation but via the hereditary transmission of the maternal germline as the basis for the "*Health of the Nations*" (Sagan 1987) as well as for those in future generations (Sören 1981, Richter 1997, Yakes 1997, Kremer 1997, Wallace 1999).

Fig. 63) Formula for the structure of Trimethoprim (above) and of sulfamethoxazole (below), i.e. the active agents contained in the chemoantibiotic Bactrim.

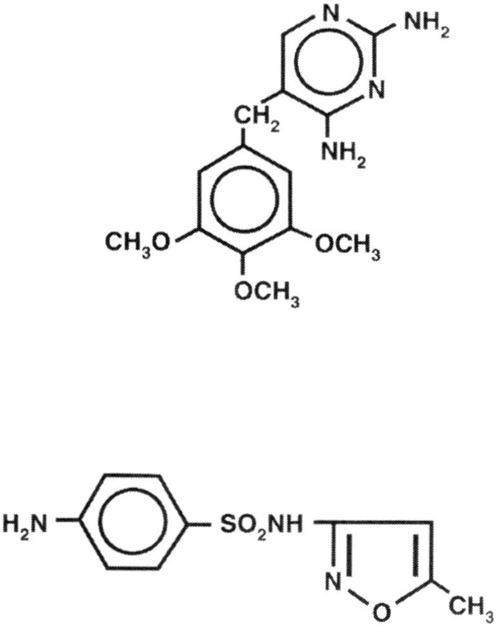
N
NH2
N
CH2
NH2
CH3O
OCH3
OCH3
H2N
SO2NH
N
O
CH3

Fig. 64) Rate of prescription of antibiotics in surgeries and clinics in Germany administered in 1995-1996. Above all the following groups of substances: Trimethoprim, tetracyclines and macrolides are seriously suspected of provoking irreparable damage to mitochondrial DNA.

Surgery prescriptions 53.2 million units, +2%

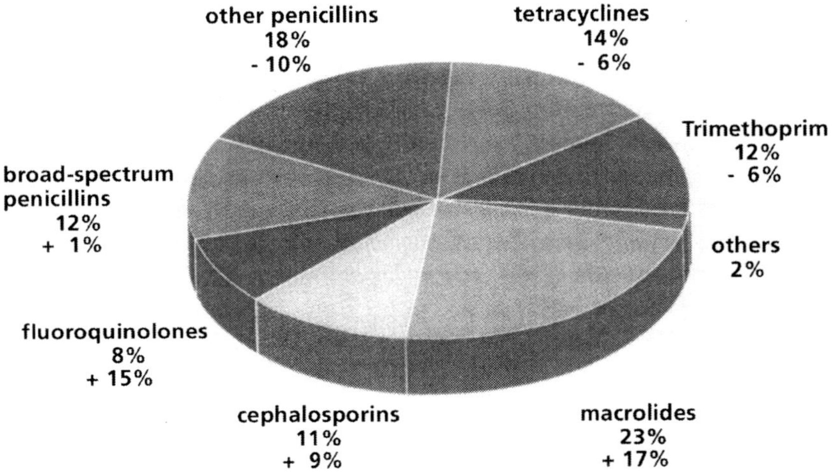
other penicillins
18%
- 10%
tetracyclines
14%
- 6%
Trimethoprim
12%
- 6%
broad-spectrum
penicillins
12%
+ 1%
others
2%
fluoroquinolones
8%
+ 15%
cephalosporins
11%
+ 9%
macrolides
23%
+ 17%

Clinic prescriptions 118.7 million units (capsules, phials), 0%

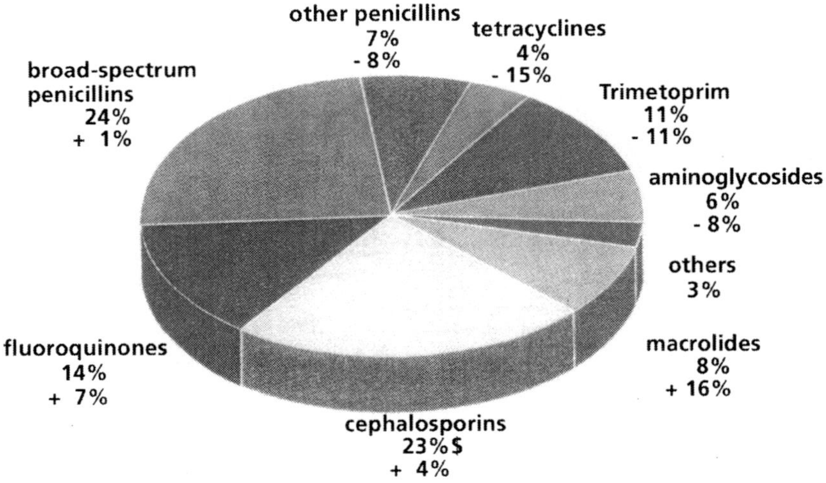
other penicillins
7%
- 8%
tetracyclines
4%
- 15%
broad-spectrum
penicillins
24%
+ 1%
Trimetoprim
11%
- 11%
aminoglycosides
6%
- 8%
others
3%
fluoroquinones
14%
+ 7%
macrolides
8%
+ 16%
cephalosporins
23%$
+ 4%

Fig. 65) **Azidothymidine (= AZT = Zidovudine/Retrovir), the "anti HIV" drug most frequently prescribed is believed to become incorporated in the chain of the proliferating "HIV" nucleic acid.**
Above: description of the DNA sequence. Below: description of the interruption of the sequence due to the supposed incorporation of AZT into the DNA sequence.

Sequence of human DNA

A single human DNA-strand is a sequence composed of more than 3 billions of A,T,C and G bases linked in a specific order

a) Normal DNA synthesis

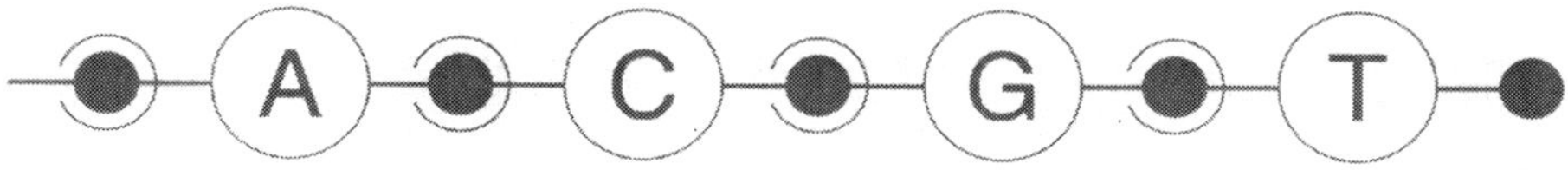
A
C
G
T

The chain continues

b) DNA synthesis with T-analog, AZT

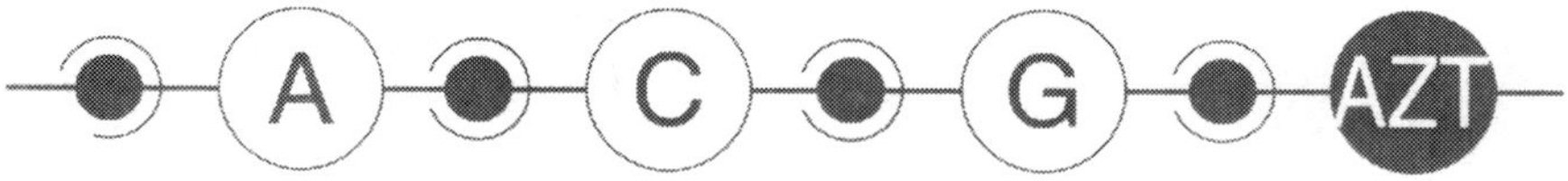
A
C
G
AZT

The chain is broken

Fig. 66) **Structural formula of AZT (right) and an AZA substance with the characteristic $N^{- - -}$ molecular groups. This nitrogen groups bond quickly to the enzyme cytochrome C oxidase in complex VI of the mitochondrial respiration chain. The consequence is the inhibition of ATPase, that can lead to an evolutionary pre-programmed counterregulation and thus to tumor transformation of the cell systems that are capable of dividing or respectively to the degeneration of muscular and nervous cells, which are not capable of dividing.**

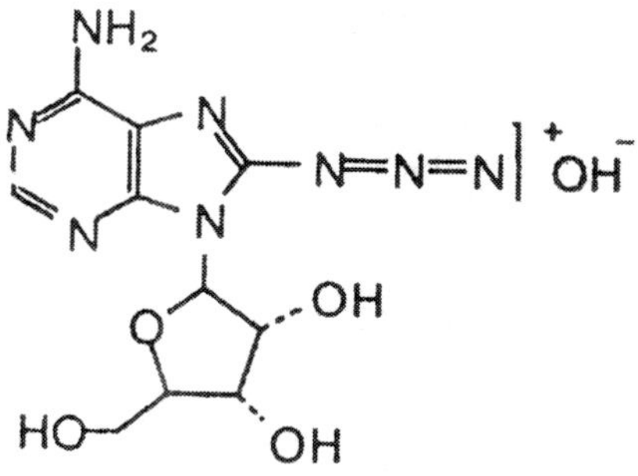
NH2
N
N
N
N
N=N=N
OH
OH
HO
OH

AZA Azidoadenosine

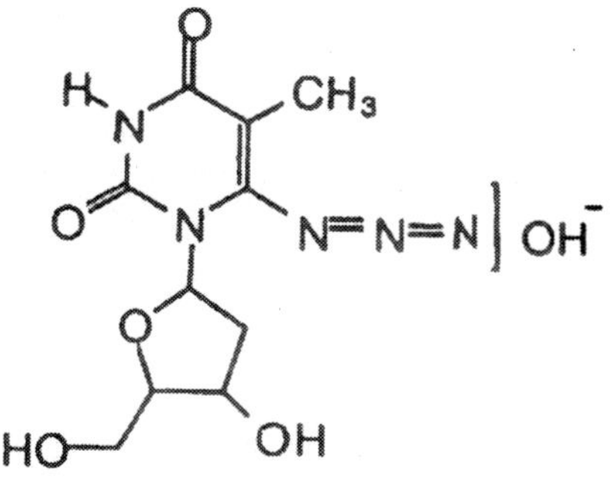
O
H
N
CH3
O
N
N=N=N
OH
O
HO
OH

AZT Azidothymidine

Fig. 67) The arsenal of "anti-HIV" substances.

Daily doses of the available antiretroviral agents		
Class/active principles	Normal daily dose for adults	Comments
Non-nucleoside reverse transcriptase inhibitors		
Nevirapine Delavirdine mesylate	1x 200mg tablet 2x a day 4x 200mg tablets 3x a day	Initial dose for the first two weeks of therapy: 1x 200mg tablet once a day. To be taken at least one hour after didanosine antacids.
Nucleoside analogs		
Lamivudine/Zidovudine	1x 150/300mg tablet 3x a day	Not to be prescribed to patients who need an adjustment to the dose.
Lamivudine aka 3TC	1x 150mg tablet 2x a day	
Stavudine aka d4T Zalcitabine aka ddC	1x 40mg capsule 2x a day 1x 0.75mg tablets 3x a day	For patients under 60 kg, the dose is 30mg 2x a day. Not to be used with didanosine. Not to be taken with antacids that contain magnesium or aluminium.
Didanosine aka ddl	2x 100mg tablets 2x a day	To be taken on an empty stomach. Alcohol could increase its toxicity. For patients under 60 kg the dose is 125mg 2x a day
Zidovudine aka ZDV or AZT	2x 100mg capsules 3x a day 1x 300mg tablet 2x a day	A wide range of doses is usually used in different countries. For instance 500 or 600mg/day given in 2 to 5 doses.
Protease inhibitors		
Indinavir	2x 400mg capsules 3x a day	To be taken on an empty stomach one hour before meals or two hours after meals. At least 1.5 litres of liquids have to be taken with it a day.
saquinavir mesylate	3x 200mg capsules 3x a day	To be taken within 2 hours of a full meal. Without intake of food there is no antiviral activity.
Nelfinavir mesylate	3x 250mg tablets 2x a day	To be taken with meals or with snacks
Ritonavir	6x 100mg capsules 2x a day	To be kept in a cool place. To be taken with meals. Dose to be increased over two weeks: 300mg (days 1-2), 400mg/ days 3-5), 500mg (days 6-13), 600mg (after day 14).
Saquinavir	6x 200mg capsules (in soft gelatine) 3x a day	To be taken within 2 hours of a full meal, without food Saquinavir could have less bioavailability.

Fig. 68) A survival specialist - a "professional pill consumer" for "HIV"/AIDS medicine:

16 REPORTAGEN

Seit zwölf Jahren kämpft Andreas Hastreiter gegen Aids

56 Pillen täglich halten das Virus in Schach

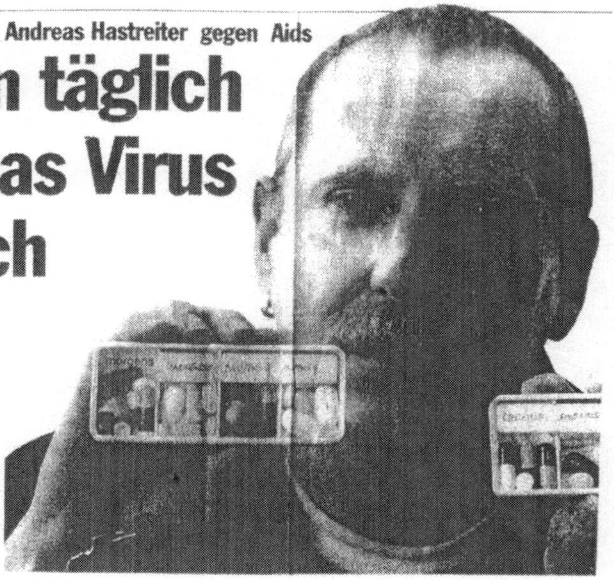

Der Münchner wehrt sich gegen einen unerbittlichen Feind in seinem Körper. Es ist ein Kampf auf Leben und Tod, denn Andreas Hastreiter ist HIV-positiv. In ihm sind Viren, die Aids verursachen. Daß er am Leben ist, verdankt er einem Cocktail von mehr als 50 Pillen, die er täglich nach einem strengen Plan einnehmen muß.

For twelve years Andreas Hastreiter has fought against AIDS

56 pills a day
keep the virus at bay

The man from Münich is fighting against the relentless enemy in his body. It is a battle of life and death because Andreas Hastreiter is HIV positive. Inside him are viruses that cause AIDS. He is alive thanks to a daily cocktail of more than 50 pills that he has to take following a strict programme.

Chapter X

The Daunting Task of Reconsideration

The elementary malpractices of AIDS and cancer medicine—why patients die by chemotherapeutic poisoning

Whoever wants to learn about the pool of knowledge of research into nitrogen, cytokine or cell symbiosis in the newer standard works on HIV/AIDS medicine, published by respected clinicians and practitioners by well-known medical publishers, will be disappointed (L'arge-Stehr 1994, Gölz 1995, Husstedt 1998). Mitochondrial cell symbionts and the crucial synthesis of cytotoxic NO gas and the essential detoxifying function of non-protein thiols (cysteine, reduced glutathione) are only mentioned incidentally, if at all. Consequentially, in one of these handbooks, aimed at "established physicians who deal with the care and provision of HIV and AIDS patients on a daily basis," it is claimed misleadingly:

"In the later stages of HIV a shift from Th1 to Th2 cells takes place, the cause of which has yet to be sufficiently explained but which is jointly responsible for the final disease progression" (Gölz 1995).

Deficits in the state of scientific/medical understanding are reflected in the standard works of HIV/AIDS medicine

The fact of the Th1-Th2 immune cell switch at the earliest possible point in time of the appearance of molecular markers of the "HIV infection" (overview Lucey 1996) in the preceding or simultaneous systemic extracellular and intracellular deficit of non-protein thiols (Buhl 1989) is either not known or ignored. Reports are largely restricted to an uncritical presentation of the HIV/AIDS theory and the practices of proof for the supposed HIV, descriptions of clinical symptoms and progressions, the administration of antimicrobial and "anti-retroviral" pharmaceutics and the superficial listing of the risks and side-effects of toxic therapy. Clinical and therapeutic demands and the medical state of knowledge diverge enormously:

"AIDS, the final stage of a chronic progressive infection has within a few years developed into a problem which all medical disciplines have to deal with. The exceptional efforts of international research have, within a very short time, led to an explosive growth in knowledge and as a result an avalanche of medical primary and secondary publications. The practising physician simply does not have the time to grasp the more profound insights of the scientific dimensions of these new themes, however, the practical applications have to be acknowledged. Everyone who is professionally confronted with these problems needs a form of code of practice to cover the suddenly emerging need for substantiated information. The necessary information has to be easy to access and to be compiled under the aspects of practical implementation and significance for particular needs (therapeutic, diagnostic, advisory, management). Everyone concerned with these topics needs information . . . and with the guidelines presented here we want to keep all interested or professionally affected physicians informed, whether in practices or clinics, so that they are in the position to optimally examine, treat and advise their patients" (L'arge-Stehr 1994).

"The HIV disease has become one of the greatest challenges to mankind. More than 11 years have passed since the first patients turned to medical treatment with signs of this immune disease. Meanwhile, medical science and research have been revolutionized. Increasing knowledge and growing experience have meant that it is one of the best-researched diseases. Today, the HIV disease appears to be able to be influenced therapeutically. It is still not possible to heal it. The increasing number of HIV infected patients and better knowledge of the clinical picture have led to a change in trends in medical research systems. In addition to specialized practices and clinical units, increasing numbers of established physicians are being confronted with this disease. The polymorphism of the disease demands a multi- or interdisciplinary approach. All medical faculties are addressed here. This book applies to all established physicians who are concerned with the care of and provision for HIV and AIDS patients on a daily basis but also those who in the future wish to come to terms with the subject. Above all practising physicians and general practitioners, internists, gynaecologists and paediatricians are being confronted with the fundamental care of HIV patients. Sometimes it is not easy for an established physician, within a short period of time, to gather sufficient experience of such a complex disease like HIV. Many colleagues remain unfamiliar with the lifestyles of those affected—mainly homosexual men and drug addicts. With this book the authors would like to contribute to a narrowing in the gaps of information and to a dismantling of existing barriers. Composition and choice of subject are aligned to the needs and questions of established physicians [Preface to the first edition] . . . On publication of the first edition in 1992 and 1993 there was still certain euphoria. A longer path with small advances seemed to be opening up. This hope was shattered by the findings of the World AIDS Conferences in Berlin and Yokohama. Well-known scientists deliberated whether the targets of the hitherto research had to be radically changed. But for all that, the continuous advances in research and clinical practice necessitated an updating of the existing handbook three years after the first edition . . . At the same time the new edition remains true to its original character: practical guidelines for established physicians based on experiences over a number of years in Berlin, where more than 20% of all Germany's HIV and AIDS patients live" (Gölz 1995).

"More than 16 years ago the human immunodeficiency virus (HIV) and the associated acquired immunodeficiency syndrome (AIDS) appeared in medical focus and introduced new challenges to clinical medicine and fundamental research, which at that time were of an inconceivable magnitude. It rapidly became clear that HIV was a virus of completely new dimensions whose clinical implications in form and gravity were equally exceptional. Pneumocystis carinii infections, brain toxoplasmosis, nontuberculous mycobacteria, cryptosporidiosis and Kaposi's sarcoma, for instance, which were previously known to the majority of physicians only in textbooks, suddenly became everyday clinical reality. It was not only the diseases that were new but also the diversity of their clinical appearance and peculiarities in acute therapy and prophylaxis. Due to the diversity of clinical manifestations virtually all medical fields are integrated in the treatment of HIV-dependent diseases, also those whose task is not the primary treatment of the HIV-infected. This makes interdisciplinary thought processes and actions necessary, as this is the only way to coordinate individual findings into a comprehensive concept. That is why practical handbooks, based on organ manifestation or clinical symptoms, which identify etiologic and clinical differential diagnostics including rational descriptions of diagnoses and therapy are helpful. In this respect the present book has been an exemplary success. Also non-specialists can find the central thread through the complexities of a multitude of etiological and diagnostic options. The half-life of our knowledge of HIV infection and AIDS is so short that textbooks will always hobble behind the latest level of awareness. Thus, publications like this one are of topical interest and are well-suited to impart the current state of knowledge. The publisher has managed to gain experienced authors from every field of medicine. All relevant clinical pictures are presented precisely and informative tabular figures and many illustrations enable a rapid transfer of information. This book is suited to facilitating and optimizing daily work with the HIV-infected in practices and clinics. So I hope that this book has a wide distribution in practices and clinics, also in the interests of the patients" (Husstedt 1998).

But, knowingly or not, these "exemplary" handbooks on "AIDS and the Preliminary Stages—Guidelines for Practices and Clinics," "HIV and AIDS Treatment, Counseling and Care" and "Specialist HIV and AIDS Diagnostic and Therapy" were not penned in the "interest of patients"—as these HIV/AIDS specialists recommend without restrictions indefinite medication for "HIV positive" and AIDS patients with pharmaceutical substances that have been proven to cause severe damage to the core of human cell systems—the mitochondrial cell symbionts.

In no way have these standard HIV/AIDS guidelines been "an exemplary success," as claimed, in keeping "interested or professionally affected physicians informed so that they are in the position to optimally examine, treat and advise their patients." Needless to say, the authors do not mention and, sadly, perhaps do not know of the existence and function of mitochondria and their dependence on a balanced micro-Gaian milieu.

"The strong suspicion persists that the disease (AIDS) is not caused by HIV but among other things by AZT and other nucleoside analogs as it cannot yet be ruled out that AZT leads to cell loss not only in the muscle but also in lymphocytes by damaging mitochondria. Evidence of such medicament-induced damage to the immune system has far-reaching political, social and economic consequences" (Richter 1997 b).

The "strong suspicion" and the "political, social and economic consequences" of a systemic toxic cell destruction were already disclosed 20 years ago as can be demonstrated by the first patients in whom the diagnosis of a *Pneumocystis carinii* pneumonia (PCP) was proposed as an AIDS-indicating disease. These five homosexual PCP patients were treated in the University Clinic in Los Angeles between October 1980 and May 1981. All were chronic consumers of inhaled nitrite gases as a "sexual doping" agent during anal sexual intercourse. The patients were treated with the folic acid inhibitor co-trimoxazole (TMP/SMX, Bactrim, Septra etc). Two patients died during treatment (CDC 1981 a). The clinical pathology and the abnormal immune status were described in the detailed treatment report of December 1981. The pros and cons of a cytomegalovirus infection were debated and an "undetected microorganism, drug or toxin" was vaguely speculated about without concrete analysis. Subsequently the university clinicians stated:

"To date there has been no indication of spontaneous recovery of cellular immunocompetence in our surviving patients. All have continued to have a severe wasting syndrome despite intensive supportive measures" (Gottlieb 1981).

The fatal mistake of confusing wasting syndrome (cachexy) with chronic states of hunger

As a result of this precise clinical observation of the progression the AIDS specialists might have been expected to recognize the primary cause of the syndrome in their homosexual patients even given the state of knowledge at that time. Instead they appeared perplexed and fixated on chemoantibiotics:

"Pneumocystis pneumonia recurred in two of the three patients who did not receive TMP-SMZ [Co-trimoxazole] prophylaxis. We therefore believe that long-term TMP-SMZ prophylaxis should be initiated in such patients after the first episode of pneumocystis. At present it is unclear whether antiviral and antifungal agents, intensive nutritional support, or immunostimulators will prove useful in the management of this syndrome" (Gottlieb 1981).

These concluding sentences of the historic clinical documentation about diagnosis and therapy of the first homosexual AIDS patients reflect the lack of knowledge about healing the causes and consequences of systemic cell dyssymbiosis. The statements were the beginning of one of the most disastrous collective blunders of modern medicine and unleashed the deadly virus hunt that continues until today.

Wasting syndrome is the key to understanding the occurrence of the disease in HIV positive and AIDS patients. Wasting syndrome is characterized by a loss of weight in the peripheral organs, especially in the skeletal muscles. There is a significant difference to undernutrition: The latter is characterized by loss of weight in virtually all organs, whilst in wasting syndrome the heart, liver and spleen do not suffer weight loss.

Practicing HIV/AIDS specialists seem to predominantly regard the energy fluxes and metabolic circulations in the cell systems of their patients as a "black box." Just as their colleagues who adopted "intensive nutritional support" (Gottlieb 1981) at the beginning of the AIDS era, they recommend today, after 14 years of clinical experience in AIDS, large supplies of calories, without qualifying which particular deficit in nutrition should be compensated.

"The central principal in the prophylaxis and treatment of wasting syndrome is a sufficient caloric intake. The majority of AIDS patients who lose weight do not nourish themselves adequately. Nutritional counseling should be initiated, the target being to devise a calorie-rich nutritional program. The substance loss is usually irreversible once the actual or final body weight has reached 60% of the ideal weight. Historical analyses of death from starvation have demonstrated that the probability of death is very high" (Gölz 1995).

Evidently the HIV/AIDS practitioners are confusing the state of chronic starvation with wasting syndrome. Both life-threatening states are indeed linked to immune cell deficiencies and a disposition to opportunistic infections but there remain significant differences in metabolism that affect the life and death of patients: In states of chronic starvation the long-term lack of proteins and other nutrients, vitamins, minerals, and trace elements is the cause of death, whereas wasting syndrome can lead to death even without opportunistic infections despite "intensive nutritional support" (Gottlieb 1981) and "sufficient caloric intake" (Gölz 1995). Therefore, it is not enough just to "devise a calorie-rich nutritional program" (Gölz 1995) in order to "optimally examine, treat and advise patients" (L'arge-Stehr 1994).

In states of chronic starvation the organism minimizes the breakup of proteins, the production of urea nitrogen in the liver is stronger inhibited than normal, whilst in wasting syndrome nitrogen expulsion by urea synthesis in the liver and the urea disposal in the kidneys is highly increased. Knowledge of the cause of this fundamental difference is decisive for life-saving therapy.

The central role of the exhaustion of the thiol pool (cysteine, glutathione)

If one assumes, based on well-founded facts, that the performance of human cell symbiosis is dependent on self-organizing regulation of gases (nitrogen oxide and reactive oxygen species) and that this system has to be counterdriven within an optimum regulatory range by sulfurous detoxifying molecules (non-protein thiols), then one has to ask what happens when the thiol pool (cysteine, reduced glutathione) becomes exhausted. This is the general rule with "HIV positives" at the earliest possible point in time of the "HIV" seroconversion.

Numerous studies have demonstrated that the glutathione level of "HIV positives," for instance within T-helper immune cells, in the blood plasma and in the mucosal fluids in the lungs, are already greatly depleted even though the test subjects had shown no clinical symptoms whatsoever (Buhl 1989, Eck 1989, Jarstrand 1990, Halliwell 1990, Baker 1992, Greenspan 1993). If the glutathione levels of the first homosexual AIDS patients in 1980/81, who had been termed "previously healthy" (Gottlieb 1981) and were chronic nitrite abusers (CDC 1981 a) had been analysed a few months or a year before their illness, then it would have been established that there was a "global deficit" (Greenspan 1993) of glutathione not only in the immune and non-immune cells but also in the blood plasma and in the mucosal fluids.

The sulfurous detoxifying molecule glutathione, synthesized from the three amino acids, glutamine acid, cysteine and glycine, represents 90% of the extracellular and intracellular non-protein thiols. The sulfhydryl groups (SH groups) for the detoxifying function of glutathione are provided by cysteine. Without sufficient amounts of cysteine, glutathione cannot be assembled. The SH groups of cysteine and glutathione bond in equal measures to NO and its derivatives (nitrosation) and to reactive oxygen species (ROS). From this process nitroso thiols are formed (SNO-cys, GSNO), respectively cystine and glutathione disulfide (GSSG). When the thiol pool is exhausted, NO and its derivatives also bond to the SH groups in proteins and enzyme proteins (nitrosylation). This process of nitrosylation can transform the function of numerous enzymes and proteins and damage DNA molecules, which in turn lead to disruptions to protein syntheses (overview Stamler 1995). Likewise deficient neutralization of ROS on an increased consumption of the thiol pool can lead to much damage to DNA and protein molecules (Sies 1985, Halliwell 1991). The ROS reaction through nitrosation and the processes triggered by nitrosylation change the redox milieu and influence transcription factors and the genetic expression for the biosynthesis of proteins. The results are evolutionary biologically programmed counterregulations of energy production and cycles of chemical compounds.

The early and late phases of thiol deficiency syndrome

It can be assumed that the first homosexual AIDS patients had a considerable thiol pool deficit a long time before their manifest AIDS illnesses. The preceding nitrosative and oxidative stress loads of this group of patients are well known:

Prolonged nitrite inhalation, uncontrolled consumption of antibiotics, chemotherapeutics, analgesics and "recreational drugs," chronic antigen stress through multi-infectiousness, alloantigen stress through resorption of foreign proteins (Overview Jaffe 1983, Pifer 1987, Root-Bernstein 1993).

Thiol deficiency syndrome in these patients can therefore be divided into three stages:

- The clinically mute phase: Reserve capacity of cell respiration at critical threshold.
- The clinically compensated phase: type 1 and type 2 cytokine dysregulation Th1 to Th2 switch, Type-I overregulation of cell dyssymbiosis and/or Type-II counterregulation of cell dyssymbiosis, the point in time of a possible "HIV" test reaction.
- The clinically manifest phase: Opportunistic diseases, Kaposi's sarcomas, lymphomas, myopathies, encephalopathies, wasting syndromes.

The ornithine-urea cycle of nitrogen transport passes through the mitochondrial cell symbionts and is controlled by cysteine

It is a serious medical malpractice to define the beginning of the prolonged process of nitrosative and oxidative triggered thiol deficiency syndrome on the basis of the immune cell anomalies of cell dyssymbiosis. Rather, thiol deficiency should be diagnosed in persons at risk before a possible "HIV" seroconversion by measuring the laboratory readings of the glutathione levels intracellularly in T-helper immune cells, in mucosal fluids of the lungs and in the blood plasma, so that "physicians in practices and clinics are in the position to optimally examine, treat and advise their patients" (L'arge-Stehr 1994).

Wasting syndrome, on the other hand, reflects the later phase of thiol deficiency. The export of nitrogen, gained from toxic ammonium from the degradation of proteins in the skeletal muscles and other peripheral organs, takes place in the liver via the ornithine cycle as urea. This metabolic cycle affects the mitochondrial cell symbionts, in which the first stage of urea synthesis is performed. Ammonium (NH_4^+) originating from the amino acids of proteins, in an intermediate step is transported to the mitochondria with glutamate as glutamine. Here it can again be separated and bond with hydrogen carbonate to carbamoyl phosphate. This building block reacts with ornithine to a new product from which, after a number of intermediate steps within this cycle, arginine is synthesized. The latter is split into urea, secreted via the kidneys, and ornithine, which returns to the cell symbionts for the next cycle. The control for the first stage of nitrogen export via the ornithine-urea cycle is executed in the mitochondria in the liver by cysteine thiol. Cysteine is split into sulfate (SO_4^{2-}) and hydrogen ions here, the latter bonding with hydrogen carbonate and in doing so inhibiting urea synthesis. Toxic ammonium instead couples with glutamate and forms glutamine, which is important for the formation of nucleic acid, the building blocks of DNA, for the regulation of the base-acid household and the energy supplies above all in intestinal cells and immune cells. If the cysteine level in the plasma is normal, controlled amounts of urea are produced. If, however, the cysteine level is too low, too much nitrogen is exported. In such cases a reflux brake engages above all between the liver and the skeletal muscles. A too-low cysteine level triggers an increased degradation of proteins in the musculature, the cysteine level and the levels of other amino acids in the plasma climbs again, the liver is again supplied with cysteine, the urea brake engages. Conversely, if through the normalization of the plasma levels of amino acids the continued degradation of proteins in skeletal muscles is again halted, the protein reserves in the muscle cells are replenished by the regeneration of amino acids from nutritional proteins.

Why the negative nitrogen balance of wasting syndrome cannot be stopped by "sufficient caloric intake"

Why can the enforced protein degradation in the skeletal muscles in wasting syndrome not be stopped by "intensive nutritional measures" (Gottlieb 1981) and "sufficient caloric intake" (Gölz 1995)? The adjustment of the cysteine levels in plasma and in the mitochondria of the liver is regulated via the lowered amino acid levels in the plasma. This supply from outside prevents the further breakup of proteins in the skeletal musculature by increasing the amino acid levels in the plasma and prevents the supply of cysteine from the degraded muscle proteins into the mitochondria of liver cells. The synthesis of urea continues and most of the nitrogen of the supplied amino acids is rapidly exported again as urea. The negative nitrogen balance remains (Dröge 1997 a). In a state of hunger the processes are reversed: The body attempts to save protein, the degradation of protein is curbed, nitrogen export via the ornithine-urea cycle is slowed down in states of hunger not by cysteine but by the ketone bodies of the acidosis (Felig 1969, Aoki 1972, Smith 1974).

The lack of thiol, increased urea synthesis via use of arginine and the associated reduction of NO synthesis, have extensive systemic consequences.

The increased turnover of arginine in the ornithine-urea cycle through splitting arginine in urea and ornithine has another decisive consequence. Arginine is the substrate for the synthesis of the nitrogen monoxide of NO gases and its derivatives. If too much arginine in the urea cycle is lost then less NO gas can be formed. The NO deficit has systemic consequences: Without sufficient NO levels the equivalence of calcium-dependent NO and superoxide anions for the regulated formation of peroxinitrite can no longer be maintained, and the mitochondrial channels close and calcium cycling between the cytoplasm and mitochondria is interrupted. The exhausted reserve capacity of cell respiration and ATP production, due to the lack of cysteine thiol, compels a switch to oxygen-independent ATP production in the cytoplasm, a state of pseudohypoxia triggers via changes in the redox milieu an activation of the promoter regions in the nuclear genomes, which are biologically conserved for the transcription signals in hypoxic and pseudohypoxic states.

This means, however, the genetic expression for biosynthesis of glycolytic enzyme proteins for aerobic glycolysis (Warburg Phenomenon). The glycolytic metabolism intensifies the export of nitrogen in several ways. On the one hand, amino acids in the skeletal musculature and other periphery organs are converted to glucose and pyruvate to satisfy the roughly 20-fold increase in glucose requirement in glycolytic energy supply. This also includes the conversion of cysteine to pyruvate. Separated amino groups (NH_2), highly toxic ammonia (NH_3) and ammonium (NH_4) form and have to be exported via the urea cycle.

Lactate, the product of aerobic glycolysis, is reinvested in the liver predominantly as glucose. This conversion uses significant amounts of hydrogen ions that are then missing as a brake for urea synthesis. Simultaneously the retrieval of glucose from lactate needs three to six times as many ATP energy molecules as are originally gained from a molecule of glucose through glycolysis. The development of wasting syndrome means, on top of a negative nitrogen balance, a simultaneously negative energy balance (Cohen 1971, Tayek 1992).

Even the addition of methionine into the protein infusions cannot compensate for the systemic cysteine deficit

To balance out the lack of cysteine methionine is added to the protein infusion solution. This sulfurous amino acid cannot be synthesized in the body and essentially has to be supplied. Methionine can be converted to cysteine, but in order to do this it needs the enzyme cystathionase, which splits cystathionine and releases cysteine. Cystathionine is formed from the methionine product, homocysteine and the glucose degradation product, serine.

Under conditions of glycolytic metabolism, however, the production of serine is impaired and the enzyme cystathionase is produced inadequately.

As a consequence of this cysteine synthesis from infused methionine cannot counterbalance the lack of cysteine (Greenspan 1993).

With cysteine/glutathione deficiency, the production of cytotoxic NO gas is inhibited, so that from the continuous prophylaxis with Bactrim etc. a vicious cycle results, which can lead to the development of counterregulated "resistant" PCP microbes.

Methionine as the source of homocysteine and cysteine can be blocked by a lack of folic acid and/or by inhibition of the biologically active folate (THF) by folic acid inhibitors like, among others, co-trimoxazole. THF transfers methyl groups to methionine. If this process is inhibited, the homocysteine reserve decreases, and the production of cysteine diminishes. Treatment and long-term prophylaxis with Bactrim, Septra, Eusaprim, Cotrim forte etc. aggravates the cysteine/glutathione deficiency without at the same time catering for the vital thiol balance.

"To date there has been no indication of spontaneous recovery of cellular immunocompetence in our surviving patients. All have continued to have a severe wasting syndrome despite intensive supportive measures. *Pneumocystis pneumonia* recurred in two of the three patients who did not receive TMP-SMZ [Co-trimoxazole] prophylaxis. We therefore believe that long-term TMP-SMZ prophylaxis should be initiated in such patients after the first episode of pneumocystis." (Gottlieb1981).

This clinical analysis demonstrates the crucial error in reasoning: The cause for the relapse to PCP is not the deficit of TMP-SMX prophylaxis but the acute systemic lack of cysteine and glutathione and thus the linked deficit of cytotoxic NO gas. As new pneumocystis fungi continuously enter the respiratory passages, a long-term prophylaxis with co-trimazole, however, contributes to the progressive depletion of thiol in the mucosal cells of the lungs and the pulmonary fluids, while pneumocysts in the cells can only be eliminated by the defense of NO gas, which again in cases of thiol depletion can no longer be sufficiently produced, then it should be obvious that a long-term prophylaxis with co-trimazole creates selectively "resistant" counterregulated pneumocysts and cannot counterbalance the root cause of the disposition for the PCP lung infection. As human cells can only survive a deficit of thiol at the expense of inhibited NO gas production the microbes will, sooner or later, be able to proliferate during long-term prophylaxis with co-trimazole, as was the case in the 1970s when, contrary to expectations, massive resistance to co-trimazole emerged (Gysling 1995).

Wasting syndrome can be intensified by deficiencies of cysteine and folic acid, as well as many other nutritional deficiencies of the absorption process of the small intestine

Deficiencies of cysteine and folic acid under conditions of a Type-II counterregulation can additionally be aggravated by absorption failures in the small intestine. There are a number of indications that the electrolytic exchange in the mucosal cells is NO-dependent (Lincoln 1997). At an early stage an achlorhydria (Achylia gastrica) appears with a diminished production of sulfates due to the lack of cysteine and a diminished sulfate bonding of acids and enzymes. These symptoms appear as changes to the intestinal flora, a decline in the activities of enzymes and absorption dysfunctions in the small intestine to essential nutrients, among others fat-soluble and other vitamins and minerals (A, E, C, B-complex, selenium, zinc, magnesium; Ulrich 1989, Keusch 1990, Javier 1990). The diversity of symptoms of malabsorption at an early stage of "HIV infection" (and likewise before this point in time!) (Gillin 1985, Dworkin 1985, Ellakany 1987, Greenspan 1993) demonstrates that systemic deficiencies of thiol are long-term processes involving intermittent phases of NO over-stimulation that are answered by an inhibition of NO synthesis in immune and non-immune cells. This cannot be explained, at such an early point in time, by an infection from "HI viruses." In fact, the adoption of a fictional causal general factor of an "HIV" infection simply explains the blatant lack of understanding of the complex illness and its preventative and therapeutic treatment. This concept is supported by the fact that despite much speculation and the most intensive efforts by researchers no convincing pathological disease mechanism has been demonstrated through "HI viruses" (Balter 1997). The assumption of an "HIV" infection apparently explains everything and at the same time nothing, as demonstrated by the fatal treatment of wasting syndrome by HIV/AIDS medicine.

Wasting syndrome develops accordingly with all systemic illnesses e.g. cancer, sepsis, surgical trauma and ulcerative colitis etc.

The clinical picture of wasting syndrome, which was included in the catalogue of "HIV-related" AIDS-indicating illnesses by the US surveillance authority, CDC, in 1987 (CDC, 1987), is to be observed in all physiological and pathophysiological conditions that are linked to strong temporary or prolonged nitrosative and/or oxidative stress to the system in immune and non-immune cells. Wasting syndrome is the mirror image on a system level—above all between the skeletal musculature and the liver—of compensation to the counterregulating processes on the level of cellular symbiosis. If under the impact of excessive nitrosative and/or oxidative stress, lasting changes to the redox milieu (ongoing electron flows and hydrogen ion gradients) do not result in programmed cell death (apoptosis) and/or necrosis, the oxidative energy production can sink so strongly, after depletion of the anti-oxidative capacity, in mitochondrial cell symbionts that the signal for a state of pseudohypoxia is triggered. On genetic and non-genetic levels the energy supply through impulse reversals of the electron flows and hydrogen ion gradients switches predominantly to oxygen-independent ATP production via glycolysis (Warburg Phenomenon). The massively increased need for glucose is compensated by an increased conversion of amino acids to glucose and pyruvate above all in the skeletal musculature.

The missing cysteine protons from the splitting of cysteine into sulfate and hydrogen ions reduce also the glutamine synthesis of glutamate and ammonia in liver mitochondria. Glutamine through oxidation becomes an additional source of energy for mitochondria via glutaminolysis. The glutamate content in skeletal musculature, however, in wasting syndrome is debased by disruption of the sodium-dependent transport systems in the cell membrane. These systemic interactions result in the characteristic main symptoms of reduced levels of cysteine, arginine and glutamine as well as increased levels of glutamate in plasma found in laboratories in all wasting syndromes (Dröge 1997 b).

Wasting syndrome can develop independently of any kind of viral infection, e.g. in healthy people after **an**aerobic exercises (Kinscherf 1996), in over-trained athletes (Janssen 1988, Parry-Billings 1990, Pedersen 1994), after serious injuries, burns and surgical traumata as well as sepsis (Long 1976, Brennan 1977, Wilmore 1978, Siegel 1979, Bergström 1981, Turinsky 1982, Roth 1985, Low 1994), cancer illnesses (Brennan 1977, De Wys 1980, Heymsfield 1985, Shaw 1987, Zhang 1992, Tajek 1992, Hack 1997), in Crohn's disease, ulcerative colitis and chronic inflammatory bowel syndrome (Erikson 1983, Lundsgaard 1996), but also in chronic fatigue syndrome (Aoki 1993), in old age (Hack 1996, 1997) and after chemotherapy (Duesberg 1996).

The thiol deficiency syndrome is associated with all wasting forms accordingly associated with cellular immune weakness (AID, pre-AIDS)

Characteristic of all forms of wasting are the redox-dependent switch to type 2 cytokines in non-immune cells, the loss of type 1 cytokine-dependent immune cells (Th1 cells), natural killer cells (NK cells), neutrophile granulocytes and the switch to Th2 dominance with increased antibody production and eosinophiles (Blazar 1986, Shanahan 1989, Lozano-Polo 1990, Puente 1991, Aoki 1993, Pedersen, 1994, Brittenden 1996, Lucey 1996, Duesberg 1996, Shearer 1997, Doria 1997).

Animal experiments have acknowledged the causal relationship between cysteine deficiency, type 2 cytokine status, inhibition of NO synthesis and wasting syndrome (cachexia) as the main cause of death from cancer

Animal experiments have demonstrated the significance of the reversion of the micro-Gaian milieu and the re-stamping of the dominant cytokine profile of type 1 to type 2 dysregulation. Normal mice were treated with the type 2 cytokine, interleukin-6. Within a few hours a wasting syndrome developed, characterized by increased urea production and reduced levels of sulfate and glutamine in the liver as indicator of a diminished contribution of protons from cysteine. These findings were identical to experimental research data of tumor-bearing mice that had developed wasting syndrome (Hack 1996). Correspondingly the experimental induction in mice of type 1 cytokine tumor necrosis factor (stimulated by ROS) and interferon-γ (iNO stimulation) was answered with the synthesis of the type 2 cytokine, interleukin-6, a massive production of lactate and wasting syndrome (Bauss 1987, Tracey 1988, Brouckaert 1989, Turksen 1992, Strassmann 1992). The causal relationship between a type 2 cytokine induction triggered by type 1 cytokine stimulation is of crucial interest as type 2 cytokines inhibit cytotoxic NO production and simultaneously type 1 cytokine synthesis (Lincoln 1997). The inhibition of NO production by a counterregulation of Type-II cell dyssymbiosis below the critical NO thresholds that are necessary for activating the mitochondrial cell symbionts, is, however, characteristic of the glycolytic energy production and the linked nitrogen and lactate disposal via the liver, and leads to the negative nitrogen and energy balance that is termed wasting syndrome. The fact that rapidly growing tumors feature a very low NO synthesis (Chinje 1997) and metastatic cells feature a very high threshold for the stimulation of cytotoxic NO (Xie 1996) supports the theory of a systemic relationship, so that cachectic patients with advanced wasting syndrome break up a large proportion of their skeletal muscle protein and convert it to glucose (including cysteine to pyruvate) and large amounts of nitrogen are released as urea, which they do as a consequence of the archaic genetic re-programming under pseudohypoxic conditions that lead to the inhibition of NO synthesis. In this respect it is of special interest that wasting syndrome triggered by type 2 cytokine 6 in normal mice could be completely normalized by administration of cysteine (Hack 1996).

"In virtually all types of cancer, weight loss is correlated with survival and a major cause of death" (Hack 1997).

This fact has been recognized for almost as long as the Warburg Phenomenon of aerobic gylcolysis (Warren 1932, Waterhouse 1979, De Wys 1980, Lawson 1982, Fein 1985, Friedman 1987). It is of vital importance to activate the complex circulatory regulating systems of fluid cellular symbiosis by rational, considered compensation and support procedures instead of initiating a deadly vicious circle in the heat of the pharmacotoxic hunt.

Outline of the characteristic laboratory findings of "HIV positives," AIDS patients, cancer patients and others suffering from systemic diseases with threatened or apparent wasting syndrome

The uniform systemic response of bioenergetic and metabolic counterregulations after previously strong and/or prolonged nitrosative and/or oxidative exposure to stress arises homologously in "HIV positives" and AIDS patients. The conceptual consensus on acquired immune cell deficiencies circumscribes only a static snapshot on the level of the immune cell network and has aroused the awareness of HIV/AIDS physicians solely about the manifestation of opportunistic infections of cell dyssymbiosis. In reality it is all about a process-like systemic event in immune and non-immune cells that had already become established before "HIV" seroconversion and by no means leads straight to death. Cell dyssymbioses, like all cellular biological regulations, are driven in a non-linear way (Waliszewski 1998). Apart from the sum of real lifetime pressures and the individual disposition of the sufferers, the crucial question is whether medical intervention is virus-fixated or non-virus fixated. "HIV positives" can have a systemic glutathione deficiency at the earliest point in time of "HIV" seroconversion without developing clinical symptoms (Buhl 1989).

Whether these findings also apply to people with the same risk profile, who did not react positive in the "HIV test," is unknown as no corresponding studies were carried out. The cysteine level in plasma can be low at the time of the positive "HIV" reaction, but it can also be slightly higher (Eck 1989, Dröge 1997 a). The findings are dependent, more or less, on the random time of the test. There is no conclusive evidence of a causal correlation that "HIV positive" equals thiol deficiency (cysteine, reduced glutathione). There is a lot to be said for the reverse—that the "HIV characteristics" are the result of counterregulation in a state of pseudohypoxia of mitochondria.

Then again, a given thiol deficiency in T-helper cells of blood or in the blood plasma can lead to an incalculable disease danger. Official statistics of HIV/AIDS medical science show that when the number of officially registered HIV positives is compared to the number of officially registered AIDS patients over the last 15 years there are, in the meantime, far more people who have tested "HIV positive" and have not developed any clinical symptoms of AIDS-indicating illnesses. During the last decade the annual incidence of newly registered "HIV positives" has remained relatively constant at a low level despite horrendous prognoses, but the annual incidence of AIDS sufferers has declined (Robert-Koch-Institute 1999). More important than the mental fixation on the "HIV infection" are the long-term readings of anti-oxidative thiol and the respective parameters, which through pronounced anomalies show the development of a wasting syndrome and the disposition to AIDS-indicating diseases. There are very few long-term studies, independent of the "HIV" parameters, which methodically cover a causal correlation between real stress factors including pharmacotoxic loads and cellular biologically programmed counterregulations. From the very little research data available, in contrast to the huge number of pharmacotoxic studies based on the HIV/AIDS theory, it can be deduced that there was a complete correlation of the immunological, metabolic and cytokine data from the "HIV positives" who were really ill and the data from other test subjects and patients who had been diagnosed to have wasting syndrome (see illustration: Characteristic Laboratory Findings in Cumulative Wasting Syndrome: Indicators of Type-II Counterregulation of Cell Dyssymbiosis in Systemic Diseases (see table XVII). (Boli 1985, Fontana 1986, Dröge 1988, Eck 1989, Staal 1990, Klebic 1991, Roederer 1991 a, 1991 b, Hommes 1991, Hortin 1994, Ullum 1995, Kinscherf 1996, Fearon 1996, Lucey 1996, Dröge 1997 a 1997 b, Hack 1997, Herzenberg 1997, Lincoln 1997, Nuttall 1998).

The fundamental understanding is that wasting syndrome had already been clinically defined in connection with immune weakness without a primary infectious cause since the discovery of the Warburg Phenomenon

The fact that wasting syndrome in connection with characteristic cellular immune weaknesses in non-infectious diseases had already been recognized fifty years ago should have led to doubts that the loss of immune cells does not have to be inevitably caused by an infectious immune cell defect and immune cell destruction. Rather it should have been taken into consideration that acquired immunodeficiency syndrome (pre-AIDS and AIDS) and likewise cancer diseases are concerned with a bioenergetic disruption to the system. It was not noticed that localized nitrosative and oxidative conditions of stress in immune cells and non-immune cells can lead to depletion of the cellular proton reserves of the thiol pool (Sies 1978, Siliprandi 1978, Le Qoc 1982, Meister 1983, 1995, Marchetti 1997) and could cause cell type and organ spanning systemic counterregulations as well as pathological feedback processes (Long 1976, Brennan 1977, Lundsgaard 1996, Dröge 1997 a).

At the beginning of the 80's clinicians and practitioners obviously had no fundamental understanding of the over—and underdriving of the fluid governing cycles of the micro-Gaian milieu of cell symbionts and ignored the importance of the modulation of the proton and electron flows via thiol. Apparently it was unclear that localized disturbances to the redox status, which can have their starting point in immune cells and/or non-immune cells, can build up systemically through evolutionary biologically programmed counterregulations with redox-dependent changes to the cytokine profile, prostaglandin levels and hormone regulations. These disturbances can trigger numerous signal cascades, metabolic pathways and biosyntheses on cellular and cell-spanning planes, which in turn retroact on the immune cell network and/or the highly complex network of the non-immune cell systems.

The fundamental principle of preventative and therapeutic interventions resulting from the key role of the non-protein thiols

The pattern of the laboratory parameters in all states of wasting syndrome as a result of Type-II cell dyssymbiosis demonstrates the key role of cysteine-thiol as proton donor at decisive points in the self-organized cellular and supracellular networks of the human organism. The basic principle of preventative and therapeutic intervention arises from this key role. An acute, chronic, deficient provision and/or availability of cysteine leads to a loss of the fluidity of cell symbiosis, to a predominantly glycolytic energy metabolism, to wasting syndrome and to cellular immune weakness through the redox-dependent type 1 to type 2 cytokine switch. Every kind of chemotherapeutic and antibiotic therapy, targeted at the elimination of microbial cells and tumor cells, attacks in diverse direct and indirect ways the metabolism of the system. All such attacks can strengthen the primary causes of the cysteine deficit and the negative mobilization of cysteine and besides the desired inhibiting or eliminating of microbial and tumor cells, encourage the survival of such cell systems through a Type-II counterregulation ("resistance" of microbial and tumor cells, formation of metastatic cells). At the same time the already existing immune cell deficits could become aggravated, cell dyssymbiosis in other cell systems still compensated could become decompensated and the systemic consequences of wasting syndrome be forced up to the point of lethal organ failure. Non-consideration of the primary and secondary causes and results of acute and chronic system deficits is a serious case of medical malpractice. Since the end of the 1980s several research groups in HIV/AIDS medical science have demonstrated the significant interaction between non-protein thiol deficit in plasma and the peripheral blood cells as well as the capabilities of cellular immunity (Dröge 1988, 1989, 1992, 1993, 1997 a, 1997 b, Buhl 1989, Eck 1989, Halliwell 1990, 1991, Staal 1990, Klebic 1991, Roederer 1991 a, 1991 b, Jarstrand 1990, Baker 1992, Kinscherf 1994, Witschi 1995, Olivier 1995, Akerlund 1996, Hack 1996, 1997, Herzenberg 1997, Peterson 1998).

Only a few clinical research groups investigated the obvious methodology of cysteine compensation therapy via cysteine derivatives

Notable are the experimental and clinical data from research groups from the Deutsches Krebsforschungszentrum (DFKZ, German Cancer Research Center) and the Stanford University in the USA, regarding preventative and therapeutic improvements after oral medication with n-acetyl cysteine (NAC). The research team from the DKFZ stated after a 10-year research phase:

"The obvious way to ameliorate the immunological consequences of cysteine and glutathione deficiency is treatment with cysteine derivatives like NAC. This strategy is supported by studies of the effects of cysteine on urea levels and hepatic/glutamine ratios in tumor-bearing mice (Hack 1996), studies on the effects of NAC on body cell mass and body fat in healthy individuals (Kinscherf 1996), and longitudinal observations of NAC-treated, HIV-infected persons (Dröge 1997 a) . . . Many longitudinal observations on a small number of HIV-infected patients over a period of more than 10 years have already revealed that NAC treatment is capable of increasing not only plasma cystine [the oxidized form of cysteine], but also glutamine, to levels that were even higher than the mean of healthy controls. The CD4+ T cells numbers did not increase during NAC treatment, but remained essentially stable" (Dröge 1997 b).

The interest of a few research groups concentrated on the fact that cysteine, also as building block for sulfurous glutathione, acted as the most important antioxidant within human cells, overriding the mitochondrial cell symbionts. The biosynthesis of glutathione in immune cells is considerably dependent on extracellular supplies of cysteine (Dröge 1994). The strength of defense of T-helper immune cells, natural killer cells, neutrophile white blood cells and others is seriously diminished in cases of low cysteine levels and reactively higher glutamate levels in the blood plasma (Eck 1989, Roederer 1991, Herzenberg 1997). Only a few clinical research groups within HIV/AIDS medicine have studied the obvious preventative and therapeutic consequence of improving the cellular immunity functions by a cysteine-stimulated increase in intracellular glutathione synthesis (Olivier 1995, Akerlund 1996, Hack 1997, Herzenberg 1997, De Rosa 2000).

Since AIDS clinicians did not measure the crucial diagnostic parameters, they could not understand the anomalies of cellular immunity in the first AIDS patients

A heavily increased concentration of glutamate in blood plasma, as is characteristic of all physiological and pathophysiological wasting forms, for instance after anaerobic exercises and in AIDS and cancer, is linked to the inhibited activities of T-lymph immune cells after stimulation with heavily oxidizing stimulating substances (mitogens like pokeweed, concanavalin A or phytohemagglutinin) (Dröge 1988). These findings explain the apparently puzzling dullness of the reaction of the T-lymph immune cells, *in vitro*, of the first homosexual AIDS patients (Gottlieb 1981, Masur 1981).

Without the buffer of substantial amounts of cysteine, glutathione, glutamine and arginine, medication with Bactrim, Pentamidine etc. will sooner or later provoke a deadly vicious circle leading to organ failure, which is explained until today erroneously by the laboratory construct of a fictitious immune-weakening virus

The AIDS clinicians, however, had not measured either the levels of cysteine, glutamine, arginine and glutamate in blood plasma or the intracellular glutathione levels. The false speculation of a "new agent" being responsible for the destruction of T-helper cells in the blood plasma is the consequence of this blatant lapse. Of the first 14 homosexual AIDS patients, who were diagnosed as having PCP, 13 patients in an acute stage of PCP were treated with TMP/SMX (Co-trimoxazole, Septra, Bactrim etc.) (Zakowski 1984).

The doubled folic acid inhibition had evidently not only inhibited the pneumocysts, but also the neosynthesis of cysteine from methionine in the liver (Newberne 1997). As the cause of acquired immunodeficiency (AIDS) was based on the result of heavy and/or chronic nitrosative and oxidative stress triggered primarily by cysteine and glutathione exhaustion and secondarily by glutamine and arginine depletion with a simultaneous increase in glutamate in plasma, medication with co-trimoxazole for acutely immune-weakened patients with pronounced wasting syndrome

(Gottlieb 1981) without adjustments to cysteine, glutamine and arginine was therapeutically a highly risky venture that inevitably would cause a vicious circle leading to failure of the vital organs. As the AIDS clinicians had failed to understand the primary cause of acquired immunodeficiency with opportunistic infections (PCP, *Candida* and other fungal infections, parasitic infections, mycobacterial, cytomegaly viral infections etc.) as secondary consequence as well as the primary cause of the development of Kaposi's sarcoma after chronic nitrosation of cysteine and glutathione in the endothelial cells in the capillaries, in some cases of homosexual nitrite consumers, the fatalities, prolonged wasting syndrome and Kaposi's sarcomas (CDC 1981 a, 1981 b, Gottlieb 1981, Masur 1981, De Wys 1982, Haverkos 1982, Friedman-Kein 1984 a) were interpreted pseudo-rationally by the construct of a fictitious, allegedly transmittable to everyone via blood or intercourse, immune-weakening virus. The highly media-effective success of the endlessly variable stories of the lethal sex and blood plague gave the failing retrovirus researchers the opportunistic chance to re-define their laboratory product—a cancer retrovirus that was supposed to trigger uninhibited cell growth—as an AIDS retrovirus that just at the right moment in time emerged from nowhere, but through new diagnostic procedures, assured PCP in homosexual men. As a result of well-known difficulties in diagnosis before the end of the 70's, pneumoncyst agents were seldom represented microbiologically differentiated, so that in the 70's atypical non-bacterial pneumonias were treated across-the-board with co-trimoxazole (Hughes 1975). This is how the vicious circle closed: The US surveillance authority, the CDC, deduced from the limited frequency of requests for pentamidine for the treatment of PCP, that PCP was an unusual disease before 1981. Pentamidine is a highly toxic antiparasitic substance that had already been adopted since 1939 against trypanosomes, the agents of sleeping sickness, and since 1958 against PCP (Lourie 1939, Ivady 1958 1967, Western 1970). Pentamidine belongs to the so-called orphan drugs, substances whose production in the USA is legally subsidized, as otherwise, due to the fact that they were seldom prescribed, they would not be produced. This was the reason that pentamidine had to be requested through the CDC. As suddenly after 1981 pentamidine was relatively often requested in the gay centers in New York, Los Angeles and San Francisco for the treatment of PCP in homosexual men, the razor-sharp public officials at the CDC decided that AIDS did not exist before 1981.

"Unfortunately, this conclusion is highly suspect. Pentamidine-treated cases represent a small minority of PCP cases. Physicians preferred (and many still prefer) to prescribe Trimethoprim (TMP) combined with the sulfa drug, sulphamethoxazole (SMX) (Rao 1977, Furio 1985, Masur 1992,

CDC 1993, Kovacs 1993). No records are kept of TMP-SMX prescriptions [co-trimoxazole] .... Thus, utilizing CDC records of pentamidine requests is not only inaccurate for the period preceding 1980, it is also grossly inaccurate for the early AIDS period. For every pentamidine-treated AIDS-like case, there may have been between ten and twenty TMP-SMX cases. Certainly, a significant proportion of AIDS-like PCP existed in the pre-AIDS era .... The Kaposi's sarcoma (KS) story is almost identical to the PCP story" (Root-Bernstein 1993).

So, in reality, AIDS patients, who as a consequence of an overly toxic and pharmacotoxic conditioned thiol deficit (cysteine and glutathione deficit) were suffering from a pronounced immune weakness and a wasting syndrome, were treated with a pharmaceutical substance that was proven to block the neosynthesis of cysteine and glutathione through the inhibition of folic acid (Greenspan 1993). The clinicians requested pentamidine from the CDC only after Septra, Bactrim etc. could no longer be tolerated or the pneumocysts proved to be resistant. In the 70's Septra, Bactrim etc. replaced pentamidine because of its after-effects (Hughes 1975). When pentamidine also failed, the therapeutic repertoire for the treatment of PCP was expanded to no less toxic pharmaceutical substances like clindamycine/primaquine, dapsone/pyrimethamine, atovaquone and immunosuppressive corticosteroids (Kovacs 1993). The "resistance" to co-trimoxazole, which according to the microbial theory through its preparation as dual substance to inhibit the formation of folic acid and thus to exclude microbial resistance, had already been demonstrated in 1977 (Grey 1977). The miracle weapon Bactrim etc. "one of the most successful agents ever developed" (Then 1993) had failed in the treatment of opportunistic infections (AIDS). Instead of this there was the strong suspicion that the substance itself, which had on its launch already been recognized as immunotoxic (Ghilchick 1970, Lehrer 1971 a, 1971 b), had considerably contributed to the primary causes of AIDS and the development of wasting syndrome.

The first long-term clinical study on N-Acetyl-Cysteine with "HIV positives" exhibiting strongly degraded values of both T4-helper cell counts and intracellular reduced glutathione (GSH), demonstrates a "dramatically improved probability of survival" despite the senseless counterproductivity of simultaneous administration of the mitochondriotoxic, glutathione-exhausting "combination therapy"

An intriguing question was whether the therapeutic administration of oral doses of cysteine could improve the capacity of cellular immunity to defend against opportunistic intracellular infections. There have been only a few studies published of clinical HIV/AIDS research about the preventative and therapeutic effects of n-acetyl cysteine, with, however, "encouraging results" (Dröge 1997 b; Olivier 1995, Akerlund 1996, Herzenberg 1997). Clinical HIV/AIDS researchers at Stanford University administered to a large number of "HIV positives" without clinically manifest opportunistic infections or tumors, 3.2 to 8 g of oral NAC per day, over a short double-blind phase of eight weeks and an additional open phase of six months. The overall reduced glutathione was measured (GSH) in whole blood (HPLC process) and in peripheral blood cells (as glutathione S-bimane (GSB) by FACS measuring process) before and regularly during the treatment phase. The survival of 204 patients was followed up for 2 to 3 years. On the basis of the theory "HIV causes AIDS" the Stanford team concluded:

"We have shown that GSH levels are lower in subjects with CD4 T cell counts below 200yml (CD4, 200) than in subjects at earlier stages of HIV disease; that among subjects with CD4, 200, lower levels of GSB (a FACS measure of GSH in CD4 T cells) predict decreased survival; and that the probability of surviving 2-3 years increases dramatically as GSB level approach normal range. In addition, we have presented preliminary evidence suggesting that oral administration of NAC, which supplies the cysteine required to replenish GSH, may be associated with improved survival of subjects with very low GSH levels.

The crucial connection revealed here between GSH deficiency and survival in HIV disease was foreshadowed by several studies that demonstrated that HIV-infected people, particularly those with low CD4 T cell counts, often have low levels of GSH in lymphocytes and at other locations. However, the demonstration here that low baseline GSB levels are associated with decreased survival 2-3 years hence provides the first clear indication that GSH deficiency plays a pivotal role in determining how quickly the final stages of HIV disease progress" (Herzenberg 1997).

Objections and contradictions between prominent cysteine research teams

The conclusion of the Stanford team that oral administration of NAC raised the GSH levels in T-helper immune cells contradicts the findings of the German team from DKFZ:

"Despite the strong sensitivity of various immunological functions against glutathione depletion, there is little evidence to support the hypothesis that the approximately 30% decrease of intracellular glutathione levels in lymphoid cells from HIV-infected patients (Eck 1989, Roederer 1991, Herzenberg

1997) is pathologically relevant. Even under conditions in which NAG treatment was found to improve the survival of HIV-infected patients, there was no evidence that this treatment had increased the intracellular glutathione level in the patients' lymphoid cells (Herzenberg 1997). This is in line with findings of others, that NAC treatment at daily doses of up to 4 g failed to induce a detectable increase of intracellular glutathione levels in lymphocytes of HIV-infected patients (Witschi 1995), healthy subjects (Kinscherf 1994), and cancer patients (Hack and Dröge, unpublished observation). The study of healthy human subjects revealed that persons with relatively low intracellular glutathione levels had low CD4 T cell numbers. Persons who moved during a 4-week observation period from a glutathione level of > 20 nmol/mg protein to a level < 20 nmol/mg protein experienced on average a 30% decrease in CD4 T cell numbers, and this decrease was prevented by NAC treatment (Kinscherf 1994). However, it is important that NAC caused this relative increase in CD4 T cell numbers in spite of decreasing intracellular glutathione levels (i.e., not by increasing the glutathione levels!), which suggests that the effect of NAC on the immune system was not related to its function as a precursor of glutathione (Kinscherf 1994)" (Dröge 1997 b).

The ideological myopia of cysteine therapy researchers leads to fatal preventative and therapeutic consequences

The controversy between the research teams of the DKFZ and Stanford University about whether the congruent proven improvement of the immune cell functions and the inhibition of wasting syndrome in "HIV positives" by high dosage cysteine compensation therapy depends on a "replenishment" (Herzenberg 1997) of the intracellular levels or whether the reduction of the intracellular level by 30% is "pathologically irrelevant" (Dröge 1997 b), demonstrates the core problem of HIV/AIDS medical science. Both research teams apparently cannot see the forest for the trees. The intracellular glutathione deficit in patients with an acquired elimination deficiency for intracellular agents and enforced glycolysis resulting in a negative nitrogen and energy balance is not pathologically irrelevant nor is the intracellular glutathione level directly replenished by cysteine administration.

An explanation of these contradictory research data would be the key to a life-saving therapy. The German research team stated:

"Because the glutathione level has a strong influence on mitochondrial functions (Meister 1995, Marchetti 1997), it is reasonable to hypothesize that the abnormally high glycolytic activity [mainly oxygen-independent energy production outside the mitochondria] in diseases with cachectic processes [wasting syndrome] may be the direct consequence of an inadequate level of oxidative energy metabolism in the mitochondria resulting from the decreased glutathione level" (Dröge 1997 b).

Although the researchers strongly emphasize that the loss of cellular immune defense is a common phenomenon in almost all diseases and states of wasting syndrome requiring no participation of any viruses, they do not mention the virus-independent causes of glycolytic energy production as a result of the exhaustion of the thiol pool in mitochondria through preceding excessive nitrosative and/or oxidative stress. On the contrary, they postulate without any differentiated substantiation.

"The development of this dysfunction does not require the virus but may result from virus-induced biochemical changes" (Dröge 1997 b). This ideological shortsightedness, characteristic of all HIV/AIDS medical research, leads to the fatal preventative and therapeutic consequences for the affected patients:

"Because antiviral treatment was usually not sufficient to raise plasma cysteine and glutamine close to normal levels in the absence of NAC treatment, it is suggested that NAC treatment and antiviral treatment should be used as complementary tools. NAC is not by itself an effective antiviral drug. These findings should be taken into consideration when clinical trials are being designed" (Dröge 1997 b).

In other words the researchers at the German Cancer Research Center explicitly admit that:

- the negative nitrogen and energy balance (wasting syndrome) is the main cause of death in patients suffering from systemic diseases like cancer, AIDS, heavy trauma, sepsis, organ transplants with exaggerated immunosuppressive therapy, colitis ulcerosa etc
- this wasting syndrome is commonly linked to a loss of the elimination of the intracellular agent (AIDS resulting from immune cell loss)
- the causes of cellular immune weaknesses and wasting syndrome must be in the virus-independent enforced glycolytic energy production outside of mitochondria
- forced glycolysis leads to increased protein degradation in the skeletal musculature and other peripheral organs and to a dysregulation of the amino acid levels, due to the conversion from degraded protein of amino acids to glucose for the increased glucose consumption of glycolysis

- the debased plasma levels of the amino acid cysteine in the liver cause a reduced synthesis of glutamine and in its place an increased glutamate plasma level and excessively increased urea production

Forced glycolysis in patients with immune weaknesses and wasting syndrome is a direct consequence of the disruption to the oxidative energy production in the mitochondrial respiratory chain

Disruption of the oxidative ATP production and the switching to aerobic glycolysis (Warburg Phenomenon) is a result of glutathione deficiencies in the mitochondria.

Since the "HIV disease" is in reality a mitochondrial illness, it is absurdly untenable to treat it with cysteine compensation and at the same time with nitrosative substances, which are demonstrated to provoke mitochondrial diseases

Despite awareness of the cause-effect relationship, however, a therapeutic somersault was performed and the use of anti-retroviral substances like AZT etc. recommended, even though they were recognized to inhibit oxidative energy production in mitochondria by blocking the enzyme cytochromoxidase in the respiratory chain (Benbrik 1997) and secondarily through mitochondrial DNA defects (Lewis 1995). This damage to mitochondria by AZT and derived substances cause the increased production of reactive oxygen species that leads to an increased glutathione consumption. After exhaustion of glutathione and mitochondrial ATP deficiency through the actions of AZT etc. the immune cells and non-immune cells switch to aerobic glycolysis, as long as programmed cell death or necrosis have not yet occurred, and initiate through intensified Type-II counterregulations of cell dyssymbiosis the whole chain of reactions in the already counterregulated or not yet counterregulated immune cells and non-immune cells, which was originally ascribed to the fictitious "HI virus." The recommendation to deploy n-acetyl cysteine for the prevention and therapy of cellular immune malfunctions and wasting syndromes merely complementarily together with "anti-retroviral" substances like AZT etc. ("cocktail therapy"), which have been shown to produce no anti-retroviral effects (Papadopulos-Eleopulos 1999), but which have been shown to cause AIDS (Rosenthal 1994, Lewis 1995, Glaxo Wellcome 1998, Giraldo 1999), defies all medical logic. *Given the well-founded fact that the "HIV disease" is in reality a mitochondrial illness it is rationally incomprehensible to treat mitochondrial illnesses with nitrosative substances that have been proven to trigger mitochondrial illnesses.*

To foil the experimentally and clinically proven beneficial effects of cysteine by a simultaneous administration of mitochondria inactivators such as AZT etc. and folic acid inhibitors such co-trimazole etc. is preventatively and therapeutically counterproductive. There have been to date no comparative studies between the "HIV positive" patients treated with toxic substances and those treated with non-toxic substances. There will be no such comparative studies for as long as the laws of cellular symbiosis are not sufficiently understood either by HIV/AIDS medical dogmatists or in orthodox oncology. The counterproductive attempts to eliminate "HI viruses" and cancer cells with pharmacotoxic substances instead of expediently compensating the elementary fundamental needs of the symbiotic cell system reflects this lack of understanding up until now.

Also the clinical studies of the Stanford research team demonstrate this dilemma in HIV/AIDS medical science based on the dogmatic "HIV causes AIDS" theory. The vital dynamics of the interplay between the fluid nitrogen gases (NO and its derivatives) and the sulfurous thiols (cysteine and the glutathione system) is just as little discussed as by the researchers from the German Cancer Research Center. The fundamental fact of the link between NO and its derivatives and non-protein thiols (nitrosation) for the function-regulating interactions in cellular control mechanisms (Stamler 1995, Hausladen 1996) is ignored. The existence of NO is only incidentally mentioned in connection with glutathione functions. There was also no reference to NO and its functions.

"Glutathione (GSH), like nitric oxide (NO), is a small ubiquitous molecule that plays a key regulatory roles in metabolic and cell-cycle-related functions. This cysteine-containing tripeptide (γ-glutamylcysteinylglycine), which is found in millimolar concentrations in all animal cells, also provides the principal intracellular defense against oxidative stress and participates in detoxification of many molecules. GSH depletion, caused for example by acetaminophen overdose, results in hepatic and renal failure and ultimately in death. HIV-infected people tend to have subnormal GSH levels in plasma, lung epithelial lining fluid, peripheral blood mononuclear cells (PBMC) and, as determined by measuring GSH as intracellular glutathione-*S*-bimane fluorescence (GSB) with the fluorescence-activated cell sorter (FACS), in individual CD4 T and other blood cells.

In vitro studies show that lowering intracellular GSH levels decreases cell survival, alters T cell functions, and increases HIV replication, NF-kB activation [protein molecules that activate the redox-dependent expression of genes for the biosynthesis of proteins], and sensitivity to tumor necrosis factor-induced cell death [a type 1 cytokine that increases the formation of superoxide anion and calcium^{2+} ions in mitochondria, Type-I overregulation]" (Herzenberg 1997).

This introductory account by the Stanford team about the functions of glutathione in human cell systems in the publication, "Glutathione deficiency is associated with impaired survival in HIV disease," is an exemplary demonstration of all clinical HIV/AIDS medical science, which one-sidedly recognizes only the overregulated mitochondrial cell symbiosis with accelerated cell death through glutathione exhaustion as a result of oxidative stress, lack of detoxifying oxidizing molecules and induction through tumor necrosis factors (apoptosis/necrosis) via Type-I overregulation of cell dyssymbiosis.

The alternative, however, namely the underdriving of mitochondrial cell symbiosis after exhaustion of the thiol pool through nitrosative and/or oxidative stress and resulting from this, the pseudohypoxic states (apparent lack of oxygen through disrupted oxygen utilization), which after a shortfall in the critical reserve capacities of oxidative energy production in mitochondria provokes the genetic switch to an archaic emergency program of oxygen-free energy production (Type-II countrregulation of cell dyssymbiosis), is not recognized.

The lack of perception of the evolutionary biological laws of the self-organizing fluid micro-Gaian milieu of cell symbiosis is disguised by the dogma of a hypothetical infection with an "HI virus." This misinterpretation of the laboratory construct of AIDS research had fatal preventative and therapeutic consequences. The correct cognition, that the supply of n-acetyl cysteine as hydrogen ion-donating natural amino acid can eventually improve deficient oxygen utilization in mitochondria and the glycolytic energy production with the systemic consequence of lessening the immune cell weakness as well as the negative energy and nitrogen balance, is accompanied by the fatal perception that for the supposed blockade of "HI viruses" the simultaneous prescription of a "cocktail therapy" from thiol-consuming pharmaceutical substances (AZT and converted nucleoside analogues and protease inhibitors) are necessary. The pharmacotoxic ingredients of "cocktail therapy" for "HIV positives" and AIDS sufferers are all mitochondrial deactivators (Dalakas 1990, Hayakama 1991, Arnaudo 1991, Tyler 1992, Hobbs 1995, Lewis 1995, Benbrik 1997, Carr 1998, Brinkman 1998, 1999).

The mitochondria-deactivating "cocktail therapy" has two crucial effects: one, the direct inhibition of enzymes of the respiratory chain (cytochromoxidase etc.) and two, the inhibition of enzymes for the replication of mitochondrial DNA (polymerase). The latter leads to damage of DNA and deficient synthesis of protein for the mitochondrial respiratory chain. The result is accelerated cell death or dysfunction of mitochondria that leads to an increased production of reactive oxygen species and increased glutathione consumption. This triggers the pseudohypoxic genetic switch of Type-II counterregulation programs. The genetic damage to mitochondria cannot be repaired and is passed on with every cell division. The consequence is that n-acetyl cysteine (NAC) does indeed compensate DNA damage, depending on dosage and time, as well as the damage already incurred by the mitochondria, for a limited period, via "cocktail therapy" but in the long run cannot prevent the mitochondrial performance from being further damaged by continued use of "cocktail therapy." The effective NAC compensation therapy, which can compensate for the glutathione deficit triggered by "HIV diseases," is absurdly counteracted by the glutathione-consuming pharmacotoxics of the therapeutically useless and extremely damaging "cocktail therapy." The results of this serious medical malpractice are projected on the fictitious HIV infection.

"Surprisingly, subjects with CD4 <200 who took NAC for 8-32 weeks in our study survived significantly longer than a comparable group (also CD4, <200) who were not offered or did not choose to take NAC . . . Subjects who took NAC were roughly twice as likely to survive for 2 years as the subjects who did not take NAC . . . Survival was not affected . . . by reverse transcriptase inhibitor usage [AZT etc., "cocktail therapy"]. The association of oral NAC administration (consequently GSH replenishment) with greater survival is consistent with the dramatically better survival of individuals with higher GSB levels" (Herzenberg 1997).

From this information it can be inferred that all "HIV" infected patients in the Stanford study with a T4 helper cell count of less than 200 per microlitre were partaking of a "cocktail therapy," as in HIV/AIDS research these T4 helper counts are the absolute indicators for "cocktail therapy." The mixture of AZT etc. could not lower the mortality rate of these thiol-depleted patients, but "surprisingly" high dosage administration of the simple sulfurous amino acid cysteine sliced the mortality rate of immune cell-weakened patients almost in half. The Stanford University researchers, fixated on the HIV/AIDS theory, could not, however, come to the simple logical conclusion that as the "cocktail therapy" had no obvious influence on mortality rates that this also could not be the case if they mixed NAC therapy with a mitochondriotoxic "cocktail." Since the Stanford researchers solely associated the "dramatic," almost-halved mortality rate with the enriched glutathione recovery after NAC administration, the compelling preventative and therapeutic logic would have been to recommend just high-dosage NAC compensation therapy to improve the glutathione balance under controlled conditions, without forcing the glutathione increase via a mixture of mitochondria-deactivating, glutathione-consuming "pharma-cocktails" from AZT etc., to new sub-normal levels and thereby actuating irreparable damage to mitochondrial DNA. Had the Stanford researchers practiced this rationally based recommendation, instead of recommending like their German colleagues, NAC treatment simply as a "complementary tool" (Dröge 1997 b) for "cocktail therapy," they could have "surprisingly" established that the mortality rate was heading towards zero. A small number of clever individual therapists have applied exactly this preventative and therapeutic treatment strategy and a number of other non-toxic measures for "HIV positive" patients for years with "surprising" success and thereby reduced the unscientific disease theory of the inevitably lethal "HIV infection" to absurdity.

The vital significance of cysteine compensation is to supply a sufficient amount of freely convertible protons, in order to reverse dysregulation of the switching-rhythm of cellular symbiosis and the resulting negative nitrogenous and energetic balance

The therapeutically beneficial working principal of the cysteine effect lies in feeding the cell systems of the organisms with compatible, freely convertible hydrogen ions (protons). This task is performed by the sulfur hydrogen groups (sulfhydryl groups, SH groups) of n-acetyl cysteine (NAC). In systemic diseases, too many protons have been involved in the preceding phase of excessive nitrosative and oxidative stress (Type-I overregulation). The proton supplies for powering the hydrogen pumps of the OXPHOS system for ATP production in mitochondria slow down. The resulting shortfall of the critical reserve capacities of mitochondrial respiratory chain (pseudohypoxia) forces, after a time lapse, the genetic switch to oxygen-independent energy production and thereby a re-distribution of the transfer of hydrogen ions to aerobic glycolysis (Warburg Phenomenon) instead of to the cell symbionts and as investment in the increased cell division cycle. The mitochondria are weakened, in contrast to the proton suppliers, by hydrogen ion diffusion into the cytoplasm via a leakage in the energetically stabilized mitochondrial membrane. The milieu of counterregulated "host cells" is highly hydrogenated and reductive (from reduction—the bonding of protons and absorption of electrons, in contrast to oxidation—the release of protons and electrons). The situation becomes aggravated by the consequential systemic process of glycolytic energy production, too-high consumption of protons in the re-supply of the glycolysis product lactate with simultaneous excess energy consumption in the liver. Therapeutically, the core problem of all systemic illnesses with a pathology of immune cell deficiency and wasting syndrome as well as the characteristic non-protein deficiency (cysteine, reduced glutathione) is to satisfy the proton hunger in cell systems and to supply a surplus of convertible hydrogen ions for vital proton floating. The understanding of this fundamental bioenergetic problem has been impeded up until now by the lack of knowledge of the hybrid character of human genomes. Since the human genome, according to more recent findings of mitochondrial research, (like genomes of all multicellular organisms) comes from a fusion of a hydrogen-fueled archaeum and a hydrogen-supplying proteobacterium (Gray 1999), one could say that in the counterregulated cells (Type-II counterregulation of cell dyssymbiosis) the archaeal genome portion had taken over command as a result of pseudohypoxic activation, and that the cooperation with the proteobacterial genome parts in the nucleus and in mitochondria had regressed to a competition for survival between the archaeal and proteobacterial cell symbionts (Kremer 1999).

The oxidative overregulation of archaic cell symbiosis has been relatively well-researched under the terminology "oxidative stress" (Sies 1985, Papadopulos-Eleopulos 1988, 1992, Halliwell 1991, 1992, Buttke 1994, Kroemer 1997, Wallace 1997, 1999). The evolutionary biologically programmed underregulation of cell symbiosis as response to excessive or prolonged nitrosative and/or oxidative stress, however, was first recognized in the course of the 1990s based on the fundamental findings of mitochondrial, NO and cytokine research (Kremer 1999). This evolutionary medical concept of understanding gleaned from a multitude of individual findings is of the most vital importance for the prevention and therapy of systemic diseases including AIDS, cancer, sepsis, traumata and colitis. The preventative and therapeutic practices, to date, in cancer and AIDS medical science, namely trying to eliminate the "HI viruses" and tumor cells through toxic chemotherapy, is bound to fail as long as the researchers and clinicians only partially understand or completely ignore the fact of hybrid cell symbiosis. The urgency to re-think is shown by the fact that according to the analysis of epidemiological process data, over many years, at the German Cancer Research Center chemotherapeutically treated cancer patients survived on average 3.5 years while non-chemotherapeutically treated patients survived on average for 12 years (Abel 1990). "HIV positive" patients, two to three years after toxic "cocktail therapy," had double the mortality rate of patients with the same unfavorable origins who in addition to "cocktail therapy" were treated with "complementary tools" of high doses of cysteine for eight months (Herzenberg 1997).

The "replenishment of intracellular glutathione" via cysteine supplementation can only occur after a complex and complete changeover, resulting from the increased availability of freely convertible protons

The controversial interpretation of the clinical research teams regarding the effects of cysteine compensation therapy and the normalizing of the intracellular glutathione levels is based on an unnoticed contraction of thought, in common with HIV/AIDS medicine on the whole, as the crucial findings of NO, cytokine and mitochondrial research were not taken into account. The oral administration of n-acetyl cysteine for patients with intracellular glutathione deficiency does not serve the direct "replenishment of glutathione" (Herzenberg 1997), but rather the absorbed cysteine initially tops up the depleted pool of convertible protons. In already pathophysiologically counterregulated cells a roughly 30% of reduction of glutathione is sufficient for the antioxidative functions, as the number and activities of mitochondria are hugely reduced (overview Pedersen 1997). The nitrosative and oxidative stress is, on the contrary, precisely as a result of the prolonged counterregulation of Type-II cell dyssymbiosis, highly subdued, as the cells have greatly reduced both the synthesis of NO and its derivatives and the production of reactive oxygen species (ROS). This situation corresponds to the limited counterregulated physiological state of the cell symbiosis of fetal cells, of cells in the late cell division cycle and during the early phases of the healing of wounds.

In addition, through the glycolytic metabolic situation increasing amounts of pyruvate as antioxidant are formed. An increased demand for intracellular glutathione develops only if, after replenishment of the proton pool, the redox milieu has been stabilized in such a way that the whole genetic and supragenetic network can again be redirected. This means that the convertible proton yield of the redox milieu must have improved correspondingly to overcome the redox-dependent "semiconductor threshold" for the electron flows of macromolecules (transcription proteins, and RNA and DNA molecules) for the genetic expression of the biosyntheses of the necessary enzyme profiles. This redirection of the enzymes and co-enzymes of the micro-Gaian regulation cycle system for renewed oxidative energy supply is a precondition for the increase in intracellular glutathione, which the Stanford team associated with the "dramatically improved survival" during NAC treatment (Herzenberg 1997). So, the provoked exhaustion of the thiol pool caused by prolonged nitrosative and oxidative shock and the regressive competition for survival of the archaeal and the proteobacterial subgenomes have to be restored to a harmonic cooperation in the fringe areas between the macromolecular and fluid phase.

The improvement in the redox potential through the supply of proton-donating cysteine reactivates, among other things:

- The enzymes of the glucose degradation pathway for the planting of the glucose degradation product, pyruvate as fuel in the citrus cycle of mitochondria and for the supply of electrons for the mitochondrial respiratory chain.
- The shift in the ratio of the oxidizing co-enzyme NAD^+ to NADH, in favor of NAD^+, and the transfer of released hydrogen ions to the proton transport molecules for transfer to the mitochondria as well as the return transfer on the co-enzymes NAD, FAD, FMN in the mitochondria which in turn stock the hydrogen ion pumps of the OXPHOS system of mitochondria for oxidative ATP energy production.
- The increase of $calcium^{2+}$ not bonded to the membrane through increased hydrolysis of NAD^+ and an increased synthesis of the calcium-dependent enzyme, NO synthase for the formation of NO gas with the assistance of NADPH, other co-enzymes and co-factors.
- The formation of peroxinitrite from the increased supplies of NO gases and the again increased superoxide anions from the reactivated respiratory chain of the mitochondria, to open, with the aid of peroxinitrite, the mitochondrial channels in the membrane of the cell symbionts for the exchange of $calcium^{2+}$ and the nuclear DNA-coded proteins for the complexes of the respiratory chain.
- The enzyme for the neosynthesis of glutathione, γ-glutamyl cysteine synthase, that is regulated through the bonding of the newly enriched NO and its derivatives to the sulfhydryl groups of enzymes.
- The inhibition of the synthesis of communication proteins of a type 2 cytokine profile in favor of a type 1 to type 2 cytokine balance.

The "replenishment of intracellular glutathione" (Herzenberg 1997) through the supply of cysteine is, thus, the consequence of a complex master switch as a result of increased convertible proton availability. The neosynthesis of glutathione can only gather momentum via the glutathione synthesis enzyme (Han 1995, Stamler 1995) once the fluid gas mixture for the OXPHOS system of mitochondria (NO, superoxide anion, peroxinitrite) is again optimized.

Subtle reductions of glutathione in antigen-presenting cells by toxic substances are sufficient to provoke the "HIV seroconversion," which in reality is simply a reprogramming of the T4-helper immune cells to the immune status of Th2-cells (type 2 cytokine profile)

In addition to the explicit findings, that the intracellular glutathione levels in immune cells are reduced in "HIV positives" already at the earliest stage of seroconversion (positive "HIV test") (Eck 1989, Buhl 1989, Roederer 1991 a, 1991 b, overview Herzenberg 1997, Dröge 1997 b) and the type 2 cytokine profile in Th2 immune cells dominates (Barcellini 1994, Meyaard 1994, Navikas 1994, overview Mosmann 1996, Abbas 1996, Lucey 1996), the Stanford team demonstrated in a new study with a research team from Chicago University that the glutathione yield of the antigen-presenting cells (APC) crucially co-determines the cytokine status of T4 helper immune cells.

"Studies presented here demonstrate that GSH levels in APC play a central role in determining whether Th1 or Th2 cytokine response patterns predominate in immune responses. Using two immunologic models and three methods to deplete GSH, we show that in all cases, GSH depletion leads to a shift away from the typical Th1 cytokine profile and toward Th2 response patterns .... Our data demonstrate that subtle changes in GSH levels may have profound effects on the immune response .... A wide range of human diseases is associated with altered levels of GSH (Uhlig 1992), including cancer (Richie 1992) and AIDS (Staal 1992). Indeed, we have recently shown that GSH deficiency in HIV-infected individuals correlates with decreased survival during a 2- to 3-year monitoring period. This diminished survival capacity could be due to any or all of the multiple metabolic and regulatory functions of GSH .... Furthermore, we have shown that treatment with NAC, a GSH prodrug, reverses the *in vivo* immunomodulating effects of low-dose CY [= one of the substances deployed to deplete glutathione; a cytostaticum that is used in cancer therapy!]; and others have shown that supplementing cultures with NAC decreases IL-4 production. Together, these findings persuasively argue for a key role for APC GSH in determining whether antigenic stimulation induced a Th1 or Th2 response pattern" (Peterson 1998).

The primary causes for the beginning of the chain reaction, thiol exhaustion → cytokine switch → NO inhibition → Type-II cell dyssymbiosis → "HIV"/AIDS, cancer, wasting syndrome, myopathy, encephalopathy and polyneuropathy, enteropathy etc. in AIDS risk groups are given through the defined risk profile:

> "Multiple mechanisms may contribute to systemic GSH deficiency in HIV disease, including excessive production of inflammatory cytokines [= type 1 cytokines that trigger an increase in cytotoxic NO gas production] and excessive use of GSH depleting drugs [= toxic and pharmacotoxic substances]" (Herzenberg 1997).

The Nobel Prize winner Mullis demands evidence of the disease theory "HIV is the cause of AIDS" that follows the "strict laws of scientific logic"

Recently in an interview, the American Nobel Prize for Chemistry winner in 1993, Mullis, responded to the question of why a man like Gallo was so successful, if in the opinion of Mullis, the dominant AIDS thesis had never been scientifically proven:

"Gallo only had success as a businessman, not as a scientist," was his response.

To the linked question:

"But how is a layman supposed to know which scientist he can believe?"

Mullis said:

"You should never believe anyone, not even me. You can only trust your own research. If you just comfortably lie on your back and let people tell you everything then you'll always get some sort of answer, mostly the wrong one."

And then Mullis defined as the most important rule of scientific methodology:

"Whoever wants to convince someone about his truth has to be able to show them what it was that had convinced him—within a scientific framework and following the strict laws of logic. Whoever wants to prove to me that the HI virus really causes AIDS has to be able to show me his experiments." (Mullis 2000).

It is incongruous with the strict laws of scientific logic to warn "HIV positives" against alcohol and acetaminophen as glutathione-exhausting drugs, yet simultaneously conceal the similar effects of the chemotherapeutic effects that are prescribed

In the reference to Gallo being "a businessman not a scientist," Mullis, among other things, is alluding to the fact that Gallo in his publications about the supposed evidence of the "HI virus" in T4-helper cells of patients had remained secretive about the use of hydrocortisone, and so had passed off the substance effect as the effect of a supposedly new retroviral HIV (Kremer 1998).

According to the "strict laws of logic" (Mullis 2000) the combination of life-saving high-dosage cysteine compensation therapy with "antiviral" substances (Dröge 1997 b, Herzenberg 1997) in "HIV"-fixated AIDS therapy cannot be justified. The Stanford team demonstrated the blind spot of "HIV"/AIDS therapy through the provident warning to minimize the glutathione deficiency in "HIV infected" patients through certain precautionary measures without considering for a moment that substances like AZT etc. put in the "anti-retroviral cocktail therapy" are "excessively GHS-depleting drugs" (Herzenberg 1997).

"It may be prudent for these individuals to avoid excessive exposure to UV irradiation and unnecessary use of drugs that can deplete GSH—e.g., alcohol and prescription or over-the-counter formulations containing acetaminophen" (Herzenberg 1997).

The medicamentous substances, acetaminophen and aminopyrine are, just like the immunosuppressive substances Azathioprine, Trimethoprime, co-trimoxazole, numerous chemotherapeutics, cytostatics, antibiotics, antiparasitics, fungistatics (fungi inhibitors), virustatics (virus inhibitors), the "cocktail therapy" of nucleoside analogue and non-nucleoside analogue reverse transcriptase inhibitors such as azidothymidine (AZT) and related substances, in addition to protease inhibitors, excessively activated NO and its derivatives, nitrites (poppers), peroxinitrites, nitrosamines, nitroso thiols etc. all "excessively GHS-depleting drugs." AZT, for instance, induces the characteristic increase of glutamate in glutathione deficiency (Greenspan 1993) and just like acetaminophen has to be detoxified in the liver by enzymatic bonding to glucuron acids (Nelson 1963, Mrochek 1974, Good 1986, Richman 1987).

"GSH depletion, caused for example by acetaminophen overdose, results in hepatic and renal failure and ultimately in death (Thomas 1993) .... The severe liver and kidney damage caused by exposure to high levels of GSH-depleting drugs such as alcohol and acetaminophen (Thomas 1993) also underscore the dangers of systemic GSH deficiency. Such damage has

> recently been shown to occur even at relatively low doses of such drugs when systemic GSH levels are compromised (Zimmerman 1995) . . . . Oral administration of *N*-acetylcysteine (NAC), a cysteine prodrug used to replenish GSH after acetaminophen overdose (Thomas 1993), increases GSH levels in HIV-infected subjects; and this GSH replenishment may be associated with prolongation of survival" (Herzenberg 1997).

It is incongruous with the strict laws of scientific logic to determine that nitrosative and oxidative substances cause life-threatening damage, even after relatively low dosages if the systemic glutathione levels are previously damaged; and at the same time "preventatively" medicate "HIV positives," who are pathognomonic for early glutathione insufficiency, with glutathione-exhausting nitrosative and oxidative drugs

These clear statements from the Stanford researchers demonstrate the shortsightedness of the medical double standards even of the most progressive HIV-fixated AIDS prevention and therapy. AZT and the various other "excessive GSH-depleting drugs" (Herzenberg 1997) of the "anti-retroviral" and antimicrobial "cocktail" long-term prophylaxis and therapy cause on the basis of their objective biochemical working mechanisms clinical symptoms analogous to acetaminophen. For "HIV positive" patients, above all, the following statement applies:

"Such damage has recently been shown to occur even at relatively low doses of such drugs when systemic GSH levels are compromised" (Herzenberg 1997). The systemic depletion of the glutathione level of "HIV positives" at the earliest stage of the "HIV infection" has been recognized by all HIV/AIDS physicians for more than a decade as the leading symptom of "seroconversion," the AZT analog toxic risks and the metabolic detoxifying process of acetaminophen for 40 years (Nelson 1963, Good 1986, Richman 1987, Buhl 1989). No serious physician would dream of treating patients who had been chronically poisoned by acetaminophen with NAC compensation therapy and simultaneously prescribe acetaminophen, unless this physician negligently wished to harm his patient with "hepatic and renal failure and ultimately death" (Herzenberg 1997).

It is incongruous with the strict laws of scientific logic to prescribe nitrosative and glutathione-exhausting chemotherapy to patients who tested "HIV positive" after chronic acetaminophen abuse due to Th1 to Th2 switch, even though the nitrosative and immunotoxic effects of acetaminophen have been known for over 40 years

In numerous cases female patients without a recognizable risk had a positive result in the "HIV test" and desperately searched for many years with their relatives and physicians for the reasons for the "HIV infection" and out of the fear of death took on "cocktail therapy" with its respective consequences. A detailed study of case histories showed a long-standing abuse of substances containing acetaminophen. None of the many HIV/AIDS physicians who had been consulted were interested in the connection between acetaminophen abuse and "HIV positivity" as a result of glutathione deficit. The patients could have been relieved of their sickening fears and the thiol pool could again have become balanced through high dosage NAC compensation therapy and treatment to protect the liver (Kremer, unpublished observations).

It is incongruous with the strict laws of scientific logic, to on the one hand stimulate via "glutathione replenishment" the proliferation of the Th1-helper immune cells, which in turn allegedly hatch millions of T-cell destructive "HIVs" daily; and on the other hand state that "HIV positives" provided with "glutathione replenishment" via cysteine supplementation show "dramatically improved survival rates" compared to those "HIV positives" that were only treated with the allegedly "HIV-inhibiting cocktail therapy"

It is an inexcusable medical aberration to subject already chronically poisoned "HIV positive" patients with a glutathione deficit status, a type 2 cytokine dominance (Th2) and an inhibition of cytotoxic NO defense gases, to immunotoxic and cytotoxic long-term treatment with AZT etc. for the prophylaxis of AIDS, since the suffering HIV-stigmatized patients have no opportunity to compensate by non-toxic means the mitochondrial illnesses caused by excessive inflammatory cytokines and excessive consumption of GSH-depleting drugs. This also applies to the administration of "complementary" NAC in simultaneous antimicrobial and "anti-retroviral cocktail therapy." It is contrary to the "strict laws of logic" (Mullis 2000) to expect to drive off the Devil "HIV" with Beelzebub AZT etc. while at the same time treating with NAC. According to the prevailing theory of the billion-fold increase in "HI viruses" (Ho 1995 a, Wei 1995 b) the replenishment of glutathione of antigen-presenting cells must increase the synthesis of type 1 cytokines (Peterson 1998) and thus stimulate the growth and proliferation of Th1 immune cells. That would mean, according to the prevailing HIV theory, that the "HI viruses" that are dependent on the division of Th1 host cells would also rapidly increase and the postulated destruction of T4 helper cells would be forced by "HI viruses." So, according to the prevailing HIV theory, the dosage of the "cocktail therapy" must be increased to check the induced virus boom. A real vicious circle for theory-fixated virus hunters! Fortunately the biological reality does not match the dogmatic theory since "the association of oral NAC administration (consequently GSH replenishment) with greater survival is consistent with the dramatically better survival of individuals with higher GSB levels" (Herzenberg 1997).

It is incongruous with the strict laws of scientific logic to claim that on the one hand wasting syndrome (cachexia) is the main cause of death in "HIV positive" AIDS patients (and similarly the main cause of death with cancer and other systemic diseases), and is "the direct consequence of an inadequate level of oxidative energy metabolism in the mitochondria resulting from the decreased glutathione level"; and on the other hand prescribe unlimited therapy with glutathione-reducing and mitochondria-inactivating AZT etc. and Bactrim etc., while at best death is held at bay with brief courses of cysteine supplementation

If this is so then the currently dominant disease theory that "HIV causes AIDS" must be wrong and the "anti-retroviral" immunotoxic "cocktail therapy" is not only a horrifically futile, but rather—as glutathione-reducing, mitochondria-inactivating treatment with or without "HI viruses"—extremely damaging and in the long term reduces life expectancy of patients. The central question on AIDS prophylaxis and therapy must be: What strengthens the vitality and performance capacities of mitochondria and what weakens the vitality and performance capacities of mitochondria?

The data from the most comprehensive clinical study on AZT and Bactrim therapy (Concorde study) with European "HIV positive" patients proved that administration of AZT and Bactrim did not reduce AIDS incidence and death rates either in the early or late stages of illness

In April 1994 the clinical Concorde Studies were published on the results of the chemotherapeutic treatment of 1749 symptom-free "HIV positive" patients. It was concerned with patients from 40 treatment centers in the UK and Ireland and 34 treatment centers in France. More than 60% of the participants were homosexual patients, 13% were intravenous drug addicts, with the remaining patients belonging to other risk groups. The patients were randomly split into 2 groups, members of the one group receiving immediately 1,000 mg of AZT daily, the other group were given a placebo and 1,000 mg of AZT daily only on developing ARC (AIDS related complex, defined according to the classification profiles for HIV/AIDS of the US authority CDC as Pre-AIDS) or once the cell count of T4 helper cells in the blood had sunk to below at least 500/μL. 613 participants (32% from the first group and 38% from the second group) received in addition co-trimoxazole as prophylaxis against PCP, most of them before the appearance of clinical symptoms.

The 3-year clinical observation period was the longest of all AZT/co-trimoxazole studies that had been carried out worldwide until that time. The clinical research hypothesis was based on the theory that AZT inhibited the proliferation of "HI viruses" by blocking the provirus DNA of the "HI viruses" and thus preventing the destruction of T-helper immune cells. It was expected that the rate of opportunistic infections, wasting syndromes, encephalopathies and myopathies among others (AIDS) would drop by roughly 30% within the 3-year observation period in the immediately treated group in comparison to the deferred group. This expectation was obviously based on the logic of the HIV/AIDS theory that the earlier AZT etc.—for inhibition of the "HI viruses" and co-trimoxazole etc.—for the inhibition of pneumocyst fungi—the agent for the most frequent AIDS-indicating disease PCP—were deployed—the lower the number of cases of ARC, AIDS and AIDS deaths there would be recorded in the early treatment group compared to the late treatment group over the 3-year observation period. In fact, the results were:

"3-year progression rates to AIDS or death were 18% in both groups, and to ARC, AIDS, or death were 29% (Imm) and 32% (Def) [immediate AZT from the time of randomization; deferred AZT until onset of ARC or AIDS] . . . . The results of Concorde do not encourage the early use of zidovudine [AZT] in symptom-free HIV-infected adults" (Concorde Coordinating Committee 1994).

The logically linked question of whether the results encouraged a deferred administration of AZT in symptom-free "HIV-infected" patients whose T4 helper cell had sunk below 500/μL, or in "HIV positives" who had developed AIDS symptoms, was not answered by the Concorde study. The international research group, who carried out the study independently of the AZT producers, however, added:

"The results also call into question the uncritical use of CD4 cell counts as a surrogate endpoint for assessment of benefit from long-term anti-retroviral therapy" (Concorde Coordinating Committee 1994).

In other words, AZT in terms of the HIV/AIDS theory cannot inhibit "HI viruses" either by early or late administration, to prevent ARC, AIDS or death. There is, however, in the Concorde study a conspicuous correlation between the number of early and late patients who were simultaneously treated with AZT and co-trimoxazole:

32% of the immediately treated AZT group were treated with AZT + co-trimoxazole after the sinking of the T4-helper count, the number of cases of ARC, AIDS and death in this group after 3 years was 29%. 38% of the deferred treatment AZT group were treated with co-trimoxazole and AZT after the sinking of the T4-helper cell count, mostly before the appearance of symptoms, the number of cases of ARC, AIDS and death amounted to 32% (Concorde Coordinating Committee 1994).

The data from the Concorde study is a compelling argument for the primarily acquired serious lack of thiol in the "HIV positive" patients, which is further worsened by treatment with AZT, Bactrim, and other glutathione-exhausting, mitochondriotoxic substances up until deadly organ failure occurs

If we assume from well-founded facts that:

- HIV positives at the earliest point in time of a positive result to the "HIV test" show signs of a systemic glutathione deficiency
- Glutathione deficiency is dependent on both the increased turnover through preceding nitrosative and oxidative stress and on the reduction in neosynthesis
- AZT is a nitrosative substance, which in the same way as acetaminophen and increased amounts of NO and its derivatives, bonds to glutathione and cysteine and thus reduces the thiol pool
- Hydroxylamin, a degradation product of co-trimoxazole, can similarly exhaust the thiol pool and co-trimoxazole impairs the regeneration of cysteine from methionin and the regeneration of glutathione from cysteine
- Glutathione deficiency in antigen-presenting cells (dendritic cells, macrophages, B-cells) activates the synthesis of type 2 cytokines in T4-helper cells
- Type 2 cytokines inhibit the synthesis of cytotoxic NO in T4-helper cells and these cannot eliminate intracellular opportunistic agents without the synthesis of NO
- Glutathione deficiency, type 2 cytokine dominance and NO inhibition through the inactivation of mitochondria and switching to glycolytic energy production can be linked to cellular immune weaknesses (AIDS), cell transformation to cancer, encephalopathy, polyneuropathy, enteropathy, myopathy and wasting syndrome

- HIV positive and AIDS patients have a type 2 cytokine dominance in T4-helper cells
- HIV and AIDS patients, in addition to a systemic glutathione deficiency show signs of a dysregulation of the amino acids cysteine, glutamine and arginine as well as an increase in glutamate and urea production
- HIV positive and AIDS patients, prior to disease show signs of "excessive production of inflammatory cytokines" through multi-infectiousity and alloantigen absorption that leads to an increased synthesis of interferon-γ, which activates cytotoxic NO and increased synthesis of tumor necrosis factors which promotes the formation of reactive oxygen species and these processes consume glutathione which triggers a Type-II counterregulation of cell dyssymbiosis as a consequence of the cell death or Warburg Phenomenon, dependent on the time span, dosage and the intensity of the prior immune suppression
- HIV positive and AIDS patients in the time prior to disease show signs of "excessive use of GSH depleting drugs [= toxic and pharmacotoxic substances]" as a result of consumption of toxic doping substances, medication abuse and a multitude of medical interventions that likewise lead to compensated or decompensated cell dyssymbiosis
- "Lower GSH levels in T4-helper cells reduce the chances of survival and the probability of surviving two to three years increase dramatically when the glutathione levels in T4-helper cells increase after high dosage eight month treatment with n-acetyl cysteine"

then the compelling logical consequence is that the patients who took part in the Concorde study and developed ARC/AIDS died not as a result of their immune weakness through non-existent "HI viruses" but as a result of the loss of the vitality and performance capacities of their mitochondrial cell symbionts, the primary cause being the serious thiol deficiency, leading to lethal organ failure via simultaneous glutathione-exhausting treatment with AZT, co-trimoxazole (Bactrim etc) and other mitochondiotoxic substances.

The results of the Concorde study and numerous other therapy trials prove that with the combination of glutathione-exhausting, mitochondriotoxic pharmaceuticals used in the treatment of HIV/AIDS, and with cancer chemotherapy, the switching-on process of Type-II counterregulation of cellular dyssymbiosis is exponentially accelerated

As a result of the Concorde study and other studies, it has to be assumed that through the combination of glutathione-exhausting substances in HIV/AIDS treatment and likewise in cancer chemotherapy, and due to the pharmacodynamic interactions of these substances that have still hardly been studied (Richman 1987, Descotes 1988, Van Meerten 1995, Brinkman 1999), the switching-on processes of Type-II counterregulations exponentially accelerate below a critically low threshold of non-protein thiols (cysteine, reduced glutathione) when the reserve capacity of the mitochondrial performance has sunk beneath the critical triggering thresholds.

The archaeal subgenome in the cell nucleus functions as the evolutionary-biological memory for the condition of a lack of freely convertible protons in the human cellular symbiosis system

In the Concorde study, as in most clinical publications and handbooks on HIV/AIDS, there are no references to intracellular or systemic glutathione levels, to plasma levels of cysteine, glutamine, arginine or glutamate, let alone to a cysteine compensation therapy.

The results of the Concorde study and numerous other "cocktail therapy studies" (overview Concorde Coordinating Committee 1994) demonstrate very clearly that from a critical threshold of the exhaustion of the thiol pool "also low doses of glutathione-depleting drugs" (Herzenberg 1997) accentuate the strong effects that the "cocktail therapy" exercises on the Type-II counterregulations of cell dyssymbiosis. As glutathione constitutes 90% of the intra—and extracellular thiols, which are not attached to a protein, the glutathione deficiency is a decisive sensor for the amounts of available freely convertible protons. Thus, when a patient is at the stage of a still to be compensated, critical threshold of a proton deficiency, then even low doses of a glutathione-depleting "cocktail therapy" without compensation therapy, forces the vitality and performance capacities of the mitochondrial cell symbionts to decompensation (state of pseudohypoxic redox status). If you make the reasonable assumption that the archaeal subgenome in the nucleus acts as evolutionary-biological memory for states of proton deficiency in cellular symbiosis in human cell systems, then the genetic switching between the host cell and the mitochondrial cell symbionts is logically justifiable. The "Warburg Phenomenon" of aerobic glycolysis that pathologically occurs as a result of critical thiol deficiency in all diseases linked to cellular immune weaknesses and wasting syndromes (AIDS, cancer etc) is the result of the reduction of the triggering threshold for the "pseudohypoxic" archaeal subgenome. The consequence is the inhibition of the transfer of protons and the supply of electron-rich fuels in mitochondria. A highly reductive cell milieu with a loss of fluidity ensues. Thus, the treatment of glutathione-deficient "HIV positive" and AIDS patients with glutathione-depleting pharmaceutical substances is definitely contraindicated.

A comparison of the different methodologies of action and thought between pharmacotoxic medicine and non-toxic medicine, speaks against the pharmacotoxic method due to the poor survival rates of chemotherapeutically treated "HIV positive" and cancer patients

In the medical reality it is a matter of the different thinking patterns and ways of operating that lead to the variously successful treatment strategies in the concrete practices of prevention and therapy of systemic illnesses. Pharmacotoxic medicine acts on the assumption of genetic and metabolic defects and predominantly attempts to eliminate "HI viruses" and cancer cells chemotherapeutically. Non-toxic medicine acts on the assumption of a bioenergetic overall analysis and attempts to compensate the fluid redox milieu and to balance out the cell symbiosis. The long-term results of the survival rates of the mostly chemotherapeutically treated cancer patients (Abel 1990) and the survival rates of the exclusively chemotherapeutically treated "HIV positives" (Concorde Coordinating Committee 1994, Herzenberg 1997), speak against pharmacotoxic practices.

After the failure of chemo-cocktails in the early and late treatment of "HIV positives" and AIDS patients, the hunt for the "virus" should have been obligatorily terminated

The failure of the antimicrobial and "anti-retroviral cocktail therapy" in early or late treatment of "HIV positive" and AIDS patients should have led to a reappraisal and an end to "*Virus Hunting*" (Gallo 1991). In the course of the decade, the retrovirus cancer researcher's question raised at the historic conference in New York in March 1983 (Thomas 1984) was answered in the clearest possible manner, both in a preventative and therapeutic sense, by the evolutionary-biologically programmed emergency reaction of cellular symbiosis of symptom-free "HIV positive" patients who were treated with mitochondriotoxic "pharma-cocktails": AIDS develops. The cause of the "intriguing puzzle of Kaposi's sarcoma" had been epidemiologically, clinically and pathophysiologically resolved for a long time. The "HIV-associated" Kaposi's sarcoma developed in Western countries almost exclusively in nitrite addicted, anal receptive homosexuals (Papadopulos-Eleopulos 1992 b, Kremer 1998 a, 1998 c). The annual incidence of Kaposi's sarcoma was in decline, contrary to the predictions of the HIV/AIDS theory, after decline in the use of nitrite inhalation as a sexual doping substance (Haverkos

1990). Kaposi's sarcoma developed in "HIV negative" and "HIV positive" patients (Friedman-Kein 1990). Kaposi's sarcoma as an "HIV disease" was also questioned by orthodox HIV/AIDS clinicians (Beral 1990). Since the discovery of the metabolism of nitrites in NO and its derivatives in the endothelial cells of the walls of blood vessels by Nobel Prize winner, Ignarro (Ignarro 1992) there is no doubt that the "HIV-associated" Kaposi's sarcomas develop as a reaction of the endothelial cells to excessive thiol-exhausting nitrite inhalation (Type-II countrregulation of cell dyssymbiosis).

Background to the abrupt modification of the "HIV" theory, after the disaster of the deadly AZT/Bactrim mass-poisonings of the mid-90s

Unimpressed by these objective data and as a result of long-standing experience in manipulating popular opinion and capital flows of research funds by ascribing to the phantom-like "HIV, virus of death" ever more insidious characteristics, the HIV/AIDS researchers suddenly changed the virus theory. For a decade the "retrovirus HIV" was sold as a lentivirus (from the Latin: *lentis* = slow) by Montagnier, Gallo and their colleagues, supposedly slumbering for many years inactive in T-helper cells before starting its works of destruction in the immune cells (overview Papadopulos-Eleopulos 1993 a, 1993 b, 1998 a). The supposedly heterosexual HIV/AIDS outside of the risk groups had, in Western countries, long turned out to be a propaganda myth of physicians and the media (Rappoport 1988, Fumento 1989, Adams 1989, Fry 1989, Nussbaum 1990, Lauritsen 1990, 1993, Kremer 1990, 1994, Willner 1994, Duesberg 1996, Hodgkinson 1996, Shenton 1998). The annual officially registered HIV/AIDS incidence, for instance, in Germany, despite numerous changes in the definition of AIDS and the extension of the catalogue of AIDS-indicatings to 29 different disease diagnoses, had levelled out at on average 0.002% of the total population with a declining tendency. Also the annual officially registered incidence of "HIV" stagnated at 0.003% of the total population. Despite all published statistical trickery the proportion of homosexual and intravenous drug addicts within the HIV-stigmatized remained dominant, although they only constituted a small proportion of the total numbers of these risk groups. The successful "businessman Gallo" (Mullis 2000) and with him the allied profiteers of the deadly business of fear must have begun to worry about the lucrative HIV/AIDS turnover. As a result of the shattering findings of the "early" AZT treatment of "HIV positives" in the Concorde study, the pharmaceutical industry was worried about heavy losses in turnover at a point in time, and the authorization of about a dozen "anti-retroviral HIV" medications were fast-tracked without sufficient clinical checks on their effectiveness (Papadopulos-Eleopulos 1999). As the incidence of the real AIDS diseases among the sum total of "HIV-infected" patients was annually about 5% in the US (about 2% in Germany) and the survival period of pharmacotoxically treated AIDS patients on average 2-3 years, the really big business could only be made using the fear factor in the long-term "early" treatment of the "HIV positives" with "anti-retroviral HIV" drugs. To this end, however, in contrast to the prevailing HIV theory up until that time, an extremely rapid proliferation had to be ascribed to the "HI viruses." In order to motivate physicians and HIV-stigmatized patients to use "anti-retroviral" drugs at the earliest possible stage, despite the findings of the Concorde study and other clinical therapy studies, it had to be suggested that the proliferation of the "HI viruses" in the blood serum could be measured as a "viral load" and that the elimination of the "HI viruses" could be quantitatively controlled after long-term medication with "anti-retroviral" drugs. Such a process promised the physicians and patients the chance of observing the "viral load" with an apparent mathematical exactitude through continuous controls in the laboratories and to be able to adjust, depending on increase or decrease of the "viral load," the "anti-retroviral" drug mixture tailor-made for individual patients.

The "kitchen sink" model of Dr. Ho as justification, after counting of the alleged "viral load," to "hit HIV hard and early" with at least three "anti-retroviral" substances (highly active anti-retroviral therapy = HAART or combination therapy)

In 1995, US laboratory researchers published the new HIV theory. From that time on they claimed that "retrovirus HIV" was not a lentivirus (= slow virus) at all but that it would proliferate by billions daily. It did not destroy the T-helper cells but the T-helper cells would mature in their billions daily and sacrifice themselves to eliminate the "HI viruses." This silent battle in "HIV-infected" patients swings back and forth until the viruses gain the upper hand and the T-helper cells are exhausted. The "anti-retroviral" substances admittedly inhibit "HI virus" proliferation, but after a few days the viruses become resistant. For that reason at least three different "anti-retroviral" substances have to be combined to prevent the development of resistance of the "HI viruses." In order to measure the "viral load" the HIV researchers deployed the method discovered by the Nobel Prize winner, Mullis, whereby individual sections from the DNA sequence can be arbitrarily increased (the polymerase chain reaction, PCR). The laboratory researchers described a mathematical formula with which they apparently had measured the dynamics of "HIV" proliferation. In order to make the new model of rapid virus proliferation and elimination more graphic, the basic image of a kitchen sink was used, in which by pulling out the plug, as much water flows out as flows in, until less flows in than drains out (Wei

1995 b, Ho 1995 a). With the battle cry "*Time to hit HIV, early and hard*" (Ho 1995 b) Ho, who was named "Man of the Year" by Time Magazine in 1996, rescued HIV/AIDS medicine after the disaster of the AZT/co-trimoxazole mass poisoning with the apparently rational justification of a chemotherapeutic treatment as early as possible and now highly active anti-retroviral therapy (HAART) or "combination therapy."

The "kitchen sink" model is lacking in any logically plausible justification

Dr. Ho's theory, gratefully and completely uncritically accepted by the HIV/AIDS physicians, has had to this day an extremely calamitous impact on affected patients. The "kitchen sink" model defies every logically comprehensible justification. The basic assumption during the first phase, of uncertain duration, after the postulated "HIV infection" that there is a balance of power between HI viruses and T4-helper immune cells, is objectively false. The characteristics of the "HIV-infected" at the earliest point in time of an "HIV seroconversion" is the striking depletion of glutathione in T4-helper cells (Eck 1989, Buhl 1989, Roederer 1991 a) and the re-programming of the cytokine profile from type 1 (Th1 cells) to type 2 (Th2 cells) (overview Lucey 1996). Every kind of intracellular virus in T4-helper cells can only be eliminated by the synthesis of NO gas, produced by Th1 cells (overview Lincoln 1997). "HI viruses" colonizing glutathione-depleted Th1 cells would be killed by NO gas attacks from other Th1 cells as a result of the apoptosis or necrosis of the Th1 cells under attack. Objectively, no "HI viruses resistant in a few days" (Ho 1995 a) could develop as neither the glutathione-depleted Th1 cells, which have a normal life of one to two days, nor the supposed virus in them would survive an NO gas attack. The "billion-fold daily proliferation" of Th1 cells and "HI viruses" according to the "kitchen sink" theory of Dr. Ho is pure science fiction (termed by critics as Ho's Intelligence-deficiency Virus theory), as the "HIV-infected" show at the earliest point in time a Th2 immune cell dominance. Th2 cells cannot, however, eliminate the "billion-fold daily" "HI viruses," as they do not produce NO gas, but stimulate the antibody production in B-cells. Whether T-cells are programmed for a type 1 cytokine profile and NO gas production or a type 2 cytokine profile and NO gas inhibition is not determined by "HI viruses" but by the glutathione content of the antigen-presenting dendritic cells, macrophages and B-cells (Peterson 1998). Aggressive HAART treatment based on the freely fantasized "kitchen sink" theory of Dr. Ho has been shown to promote advanced depletion of glutathione and a loss of the vitality and performance capacities of mitochondria (Hässig 1998, Brinkman 1999).

With the addition of a protease inhibitor, the HAART combination became an enriched substance that was supposed to blunt the imaginary enzyme-scissors of "HIV" and the involved parties promised the "Lazarus effect" of curing "HIV" in three to four years

As unintelligent and free from all competence in understanding self-organizing cellular symbiosis in human cell systems as the aggression therapy of Dr Ho ("Time to hit HIV, early and hard") may seem, in a commercial sense HAART treatment has up until today been an extremely successful method of treatment. Through the expensive HAART-combination therapy and the expensive PCR laboratory controls the therapy costs for HIV/AIDS patients, with the full involvement of asymptomatic "HIV positives," have multiplied since 1996 with the help of "The Man of the Year." After a new group of substances—protease inhibitors—were added to the combination cocktail, the specialist journals and the mass media celebrated the impact of the lethal poisoning of the already poisoned as the "Lazarus effect of the doomed." Proteases are enzyme proteins in all human cells, which as enzyme "scissors," cut the longer protein chains into suitable individual sections. The new protease inhibitors were credited with exclusively inhibiting proteases that the "HI viruses" need to tailor-make a new protein shell after replication in the host cell. Nobody had actually produced such a natural cutting tool of the "HI virus," so genetic protein molecules were designed as protease inhibitors, which were supposed to "sacrifice" themselves to the imaginary "HIV" enzyme "scissors" and so to say make them blunt. The objections of protease specialists that such molecular clamps for the postulated HIV enzyme "scissors" had to be highly specific or else the natural protease "scissors" could clamp in all kinds of cell in an incalculable manner were completely ignored (Rasnick 1996, Hässig 1998 a).

The arbitrary contentions of the HIV/AIDS theory that by employing long-term medication with the new combined mix, the deadly HI viruses could be expelled, even from hidden cell nests and completely annihilated in 3 to 4 years (Perelson 1997, Saag 1999) were spread by a huge propaganda campaign. The time span of 3 to 4 years roughly corresponds to the average survival times of chemotherapeutically treated AIDS patients.

The "early and hard" bombardment with the toxic combination therapy, irreparably damages the DNA and mitochondrial respiratory chain; risk of deadly organ failure remains even years after ending HAART treatment, since damage to mitochondrial DNA is cumulative (chemo late-consequence syndrome)

Steered by the "invisible hand of the market" the protease-inhibiting enzyme blockers on offer by the leading pharmaceutical concerns were fast-tracked, as already was the case with the approval of the enzyme blockers AZT etc. for the inhibition of the alleged HIV transcription enzyme, reverse transcriptase (RT), by the US authorizing authority FDA and approved in 1996. The idea was to combine the RT enzyme blocker with the protease enzyme blocker to hit the "HI viruses" "early and hard" (Ho 1995 b) with the dual strategy of HAART and combination therapy. Under the motto "double stitching lasts longer" the pharmaceutical mixture from two respective RT enzyme blockers (nucleoside analog reverse transcriptase inhibitors, NRTI) and one or more protease enzyme blockers (protease inhibitors, PI) were recommended by the highest health authority in the USA, the Department of Health and Human Services (HHS).

The man responsible for the policy of the HHS on HAART combination therapy for symptom-free "HIV positive" and AIDS patients was, as in 1989 on the approval of AZT for "anti-retroviral" therapy for asymptomatic "HIV positives," the already quoted director of the National Institute of Allergy and Infectious Diseases, Dr. Fauci, who avoided answering critical questions about the clinical consequences of AZT treatment by storming out of the interview (see last chapter). Compensation therapy with cysteine and other compensatory measures were not worthy of mention in the HHS guidelines (Bartlett 1997). Obviously Fauci, Ho and their colleagues had learned nothing from the toxic effects of increased glutathione consumption and mitochondrial deactivation from a "cocktail therapy" (AZT etc. + co-trimoxazole etc.) on "HIV positives" with a primary glutathione deficit and NO gas inhibition from a cytokine switch, except that, similarly to combined chemotherapy in cancer treatment, toxic agents have to be tried out until such a time that the microbial and tumor cells have been annihilated or the patients die from the "side effects."

The "planned experiments on humans" (Thomas 1984) of the virus hunters push the principal of aggression of microbial and cancer chemotherapy to extremes in that even before the appearance of microbial and tumor cells in symptom-free patients, on the basis of the arcane "HIV antibody test," they aggravate the primary causes of the increase in polyspecific amounts of antibodies as measured by the "AIDS test." Under the influence of a type 2 cytokine dominance, polyspecific self-reactive antibodies of class G immunoglobulins are formed that are not normally available in blood serum and in extracellular fluids. The polyspecific self-reactive antibodies inhibit regenerative type 1 cytokine stimulated cellular immunity (Peterson 1998, Wang 1999). The aggressive HAART combination therapy thus, in contrast to the official propaganda of HIV/AIDS researchers, must inevitably and counterproductively accelerate disruption to the enzymes of the respiratory chain and damage to the DNA in mitochondria, the primary causes of the "HIV" characteristics, by increasing glutathione consumption. The opportunistic infections provoked by "early and hard hitting" substance HAART (2 NRTI + 1 or 2 PI +TMP/SMX etc.) necessitate additionally the use of an always greater variety of combined chemotherapeutics and chemoantibiotics that is difficult to keep track of. A host of HIV/AIDS physicians is thus employed, in projecting onto the apparently chameleon-like mutating "HI viruses" their own preventative and therapeutic malpractice in most of the clinical studies which are sponsored by the pharmaceutical industry (Marco 1998, Cox 1998) instead of grappling with the problem at its bioenergetic roots, namely compensating for the obvious proton deficiency and balancing out the micro-Gaian milieu of cellular symbiosis. The more toxic bombardments that the HAART patients have to suffer, however, the greater the danger that the mitochondrial DNA and thus the biosyntheses for the complexes of the respiratory chain become irreparably damaged and that the equilibrium of the fluid cell symbioses will become more difficult or indeed impossible to maintain. Mitochondrial DNA damage is cumulative because of insufficient repair mechanisms and develops much more frequently than in nuclear DNA (Johns 1996, Yakes 1997, Wallace 1999).

The extraordinary variety of short—and long-term cellular, organ and metabolic disturbances from combination therapy with protease inhibitors

The HIV/AIDS clinicians observed under HAART treatment a disturbance of fat metabolism (lipodystrophy), which since the beginning of the 1990s was associated in non-HIV stigmatized patients with a functional disruption of the enzyme cytochrome oxidase in complex IV of the respiratory chain and damage to mitochondrial DNA and is termed multiple symmetric lipomatosis (MSL) (Berkovic 1991, Klopstock 1994, Campos 1996, Becker-Wegerich 1998, Brinkman 1998). In HAART patients it was mostly concerned with fat wasting in the distal extremities and facial region as well as an accumulation of fat in the dorsocervical area ("buffalo hump") and in the thoracic and abdominal cavities. This syndrome is linked to insulin resistance, diabetic metabolism disruptions, increased plasma levels of fat building blocks (hypertriglyceridaemia), increased lactates in the plasma, neuropathy, cytomegaly retinitis of the retina, haemolytic anaemia, liver damage, kidney stones etc. (Hengel 1997, Carr 1998 a, 1998 b, 1999, Miller 1998, Lo 1998, Roth 1998, Hässig 1998 a, Gervasoni 1999, Mallal 1999, Viard 1999, Galli 1999, Saint-Marc 1999 a, 1999 b, Brinkman 1998, 1999).

Almost all of the proven toxic effects of HAART and protease inhibitors result in mitochondrial dysfunction and strongly resemble the spectrum of congenital mitochondrial diseases

> "Since HAART almost always includes at least two NRTIs and since HAART-related lipodystrophy has been described in patients not taking protease inhibitors, but only NRTIs, we hypothesise that NRTIs have a key role in the pathogenesis of this syndrome. We propose that the mitochondrial toxicity of these drugs is the responsible mechanism, leading to similar metabolic disturbances as those found in MSL type 1. Protease inhibitors may very well aggravate this metabolic process through additional mechanisms, as suggested by others (Carr 1998). The use of NRTIs might even turn out to be the initiating essential factor, since HAART-related lipodystrophy was only observed in patients treated with protease inhibitors when they received NRTIs at the same time. The cause of HAART-related lipodystrophy would then be based on a multifactoral, cascadic process, in which both NRTIs and protease inhibitors play a deleterious part .... The only enzyme that is responsible for mtDNA replication, DNA polymerase γ, is inhibited to a varying extent by NRTIs used in HAART (Lewis 1995, Brinkman 1998). Through this mechanism, NRTIs can easily induce depletion of mtDNA, resulting also in depletion of mtDNA-encoded mitochondrial enzymes and this will finally lead to mitochondrial dysfunction. In fact, nearly all side-effects that have been attributed to the use of NRTIs, such as polyneuropathy, myopathy, cardiomyopathy, pancreatitis, bone-marrow suppression, and lactic acidosis, greatly resemble the spectrum of clinical manifestations seen in inherited mitochondrial diseases (Brinkman 1998). Few studies have shown (with muscle biopsies) the occurrence of mitochondrial dysfunction during zidovudine monotherapy in selected patients with drug-induced myopathy (Dalakas 1990, Arnaudo 1991). Of the other NRTIs, mitochondrial toxicity has only been shown in vitro, when tested as single agents (Brinkman 1998). So far, there are no studies that have addressed this issue in clinical practice, but it is likely that a combination of NRTIs will synergistically give rise to any form of mitochondrial dysfunction .... Recently, Saint-Marc and colleagues claimed a special role for stavudine [an AZT-related nucleoside analog substance] over and above other NRTIs in the development of lipodystrophy (Saint-Marc 1999 a). During the 1st International Workshop on Adverse Drug Reactions and Lipodystrophy in HIV (June 26-28, 1999, San Diego, USA) the reversibility of peripheral fat wasting only upon interruption of stavudine therapy was described (Saint-Marc 1999 b)" (Brinkman 1999).

The quasi-statistical postulations of the "kitchen sink" model, which form the basis of using the allegedly quantitative PCR "viral load" in the individual administration of chemo-cocktails, were disproven by mathematical analysis as objectively incorrect

The statement that the effects of AZT etc. "greatly resemble the spectrum of clinical manifestations seen in inherited mitochondrial diseases" (Brinkman 1998) is absolutely clear. These findings were, however, still ignored by the HIV/AIDS medical community. The rationale of the "early and hard" HAART treatment of "HIV positives" by means of a combination of AZT and related substances + protease inhibiting substances was restated in the publications of the research groups of Ho (Ho 1995 a) and Shaw (Wei 1995 b) in a quasi-mathematical and quasi-statistical manner. The core of their declaration was the inhibition of the apparently daily billion-fold reproduced "HI viruses" could be controlled in laboratories with HAART medication by using the modified genetic DNA reproduction methods of the polymerase chain reaction (PCR). The administration and respective adaptation of the dosage schemata of combination therapy with "anti-retroviral" and protease inhibiting chemotherapeutics is based, to this day, on this speculative change in the theory of the HIV doctrine and the laboratory readings of the so-called "viral load" in the blood plasma of "HIV positives" and AIDS patients, as a laboratory finding expressed in logarithmic scales. Mathematicians have analyzed the assumptions, predictions, formulae, projections and result data, derived from calculations in the publications of the research teams of Ho and Shaw (Craddock 1995, 1996 a, 1996 b, 1997, Lang 1998). After discussing the special mathematical problems in an abstract symbolic language, the Australian mathematician Craddock declared:

"If there is so much HIV present, and it's replicating so fast, why does 'HIV disease' take ten years to progress to AIDS? In the publications of Ho *et al.*, they use the analogy of a sink with the drain open, and the water pouring in from a tap at a slightly slower rate than it drains away. So you get a slow steady decline in CD4 cells. Ho *et al.* have a few equations that are supposed to describe the changes in virus levels and CD4 cells over time. What do these equations actually predict, as opposed to what Ho *et al.* say they predict? In order to make them work you have to correctly formulate them, which Ho et al. do not. When correctly formulated what emerges is stunning. Ho *et al.*'s observations combined with their simple model for T cells and virus, predict that the T cell count should reach an equilibrium state quickly. Meaning exponentially fast. It is actually difficult to understand exactly what the equation on p.126 of Ho *et al.* is supposed to mean but it definitely predicts that equilibrium is approached exponentially. When you add terms to the equation to describe the effects of Virus (inexplicably, they do not include the effects of the virus on the T cell population in their model. I thought HIV was supposed to be killing these cells somehow), then include the expression for the amount of virus that they give on p. 124, you get a picture of 'HIV disease' that bears no relation to what happens in actual patients. AIDS should develop in days or weeks. There is no possible way it can take ten years. This emerges from Ho *et al.*'s own model. They seem blissfully unaware of the prediction that their own results give. They have not bothered to look at tedious questions like 'do our results correspond with what we have observed in our patients? . . . In fact, if we submit the possibility that the number of actively proliferating viruses increases as the diseases progresses, which is probable, then the death of T-4 cells should also accelerate as the disease progresses. Rigorous analysis would surely predict that it is simply impossible for a virus, which is actively increasing and available in large numbers to take years to cause a disease. Such a virus should quickly cause a disease or not at all. So we have to question the claim that HIV is available in large quantities, in all stages of the disease, is active and still takes ten to twelve years (or even more) to produce AIDS in an "HIV" positive. In 1993 Piatak *et al.* (Piatak 1993) claimed to have devised a technique, called the quantative polymer chain reaction (QC-PRC), to demonstrate very large amounts of HIV RNA in the plasma of "HIV" positive patients. The basis of this technique was quantifying the HIV amounts in a sample (wild-type HIV). A control sample, which differed from the wild-type only through a small internal variation, competed with PCR-amplified wild-type. The ratio of wild-type to control sample could be calculated according to the number of PCR-amplified cycles. Knowledge of the initially available control amounts allowed the estimation of the total amounts of wild-type in the original sample. The method is based on the assumption that the ratio of wild-type to control remains constant throughout the amplifying cycle. The justification for this was that the wild-type and control only differed in a small internal variation and the efficiency of the amplification should be the same for both and therefore the ratio would remain the same. For every sample in the PCR process, replication is essentially a matter of chance (Brock 1994). A DNA strand can either replicate or not. So we have a process governed by a binomial probability distribution. Remarkably, in Piatak *et al.'s* publication a statistical error analysis is missing. It is not my intention to carry one out here, but rather to show a method through which the problem of the mistake can be approached. This method shows that the QC-PCR technique is highly suspect and its readings should be treated with extreme caution" (Craddock 1996 b; 1996 a, 1997).

Practicing physicians and their "HIV patients" let themselves be impressed by pseudo-mathematical values (in log scale) of the laboratory numbers gained by the alleged PCR "viral load" measurement, which cannot rationally justify the guidance of treatment in individual chemotherapy

Numerous clinical and experimental studies before the introduction of aggressive HAART chemotherapy had demonstrated that the PCR method did not allow any conclusions to be drawn about the success of combined chemotherapeutic inhibition of "HI viruses." Nobody could produce a single piece of evidence that the RNA fragments in blood plasma, shown in the modified PCR reproduction processes (QC-PCR, bDNA) as DNA enrichment and presented in log scales, actually originated from "HIV-RNA." So far the HIV/AIDS researchers have not been able to conclusively answer the logical question of how by means of an RNA fragment they were able to determine the original (the complete "HIV" genome), without actually having to isolate the original "HIV" genome. Only by means of such a gold standard—the actual isolation of "HI viruses"—could it be proved that the special PCR method only enriched HIV RNA-DNA and not any other RNA sequence. Only with these gold standard methods can you guarantee that a positive "HIV-PCR" result was ever exclusively found in the presence of an actual "HIV infection," and that the "HIV-PCR tests" are highly specific for an "HIV infection."

But nobody has ever been able to demonstrate the gold standard of real isolation (Blattner 1989, overview Papadopulos-Eleopulos 1993 a, 1998 a, Philpot 1997) of an "HI virus" as independent yardstick for all indirect verification processes. The exclusive specificity of RNA-DNA enrichment on the basis of PCR as "HIV-RNA" has also never been proven. Positive "HIV-PCR" results have been demonstrated in "HIV positives" and "HIV negatives," healthy and unhealthy. The starting sequences, necessary for regulating the process of PCR-DNA enrichment (as proof of an "HIV-RNA") are also not specific for a certain RNA-DNA; they could exponentially reproduce completely different DNA fragments. There are many other laboratory inconsistencies in the HIV-PCR confirmation method, most of which have been detected and published by orthodox, mainstream HIV researchers (overview Johnson 1996, Hässig 1998 a).

Thus, the "early and hard" HAART treatment (Ho 1995 b) was defined by means of the unholy alliance of a non-specifically confirmed procedure for gathering evidence of a "viral load" combined with a pseudomathematical HIV theory. The destiny of the "HIV-infected" patients was subjected to medical practices that were not much better than reading tea leaves. If the log readings of the PCR measurements lay above the confirmation limit, then the

"HIV positive" patients were prescribed a "HAART combination therapy." If the control readings of the log values were lower, then an inhibition of the "HI viruses" was claimed and treatment indefinitely continued. If the log control readings were as high or higher, then a "resistance" to HAART combinations was postulated and the toxic pharmaceutical mixture was rearranged for the individual patient. In fact both these treatments were wrong. Even without HAART, varying log values were measured in the blood plasma of "HIV positives" and "HIV negatives" in samples of the same patients in different laboratories using the PCR technique. Likewise varying log values were measured in the same laboratories on samples of the same patients at different measurement times. Therefore, completely contradictory "HIV PCR" log values are to be expected, independent of HAART, which cannot justify a rational directive for chemotherapeutic treatment for HIV positives. Practicing physicians and affected patients, however, allowed themselves to be impressed with the pseudomathematical log scales on the laboratory print-outs. The practicing physicians trusted the laboratory staff who in turn trusted the groundwork researchers like Ho, Shaw, *et al* (Ho 1995 a, 1995 b, Wei 1995 b). In reality it was just a pseudoscientific chain of evidence:

"bDNA uses QC-PCR as a gold standard; QC-PCR uses regular PCR as a gold standard; regular PCR uses antibody tests as a gold standard, and antibody tests use each other .... Kary Mullis, inventor of PCR, won a 1993 Nobel Prize for his billion-dollar invention, which has become indispensable to any genetics lab. It is ironic that one of the first applications of PCR was to detect HIV, considering that Mullis himself doesn't believe his invention is capable of this. Mullis states: the problem is PCR is too efficient—it will amplify whatever DNA is in the sample, regardless of whether that DNA belongs to HIV or a contaminant. And how do you decide which part of the amplified material could be HIV and which part the contaminant(s), if you couldn't detect HIV in the sample without using PCR?" (Johnson 1996)

Apart from the methodical measurement of errors of the PCR technique, a reduction of RNA in the blood plasma is not due to inhibition of "HIV" by combination therapy, but on the contrary is from the increased DNA repair set in motion by such damaging therapy; furthermore, an increase of RNA in the blood plasma is not from "HIV resistance" but rather from the disturbed repair of the DNA defects resulting from combination therapy

However, another crucial fact relating to the interactions between:

- glutathione (GSH) as sensor for the redox milieu
- the number of T-helper immune cells (Th1 or Th2 immune cells) as effectors of the balance of the redox milieu
- and the amounts of RNA in the blood plasma as indicator for the repair of the DNA software
- as well as the HAART treatment as stressor of the counterregulation via the GSH sensor, the immune cell effectors and the RNA-DNA software

that could explain, consistently and without any exceptions, all the observed phenomena of an "HI virus" infection, was not considered by the HIV researchers.

"HIV positives," at an early stage, feature a systemic glutathione deficiency in immune and non-immune cells as well as in the mucous membranes. Glutathione (GSH) deficiency in the antigen-presenting cells clearly triggers a cytokine switch in T4 helper cells and causes Th2 immune cell dominance with a type 2 cytokine profile. However, the latter induces, among other things, the increased production of prostaglandin (PGE2) and transforming growth factors (TGF). These stimulate the increased ornithine production from arginine and in further steps the formation of polyamine. Polyamines stimulate repair procedures and the regeneration of DNA.

If we assume that "retroviral" substances (HAART), on the basis of their biochemical characteristics, cannot inhibit "HI viruses," but as prooxidative substances very certainly do aggravate the already existing GSH deficiency, HAART treatment can intensify the characteristic type 1 to type 2 cytokine switch. The repair procedures stimulated by a type 2 cytokine profile and DNA syntheses use RNA also from blood plasma as building blocks for synthesis. If we assume that the modified PCR technique (bDNA, QC PCR), regardless of all of its methodological failings, can measure the RNA level in blood plasma, then it follows that the decreased RNA readings in HAART treatment can be explained not as inhibition of "HI viruses" but as intracellular usage of RNA. As a result of HAART treatment the glutathione deficiency is aggravated, type 2 cytokine synthesis increased and the RNA usage in immune and non-immune cells is considerably raised.

This point of view is supported by experimental findings that the extra RNA can countermand an induced immune cell suppression (Kulkarni 1984, 1986, 1987, Van Buren 1990). "T-4 immune cells and macrophages seem to profit from nutritional supplement with RNA" (Van Buren 1990, Bower 1990).

RNA and DNA differ in one of the two pyrimidine bases, which together with two purine bases form the building blocks for RNA and DNA. RNA contains the pyrimidine base uracil and whilst DNA contains thymine. With the addition of a methyl group (CH3) the RNA building block uracil becomes the DNA building block thymine. Uracil appears to be the decisive building block to prevent the inhibition of the maturation of T4 helper cells and the inhibition of production of the T-cell growth factor interleukin-2 (assigned to a type 1 cytokine profile) (Kulkarni 1984). The methylation of uracil to thymine can be inhibited by the blockade of biologically active tetrahydrofolate (THF). This disruption mechanism is effected by long-term medication with folic acid inhibitors co-trimoxazole (Bactrim, Septra, Eusaprim etc.), pyrimethamine, dapsone, pentamidine etc. as standard long-term prophylaxis against the opportunistic fungal infection *Pneumocystis carinii* pneumonia (PCP), the most frequent AIDS-indicating disease.

The little-researched potentiating effects of combined HAART treatment plus long-term prophylaxis with co-trimoxazole rank as especially critical (Kremer 1999). A precise analysis of the findings of the Concorde study demonstrated that the immediate as well as the deferred AZT treatment led to adaptation of the clinical ARC/AIDS manifestations and death as the immunotoxic and other cytotoxic effects of both individual substances were combined in the immediately treated group AZT with co-trimoxazole etc. or the other way round in the deferred treated group co-trimoxazole with AZT (Concord Coordinating Committee 1994). Both substance groups provoke mitochondrial illness as the intensified type 2 cytokine switch due to the substance-induced glutathione deficiency triggers an increase in glycolytic biosynthesis activities via regenerative effects. These use RNA so that the RNA decrease in blood plasma assumed in the PCR controls by no means has to be attributed to the inhibition of "HI viruses." The remaining or increased RNA levels under HAART treatment must be construed not by resistance to "HI viruses" but can be explained much more plausibly by increased substance-induced disruptions to nucleic acid synthesis and secondary RNA/DNA defects that lead to the deficient transformation of RNA and effect a backlog in blood plasma. HAART treatment without cysteine compensation causes a rapid glutathione deficiency, which leads to defects in mitochondrial RNA/DNA (Lewis 1995, Herzenberg 1997, Peterson 1998). Prophylaxis with co-trimoxazole etc. also provokes considerable glutathione consumption (Cribb 1992) and DNA defects (Sörensen 1981) by the formation of hydroxylamine.

The increased serum levels of niacin seen during AIDS progression, due to a lack of glutathione, cannot be explained by HIV/AIDS research; this increase is also characteristic following cancer chemotherapy, proving that the fluctuating plasma RNA levels are due to the DNA-toxic effects of combination therapy

The concept that the relative decline in RNA concentrations in blood serum after HAART treatment is caused by increased RNA usage for the repair of DNA defects induced by HAART and not proof of an "HIV" provirus DNA blockade is supported by findings of increased niacin values in the serum of "HIV positives" and AIDS patients. These findings cannot be explained by HIV/AIDS medical science to this day:

"Niacin levels were higher among HIV-infected subjects, both on average and in proportion with above-normal levels. Furthermore, higher niacin levels were highly correlated with lower CD4+ counts. The significance of this inverse relationship is not clear" (Skurnick 1996).

The vitamin niacin, however, is characteristically released in increasing amounts after treatment of cancer patients with DNA-toxic chemotherapeutics.

Niacin is a component of the co-enzyme NAD that is enzymatically split for DNA repair (overview Mazurek 1997). In HIV positives and AIDS patients the increased niacin level is associated with the progression of clinical symptoms and the decline in RNA values in serum (Murray 1999). These findings clearly contradict the HIV/AIDS disease theory and support the fact of a Type-II cell dyssymbiosis resulting from toxic and pharmacotoxic prooxidative glutathione deficiency with a primary inhibition of the mitochondrial respiratory chain leading to DNA defects.

The relative increase of T4 cells in blood serum after combination therapy is also deceiving the physician and the patient, because Th1 and Th2 cells are not differentiated in routine laboratory tests; due to maturation-inhibition of the B-cells as interaction partners, the Th2 cells migrate back into the bloodstream, yet the crucial Th1/Th2 immune balance has not actually improved

On the other hand "HIV positives" feature, at a very early stage, a systemic glutathione deficiency as well as a type 2 cytokine dominance. This is why the observed intermittent and relative increase in T4 helper cells in blood serum during HAART therapy cannot be assessed as an improvement of the cellular defense resulting from the inhibition of "HI viruses." In fact the well-founded assumption persists that it is a question of an increase resulting from glutathione deficiency in the antigen-presenting cells of the type 2 cytokine-driven Th2 cells (Peterson 1998), which produce no cytotoxic NO gas and therefore cannot improve the intracellular pathogen defense. In clinical routine laboratory practice, however, Th1 cells, which feature a type 1 cytokine profile and form cytotoxic NO gas for defense, are not differentiated from Th2 cells. Specification of a relatively increased gain in T-4 immune cells during HAART treatment carries no diagnostic or prognostic weight without this differentiation, but is still used to claim the apparent effectiveness of aggressive chemotherapy against "HI viruses." No studies have been published analysing the ratio of Th1 cells to Th2 cells during HAART treatment. This lack of written evidence of the relative increase in T4 cells on the print-outs of the laboratory results after HAART treatment deceives physicians and patients about the fact that the crucial improvement in the balance of the Th1/Th2 immune cells has not been reached.

In order to prevent death by poisoning from combination therapy, patients and their physicians must learn to understand why and how mitochondrial diseases develop and how they can be treated by non-toxic compensation therapy

The "HIV positive" stigmatized patients or the parents of "HIV positive" stigmatized babies or children have only two alternatives. The first alternative is to blindly trust that the attending physician has rationally and thoroughly checked why the HAART treatment was prescribed "early and hard." This trust of "HIV positive" patients is repaid with the clinical consequences of diseases like "inherited mitochondrial diseases" (Brinkman 1998, 1999). The attending physician, however, will explain that all consequential symptoms of the "cocktail-, combination-, chemo-therapies" are regrettable progressions of the lethal "HIV infection."

The second alternative is to say no to blind faith and resist "early and hard" the HIV/AIDS physicians and their practises despite the fear of death scenario and massive psychological pressure. In order to realize this chance of survival, the therapists and those affected have to have understood how mitochondrial diseases originally develop and how they can be non-toxically treated.

The elegant refutation by orthodox HIV/AIDS researchers of the "kitchen sink model," the basis for aggressive mitochondriotoxic combination therapy, furnishes proof that the entire construction of the official disease theory "HIV causes AIDS" is objectively false

The research findings of the leading immunologists and HIV researchers support the rejection of HAART combination and "cocktail therapy." The abruptly transformed theoretical concept (Ho 1995 a, Wei 1995 b) created because of the numerous contradictions in the previously asserted disease theory "HIV causes AIDS" was shaken by an elegant research procedure. The Ho/Shaw concept postulated the daily billion-fold infection of T-4 immune cells by "HI viruses," the daily, billion-fold destruction of "HIV-infected" T-4 immune cells by non-infected immune cells (the open drain of the "kitchen sink model") and the daily, billion-fold new maturation of T-4 immune cells (the running tap of the "kitchen sink model").

In the course of time according to the Ho/Shaw theory the new maturation and proliferation of T-4 immune cells becomes exhausted and the elimination of the "HIV-infected" T-4 immune cells can no longer be sufficiently performed. The number of T-4 immune cells drops towards zero and a state of acquired immune weakness with clinical manifestations (AIDS) is reached. The proliferation of "HI viruses" is stopped by "early and hard" HAART treatment and the T-4 immune cells are saved from destruction. The success of HAART treatment could be measured by the PCR technique on the basis of the diminished "HIV RNA" levels in the blood plasma. Failure of the "HIV RNA" levels in the blood to sink during HAART treatment is a sign that the "HI viruses" are "resistant."

Which subgroup of T-4 immune cells, the Th1 cells (type 1 cytokine profile) or the Th2 cells (type 2 cytokine profile), that are supposed to be infected, destroyed or matured in their billions every day is curiously not investigated by the HIV laboratory researchers. Many HIV research groups have checked the validity of the central assertion of the Ho/Shaw theory, namely the rapid daily turnover of cells of T-4 immune cells resulting from the daily mass destruction of the "HIV-infected" T-4 immune cells and their daily mass maturation. To this purpose they examined the wear on telomeres (from the Greek: *telos* = end + *meros* = part), the tail of chromosomes (from the Greek: *chroma* = color + *soma* = body). Chromosomes are the visible bearers of genetic information. The genes are arranged linearly on the chromosome. These packages of genes are present in a doubled format. However, before cell division chromosomes have to be reproduced so that the daughter cells each contain a doubled set of chromosomes. This replication process is rendered by a special enzyme which separates the coiled double spiral of the DNA chain. A different enzyme then replicates the individual strands of the DNA chain. Thereby there are always two particular bases of the four DNA bases opposite each other—the base pairs (bp). This enzyme needs a starting point without any genetic information. With every division (altogether there are about 50 possible division cycles) a piece of the starting point of the telomeres goes missing. The telomeres are assembled by the enzyme, telomerase. This enzyme regulates the transcription of an RNA template in a DNA sequence (reverse transcriptase) (Temin 1970, 1972,

1974, 1985, Baltimore 1985, Greider 1996, Boeke 1996, Teng 1996, 1997, Hässig 1998 a). Telomerase is, therefore, a reverse transcriptase, the enzyme whose postulated availability in T-4 immune cells from the blood serum of homosexual patients, Montagnier, Gallo and their colleagues misinterpreted as exclusive evidence for the existence of "HI viruses" (Barré-Sinoussi 1983, Popovic 1984, Papadopulos-Eleopulos 1993 a).

Researchers at the Netherlands Red Cross Blood Transfusion Service and the Academic Medical Center of Amsterdam University have measured the wear on the telomeres of chromosomes in T-4 immune cells of "HIV positive" patients:

"If T-4 immune cells have a rapid turnover and thus a high proliferation rate during an HIV infection this must be reflected in an accelerated loss in the length of the telomeric terminal restriction fragments (TRF). Telomeres are the extreme ends of chromosomes that consist of TTAGGG repeats [linear sequences of the pyrimidine base, thymine (T) and the purine bases, adenine (A) and guanosine (G)], ~10.000 bases long in humans. Some findings have led to the belief that telomeric length can be used as a marker of the replicative history of cells and can indicate the accelerated deterioration or increased cell division rates. Firstly, body cell telomers shorten with increasing age (roughly 30 to 50 base pairs (bp) per year) and after *in vitro* cultivation. Secondly, telomeric length in *in vitro* lymph cells and fibroblasts dictates the division capacity. Thirdly, just like tumor cells and germ cells, the telomeric length in cultivated cells that continuously divide and are immortal is maintained by the enzyme telomerase. These cells display an elevated telomerase activity, while body cells show limited or no telomerase activity .... Longitudinal analysis of samples of lymph cells showed no accelerated loss of TRF length during the [alleged] HIV infection phase before the clinical diagnosis of AIDS. Other research teams have also observed no loss in TRF length of T-4 immune cells of HIV-infected individuals .... Consequently, telomeric length is not impaired by HIV infection .... There is no evidence of increased turnover in T-4 immune cells and thus the reduction in numbers of T-4 immune cells [in the bloodstream] cannot be accounted for by depletion of regeneration as a consequence of continued HIV-induced cell destruction .... New research data indicates another cause for the reduction of T-4 immune cells in HIV infections. The depletion in regeneration driven by a rapid turnover in T-4 immune cells no longer seems a plausible cause for the loss of T-4 immune cells" (Wolthers 1998, Rosenberg 1998). In other words: there is no billion-fold destruction of T-4 immune cells every day by "HI viruses." The whole construction of the official disease theory that "HIV causes AIDS" is objectively false. This fact means "early and hard" chemotherapeutic HAART treatment is also counterproductive and harmful and that the supposed inhibition of HIV RNA, measured by the PCR technique, is a fundamental misinterpretation.

The Dutch research team also made no mention of whether the T-4 immune cells that they examined were Th1 or Th2 immune cells. However, it can be logically assumed that it was Th2 immune cells that were analyzed as "HIV positives" from the earliest point in time of an "HIV infection" that have a Th2 immune cell dominance (overview Lucey 1996). This fact explains why AIDS patients have been wrongly treated for 20 years and "HIV positives" for 17 years. This blatant failure of modern medical science shows the extent of rethinking necessary to learn to understand the most elementary laws of cellular biology as the basis of rationally founded prevention and therapy.

The mainstream HIV/AIDS physicians, however, refused to learn to understand the most elementary principals of cellular biology, as the foundation of rationally justified methods of prevention and therapy; ironically they concluded that the patients who deceased (due to primary and secondary mitochondrial inactivation) did not die from too many toxic drugs but rather from an insufficient prescription of toxic drugs

The aggressive treatment motto of the virus hunters, "hit HIV, early and hard" (Ho 1995 b) had yet another fateful delayed-action effect on RNA/DNA transcription. The therapy with the prooxidative cytotoxins of the HAART cocktail on asymptomatic "HIV positives"—patients with a still compensated constraint of detoxifying capacity—initially has an activating effect on the RNA/DNA turnover of DNA repair in order to balance out disruptions to the redox milieu by slowing down the proton and electron transfer in mitochondria.

But, after enrichment of the pharmacotoxins in prolonged medication, just like DNA-toxic chemotherapeutics in the treatment of cancer, disturbances in the interplay within the natural base pools arise. The results are changes in the coding profiles of DNA in mitochondrial DNA and in the nuclear genomes that lead to a diversity of disturbances to the biosyntheses of proteins and enzyme proteins (Strahl 1996, Yegorov 1996, Hässig 1998 a). When in this phase, due to the diminishing T-helper immune cells, which are simply measured across-the-board as "T4 cells" in the bloodstream, and because of the early symptoms, folic acid-inhibitors are additionally deployed for PCP prophylaxis (Bactrim, Pentamidine, Pyrimethamine etc.), then the effects in the redox milieu multiply due to the accelerated thiol deficiency.

The inhibition of the biologically active form of folic acid disrupts the transformation of the RNA base, uracil to the DNA base, thymine. DNA repair is impaired, the conversion of RNA sequences are reduced. The HIV/AIDS physicians misinterpreted these processes as an increase in the "RNA HI viral load" and increasing "HIV resistance." In fact the folic acid inhibitors implement additional DNA defects and the RNA/DNA transcription (reverse transcription) is blocked (Sörensen 1981, Lambie 1985, Lacey 1985, Steen 1985, Committee on the Safety of Medicines 1985, 1995, Zimmermann 1987, Jick 1995, Gysling 1995, Kremer 1996 a, 1996 b).

The authors of the first clinical AZT study were very aware of the incalculable interaction between AZT etc. and Bactrim etc., but in the "planned experiments on human beings" (Thomas 1984) they were tacitly accepted:

"The safety of such drugs and their interactions with AZT are largely unknown .... The study documented the potential for serious hematologic toxicity, but only further experience will permit assessment of the long-term toxicity of AZT. In addition, only well-controlled studies will provide data to assess the relative benefits and risks associated with AZT in other patient populations .... AZT should be administered with caution because of its toxicity and the limited experience with it to date" (Richman 1987).

After numerous "well-controlled studies" had proven the massive mitochondriotoxic effects of AZT (overview Rosenthal 1994, Lewis 1995) and the clearly mitochondriotoxic exponential effects of interaction between AZT and co-trimoxazole (overview Concorde Coordinating Committee 1994), the ignorant HIV/AIDS physicians still could not draw the irrefutable conclusion that mitochondriotoxic pharmaceutical substances for already mitochondria-damaged, glutathione-depleted patients could not be the preventative and therapeutic resource of choice. Rather they rejected all experimental and clinical data clearly showing that "HIV infections" and AIDS-indicating diseases were without doubt the results of primary and secondary mitochondrial damage (Kremer 1996 a). Instead, on the basis of the objectively false disease theory (Wolthers 1996, 1998), it was postulated that the "HI viruses" had to be attacked even earlier and even harder with a combination of pharmaceutical substances that had been shown to be mitochondriotoxic, while at the same time attacking the cell membrane of "HI viruses" with protease-inhibitors (Carpenter 1996, 1997, British HIV Association 1997, Harry J. Kaiser Family Foundation 1997, CDC 1998, Cox 1998, Cooper 1999).

"Extended follow-up of patients in one trial, the Concorde study, has shown a significantly increased risk of death among the patients treated early. The trials mainly involve monotherapy with AZT. The suggestion is that the situation is different for combination therapy" (Philips 1997).

In other words, from clear-cut results of numerous clinical research data the HIV/AIDS physicians drew the conclusion that "HIV positives" and AIDS patients with primary and secondary toxic-conditioned constraints on the detoxifying capacities of cell symbioses (Type-II counterregulation of cell symbiosis) did not die from being prescribed too many toxic drugs but from being prescribed too few!

Background to the empty promise of salvation: to be able to exterminate "HIV" in three to four years via combination therapy

In 1996 HIV/AIDS physicians seriously discussed the possibility of an "HIV cure" with the introduction of highly active anti-retroviral therapy (HAART), based on trial and error, with a combination of:

- 1-2 so-called nucleoside analog reverse transcriptase inhibitors (AZT = zidovudine, didanosine, lamivudine, stavudine, zalcitabine, adefovir, abacavir) (NRTI)
- 1 so-called non-nucleoside analog reverse transcriptase inhibitor (delavirdine, nevirapine, efavirenz) (non-NRTI)
- 1-2 so-called HIV protease inhibitor (indinavir, nelfinavir, ritonavir, saquinavir, amprenavir) (PI).

It was propagated that via prolonged medication with HAART it would be possible to completely wipe out "HI viruses" within three to four years (Perelson 1997, Saag 1999). The claim of an "HIV cure" was highly speculative even in the opinion of most orthodox HIV laboratory researchers, as such a statement could only actually be judged on the basis of clinical progress studies after three to four years. The leading lights of HIV/AIDS research sold, against their better knowledge, apparently trusted scientific perceptions about analyses that nobody in fact had carried out, for instance the effects of the new class of substances of synthetic protease-inhibitors (PI) on the natural proteases in human cells, the exponential effects of PIs on the pharmacotoxins of the "cocktail therapy," the intrusion of PIs in mitochondrial activities, the possible carcinogenic characteristics of PIs etc. The mass media celebrated the apparent break-through in HIV/AIDS therapy with buzzwords like the

"Lazarus effect" and the "resurrection of the doomed" (Ostrom 1996, Philpott 1996, Rasnick 1996, Lauritsen 1997, Christie 1997).

Many HIV positives had become critical of the highly toxic "cocktail therapy." A considerable number of "HIV positive" and AIDS patients, on the basis of their experiences with their own bodies or because of the horrific deaths of their fellow sufferers both young and old, whose causes of death were "similar to the symptoms of the HIV disease associated with AZT," refused administration of "cocktail therapy" or simply stopped taking the prescribed "anti-retroviral" drugs, naturally without the knowledge of their physicians. Many patients were increasingly put under pressure to participate, for their own good and for the protection of their fellow men, in new clinical studies on prolonged medication with combined HAART chemotherapy. The official promises of a cure, which would within three to four years completely eliminate the lethal "HI viruses" via combined chemotherapy with AZT etc. plus protease inhibitors, was free of risk for the HIV/AIDS establishment. Three of the world's largest pharmaceutical concerns, Abbott, Merck and Hoffmann-LaRoche, rapidly pushed through the approval of the new synthetic protease inhibitors as "anti-HIV" medication, before the first findings of the clinical studies, sponsored by the National Institute for Allergy and Infectious Diseases in the USA (NIAID), under the directorship of Dr. Fauci, had been published. The drug companies hoped, according to "*The Economist*" from 12th of October 1996, to be able "to siphon off a billion dollars" with the new chemotherapeutics (Christie 1997). The financial newspaper "*The Wallstreet Journal*" warned shareholders on the 10th of October 1996:

"The new AIDS medications have gained the approval of the Food and Drug Administration so quickly that the researchers still have no clear perception [about the working mechanisms of the drugs] . . . Protease patients are, in fact, the guinea pigs in one of the largest and most expensive medical experiments of our time" (Christie 1997). The findings of the official NIAID study were delivered via a press release after only a 9-12 month period of treatment in February 1997. The impression was given that it provided "evidence that combination treatments that include protease inhibitors can reduce the risk of death" (Knox 1997).

1,156 patients diagnosed with AIDS were treated either with AZT plus one of two further nucleoside analog substances, or with AZT plus one of two further non-nucleoside analog substances plus a protease inhibitor. The supposed inhibition of the "HIV RNA" was measured by means of the PCR technique, although the US Centers for Disease Control (CDC) had disclosed that: "PCR is not recommended or approved for the purpose of routine diagnosis . . . neither the specificity [the PCR readings of the "HIV RNA" have to also be negative in "HIV test" negatives blood samples] nor the sensitivity [the PCR readings must measure the "HIV RNA" in blood samples of "HIV positives"] is known" (CDC 1993, Johnson 1996). In the official medical publication it was stated that it was not possible to say that difference in the deaths in both treatment groups was statistically significant (Knox 1997, Christie 1997). The FDA adopted a similar dual strategy of official press releases and differentiated statements in medical publications concerning the manipulated rapid approval of AZT ten years previously (Richman 1987, Lauritsen 1990, 1993).

The subsequent appearance of massive mitochondrial damage and metabolic disturbances due to intensified "planned human poison-experiments" is answered by the HIV/AIDS profession with the absurd new promise: the elimination of "HIV characteristics in latently infected cells" would take 10 to 60 (!) years of continuous chemotherapeutic poisoning

The feigned promises of HIV/AIDS physicians of a cure in three to four years (the average time of survival of patients with critical thiol deficiencies when treated with glutathione-reducing chemotherapy instead of supplementing the life-threatening shortages of cysteine and glutathione) via chemotherapeutic long-term medication with a highly toxic combination therapy with AZT, one to two further nucleoside analogs and protease inhibitors that could release "HIV positives" from their "viral load," were revised very soon. The projected time span of three to four years bore a striking resemblance to survival time of cancer patients after combined chemotherapy (Abel 1990). Also in oncology the expectations of success, in regard to the dozens of chemotherapy schemata, had a short shelf life.

The mock claims of the HIV/AIDS profession to be able to completely eliminate the "HI viruses" through aggressive HAART treatment, very quickly turned out to be illusionary. From 1997 many research groups demonstrated that the "anti-retroviral" chemical cocktails measured by PCR techniques, produced varyingly fluctuating "HIV RNA" values in long-term treated patients. These findings led to a revised claim that a long-term HAART treatment of between 10 and 60 years would be necessary to eliminate "HI viruses." The findings, which did not fit in with the theory, were explained by "HIV" activity in latently infected cells (overview Saag 1999). Other clinical research teams treated "HIV positives" with the type 1 cytokine, interleukin-2 (IL-2) with the idea of flushing "HI viruses" out of latently infected cells, while at the same time eliminating them with a potent anti-retroviral chemotherapy (overview Cooper 1999). This approach demonstrated most clearly the clumsy template of the perceptions of the world of the HIV/AIDS professionals. IL-2 is strong growth factor for T-4 immune cells and stimulates the synthesis of cytotoxic NO via the activation of interferon-γ, as well as the production of reactive oxygen species (ROS) via the formation of tumor necrosis factors. Increased amounts of these prooxidative cocktails from IL-2 + NO + AZT etc. + Bactrim were supposed to prompt the already activated ephemeral effector T-4 cells and long-living dormant and memory T-4 cells to increased division.

According to the HIV theory, in addition to the thus enforced effector and the previously dormant T-4 cells that are supposed to be infected with HI viruses, the proliferation of hypothetical HI viruses, which are anyway supposed to be dividing by the billions daily, also increases. These are now supposed to be blocked at decisive stages in their proliferation cycle by HAART substances. In fact, the active and latent "HIV-infected" T-4 cells are glutathione-depleted cells, the vast majority of which have switched to a type 2 cytokine profile (Th2 cells) (overview Lucey 1996, Dröge 1997 a, Herzenberg 1997, Peterson 1998). As interleukin-2 (a type 1 cytokine) and interleukin-4 (a type 2 cytokine) mutually suppress each other, some of the T-4 immune cells will quickly overreact via prooxidative overstimulation due to an antioxidative deficit and die through apoptosis/necrosis while others will underreact through counterregulations (Th2 cells). As, according to the HIV theory, the "HI viruses" cannot be eliminated quickly, but with prolonged therapy with HAART requiring three to four years (Ho 1995 a) or as the case may be 10 to 60 years (Saag 1999), prooxidative HAART treatment plus interleukin-2 will further aggravate the glutathione deficiency in surviving Th2 cells that are already GSH-depleted through counterregulations. This means that, in a short time the Th2 immune cells, which are unable to produce cytotoxic NO gas against intracellular fungi, parasites, mycobacteria, cytomegalo viruses etc. (overview Lucey 1997), will be highly selected by HAART, independently of whether the "HI viruses" exist or not. In other words the proliferation of the "HI viruses," according to the HIV theory, would indeed be prevented by HAART and interleukin-2 treatment, but the organism would be made incapable of defense against opportunistic agents (AIDS).

Addition of protease-inhibitors to the HAART cocktail only aggravates the problem. As HAART + protease-inhibitors have been shown to cause mitochondrial damage and metabolic disruption (overview Brinkman 1999), the claim that protease-inhibitors exclusively target the protein-splitting proteases of "HI viruses," even if they were to exist, is objectively false. It is quite obvious that the synthetic protease-inhibitors are not specific for the never isolated "HIV" protease enzyme that was genetically reconstructed along the lines of a theoretical requirement. These enzymes were strikingly similar to a human digestive enzyme of the sour aspartate proteases (Hässig 1998 a). Natural proteases crucially participate in the biochemical cascade of reactions triggered by mitochondria on programmed cell death (Kroemer 1997, Zamzami 1997). The aggressive and prolonged treatment of "HIV positives" with interleukin-2 and/or HAART and/or PCP long-term prophylaxis plus protease-inhibitors can, thus, slow down programmed cell death initiated by the prooxidative targeted attack on the glutathione-depleted, type 2 cytokine-programmed T-4 cells, and force the selection of counterregulated T-4 immune cells, as the cells can only survive via a Type-II counterregulation of cell dyssymbiosis.

The demand of RNA of counterregulated cells fluctuates in the various stages of long-term intoxication of "HIV positives" and the available quantities of RNA sequences in the blood plasma of every human being increase and decrease. If the theoretical amounts of unspecific RNA, measured by the PCR technique, decrease under prolonged HAART treatment, then the HIV/AIDS physicians gauge this as a sign of medication-based inhibition of "HI viruses" and if the amounts of RNA increase it is taken as a sign of "HIV resistance." Even if the "HI viruses" were to exist, the quantitative PCR technique would not be diagnostically or prognostically suitable for proving "HIV RNA" (viral load) due to the high susceptibility to error and lack of specificity (CDC 1993, Hagen-Mann 1994, overview Johnson 1996, Hässig 1998 a).

That "[a] cluster of false-positive results by RT-PCR" is "a well-recognized phenomenon" is even admitted by orthodox HIV physicians (Weber 1997).

The results of numerous clinical studies performed in Western countries substantiate that on the basis of the objectively culpable non-treatment of the primary cause of their disease, the "HIV positive" patients paid with their lives for the absolutely pointless aggressive chemotherapy

The findings of the Concorde study, the Stanford study and many further clinical studies in all Western countries substantiate the claims represented here, that as a result of an objectively false disease theory, an objectively misleading HIV test and the objectively culpable non-treatment of the primary cause of the disease that "HIV positive" patients have paid for the absolutely pointless aggressive chemotherapeutic treatment with their lives. The patients in the Concorde study who were treated "early and hard" with AZT and simultaneously sooner or later with Bactrim etc. had a higher mortality rate than the patients with deferred treatment with AZT and simultaneously sooner or later with Bactrim etc. (Concorde Coordinating Committee 1994, Philips 1997). There was no significant inhibition of "HI viruses" in either of the patient groups. In both patient groups the objectively necessary compensation therapy of the primary thiol-deficiency syndrome was neglected. In the Stanford study the mortality rate in the patient group treated with AZT etc. without compensation therapy was "dramatically" higher, in the patient group treated with AZT etc. and simultaneous compensation therapy "dramatically" lower, despite a lower T-4 cell count of under 200 per µL. In both patient groups a critically low intracellular glutathione level (GSH value) was a reliable predictive factor for AIDS diseases and mortality (Herzenberg 1997). In the Stanford study it was explicitly stated that the "excessive production of inflammatory cytokines and excessive use of GSH depleting drugs may contribute to systemic GSH deficiency in HIV disease" (Herzenberg 1997). However, they failed to draw the obvious conclusion, that the "HIV characteristics" observed by Gallo, Montagnier and others in *in vitro* cell cultures of glutathione-depleted T-4 cells likewise have to be traced back to the glutathione depletion in these clearly Th2 cells. To date it has not been rationally explained, why in the T-4 cells of "HIV positive" and AIDS patients in a primary systemic glutathione depletion (Buhl 1989), the cellular biological laws of counterregulation should to be overridden after provocation by prooxidative stress.

At the World AIDS Congress of 2000 in South Africa, the US chemotherapists involuntarily declare their clinical bankruptcy

At the World AIDS Congress of 2000 in South Africa, the US surveillance authority for disease control and prevention, the CDC, reported about the clinical results of standard chemotherapeutic treatment of a large collection of "HIV positive" patients (CDC 2000). The data from 1,600 "HIV-infected" people were assessed. All patients were treated with the standard HAART chemotherapy (AZT and a second NRTI plus a protease inhibitor). The aim of the treatment was the total extermination of "HI viruses" in three to four years. As control for the success of the therapy the "HIV RNA" values in the blood plasma were measured by the unspecific PCR method. Even after a year of chemotherapeutic treatment this aim proved to be illusory, 64% of patients chemotherapeutically treated showed no signs of the desired decrease in PCR values as apparent indicator of the activity of reverse transcription (RNA-DNA transcription). There was a clear correlation between the total doses of prescribed chemotherapeutics before and during the clinical study.

- If HAART was the first chemotherapeutic plan of action, then during the twelve-month treatment period the PCR values sank below 10% of their initial readings in 49% of the patients, if HAART was the second option the respective PCR values dropped in 30% of patients.
- If HAART was the third or fourth chemotherapeutic option then the PCR values dropped only in 15% of the cases (CDC 2000).

As there is neither theoretical nor experimental evidence that the chemotherapeutic substances of the HAART combination could be integrated into an "HIV" provirus DNA chain or that the protease inhibitors are able to disrupt the design at the formation of "HIV" protein shells, as claimed by the HIV/AIDS researchers (overview Papadopulos-Eleopulos 1999), the CDC study demonstrates the counter-evidence of progressive mitochondrial inactivation through the prooxidative substances of HAART treatment. If we leave the susceptibility to error of the modified PCR measuring method out of the equation, the CDC data can only be interpreted as being the increasing impact of the HAART substances progressively deactivating mitochondrial vitality via inhibition of the mitochondrial respiratory chain going on to cause RNA and DNA defects. The primary glutathione-deficiency is in turn increased and a type 2 cytokine switch forced. NO production as required fuel for cellular respiration and intracellular defense is inhibited. The reverse transcription as expression of the natural response of repair processes and DNA regeneration under prooxidative cell stress (and not as expression of the activity of "HI viruses") is progressively blocked, RNA turnover, especially the turnover of the RNA-specific pyrimidine base uracil, is reduced and the RNA values rise in blood plasma as measured by the PCR method. The HAART treatment of the HIV/AIDS physicians fights the natural healing processes of immune and non-immune cells that have been imbalanced by the glutathione deficits with aggressive chemotherapy, while the necessary compensation therapy is neglected. On the basis of the progression of the data from the one-year study of the CDC it is easy to work out how high the percentage of victims of the dangerous HAART treatment would be on continuation of chemotherapy. Instead of the "complete HIV cure in three to four years" promised to affected patients and the world press in 1996, the CDC study confirms the conclusions from HIV/AIDS researchers from Alabama University in the USA published at the beginning of the study:

> "An apparent nail was driven in the 'cure' coffin in the past month with the publication of two articles by independent research groups at John Hopkins University and the Aaron Diamond AIDS Research Center " . . ." (Saag 1999)

The traditional HIV research had submitted data that had already in June 1999 provoked the following statement:

> "Two clinical studies show the failure of conventional anti-retroviral therapy in achieving complete HIV eradication; 10-60 years are deemed necessary to eliminate HIV" (Saag 1999).

For thousands of "HIV" specialists, it is forbidden to think that the glutathione level can be systemically balanced with a daily dose of three to eight grams of the natural amino acid cysteine, for six to eight months, and the AIDS mortality rates would become "dramatically lower"

Affected patients and the world press did not learn about these findings at the World AIDS Congress in South Africa. It would no longer have been possible to sell AZT etc. to the developing countries. In fact the CDC's one-year study reveals that hardly any AIDS patients would survive three to four years of prolonged HAART treatment as the toxic effects of the useless mitochondriotoxic, glutathione-reducing HAART substances would accumulate (Herzenberg 1997, Brinkman 1998,1999).

Every physician since Paracelsus knows that it is the dose that makes the poison. As by systemic glutathione-deficiency even relatively small doses of a nitrosative substance like acetaminophen overextends the detoxifying capacities of mitochondria (Herzenberg 1997), the logic of HIV/AIDS physicians seeking to "cure" patients who have been shown to suffer from a systemic glutathione-deficiency with ever-increasing combinations of nitrosative substances like AZT and other HAART drugs is rationally incomprehensible. The commentator of the CDC study at the World AIDS Congress ignored, however, the causal links between the bioenergetic characteristics of HAART substances and the concurrently prescribed folic acid inhibitors etc. and the diminishing detoxification capacities of cellular symbiosis confronted with the accumulated dosage. The conclusions of the CDC researchers after 20 years of AIDS research, unchallenged by 12,000 conference participants, betrays the simplicity of the medical mind:

"Reasons for a non-optimal assessment of HAART are incompatibility, non-compliance [patients not following the physician's prescription], and lack of effectivity due to resistance" (CDC 2000)

But the reasons for the "resistance" do not lie in the nature of the phantom-like "HI viruses," but in the collective resistance of HIV/AIDS physicians against new research insights. The American Nobel Prize winner for chemistry Mullis, who has continuously hinted at the dubiousness of measuring "HIV RNA" in blood plasma using his discovery of the PCR method (Null 1997), encapsulated the collective mentality of the HIV/AIDS researcher:

"Where is the research that proves HIV is the cause of AIDS? We now know everything in the world about HIV. There are now 10,000 researchers in the world specialized on HIV. Nobody has shown any interest in the possibility that HIV doesn't cause AIDS as their special knowledge is of no use if HIV isn't the cause" (Mullis 1993).

For all these "HIV" specialists it is a forbidden thought even to imagine that the systemic glutathione-deficiency of "HIV positives," like a serious vitamin deficiency, could be balanced by "3 to 8 grams of the natural amino acid cysteine for six to eight months and that the AIDS and mortality rates could become "dramatically lower" (Herzenberg 1997). Even the Stanford researchers do not dare to utter this conclusion. They cautiously state:

"The preliminary evidence of improved survival associated with oral NAC administration that we report here is consistent both with GSH deficiency being an important determinant of survival in AIDS and with GSH restoration potentially being beneficial" (Herzenberg 1997).

One year after the report of clinical success in the "dramatic" drop in disease and mortality rates in glutathione-depleted HIV positives through cysteine compensation therapy, the researchers from the Stanford team together with researchers from the Northwestern University in Chicago demonstrated the cause of the disappearance of Th1 immune cells and the lack of production of cytotoxic NO defense gas:

"By using three different methods to deplete glutathione from T cell receptor transgenic and conventional mice and studying *in vivo* and/or *in vitro* responses to three distinct antigens, we show that glutathione levels [GSH] in antigen-presenting cells determine whether Th1 [type 1 cytokine] or Th2 [type 2 cytokine] response patterns predominate. These findings present new insights into immune response alterations in HIV and other diseases" (Peterson 1998).

The hysteria surrounding the AIDS problem (like the demonizing of the cancer problem) reflected a foreboding development in modern medicine; the sales volume of expensive chemotherapeutic agents determines the flow of research funds to laboratories, hospital clinics and specialist practices

In other words, the toxic, pharmacotoxic, infectious, alloantigen or nutritive-caused systemic glutathione-deficiency (GSH) of "HIV positives" provokes the redox-dependent reprogramming of T-4 immune cells to a type 2 cytokine profile, the characteristic of the "HIV infection" at the early stage (overview Lucey 1996). As type 2 cytokines suppress the production of cytotoxic NO gas, the T-4 immune cells can no longer sufficiently eliminate intracellular agents (overview Mosmann 1996). As a result the patients are susceptible to opportunistic infections (AIDS).

The hysteria surrounding the AIDS problem (like the demonizing of the cancer problem) reflected a foreboding development in modern medicine. There exists an immense circulation of capital between physicians, the media, politics, the pharmaceutical industry as well as the affected patients and the general public that in the end can only remain in motion and be financed by the public at large as long as the stage-managing of the sham lethal sex and blood plague is maintained. The sales volume of expensive toxic chemotherapeutics affects the evaluation of shares of the drug companies and thus the flow of research funds to the laboratories, hospital clinics and specialist practices of all the HIV specialists (Rappoport 1988, Adams 1989, Lauritsen 1990, 1993, Miller 1992, Berridge 1993, Willner 1994, Epstein 1996, Duesberg 1996, Hodgkinson 1996, Lang 1998, Shenton 1998).

The HIV researchers continually discover new quirky characteristics of the "insidious HIV agent" (Cooper 1999) while at the same time continually announcing new promises of an "HIV cure" (Saag 1999) with ever-increasing pharmacotoxins in chemotherapeutic cocktails not only because their specialist knowledge would be useless without them, but because of the logic of the laws of the market, funding would be axed and "*virus hunting*" (Gallo 1991) be finished if the objective research data were known to the world at large.

The chief instigators of the excessive chemotherapeutic poisoning are likely to be aware of the fact that "HIV characteristics" are nothing more than decay products of the type 2 cytokine shift of T4-helper immune cells in response to glutathione depletion

Dr. Fauci, director of the National Institute for Allergy and Infectious Diseases, one of the chief instigators of chemotherapeutic research and practice in addition to the therapy guidelines and the appraisal and approval for the market of so-called highly active anti-retroviral chemotherapeutics (HAART), explained at the World AIDS Congress of July 2000 in South Africa, that an elimination of "HI viruses" by HAART chemotherapy could not be achieved (Fauci 2000). This admission, in contrast to the widely propagated promises, also from Fauci, of an "HIV cure" (Saag 1999) since 1996, can be seen as indirect confirmation that Fauci and his colleagues were very much aware of the nature of "HIV characteristics" as decay product of the type 2 cytokine shift of the effectors of T-4 immune cells as a result of glutathione depletion as sensor for the genetic software of the biosynthesis of cytokine protein. The immunologist Fauci and his colleagues had demonstrated since 1974 that certain T4 immune lymph cells, under the influence of hydrocortisone in the bloodstream, decrease and this subgroup of T cells accumulate in the bone marrow to support B-cells in the production of polyclonal antibodies (Fauci 1974, 1975, 1976 a, 1977, Haynes 1977). In acute states of stress, for example injuries and burns, the decay of T-4 immune cells in the bloodstream has been shown to be likewise dependent on the cortisol levels (Calvano 1986). After the appearance of the first AIDS cases in homosexual patients, whose immune status was characterized by a decline in numbers and also the capacity of T-4 lymph cells in the bloodstream to be prooxidatively stimulated (CDC 1981 a, Gottlieb 1981, Masur 1981), the findings from the 1970s suddenly no longer counted. In interplay between retrovirus researchers, immunologists and clinicians the lower T-4 cell values were causally traced back to the hypothetical retrovirus HIV, although the characteristically simultaneous increase in antibody production supported the validity of the findings of Fauci and colleagues from the 1970s. It is revealing that Fauci, who must have known better, remained silent about and deliberately chose not publish the fact that Gallo could especially effectively prove "HIV characteristics" (Sarngadharan 1987, Montagnier; Tahi 1997) on addition of hydrocortisone to the T-4 cell culture of AIDS patients (Kremer 1998 a, 1998 c). *With his test-tube trickery on T4 cells extracted from AIDS patients—first the forcing of reverse transcription by the addition of hydrocortisone, and second, overcoming the hydrocortisone-induced blockade of cytokine synthesis with the addition of interleukin-2, which accordingly activates interferon-γ (Luedke 1990)and in turn stimulates cytotoxic NO—Gallo produced two crucial "HIV characteristics": RT, and the apparent destruction of T4 cells by the "retroviral HIV" (Popovic 1984, Gallo 1984).*

"It is completely incomprehensible why Fauci, after transferring to AIDS research, no longer mentioned his own studies" (Hässig 1998 a).

The statement of the alleged lowering of mortality rates from "HIV infections" is based on tentative medical assertions that violate the logic of Epimenides, and cannot be accepted as enhanced survival due to combination therapy

Fauci demonstrated to his colleagues at the World AIDS Conference in July 2000 in South Africa the customary practices of how to convert the failure of "early and hard" chemotherapy into a therapeutic pseudo-success in front of representatives of the international media:

"We have managed to lower considerably the mortality rate of the HIV-infected with the anti-retroviral therapy to date. That is progress" (Fauci 2000). This statement is misleading: In a larger patient group of "HIV positives," gradually, different glutathione depletion could be measured (Herzenberg 1997). If these patients were chemotherapeutically treated without cysteine compensation therapy, the patients with the lowest glutathione values after crossing the critical threshold would first of all develop AIDS symptoms and a certain high percentage would die. The patients with relatively favorable initial glutathione values would be able to tolerate long-term HAART therapy considerably longer. Thus, from the starting point of HAART chemotherapy in 1996 until the year of the report in 2000, there would be a sink in the annual mortality rate with a time-delay. After a mortality peak of the most obviously seriously glutathione-depleted "HIV positive" patients after aggressive chemotherapy the duration of illness and death of the patients with relatively better glutathione values become extended over a period of time giving the impression that the long-term chemotherapeutic treatment has extended the life of the patient or, as the case may be, led to a decline in the annual mortality rate. This self-deception and deception of others is based on the false premise of "HIV infection." Even the Cretan philosopher, Epimenides had taught people at the marketplace in ancient Greece that proof should not be deduced from a false premise. His paradox was:

"All Cretans are liars, he is a Cretan and therefore, he must be a liar".

Just as anomalously, the paradox of HIV/AIDS medicine contravened the laws of logic:

"All HIV positives must die, the patient is HIV positive and therefore he will die." The premise cannot anticipate the reasoning. Proof of the premise is rather dependent on intervening conditions, in the case of the HIV positives the premise of the mortality rate (Fauci 2000) depends on causal factors of primary glutathione deficiency and the non-treatment of the glutathione deficiency or as the case may be on the aggravation of the glutathione deficiency through long-term chemotherapeutical treatment dependent on dose and duration as well as the patient's disposition. Nobody has proven that the premise "HIV positive" is an independent variable, as this appears simultaneously with the variable glutathione deficiency (Buhl 1989, Roederer 1991) and the variable type 2 cytokines (Clerici 1994, Lucey 1996), while it has been shown that the variable type 2 cytokines are dependent on variable glutathione deficiency and this varies with prooxidative stress (Peterson 1998).

The first proposition of proof of the HIV/AIDS theory: The HIV infection causes as independent variable the dependent variable prooxidative overstimulation, which causes the dependent variable glutathione deficiency, which causes the dependent variable type 2 cytokine profile, which causes the dependent variable cytotoxic NO inhibition, which causes as dependent variable the inadequate elimination of intracellular agents (AIDS), and this finally causes as dependent variable the unavoidable death of the HIV sufferer. But this proposition of proof of the HIV/AIDS theory is objectively refuted:

The indirect molecular marker of "HIV characteristics" (Montagnier; Tahi 1997) could be proven exclusively only after stimulation of T-4 immune cells and leukaemia cells with interleukin-2 and oxidizing substances (mitogens) like phytohemagglutinin, concanavalin A etc., and never without stimulation by interleukin-2 and oxidizing mitogens etc. (overview Papadopulos-Eleopulos 1993 a, 1998 a).

In other words, the prooxidative stimulation as independent variable caused as a consequence the dependent variable "HIV characteristics" in cell types like Th2 cells of AIDS patients and leukaemia cells which are already reprogrammed before the prooxidative stimulation *in vitro* (as a result of the independent variables of the primary prooxidative overstimulation as a result of toxic, pharmacotoxic, chronic inflammatory and/or infectious, nutritional, alloantigenic, radiative and other causes) via the dependent variable chain: glutathione deficiency → type 2 cytokine profile → cytotoxic NO inhibition → Th2 immune cell dominance and opportunistic tumor cell growth (overview Lucey 1996, Lincoln 1997, Peterson 1998, Hässig 1998 b, Kremer 1999).

This chain of evidence asserts that "HI viruses" are not the cause of AIDS, and that the mortality rate of "HIV positives" is increased by prooxidative chemotherapeutics like AZT etc. (with co-trimoxazole as secondary cause), if the first link in the dependent variable chain, the glutathione deficiency, is not compensated (Herzenberg 1997, De Rosa 2000).

The primary mortality peak of "HIV positives" is, thus, dependent on the trusting consumption of cocktails from prooxidative pharmacotoxins by the most seriously glutathione-depleted HIV positives. The time-delayed drop in the annual incidence of mortality rate of HIV positives is a reflection of the effects of the prooxidative chemotherapeutics on the HIV positives with relatively high initial glutathione values. The drop in the mortality rate of "HIV positives" benefits from the fact that ever-increasing numbers of them either openly or secretly refused aggressive chemotherapy. This survival strategy counts especially for the largest patient group, the homosexual men in Western cities, who due to the channels of communication in the gay scene are relatively well-informed about the risks and side-effects of the changing chemotherapeutic strategies of HIV/AIDS medicine after 15 years of "planned experiments on humans" (Thomas 1984), despite psychological pressure from HIV/AIDS physicians and the continuous disinformation and hindrance from the media. *The HIV/AIDS establishment, however, took credit for the relatively improved survival rates—due to open or secretive refusal of chemotherapy—by claiming the supposed success of HAART treatment. The pharmaceutical companies tried to recoup the drop in sales of chemotherapeutics by increasing sales volume in developing nations.*

The proven correlation between glutathione level and the incidence of disease in elderly patients, shows that "HIV positives" can be regarded cellular-biologically as prematurely aged patients, due to their preceding long-term prooxidative (nitrosative and oxidative) overload of the cellular symbiosis

The medical-statistical effect of time-delayed mortality, termed by Dr. Fauci as progress, thus, does not prove the effectiveness against "HI viruses," but merely proves the correlation, demonstrated by the Stanford team, between the degree of dependent variables of the lower glutathione level and the rate of survival (Herzenberg 1997).

The correlation between the glutathione level and disease rates in elderly patients was shown by a study from Birmingham University in England. The glutathione values were measured in evenly sized groups of young healthy and elderly healthy test subjects, chronically ill elderly out-patients and elderly patients acutely in need of treatment in hospital (all elderly patients were over 70). The glutathione values of the 70+ year-olds were more than 50% lower than their healthy young counterparts. The glutathione levels of the hospital patients were the lowest, and the glutathione levels of the out-patients were lower than the healthy elderly subjects. Likewise, the lipid hydroperoxide (LHP) values as expression of prooxidative cell damage were at their highest in the acute elderly patients in hospital and at their lowest in healthy young test subjects (Nuttall 1998).

In this respect, "HIV positives" can be considered as prematurely aged patients, as a result of the preceding long-term prooxidative overload of the cellular symbiosis. Therapeutic progress, in Dr. Fauci's sense, could only be conceded if in controlled studies the "HIV positives" were treated comparatively:

- one treatment group of thiol-depleted patients with thiol compensation therapy but without any anti-retroviral chemotherapy, nor any long-term chemotherapeutic PCP prophylaxis;,
- a second treatment group of thiol-depleted patients with both a compensation therapy and simultaneous HAART chemotherapy etc. plus long-term co-trimoxazole (Herzenberg 1997); and a third treatment group solely with long-term HAART etc. and co-trimoxazole etc.

Unlike the countless clinical chemotherapy studies, there are no such controlled comparative studies of "HIV positives" who were exclusively treated by biological compensation methods, as clinical therapy studies have yet to be carried out and financed. The declining progression of the "responsiveness" to HAART even after nine to twelve months in correlation to the dosage of amounts of chemotherapeutical substances as a whole before and during the clinical CDC study (CDC 2000) demonstrate indirectly, however, the causal connection between the declining glutathione-dependent detoxifying capacity of patients and the toleration of glutathione-reducing chemotherapy. This crucial correlation to natural laws must be known to every physician on the basis of the data from findings in oncology: three and a half years average survival time after chemotherapy, twelve years average survival time without chemotherapy (Abel 1990).

As a final irrational evasion from responsibility for the deadly consequences of the objectively false disease theory, the virus hunters at the World AIDS Congress of 2000 called for the use of still more chemotherapeutic agents, in the absurd combination with vaccines against non-infectious human stress proteins, which are decay products and not the cause of systemic disturbances to the cellular symbiosis

HIV/AIDS medical science is, like oncology, far from being able to draw consequences from these concepts.

With the following words Fauci appealed to his colleagues to spur on intensive research against HIV, at the 13th International AIDS Conference in Durban: "The present possibilities of treatment cannot remain our response to the AIDS agent. We need new substances . . . a concept for the future could be, for example, to combine medicamentous treatment with vaccinations" (Fauci 2000).

The fact that "HIV positive" long-term survivors were without exception not treated with AZT etc., Bactrim etc., proves that "HIV" stigmatized patients die as victims of the elementary malpractices of Retrovirus-AIDS-Cancer medicine

So Dr. Fauci made demands for vaccines against the human stress proteins that are released in prooxidative activated T4 cell cultures of AIDS patients and in human leukaemia cells and which are attributed to phantom-like HI viruses, and then advocated combining these vaccines with even more prooxidative chemotherapeutics. The perverted scientific curiosity has apparently still not been satisfied, namely to find out in "a planned series of human experiment . . . what would happen if you were to remove the putative defense mechanism of cellular immunity in human beings?" (Thomas 1984). After twenty years of AIDS therapy, despite all kinds of clear immunological and cytotoxic effects as a consequence of chemotherapeutic and chemo-antibiotic prolonged treatment on "HIV positives" and AIDS patients on the basis of the objectively false disease theory and the failure of long-term HAART treatment, the HIV/AIDS physicians are apparently still "very confused about the mechanisms that lead to higher T-4 immune cell depletion, . . . but at least we are now confused at a higher level of understanding" (Balter 1997) and still claim that "the riddle of T-4 immune cell loss remains unresolved" (Balter 1997).

The available medical publications about so-called long-term survivors in Western countries (defined in the sense of the objectively false disease theory of the sooner or later apparently unavoidably lethal "HIV infection") showed that "HIV-induced" acquired immunodeficiency (AIDS) is primarily to do with glutathione-depleted patients whose untreated glutathione deficiency progressed to chemotherapeutically induced "pharmaceutical" AIDS:

"On reviewing the eight studies on HIV positive 'long-term non-progressors', who have remained symptom-free over ten years, we were struck that without exception they were not treated with nucleoside analog substances (AZT etc.) (Buchbinder 1994, Hoover 1995, Hogervorst 1995, Cho 1995, Pantaleo 1995, Harrer 1996, Montefiori 1996, Garbuglia 1996). We consider this observation as confirmation of the warning, described in this study, about the prophylactic and therapeutic adoption of these cytotoxins originally designed for the treatment of cancer" (Hässig 1998 a).

Chapter XI

The Lifesaving Knowledge of Healing

On the practice of diagnosing, preventing and treating AIDS, cancer and other systemic diseases—equilibrating rather than eliminating

The prevailing AIDS and cancer medicine has mostly been unsuccessful through ignorance, or failing to take notice, of the evolutionarily conserved bioenergetic, genetic and metabolic fundamental principles of the intact or disrupted alternating switch of cellular symbioses. The one-sided medical intervention of attempting to eliminate the "HI viruses" and the eradication of cancer cells and metastases through prooxidative chemotherapy has by its nature caused more harm than good.

The disease theory "HIV causes AIDS," as the resulting construction of retrovirus cancer research, has more than clearly demonstrated the meanderings of modern hi-tech laboratory research. Experimental and clinical research data since the historical statement by Warburg that the causes of no other disease are better known than the causes of cancer, however, show a way out of this diagnostic, preventative and therapeutic dead-end.

The "anti-HIV antibody test" as non-specific indicator (not a test for actual HIV antibodies)

The diagnosis of HIV-positive from a laboratory reading—the identification of a positive test result in the "anti-HIV antibody test"—cannot be the guideline, as there is no such thing as an HIV test that contains proteins of a "retrovirus HIV" as test antigen, either in the ELISA test process or in the Western blot process (overview Papadopulos-Eleopulos 1993 a). The test contains proteins from a human cell culture and is adjusted in such a way that it displays the availability of higher than average amounts of antibodies. Such antibodies are not specific and in a Th2 cell dominance could have been generated against all sorts of innate or microbial antigen proteins (Hässig 1996 c, 1998 a, 1998 b, 1998 c, Papadopulos-Eleopulos 1997 c, Wang 1999). The "HIV test" also tells us nothing about the point in time of increased antibody formation. Since antibodies survive for a long time in blood serum, the increase of antibody levels could have happened at some time in the past or the cause for this rise in antibodies could still be given at the time of the test.

The DHT skin reaction as test for immune cell status and indicator of Th2 dominance

The easily conducted delayed-type hypersensitivity (DTH) skin test with recall antigens is suitable for measuring the T-cell reactivity (Christie 1986, 1995). Weak or anergic reactions permit the supposition of Th2 immune cell dominance.

Measuring the Th immune cells (T4 cells or CD4+ cells) in the blood does not reveal the relation between Th1 and Th2 cells, as no reliable surface markers were shown in order to routinely differentiate the proportions of the Th1 and Th2 cells subgroups. This is only possible via special measurements of type 1 and type 2 cytokine profiles in T-helper immune cells. A Th2 immune cell dominance can be expected with a high degree of certainty if the numbers of T-helper cells and the ratio of the numbers of T4 to T8 cells clearly drop with a simultaneously decrease in natural killer cells (NK), neutropenia (a decrease below the norm of neutrophile granulocytes) and simultaneous eosinophilia (an increase in eosinophilic granulocytes) and an increase in antibody levels (especially immune globuline G and E).

The intracellular and plasma levels of reduced glutathione, in connection with plasma levels of cysteine, glutamine, arginine and glutamate as well as the immune status, as indicators for preventative and therapeutic intervention

The measuring of glutathione (GSH) values in plasma and the intracellular GSH values in T4 cells are crucial for preventative and therapeutic intervention in "HIV-positives" as indicators of the status of the redox balance and thus the performance capacities of the whole immune cell network. "HIV positives" with normal GSH values in the plasma and in T4 cells and other peripheral blood cells, and normal cysteine, glutamine, arginine and glutamate values in plasma as well as other balanced readings of T4 cells, NK cells, neutrophiles and eosinophiles within normal fluctuations are not threatened by opportunistic infections. They require a detailed clarification about the clinical insignificance of an isolated "HIV positive" test result.

Even orthodox HIV/AIDS medicine admits that 5% of the "HIV positive" test results are "false positive," and thus 5% of the "HIV positives," even within the bounds of the HIV/AIDS theory, are confronted with a medical death sentence for no reason. The disability to differentiate between a "false positive" and a "real positive" is a tragedy on top of a tragedy. It shows, too, how irrational the approach of HIV/AIDS physicians is in diagnosing and predicting the possible dangers to a symptom-free patient on the basis of a more-than-arcane antibody test, the measuring of the T4 cell status and the non-standardized unspecific measurements of "HIV RNA" as viral load by means of the error-prone PCR method.

A proven deficit of reduced glutathione (GSH) calls for mandatory treatment

If you stand back from the obsession with an "HIV infection" as the cause of AIDS and assume from the firm facts that in all immune and non immune cells glutathione levels, conforming to the norm, are of central importance to the vitality and performance of intact cellular symbiosis as well as a stable redox balance, then it should be mandatory to treat a proven glutathione deficiency. This medical principle applies completely independently of any "HIV characteristics" for symptom-free and symptomatic patients with known or unknown prooxidative stress risks (Ohlenschläger 1991, 1992, 1994, Scandalios 1992, Meister 1995).

The independent variable of strong and/or long-lasting prooxidative stress and the dependent variable of glutathione depletion, activate the causal chain of Type-II counterregulation of cellular dyssymbiosis

The causal chain of a Type-II counterregulation of cellular dyssymbiosis in immune cells or non-immune cells in risk patients with a recognized excessive prooxidative burden has clearly shown:

- Strong or long-standing prooxidative stress → glutathione depletion → loss of the redox balance → type 1 to type 2 cytokine switch (Th1-Th2 switch) → inhibition of the synthesis of cytotoxic NO → opportunistic infections → organ failure (AIDS)
- Strong or long-standing prooxidative stress → glutathione depletion → loss of redox balance → type 1 to type 2 cytokine switch → mitochondrial inactivation → aerobic glycolysis → re-fetalization → wasting syndrome → organ failure (AIDS, cancer, nerve and muscle degeneration among other systemic diseases).

The core concept of restoring the redox balance

If the suppositions of glutathione depletion and cysteine deficits are confirmed through laboratory diagnoses and Th1 to Th2 dysbalances are confirmed immunologically, non-toxic balancing measures are always necessary and effective to even up the redox performance:

- Minimization of prooxidative loads
- Balancing of the thiol deficit
- Balancing of the amino acid dysregulation
- Liver protection to relieve the systemic thiol deficiency
- Modulation of Type-II counterregulation
- Balance of the micronutrients
- Strengthening of the extracellular matrix
- Mitochondrial activation
- Curbing of hormonal stress state
- Reduction of fear and 'psychagogic' aid

The glutathione system of the cellular symbiosis must intercept and convert an enormous amount of poisonous materials and potentially carcinogenic substances, via coupling with cysteine, to form the kidney-excreted mercapturic acid

The military metaphor of an "ongoing titanic struggle between HI viruses and the immune system" (Ho 1995 a, 1995 b) used by HIV/AIDS medicine has obstructed the view of what the time-delayed prooxidative stress in general and specifically for the glutathione-protected cellular symbioses in immune and non-immune cells really means. The human organism is exposed, in daily life, to the effects of almost 60,000 chemical compounds, of which 4,000-6,000 display carcinogenic characteristics. Alone the skin macrophages and the T immune cells of the outer skin in dealing with the immune cell network as a whole have to perform enormous glutathione-consuming detoxification activities to stabilize the redox status. A vast number of preservatives (lindane, pentachlorophenol, halogenated fungicide), 8,000 dyes, of which roughly 2,000 are nitrosative azodyes and 6,000 textile additives (halogenated hydrocarbons, phosphoric acid esters, formaldehyde, ammonia etc), penetrate mostly through the skin and continuously have to be prevented from triggering uncontrollable chain reactions that would overtax the reserve capacities of cellular symbiosis either directly via reduced glutathione (GSH) in immune and non-immune cells or enzymatically with support from the enzymes of the multifunctional oxygenases of the cytochrome system.

Additionally, there is the increased inhalation of aerosols (nitrogen oxides, nitrosamines, ozone, aromatic hydrocarbons like benzopyrenes, benzanthracenes etc., metallic dusts, organic solvents, plutonium, radon etc.). These nitrosative and oxidative stressors also have to be neutralized by GSH to prevent damage to bronchial and lung epithelial cells as well as lung macrophages and T-helper cells and the especially vulnerable surfactant factors. GSH consumption is at the same time strained by a diversity of more than 1,000 toxins in conventional agricultural and industrial foodstuffs (heavy metals, insecticides, pesticides, nitrates, nitrosamines, aliphatic and aromatic hydrocarbons, monomers and oligomers as well as softening agents of plastics, dyes, preservatives, aldehydes etc.). These nutrition toxins contaminate not only intestinal, hepatic and pancreatic cells, but also directly burden the T-helper immune cells in the lining of the intestines and in the spleen, which form the largest proportion of the T-cell reservoir in the organism (overview Ohlenschläger 1992).

The total of electrophile (electron-receiving) toxins have to be decontaminated in a number of stages by nucleophile (electron-donating) GSH via conjugation with the aid of special enzymes (glutathione S-tranferase). After conjugation of the foreign matter with GSH, enzymes separate the amino acids glutamine and glycine from the glutathione tripeptides, a cysteine conjugate is produced that is acetylated and releases water. The stable end-product mercapturic acid is produced, which is readily soluble in water and can be excreted by the kidneys and liver (overview Ohlenschläger 1992).

The continual binding of toxic foreign molecules by the glutathione system consumes an enormous quantity of cysteine, which puts cellular symbiosis at risk of systemic glutathione deficiency syndrome

This outline of the fundamental workings of the decontamination of prooxidative foreign matter by the unique and most important nucleophilic molecule in all cell systems and cell symbionts in the human organism—glutathione—is of vital importance for understanding therapy. It demonstrates that on top of the continuing task of glutathione to balance out countless redox oscillations with nitrogen oxides and radical oxygen species, to limit radical chain reactions and to regenerate radical intermediate stages of ascorbic acid (vitamin C) and ß-carotene, vitamin E etc., cysteine is permanently withdrawn through the forced conjugation of toxic foreign molecules to GSH. The consequence is that the increased demand for the balancing neosynthesis of glutathione can no longer be covered when additional excessive prooxidative pressures overtax the capacity for the biosyntheses of GSH. The redox balance is in danger of tipping when the critical reserve capacities of the mitochondrial OXPHOS system become exhausted and an optimum gas mixture from NO/O_2- for regulating cellular symbioses can no longer maintain the fluidity of the micro-Gaian milieu. Depending on how quickly and how steeply the exponential increase in the gas components takes place, inflammatory cytokine profiles are synthesized, which trigger apoptosis or necrosis, or immune cell weakening cytokine profiles are synthesized, which could lead to pre-AIDS and AIDS, cancer and nerve and muscle cell degeneration.

Despite proof of the effective reduction of "HIV characteristics" by N-acetyl-Cysteine, "HIV positives" and AIDS patients were not obligatorily treated with the reducing substances cysteine, and glutathione, which are "cheap, readily available and virtually devoid of any serious side effects."

It is rationally incomprehensible why, ever since the proof of the systemic and intracellular glutathione depletion in immune and non-immune cells of "HIV positives" at an early point in time of the "HIV seroconversion" (Buhl 1989, Eck 1989, Roederer 1991), HIV/AIDS physicians did not obligatorily treat the glutathione deficit of "HIV" infected individuals, despite very detailed and differentiated knowledge about the essential importance of the glutathione system for the vitality of all cell systems (Ohlenschläger 1991). Already in 1985, the research team at the Royal Hospital in Perth, Australia, had discussed the obvious hypothesis that the oxidative stress of the risk factors was the primary cause of AIDS and could be counteracted by glutathione and N-acetyl cysteine (Papadopulos-Eleopulos 1998). One of the Perth Group posed the adjuratory question:

"Reducing agents and AIDS—why are we waiting? . . . There is now abundant evidence that HIV-positive individuals as well as AIDS patients have an altered redox state and that this may be an important factor in their disease process. For example, in February 1989 Eck and his colleagues showed that plasma levels of acid-soluble thiols (cysteine) and glutathione levels in peripheral blood mononuclear cells and monocytes [precursor cells of macrophages] are significantly decreased in the various AIDS groups (Eck 1989). Their *in vitro* studies also showed a strong dependence of intracellular glutathione concentration on extracellular cysteine with an accompanying strong correlation between the glutathione concentration and the viability and functional activities of T cells. In December 1989, Buhl *et al.* described systemic and lung epithelial lining fluid glutathione deficiency in symptom-free HIV-positive individuals (Buhl 1989). The levels reported were respectively 30% and 60% of the levels in healthy controls. These authors also pointed out that, although unexplained, the glutathione deficiency might be a direct causative factor in the reduced immune function observed in patients with HIV infection. Glutathione is the major transport system in plasma for the sulphydryl-containing amino acid cysteine which itself is a major antioxidant. Oxidants cause breaks in the DNA strands of lymphocytes and damage many of their innate functions. Sulphydryl compounds also augment a number of lymphocyte functions *in vitro*, including mitogenic T cell proliferation and T and B cell differentiation. The fact that glutathione deficiency is clearly demonstrated in the lungs of HIV-positive patients may be of importance in understanding the genesis of opportunistic pulmonary infection that characterises AIDS [pneumonia caused by the *Pneumocystis carinii* fungal pathogens = PCP, the most frequent AIDS-indicating illness up until now] . . . . There are at least two reducing substances that are cheap, readily available and virtually devoid of any serious side effects. These are glutathione and N-acetyl cysteine. The latter is familiar to clinicians as an agent originally used in the treatment of chronic bronchitis and probably more recently used as an antidote for paracetamol poisoning. Herzenberg from Stanford University has recently documented reversal of low systemic glutathione levels in HIV-positive individuals by use of N-acetyl cysteine (Roederer 1990); experiments *in vitro* indicate that N-acetyl cysteine can produce highly desirable effects on HIV replication including a reduction in the appearance of p24 antigen (Clayton 1990). An Italian company, Zambon, will be assigned a patent on this drug for the purposes of treating AIDS when the United States Food and Drug Authority approves the first clinical trials. Oxidative stress as an important mechanism in AIDS and its possible reversal by reducing agents was hypothesized as long ago as 1985 by another Australian researcher (Papadopulos-Eleopulos 1988, 1989). Surely it is time someone carries out trials of therapy with reducing agents." (Turner 1990).

In place of the effective, non-toxic compensation therapy, the medical-industrial cartel unlawfully manipulated the fast-track approval of the expensive, highly toxic and carcinogenic AZT chemotherapy for symptomatic and symptom-free "HIV positives."

The research data were clear. In addition to the presence of the repair enzyme reverse transcriptase (RT), Montagnier and Gallo had misinterpreted the presence of the protein molecule p24 as the second "molecular marker" of "HI viruses". Proof of the inhibition of these cellular prooxidative stress products, p24 and RT, in glutathione-depleted immune cell cultures by the application of reducing substance that are "cheap, readily available and virtually devoid of any serious side effects—glutathione and N-acetyl cysteine" (Turner

1990) endangered, however, the interests of the pharmaceutical industry and the industry-dependent laboratory researchers and clinicians, whose research budgets were financed and re-financed by the revenues from sales of expensive chemotherapeutics. The reducing substances glutathione and cysteine are unpatentable. From a background of knowledge established since the end of the 1980s of the evolutionary biologically programmed laws of the interactions between the essential redox balance provided by the central cysteine/glutathione system, in addition to the mitochondrial vitality, NO/ROS production and the balance of cytokine profiles loomed the fiasco of the aggressive therapy strategies of AIDS and cancer treatment. The confession of the fateful scientific errors and the clear role of toxic and pharmacotoxic industrial products in the development of AIDS, cancer and other systemic diseases as well as the lethal failure of AIDS and cancer therapy via toxic chemotherapeutics could have triggered incalculable political, social, economic, scientific and medical consequences (Epstein 1998).

The response of the AIDS establishment dominated by retrovirus cancer researchers was clear: the revolutionary findings of the more recent cellular symbiosis research were ignored and the world public and the media were deliberately misled with the infinitely variable claims about the supposed effectiveness of "anti-retroviral" AIDS therapy. The clear-cut question of the Australian research team: "As AIDS has a 100% fatality rate and 60% of HIV-positive individuals are said to develop AIDS in five years, would it not be reasonable to give urgent consideration to trials of therapy and prevention with reducing agents?" (Turner 1990), was answered by the US drug approval authority, the FDA, by fast-tracking authorization for glutathione-consuming AZT for asymptomatic HIV positives (Friedland 1990).

Compensation therapy with cysteine/glutathione, proven to be non-toxic, was not promoted.

The sufficient dosage, and the improved bioavailability of cysteine (NAC) and glutathione (GSH) in combination with coenzyme 1 (NAD) and plant polyphenols

Generally, cysteine demands in systemic disruptions of the redox balance are considerably underestimated, for instance, the increased proton consumption in oxygen-independent sugar degradation for ATP energy acquisition for the reprocessing of the dropping amounts of lactate is calculated to a respective proton contribution of 23 g cysteine per day in patients with Crohn's disease or ulcerative colitis (Erikson 1983, Dröge 1997 a). These patients have a dysregulation of non-protein thiols and amino acids, cellular weaknesses and wasting syndromes similar to "HIV positives," cancer sufferers, sepsis and trauma patients, overtrained athletes and ill elderly people (Dröge 1997 a). The Birmingham study of 1998 demonstrated, for instance, that lower glutathione levels correlated exactly to disease stages of the elderly patients but the appropriate compensation therapy is by no means agreed upon in standard clinical practice (Nuttall 1998).

Cysteine compensation therapy requires, however, medical laboratory controls in order to avoid possible under—or overdoses. Small doses of NAD are quickly used without penetrating the deeper cellular compartments of mitochondria for the regeneration of glutathione. Overdoses can cause disruption in the gastrointestinal regions in prolonged usage. The cysteine levels can vary, even independently of nutrition and in correlation to intermittent intake of foreign matter.

Astonishingly, the authors of the NAC-substitution studies did not consider the direct prescription of glutathione treatment, which the Perth research team had also brought into the discussion. As cysteine requirement is necessary for numerous molecular compounds. It cannot be implicitly guaranteed that cysteine compensation therapy will be predominantly implemented in glutathione neosynthesis. Particularly in the metallothionines, which play an important role in all cell systems, there is a high cysteine requirement. Glutathione values could already be lower when the cysteine level is still using muscle protein reserves. In these cases, depending on the readings of T4 cells in the plasma and inside cells or other peripheral blood cells, an oral glutathione therapy of 2-5 g per day or higher is indicated. The form of presentation, under certain circumstances, determines the dosage; the intake of gastric juice resistant capsules can save glutathione.

Glutathione prescriptions should be controlled in medical laboratories at fortnightly intervals in order to undertake any necessary adjustments to the dosage. Glutathione can be combined with cysteine, selenium, and antioxidative vitamins. Recently, a combination with the coenzyme NADH, which plays a decisive role in numerous biosyntheses as a hydrogen-carrier, has been discussed. NADH and NADPH, the oxidized form of NAD^+, are synthesized in glucose metabolism via the pentose phosphate metabolic pathway. As NADH cannot be directly channelled into the mitochondria, hydrogen ions have to be transported to the cell symbionts by molecular ferries in order to be absorbed by NAD, FAD and FMN. This transport pathway is disturbed by aerobic glycolysis through the switch to glycolytic isoenzymes and the influence of Bcl 2 protein family on the ratio of NAD^+

to NADH. A relative NADH surplus through oral intake of NADH or coenzyme 1 (for instance, 5mg tablets of yeast NAD, once or twice a day) appears to have a vitalizing effect in diseases associated with mitochondrial inactivation, like Parkinson's disease, Alzheimer, depression etc. Previous clinical studies, however, are contradictory (Birkmayer 1993, Swerdlow 1998). The mobilization of NADH-dependent enzymes is apparently dependent on the stabilization of the redox balance via the glutathione system. This is of importance in connection with the glutathione balance, as in order to preserve orderliness and information in the "fundamental regulation of living systems" (Ohlenschläger 1991) the ratio of reduced to oxidized glutathione (GSH to GSSG, roughly 400:1) is decisive for the redox performance. The continuous reduction of GSSG to antioxidative GSH happens with the aid of the glutathione reductase enzymes, and requires NADH as coenzyme. At the same time the NADH concentrations of mitochondria are needed for the revitalization of the respiratory chain.

Besides the combination of GSH/NADH, another combined supplement, made up from reduced glutathione (GSH), l-cysteine and anthocyanins (trade name Recancostat), is regarded as "superior to all other natural oxidative protective functions" and "superordinated protection against antioxidation and radicals" (Ohlenschläger 1992), because of its special Galenic mode of preparation, which ensures infiltration into mitochondria. Since Recancostat as a speciality remains relatively expensive, reduced glutathione/cysteine (e.g. curantox 1) and anthocyanins (e.g. curantox 2), can also be taken individually. Anthocyanins, plant pigments, belong to the over 5,000 phenolic flavonoids in plants (fruits, vegetables, seeds, skins, tubers and blossoms) (Strack 1997). These are potent antioxidants and metal chelators and have anti-inflammatory, anti-allergic, antiviral and anticarcinogenic effects (overview Ono 1990, Herzog 1992, Stoner 1995, Rice-Evans 1996, Cotelle 1996). There are beneficial synergistic interactions between GSH and anthocyanins (likewise between vitamin C and E) through redox cycle exchange programs. The argument against the combination of GSH/anthocyanin is that some phenolic flavonoids can cause DNA base oxidation and inhibition of cell division in high micromolecular concentrations. However, such concentrations are not reached in circulating flavonoid levels in human organisms so this assumption, in view of the high absorption of plant flavonoids, is unrealistic (overview Duthie 1997). Just as effective is the combination of glutathione and the polyphenol gingko biloba known as S-acetyl glutathione (SAG), which has recently become available. The alternative of SAG therapy is of practical importance when there are doubts about the sufficiency of other Galenic glutathione supplements.

In light of the "extremely few attempts at antioxidant therapy," even the "HIV"-believing therapists criticize that "the system of therapeutic clinical trials uses a surplus of cash, resources and time on highly toxic, insignificantly profitable and worthless medicines (AZT etc)"

However, HIV/AIDS physicians have to permit the question of how, without cysteine/glutathione compensation, they plan to honor the promises of an "HIV cure" (Ho 1995 b, Saag 1999, Cooper 1999, Fauci 2000), which they have been restating for 15 years with massive propaganda campaigns and the largest capital investment in the history of medicine, by treatment with glutathione-consuming, mitochondriotoxic, type 2 cytokine stimulating chemotherapeutics which, even if we assume the objectively non-existent "HIV infection" to be the cause of AIDS, could not inhibit either theoretically or experimentally the "HI viruses." In principle, this question was self-critically posed, even among "HIV"-believing therapists years ago under the restrictive perspective of oxidative stress:

"Oxidative stress can be improved through a balanced combination of antioxidants. Naturally, some antioxidants cannot be patented. That's why there are no profits in them. Despite plenty of evidence and the widespread need among the population very few therapy trials have been attempted with such compounds .... Ideally, the government should have a well-founded interest in such antioxidants. When you consider that many patients who live with AIDS belong to the lower income groups, it means that they are dependent on public health care. That is why such relatively cost-effective treatment forms should be high on the government's priority list for the prevention of opportunistic infections, the delaying of progressions and reducing the time spent in hospitals. Instead, the system of therapeutic clinical trials uses surplus cash, resources and time on highly toxic, insignificantly profitable and worthless medicines for the treatment of HIV: nucleoside analog substances [AZT etc.] and soon the highly dubious vaccines against HIV. (According to recent figures, 98 AZT therapy studies have been carried out by the National Institute of Allergy and Infectious Diseases, over 30 by the FDA and a dozen by the National Cancer Institute" (Act Up New York 1993).

The glutathione system uses unique quantum physical properties, not limited to antioxidative functions, but controls the disturbance of glutathione equilibrium, the "weak interactions" of all bioenergetic and biochemical processes of cellular symbiosis via the requisite strongly negative redox potential.

The inconclusive treatment strategies of the research teams from the Deutsches Krebsforschungszentrum (Dröge 1997 a), Stanford University (Herzenberg 1997) and other clinicians of "additional cysteine monotherapy" for "HIV positives," cancer patients and others with systemic diseases will be contrasted here with extracts from a very graphic and insistent lecture from the German physician and biochemist Ohlenschläger on treatment with reduced glutathione in special Galenism with l-cysteine and anthocyanins:

"Also in the compartments of living systems where everything is in flow, there are flow balancing systems; proton, electron, ion, matter, energy and information flows. All these flows as well as many other molecular states of orderliness, like for example the 3-dimensional shape of protein and enzyme molecules, underlie the also in flux balanced glutathione system as non-balanced system. Glutathione molecules consist of three amino acids: glutamine, cysteine with a free SH group (sulfhydryl group) and glycin. This is the reduced form of glutathione. And this glutathione together with another glutathione molecule, via the release of hydrogen and thus oxidative, can merge into a double form—a double molecule. Now you have to imagine the following: Form and function are nowhere in biology so closely related as in this situation of free SH groups and the disulfide bridge: Anywhere in cells.

Proteins are available either in one form with a free SH group or in another looped form linked by the sulfide bridge. The redox potential of glutathione ensures that this system is maintained. And nature has—and now we are back to non-balance—set an imbalance in this glutathione system in all cells, in all locations of reactions and in all mitochondria. We have a stronger representation of reduced glutathione to its oxidized form with a ratio of 400 to 1, in all cells . . . . There is not one chemical step in cells that is not catalyzed enzymatically, and these enzymes need a particular 3-dimennsional form, and they get this only from a corresponding negative redox potential through a highly current concentration of reduced glutathione. The normal cell division process that a cell splits when it is permitted to split, this whole regulated, orderly genetic program is performed by all of us—all our lives! Even protection from overoxidation and maintenance of important detoxification functions depend on the glutathione system. Also the development, for the adaptation, regulation and kinetics of all biochemical reactions of a living system's important "weak interactions" depend on glutathione balance . . . . Antigen-antibodies are bonded through weak interactions; a receptor on the surface of the membrane of a cell and a signal molecule are bonded by weak interactions, or a transport molecule that needs to carry a substance through the cell membrane are bonded for a short time by weak interactions, or a molecule that has to convert another molecule, its substrate, is bonded via weak interaction for a short time as enzyme substrate complex. Molecules nourish themselves, fall under the quantum physical influence of their, partially overlapping, outer orbitors [outer orbits of electrons]. Molecules congregate, ally themselves and again separate. Thus the reversibility and thereby the whole dynamics of cellular metabolism, phenomena of continual change, are linked to these weak interactions and these weak interactions stand and fall physiologically with the redox potential in cells, that is strongly negative and has to be; stand and fall with a thermodynamic imbalance of the glutathione system" (Ohlenschläger 1994).

The crucial question for the HIV/AIDS medical profession (and likewise for oncologists): why for over 20 years have they actively ignored the available discoveries as to the vital importance of cysteine/glutathione compensation in systemic diseases and, instead, counterproductively prescribed prooxidative chemo-cocktails?

Thus the question, which up until now has been avoided, has to be asked of the HIV/AIDS physicians as to how they envisage their propagated "HIV healing" without cysteine/glutathione compensation. For the crucial type 1 to type 2 cytokine balance for intact cellular immunity via appropriate cytotoxic NO gas production also depends on the fine tuning of the redox potential through the glutathione system of antigen-presenting cells and their double signal to the T-4 immune cells after stimulation by intracellular microbes or toxins.

Secondly, a question has to be asked of clinical researchers, who combined cysteine substitution with chemotherapeutics like AZT etc. that need glutathione or with cysteine neosynthesis-inhibiting folic acid antagonists like co-trimoxazole etc. What sense does it makes to give with the one hand and take with the other, paradoxically with substances which objectively cannot accomplish what they are meant to accomplish; namely the inhibition of HI viruses? Thirdly, why does the HIV/AIDS medical profession still believe that a systemic disease linked to opportunistic infections and wasting syndrome that should and must have been recognized 20 years ago as the prooxidative cause of the deficiency of freely convertible protons, has to be counterproductively treated with chemotherapeutics, although the cause of the cellular immune weaknesses and wasting syndromes has long been clarified by evidence of glutathione and cysteine deficits, mitochondrial inactivation, type 2 cytokine switch, cytotoxic NO inhibition, glycolytic metabolic situation, amino acid dysregulation, increased urea production etc?

Finally, 20 years after the first AIDS diagnoses, comes the publication of the first successful clinical trial for the treatment of wasting syndrome with high-dose glutathione/cysteine compensation (Shabert 1999).

The first publicized randomized double-blind study (randomly selected patients in treatment and control groups) demonstrated how hard it is for even the most progressive HIV/AIDS physicians to transform the simplest findings about the "weak interactions" in cellular biology to rational clinical actions. A small group of "HIV positive" patients with wasting syndrome were treated with cysteine and other antioxidants plus glutamine. The 21 patients who completed the clinical study, with the exception of 3, were all treated chemotherapeutically following the HAART procedure.

Simultaneously these patients received every day for 12 weeks, 2.4 g N-acetyl cysteine, 0.8 g ascorbic acid (vitamin C), 500 international units (IU) alpha tocopherol (vitamin E), 27,000 IU ß-carotene, 280 mg selenium and 40 g glutamine. The supplementary medications—supplementary to 'proper' medication with "anti-retroviral" chemotherapeutics—were taken four times daily and the patients were given new packets every two weeks. The body weight (BW) of the patients increased within three months on average by 2 kg and the body cell mass (BCM = metabolically active body tissues) by 1.8 kg. Side effects of the "supplementary agent" were not reported or not observed. In the control group after three months the increase in BW was on average 0.3 kg and the BCM 0.4 kg. The clinicians concluded:

"This randomized, double-blind, placebo-controlled therapy trial demonstrates for the first time [20 years after the first diagnosis of an AIDS-indicating disease in homosexual patients!] that supplementation of the amino acid L-glutamine and the provision of adequate antioxidants and nutritional counseling can improve body weight and restore BCM. This low-cost and low-risk supplement may be the preferred method of initial nutritional support in patients with weight loss of > 5%. Larger trials are needed to evaluate the clinical impact of this approach on reducing opportunistic infections and possibly long-term mortality" (Shabert 1999).

Experimental and clinical evidence for the systemic interactions between cysteine/glutathione, glutamine, glutamate and arginine, as well as the synthesis of urea and NO in wasting syndrome (Type-II counterregulation of cellular dyssymbiosis)

The million-dollar question is: how much more could the BW and BCM of patients have improved without HAART treatment? The clinicians at the Harvard Medical School in Boston misjudged decisive correlations: Healthy test subjects after anaerobic exercise programs resulting in increased aerobic glycolysis after 5 to 8 weeks had a loss of BCM, which correlated to lower cystine (oxidized cysteine) and glutamine values in the plasma. Furthermore, a placebo-controlled, double-blind study demonstrated that the reduction of BCM was impeded by treatment with N-acetyl cysteine. During the observation time, changes of glutamine levels in plasma strongly correlated to changes in the cystine levels in plasma (Kinscherf 1996). Similar to these studies on healthy people the treatment of "HIV"-infected people with N-acetyl cysteine resulted in a steep climb not only of cyst[e]ine values in the plasma but also the glutamine and arginine values (Dröge 1997 b).

The studies prove the following: As even a short-term shortage of oxygen (hypoxia or pseudohypoxia) in anaerobic exercise programs of healthy test subjects leads to an inactivation of the respiratory chain (ATP cannot be stored, so there has to be a switch to aerobic glycolysis, oxygen-independent enzymatic ATP production), the archaeal genetic emergency program is triggered resulting in the mobilization of the proton reserves in the skeletal musculature for the conversion of amino acids to pyruvate/glucose to feed the increased needs for sugar of glycolysis. The result is the observed loss of body cell mass and the exchange of cysteine and glutamine from the skeletal musculature for glutamate from the plasma is blocked. At the same time the splitting of cysteine to sulfate and protons in the liver is reduced because of the lower cysteine levels. The protons for inhibiting the first step of urea formation from arginine in the liver are missing. Therefore, the export of urea rises and levels of arginine sink. However, as the formation of glutamine in the liver without the help of protons from the splitting of cysteine is also heavily impeded, the glutamine level in plasma drops. Reduced levels of cysteine, glutamine and arginine in the plasma and higher levels of glutamate and urea are the characteristic laboratory findings of wasting syndrome analogous to the state of cachexia of cancer patients (Dröge 1997 b).

Simultaneously glutathione levels are reduced by the increased demand through prooxidative stress from initially increased NO and ROS formation in hypoxia and pseudohypoxia, from reduced neosynthesis as a result of cysteine and glutamine deficits and through disruption of the enzyme glutathione reductase from a shift in the ratio $NAD^+/NADH$. The consequences are a switch from type 1 cytokines to type 2 cytokines, the inhibition of cytotoxic NO production and a total Type-II counterregulation of cellular dyssymbiosis (still reversible). This dysregulation of the redox potential by overloading the glutathione system after prolonged hypoxia or pseudohypoxia is represented symptomatically by over-trained athletes with a disposition to opportunistic infections and wasting syndrome (Pedersen 1994).

Counterregulations after strong and prolonged prooxidative stress in "HIV positives" proceed in a similar fashion with the inhibition of the respiratory chain in mitochondria and pseudohypoxia (as a result of an alleged oxygen deficit through the blockade of the utilization of O_2). Here too the lowering of the cysteine/glutamine level strongly correlates with the after-effects of the sinking levels of glutamine and arginine. A too-low arginine level also means a reduction of cytotoxic NO synthesis in T-4 cells, as NO is formed from arginine (overview Lincoln 1997). A too-low glutamine level means on the one hand an overly strong glutamine decay in the protein reserves of the skeletal musculature and conversion to sugar (Dröge 1997 b), and on the other hand that glutamine as oxidation substrate is missing in the mitochondria of intestinal cells (Van der Hulst 1993, Welbourne 1994), in the immune cells and in the liver cells (Häussinger 1989) and as substrate for the acid-base balance in the kidneys (Brosman 1987, Welbourne 1994). However glutamine also supplies the necessary glutamates for glutathione regeneration (Hong 1992), so a glutamine deficit aggravates the glycolytic metabolic situation and provokes a type 2 cytokine switch (Hammarqist 1989, Hack 1996). Glutamine is, however, also a building block for the nucleic acid synthesis from RNA/DNA bases for DNA neosynthesis and repair procedures.

All these processes of the quantum dynamic regression from the fluid oxidative phase to the contra fluid reductive phase, triggered by the missing fine tuning of the redox imbalance resulting from a loss of freely convertible protons through prooxidative weakness of the cysteine-glutathione system, explain the wasting syndrome of "HIV positives" (Grünfeld 1992), cancer sufferers, sepsis and trauma patients, colitis patients, overtrained athletes and other people with systemic illnesses (overview Dröge 1997 b).

Treatment with sufficient dosages of N-acetyl cysteine simultaneously increases via "weak interactions" (Ohlenschläger 1994) both the glutamine and arginine levels (Dröge 1997 b) and thus improves the regeneration of both the glutathione level and the cytokine balance (Peterson 1998) as well as NO synthesis (overview Richter 1996, Lincoln 1997). Secondary glutathione deficiency as a result of primary deficits of freely convertible protons due to the prooxidative usage of the cysteine/glutathione supply has a massive influence on the maturation and functioning capacity of immune cells ready for defense. Glutamine serves as oxidation substrate for the energy metabolism of immune cells and as substrate for the biosynthesis of nucleosides as building blocks for RNA/DNA regeneration of immune cells. Glutamine deficits inhibit the production of the growth factor interleukin-2 of T-4 cells and reduce the numbers of T-4 cells in the plasma (immunological indicators of the acquired immune weaknesses of "HIV positive" and AIDS patients) (Newsholme 1990, 1996, Calder 1994, Rohde 1995, 1996, Hack 1997).

The interaction between the normal and lower cysteine levels on the one hand and the normal or lower glutamine values and synchronously the arginine values in plasma on the other hand derive from the ornithine-urea cycle in the liver and the regulation or, as the case may be, dysregulation of protein synthesis and decay in the musculature. This interplay is of great importance for the understanding of wasting syndrome and acquired immune weakness as well as for the therapy of these syndromes. Normally surplus amino acids that are not required for protein synthesis are converted to sugar, glycogen or fatty acids or are oxidized for ATP production. The nitrogen released by this process in the form of highly toxic ammonia (NH_4) is transferred to a-ketoglutarate and fed into the ornithine-urea cycle as glutamate.

In this metabolic cycle glutamate is routed in two ways. The first is directly into the cell symbionts where the ammonia of the glutamate is transferred to a substrate as the first step of the cyclic formation of urea, which via a number of stations in the cycle from the amino acid arginine is synthesized in the cytoplasm in the kidneys. In the second, alternative route, glutamate transfers an amino group to an intermediate product, which reacts to substrates in the ornithine-urea cycle. Finally, it is split into urea and ornithine in the kidneys. Ornithine is then available for a new passage through the cycle in the mitochondria. In this step of the cycle cysteine attacks, by making protons available through division in order to incorporate ammonia in glutamine with the aid of a special enzyme. If proton-donating cysteine is missing, less glutamine and more urea is produced and at the same time more arginine used. This is the reason why a lower cysteine level causes simultaneous lower glutamine and arginine values and explains why the N-acetyl cysteine substitution for the treatment of wasting syndrome in "HIV positives" and cancer sufferers raises levels of glutamine and arginine (Dröge 1997 b).

The crucial consequences for the prevention and therapy of cellular immune weakness and wasting syndrome arise from a multitude of networked interactions whose starting point is a profound disruption of the redox milieu (nutritional AIDS, pharmaceutical AIDS, intoxication AIDS, inflammation AIDS, alloantigen AIDS, radiation AIDS, athletes AIDS etc.).

The explanation for the favorable therapeutic effects of the high-dose arginine supply against cellular immune weakness and cancer, and the complementary combination with cysteine/glutathione/glutamine compensation

The role of arginine in cellular immunity of humans has been known through animal experiments for more than 20 years (Seifter 1978, Barbul 1980, 1981), but has not been given enough attention in HIV/AIDS medical science (Kinscherf 1996, Dröge 1997 b). Arginine substitution has shown favorable effects on the maturation and the capacity for stimulation of T-cells in healthy animals and humans. What was remarkable was the heavy increase in natural killer cells (NK cells) after daily intake of 30 g of arginine by voluntary test subjects (Barbul 1980, 1981, 1986, Daly 1988, Park 1991). The activity and number of NK cells is characteristically low in HIV positives, cancer and other systemic diseases (Dröge 1997 b). Recovery of a type 1 to type 2 cytokine balance after a type 2 cytokine dominance due to burns was shown in animal experiments when total intake of calories was enriched with 2% of arginine by improved reactivity to the DTH skin test and through inhibition of bacterial infections (Saito 1987). Likewise, there were improvements in the wound-healing processes, collagen regeneration and T4 cell functions after experiments on animals with injuries (Seifter 1978, Barbul 1980, 1985). The same favorable effects were found on recovery of the type 1/type 2 balance in patients after cancer operations in the gastrointestinal regions who were given 25 g of arginine daily and in sepsis patients one week after operations (Daly 1988, 1990, Barbul 1990).

In animal experiments anti-tumor effects were also demonstrated after arginine intake. The appearance of tumors after contact with carcinogenic substances could be reduced, the growth of cancer cells and the spreading of metastases could be delayed, the time span until tumor regression reduced and survival rates increased (Barbul 1990, Lowell 1990). In immunogenic tumors, both the unspecific cellular immunity of the macrophages and the specific T-4 cell immune response could be increased through arginine dosage (Tachibana 1985, Reynolds 1987, 1988). The favorable effects via arginine administration with nutrition for the modulation of the immune cell functions as well as the inhibition of the induction and development of malignant tumors through an improvement in the type 1 to type 2 cytokine balance are rationally understood by the fact that arginine not only acts as a semi-essential building block for countless proteins and enzymes and disposes of surplus nitrogen in the liver by splitting into urea and ornithine, but that arginine as crucial substrate for calcium-dependent and non-calcium-dependent NO synthesis enzymes also works on the production of the nitrogen monoxide gases NO (Palmer 1988, Wu 1998).

Evidence of the activation of cytotoxic NO in numerous immune cells and non-immune cells via a type 1 cytokine profile (Nussler 1993, Murphy 1993, Kröncke 1995, overview Lincoln 1997) clearly demonstrates the direct causal link between the reduced arginine levels through increased urea export and the inhibited immune cell activities due to a lack of synthesis of cytotoxic NO after a type 2 cytokine switch (AIDS) resulting from excessive prooxidative loss of the balancing functions for the fluid micro-Gaian milieu after the breakdown of the cysteine/glutathione system.

This also explains the inhibition of glycolytic, re-fetalized tumor cells, and metastatic after resettlement viable cancer cells due to the supply of arginine (Brüne 1998). The characteristic NO synthesis inhibition of tumor cells as a consequence of Type-II counterregulations is intensified by a shortage of arginine. Rapidly growing cancer cells have low NO values, slow growing tumors relatively high NO levels (Chinje 1997). From roughly 10,000 colonizing tumor cells, however, only about one survives as a metastatic cell as the exogenous stimulation by cytokines of non tumor cells (interleukin-12 from macrophages, interleukin-2, interferon-γ and tumor necrosis factors from T-helper cells and other immune and non-immune cells) can activate the cancer cells' own NO synthesis and ROS production so that regression, and cell death of tumor cells can be triggered via apoptosis/necrosis. The inducible threshold for the exogenous stimulated production of the cancer cells' own cytotoxic NO gases, which in cancer cells cannot be easily neutralized because of the depleted thiol pool, is higher in metastatic cells than in most tumor cells, above all because of prooxidative selection through chemotherapeutic treatments.

However, through arginine administration the incidence and growth rate of induced tumors could be reduced as well as the regression of these tumors improved and, at least in animal experiments, the apoptosis/necrosis rates of metastatic cells increased by repeated cytokine stimulation (Barbul 1990, Xie 1996).

The clinical results with the type 1 cytokine interleukin-2 showed an increase in the NO levels in the serum of cancer patients (Hibbs 1992, Ochoa 1992), although an increase in the permeability of capillaries was observed (Orucevic 1998). This phenomenon of unstemmable, lethal haemorrhaging was also diagnosed in Azathioprine-treated organ-transplant patients with Kaposi's sarcoma of the bowels after stopping immunosuppressive Azathioprine treatment (Penn 1979). Obviously the sudden change from a type 2 cytokine status to a type 1 cytokine status without prior compensation therapy with cysteine or glutathione (GSH) is risky. These risks, however, do not speak against the correct dosage of the arginine substitution for "HIV positives" in acquired cellular immune weaknesses, wasting syndrome and above all Kaposi's sarcoma. If the glutathione, cysteine, glutamine, and arginine compensations are correctly combined,and the right dosages prescribed, higher concentrations of NO accordingly act in an inhibitory manner whereas lower concentrations of NO force tumor growth rate and regeneration of blood capillaries in tumor cell clusters.

A number of clinical research teams have attempted to bypass the unwanted effects of interleukin-2 therapy in the treatment of cancer, namely capillary leakage (Orucevic 1998), and a drop in blood pressure (Shahidi 1998), by the selective inhibition of NO with NO-inhibitors and the exclusive stimulation of ROS production through an interleukin-2-induced stimulation of tumor necrosis factor. The aim is apoptosis/necrosis of the tumor cells through oxidative stress and the inhibition of nitrosative stress (Chinje 1997, Orucevic 1998). This one-sided process, however, is to be viewed just as critically as the use of interleukin-2 in HIV/AIDS medicine for the "flushing" of "HI viruses" in dormant T4 cells (Cooper 1999). Just as with prooxidative chemotherapeutics, compensated mitochondria in non-tumor cells could be forced to a decompensated Type-II counterregulation (secondary AIDS and secondary cancer) or active tumor cells could be selected to metastatic cells.

The confusion "at a higher level of understanding" of HIV/AIDS and cancer medicine: "At present, standard parenteral nutrition solutions and most enteral feeding formulas do not contain L-glutamine; therefore, repletion is not possible"

It is rationally difficult to comprehend why so few controlled studies have been carried out over the last twenty years in HIV/AIDS medicine on the compensation of the glutathione system and the amino acid dysregulation of "HIV positives," AIDS and Kaposi's sarcoma patients in view of the immense advances in knowledge outside of HIV/AIDS medicine. Even if you assume from the (objectively false) disease theory that "HIV causes AIDS," such treatments should still be mandatory as viruses also use up sulfhydryl groups (SH groups) for replication (Papadopulos-Eleopulos 1988). The fixation on the "HIV infection" and the treatment of the "HIV positive" stigmatized patients with a diversity of counterproductive combinations of aggressive chemotherapeutics that are difficult to keep track of, had led to inadequate and unsatisfactory attempts at therapy resulting in cellular dyssymbiosis in the immune and non-immune cells of these patients. The survey of the clinical researchers at Harvard Medical School reflects the consequence of the "confusion at a higher level of understanding" (Balter 1997):

"Significant weight loss commonly occurs in patients with human immunodeficiency virus (HIV) infection. The extent of loss of body cell mass (BCM), which is the metabolically active tissue of the body, correlates with the length of survival. Attempts to reverse this erosion of protein-rich tissue with appetite stimulants, oral nutritional supplements and enteral or parenteral nutrition have resulted in deposition of adipose tissue, with variable or no restoration of BCM (Kotler 1990, 1991, Chlebowski 1993, Van Roenn 1994). Recombinant human growth hormone administration resulted in gain in lean tissue, but the effects were not sustainable once treatment was terminated (Krentz 1993) .... At present, standard parenteral nutrition solutions and most enteral feeding formulas do not contain L-glutamine (GLN); therefore, repletion is not possible .... This study demonstrates for the first time that the provision of a specific nutrient supplement, when coupled with nutritional counseling, can improve weight and restore BCM .... The 40.0 g GLN dose was selected because open label studies providing 30.0 and 40.0 g GLN/d have demonstrated marked weight gain and improvement in BCM, and a blinded pilot study using 20.0 g GLN/d failed to demonstrate consistent results (Young 1992) .... Larger multicenter studies [a pooling of research between a number of clinics] are needed to determine whether GLN-antioxidants will support BCM and reduce the incidence of infection over the long term, as has been observed in other populations like bone marrow transplant patients (Ziegler 1992), low birth weight infants (Neu 1997) and surgical patients with multiple trauma (Houdijk 1998)" (Shabert 1999).

A comparative analysis of the experimental and clinical data for the prophylaxis and treatment of wasting syndrome (cachexia) combined with cellular immune weakness by means of prooxidative chemotherapy versus antioxidative supplementation therapy

The reference to "other patient groups" demonstrates that 20 years after the beginning of the so-called AIDS era, the clinical researchers of the Harvard Medical School still have not quite mastered the synergistic interactions of wasting syndrome in systemic diseases like AIDS and cancer. To this end there is no need of elaborate multicenter studies, just a simple balance sheet. The elite scientists at the Deutsches Krebsforschungzentrum, Stanford University and the Harvard Medical School are all agreed that the chances of survival from AIDS, cancer and other systemic diseases are dependent on the degree of development of wasting syndrome (cachexia) and that this is the main cause of death. At the same time there is also agreement that all systemic diseases involve a massive disruption to cellular immunity (AIDS) and that wasting syndrome and cellular immunity disruptions have the same fundamental origins. There is yet further agreement that in contrast to all other systemic diseases, the sole primary cause of HIV/AIDS is of an infectious nature ("retroviral HIV infection"). Thus there is also consensus among the clinical research teams that the "HIV positive" patients have to be treated indefinitely with prooxidative "anti-retroviral" chemotherapy and at the same time an antioxidative "supplementation therapy" (Hack 1997, Dröge 1997 b, Herzenberg 1997, Shabert 1999). The disagreement lies in the combination and dosage of the antioxidative "supplementation therapy" in "HIV positives."

Consensus, illogic, deficits and suppression of research regarding individual disposition factors in the preventive and therapeutic study of wasting syndrome

The synoptic analysis of these, at least, differentiated clinical publications on preventative and therapeutic cysteine and glutamine compensation therapy of patients with cellular immunity weakness and wasting syndrome demonstrate:

- The clinical research team prescribed prooxidative chemotherapy to patients with weakened immunity and Type-II cellular dyssymbiosis without clinical or experimental evidence that these substances could inhibit cellular immunity weaknesses, wasting syndrome, Kaposi's sarcoma, lymphoma, muscle and nerve cell degradation, inflammatory bowel syndrome and other serious infectious and non-infectious symptoms.
- The many publications about certain evidence that these prooxidative substances are mitochondriotoxic, genotoxic and thiol-consuming and cause AIDS, cancer and muscle and nerve cell degradation etc. were not referenced by any of the research teams.
- None of the research teams published an overview of the important immunological parameters and the cytokine status of the patients before, during or after the controlled treatment phases.
- None of the research teams reported about the combined use of immune-modulating and redox-stabilizing non-protein thiols, cysteine and glutathione or about the synergistic amino acids, glutamine and arginine.

- None of the research teams discussed a specific use of synergistic compensation therapy regarding the particular detoxification and elimination capacities of the individual patients.

The alleged "risk of infection" in risk groups was falsely and excessively overestimated for propaganda reasons, since in addition to the risk-exposure, individual illness-disposing factors are crucial to the incidence of "HIV characteristics" (similarly so with cancer and other systemic illnesses)

Knowledge of the factors involved in the individual disposition to illness have an especially important bearing on fundamental understanding of the diagnosis and the preventative and therapeutic necessity in pre-AIDS and AIDS and other systemic diseases. *The "HIV characteristics" are real, bioenergetic, biochemical and immunologic phenomena, which can be precisely and extensively explained by means of more recent insights in research on cellular symbiosis, glutathione, cytokines, NO and immunity, without the effects of any "HI viruses."* These insights also supply an answer to the crucial question of why precisely the antibodies of patients from so-called risk groups, in Western countries, react to the proteins in the "HIV test."

The term risk group means that the people are exposed to an exceptional load of risks or were exposed to them at an earlier point in time before the "anti-HIV antibody test." Closer examination, however, shows that the exposure to risk is not the only determining factor as to whether the number of antibodies in blood serum is sufficiently high to cross the highly contrived sensitivity threshold for a positive reaction in "HIV tests."

"HIV positive" homosexual men are indeed numerically the largest risk group of all "HIV positives" in Western countries, but in relation to the total homosexual population their number has remained relatively small. At the end of 1985, 50% of homosexual men were quoted to be HIV-infected. This claim turned out to be completely wrong. In the space of 20 years, conservative estimates of the proportion of homosexual men within the population as a whole amount to 3% and the number of "HIV" infected homosexuals within that group amounts to about 3% to 5% (the smaller the assumed size of the total homosexual population the higher the percentage of officially registered "HIV positives" among homosexuals).

The proportion of "HIV positives" within the second largest group of "HIV infected" individuals, the intravenous drug addicts, was given as about 75%.

This claim was also completely wrong. A constant proportion of between 3 and 5% “HIV positives” was also found after autopsies on dead heroin addicts and in detoxification units.

In contrast, in the numerically smaller groups with congenital coagulation defects, almost exclusively male hemophiliacs, roughly 50% were diagnosed HIV-positive in Germany and about 75% in the USA, although in Germany about ten times the amount of coagulating proteins were substituted and more than 80% of the coagulating protein preparations were imported from the USA. However, in Germany the proportion of AIDS patients among the “HIV positive” hemophiliacs in the six cities with the highest “HIV” loads (Berlin, Hamburg, Düsseldorf, Cologne, Frankfurt, Munich) is twice that of other cities although the percentage of AIDS incidence among “HIV infected” hemophiliacs cannot be dependent on place of residence.

All these figures show that the claims of an “HIV infection” are completely wrong and thus the numerical data of HIV/AIDS medicine in Western countries, and likewise in developing countries, completely lose track of the biological reality (CDC 1999, WHO 1998, Robert-Koch-Institute 1999, Fiala 1998, 2000, Duesberg 2000).

The exposure factor primarily comes from specific risks through excessive prooxidative stress, and secondarily through chemotherapy against the alleged HIV infection (as shown by the example of the doubled number of AIDS cases of hemophiliacs, who in the named cities were increasingly involved in clinical studies with chemotherapeutics (Kremer 1998 a, 1998 c)).

The variability of the blood types, serum proteins, enzyme groups and tissue-typing cell proteins, cause among other things individual disposition factors (genotypic and phenotypic multiformity = polymorphism, Gr. poly = many, morphe = shape)

Evidently a genetic disposition factor is included. For a long time the correlation between the blood group and certain illnesses like cancer, asthma, rheumatoid arthritis etc. has been known. Blood group characteristics in red blood cells are carbohydrates that can be differentiated in individuals but also in races, and they are determined by means of a certain genetic variability (multiformity of the genotype, polymorphism). This polymorphism, however, simultaneously corresponds to the inherited polymorphism of serum protein groups, of intracellular enzyme groups and of the human leucocyte antigen, locus A (HLA) systems. The latter are present in differing numbers as sugar proteins on the surface of the cells of almost all tissues. The HLA gene complex, the major histocompatibility complex (MHC) located on chromosome 6, which covers about a thousandth of the human genome, provides an extraordinary number of HLA phenotypes and is divided into four main areas. There are interactions between the various HLA types and certain illnesses. HLA-D region antigens appear only in certain cells, above all activated T-cells, B-cells, macrophages and their precursor cells—the monocytes. They play an important role in the interaction between the antigen-presenting cells and the cells operating the immune response.

Already in the 1970s it was recognized in the USA and Canada that kidney patients, who developed opportunistic infections and Kaposi's sarcoma during immunosuppressive treatment with Azathioprine, were overproportionally of Jewish, Italian or African descent and that in these patients the HLA-DR5 locus was dominant. It was assumed that as a result of genetic deviation of HLA-DR5 locus even a relatively low immunosuppression could trigger Kaposi's sarcoma:

"Moreover, it has not escaped our notice that X-linkage [an abnormal constellation of male X chromosomes] is frequent among the congenital immune deficiency disorders, and that the male: female ratio is high both in renal transplant and in AIDS patients (including nonhomosexual patients). These observations suggest both DR-5 and X-linkage as important factors in the etiology of AIDS" (Levine 1984; O'Harra 1982, Harwood 1984).

Various proofs for the exemplary interaction of exposure and disposition factors with "HIV positive" hemophiliacs and the refutation of "HIV infection" from cell-free blood clotting proteins

The only group of patients at risk from "HIV"/AIDS who have unquestionable congenital disposition factors are male hemophiliacs. These patients with deficient factor VIII (more unusually factor IX) of the coagulation cascade due to a congenital defect have to regularly inject individual doses of these clotting factors, depending on the degree of severity, to prevent continuous bleeding. In these patients the interplay between exposition and disposition is obvious:

"As Levine has pointed out: "To understand the occurrence of AIDS in hemophilia, it is important to recognize that each vial of factor VIII concentrate will contain, depending on manufacturer and lot number, a distillate of clotting factors, alloantigenic proteins, and infectious agents obtained from between 2500 and 25,000 blood or plasma donors". Until recently, of all the protein injected in factor VIII preparations, factor VIII accounted for only about 0.03-0.05% of the total. The rest included: albumin, fibrin(ogen), immunoglobulins and immune complexes (Eyster, 1978, Mannucci, 1992). Even the recent 'high-purity' factor VIII contains 'potentially harming proteins' such as isoagglutinins, fibrin(ogen), split products, immunoglobulins and, when monoclonal antibodies are used for factor VIII preparation, murine proteins in addition to albumin." (Papadopulos-Eleopulos 1995 b).

Strangely enough, nobody could discover any molecular evidence of "HI viruses" in the clotting proteins, and yet still it was suggested to the "HIV positive" hemophiliacs that they were infected with the apparently deadly HI viruses through the clotting protein injection. Logically, "HIV characteristics" can be provoked *exclusively in cell cultures* through prooxidative stress and cytokine stimulation as a result of Type-II counterregulations. Therefore this laboratory trick will not work in *cell-free* clotting protein concentrates. The lack of evidence of "HIV characteristics" in the factor VIII preparations conclusively rebuts the supposed "HIV transmission," as well as the laboratory findings of "HIV positivity" in hemophiliacs as apparent evidence that the positive test reaction must have been caused by an "HIV infection" through injection of clotting protein concentrates. *According to the logic of the HIV/AIDS theory, the wives or partners of hemophiliacs must have infected themselves with "HI viruses" through unprotected intercourse before the introduction of the "HIV tests" at the end of 1984, however, there is no evidence for this. It was proven, however, in a number of studies that the "HIV positivity" of hemophiliacs depends on the total amount of foreign proteins received in a lifetime.* After introduction of genetically-produced (recombinant) factor VIII preparations, the number of new "HIV" infections abruptly dropped to levels below those of HIV negative hemophiliacs (overview Papadopulos-Eleopulos 1995 b, Duesberg 1995).

The findings of these studies answer the question of why precisely these patients had an "HIV seroconversion," that is to say a reversal of the "HIV test" result from "HIV negative" to "HIV positive" as reaction to the human cell proteins of the test antigens of the "HIV test." There is a logical link between disposition and exposure which is completely independent of the impact of "HI viruses" given that the "HIV positives" at the time of the "HIV seroconversion" have a systemic glutathione deficiency (Eck 1989, Buhl 1989, Roederer 1990) and feature a reprogramming from a type 1 cytokine profile to a type 2 cytokine profile (Clerici 1994, overview Lucey 1996), and that a long-term type 2 cytokine profile effects a long-term inhibition of cytotoxic NO production (overview Lincoln 1997). It can be assumed that the hemophiliacs, as a consequence of their genetic disposition, belong to the group of people whose redox status is more sensitive, who even with a relatively minor reduction in the thiol pool (reduced glutathione, cysteine) react with a shift in the type 1 to type 2 cytokine balance. The constant irritation to the antigen-presenting cells and the T-4 cell systems through injection of a diversity of foreign proteins (alloantigens) and the prooxidative effect of the increased amounts of prophylactic factor VIII in themselves cause a continuously increasing consumption of thiol. Beyond a critical threshold of the glutathione levels in the antigen-presenting cells, depending on the redox status, a shift to the dominant biosynthesis of type 2 cytokine profile in T-4 cells is provoked (Peterson 1998). The result is an inhibition of cytotoxic NO gas production and the increased production of polyspecific and autoantibodies (Hässig 1996 c, Wang 1999). Above a certain number of antibodies the sensitivity threshold of the "HIV test" is exceeded and the quantative intensity of the reaction of antibodies in the blood serum of hemophiliacs to the human cell proteins of the so-called "HIV test" registers an "HIV positive" result.

Political hush money for the hemophiliac "victims" and the show trial against transfusion doctors strengthened the suggestive belief in the "deadly HIV mass-contagion" (During the 1993-1994 chemotherapy disaster, it was scientifically and medically undeniable that the main cause of illness and death for AIDS and wasting syndrome was the standard administration of AZT etc. and Bactrim etc. in lieu of redox compensation)

As the first "HIV positive" hemophiliacs, in the belief of a supposed deadly HIV infection, submitted a lawsuit against the German government concerning violation of the legal provisions of the German drug laws on surveillance of the production of factor VIII, a spectacular parliamentary board of enquiry was organized. On the basis of the board's report, the German parliament decided to pay 2,000 DM per month to "HIV positive" hemophiliacs and 3,000 DM per month to hemophiliac AIDS sufferers from taxpayer's money. But the pharmaceutical companies, the producers of the factor VIII concentrate, were exempted from payment. The international experts, who had been questioned by the board, had remained reticent in full knowledge and willful of the medical facts, which very definitely spoke against an "HIV infection" of hemophiliacs (Deutsches Bundestag 1994). The hemophiliacs accepted the material compensation and carried on being treated "prophylactically" with aggressive chemotherapy that had already cost many of their lives. At the same time show trials were staged in a number of countries against doctors who, either belatedly or inadequately, should have sterilized blood and blood products against "HI viruses" that nobody had actually isolated and against the "HIV characteristics" in factor VIII preparations that nobody had been able to find. With this strategy the belief in a deadly HIV mass contagion was consolidated by those affected and in the public consciousness with the help of a media who, just like doctors, politicians and pharmaceutical companies feared a loss of credibility and lawsuits for damages if the blatant research errors and resulting treatment were to become known. The silent majority of ethically aware but ill-informed doctors acted passively; the dimensions of the organized scientific swindle obviously transcended their power of imagination.

The individual disposition for quicker and long-lasting glutathione depletion explains why in the homosexual and drug-injecting risk groups, given the same or higher risk exposure, only a consistently low percentage of the exposed individuals develop a strong and/or persistent type 2 cytokine shift (Th1-Th2 switch) that activates the production of higher quantities of polyspecific antibodies ("HIV positive" test result)

The evolutionary-biologically programmed interplay between disposition and exposure also explains much of what is puzzling in the risk groups of homosexuals and intravenous drug addicts, for instance why with the same excessive prooxidative exposure only a small percentage of those affected, contrary to the speculative claims of HIV/AIDS physicians, had developed an "HIV seroconversion." In principle, everyone can have polyspecific antibodies and autoantibodies in blood serum that can react to the human cellular proteins of the test antigens of the "HIV test."

Additionally the patients have to be genetically predisposed in such a way that the average glutathione depletion of 30%, apparent in "HIV positives," is sufficient to trigger a type 2 cytokine dominance that in turn stimulates an unusually high number of antibodies. Thus, besides the prooxidative exposure, there must be a genetic disposition that activates the redox-dependent genetic expression for the biosynthesis of type 2 cytokine proteins more quickly and for a longer time span than people with the same prooxidative glutathione depletion. *As the disposition to early type 2 cytokine stimulation leads simultaneously to the inhibition of cytotoxic NO gas production, these people will not be sufficiently capable to eliminate intracellular fungi, mycobacteria, and other opportunistic agents, therefore the antibody levels will continue to rise via antibody production against the "opportunistic agents" that are usually easy to repel with NO gas. Even* in cases of a relatively low glutathione depletion, such people genetically predisposed to greater redox sensitivity will switch to a type 2 cytokine dominance, which chokes NO gas production and forms a high number of polyspecific and autoreactive antibodies (i.e. "HIV positivity"), while those with a less sensitive predisposition either will not adjust the cytokine balance, or alter it only temporarily. Precisely the same reaction over-readiness is observed in both organ transplant and surgical patients. The majority of transplant patients exhibited a variable cytokine balance without developing Kaposi's sarcoma (KS) and opportunistic infections (OI), while roughly 6% had a particular immune status corresponding to a persistent type 2 cytokine dominance and suffered from KS and OI. Similarly the surgical patients, of whom more than 50% had weak or anergic DTH skin reactions (as expression of a deficient Th1 reactivity) before operations, switched from a type 1 cytokine to type 2 cytokine balance, which in most cases normalized on the seventh day after the operation. However, those patients who maintained a dominant type 2 cytokine reaction (roughly 5% of the preoperative anergic patients) developed a significant sepsis (microbial proliferation) with a high mortality rate.

There is a striking similarity between the percentage of patients with primary persistent cellular immune weaknesses of a type 2 cytokine dominance in both organ transplant and sepsis patients, and the percentage of patients in the homosexual and drug-abusing subpopulations (in the USA annually 5% of all "HIV positives" are registered as AIDS cases, including the symptom-free "HIV positives" with a T-4 cell count in the bloodstream under 200 per microliter) (CDC 1999). This supports the view that disposition factors also play an integral role in determining whether a thiol deficit caused by primary prooxidative stress, triggers such a sustained Type-II counterregulation of cellular dyssymbiosis that the associated glutathione depletion, in cases of persistent prooxidative exposure to risk and/or secondary prooxidative chemotherapy without compensatory therapy, advances until clinically the procedural events of symptom-free "HIV positives" move from the transitory phase of pre-AIDS to the phase of a T-4 cell count of below 200 per microliter or to the manifest stage of opportunistic infections, wasting syndrome, muscle and nerve cell degeneration, and/or tumorigenesis.

The information gathered in the 1970s that organ transplant patients with OI and/or KS (AIDS) predominantly showed signs of a particular anomaly in the HLA system (MHC class II) (O'Hara 1982), did not interest the virus hunters anymore after the disease theory "HIV causes AIDS" was proclaimed as the official global doctrine. The fact that the only common grounds of the risk groups that precede the later appearance of clinical AIDS are the early systemic glutathione deficit, the type 2 cytokine switch, the inhibition of cytotoxic NO gas production, the mitochondrial deactivation and the glycolytic energy production of an increasing wasting syndrome, was largely ignored by the HIV/AIDS establishment. *Similarly, the only genetically homogenous risk group, the hemophiliacs—dependent on exposure to highly contaminated clotting factor preparations for life, as a subpopulation—had by far the highest "HIV" incidence (10 to 15 times higher than the genetically inhomogenous subpopulations of homosexuals and drug abusers), although, even within the framework of the HIV/AIDS theory, there was no evidence of "HIV characteristics" in the only possible medium of transmission: the cell-free (!) clotting protein preparations* (overview Papadopulos-Eleopulos 1995 b).

In striking contrast, in the homosexual and intravenous drug abuser risk groups, the anal passageway via semen, and the bloodstream contaminated via dirty needles were considered ideal modes of transmission by HIV/AIDS scientists. However, the propagandists of HIV transmission could not explain why, in sharp contrast to their forecasts that have never been revised, with the same potential transmission risks in the homosexual and intravenous drug abuser risk groups, only a relatively small and constant percentage of homosexuals and drug abusers developed an "HIV seroconversion" over the last 15 years in comparison to the total population of these risk groups.

The dogmatically submitted prognoses over the last fifteen years were 10 to 15 times higher than the actual number of "HIV" cases among homosexuals and intravenous drug abusers (CDC 1999, WHO 1998, Robert Koch Institute 1999, Duesberg, 1998, 2000, Fiala 2000).

For instance, there are some 20,000 intravenous drug abusers in Germany's prisons. The legal authorities have repeatedly claimed in public that they cannot prevent the injection of heroin and other substances, above all the multiple use of needles, in prisons. If we assume that only every other imprisoned drug addict uses a used needle per day, then over 15 years there would have been roughly 55 million opportunities to transmit the "HI viruses." Experts and politicians from all parties have denounced prisons as the most dangerous places for the spreading of the "deadly mass contagion of HIV." Upon arrival in prison every drug abuser is routinely tested for syphilis, hepatitis B and for "HIV positivity." The number of people refusing the tests is small. The quota of "HIV positive" drug abusers has remained constantly low for 15 years. For many years there was also a test upon release of drug abusers to see whether there had been an "HIV seroconversion" from "HIV negative" to "HIV positive" during the time in prison. The penal laws stipulate that the "health of prisoners has to be provided for" and that "dangers to the public have to be averted."

The fact that in places with the highest density of drug injection, not a single "HIV seroconversion" during the time in prison could be found in 15 years (in contrast to proven hepatitis B seroconversions), proves the fiction of "HIV transmission" and the individual dependency of disposition factors for the development of a persistent Th2 immune cell dominance ("HIV positive" test result)

The results were always the same: not one single case of an "HIV seroconversion" was found during a drug abuser's time in prison, however, there certainly were hepatitis B seroconversions. These findings completely contradict the HIV/AIDS theory. Seemingly puzzling, they are easy to explain. In 1988, the author had predicted precisely these results—that there would not be a single HIV seroconversion in prison—and suggested that after 10 years the collected data should be analyzed, as this would have been an involuntary mass experiment, carried out in the largest possible closed society in a public building maintained and controlled by the state, with a high percentage of drug abusers and thus a high risk of infections with "HI viruses."

In 1998 the leading representatives of HIV/AIDS medicine of public health systems were not even willing just to discuss the results. They simply disclaimed the indubitable facts and continued selling the transmission of the supposed deadly mass contagion in prisons to the unsuspecting public. The affected "HIV positive" drug abusers continued being prescribed combined chemotherapy. As a large proportion of the drug abusers shuttled between various drug scenes, outpatient and inpatient therapy, as well as prison over the last 15 years, the cases of transmission of "HI viruses" among "HIV positive" drug abusers, according to the official predictions of HIV/AIDS medical community must have increased in terms of percentage. But this is simply not the case: the incidence of "HIV infection" in test studies at ambulatory and inpatient drug centers and during drug therapy, in prisons and of autopsies after drug-related deaths, remains constantly low. These data and facts clearly refute the theory of rampant "HIV" transmission by used needles.

Longitudinal studies of "HIV positive" drug abusers who had stopped their intravenous drug consumption or were accepted for an oral methadone substitution program, also contest HIV transmission through used needles. In these cases the immune cell status improved quickly in comparison to drug abusers who had continued with intravenous drug consumption, despite the "HIV infection" (Des Jarlais 1987, Weber 1990, overview Duesberg 1996, 1998). In these cases the "HIV test" remained positive because of the continuously available sustained numbers of polyspecific antibodies in the blood serum of the now drug-free former drug abusers. This fact is one of the many fundamental pieces of evidence that "HIV infection" does not exist.

If we assume, however, that there are genetic and non-genetic disposition factors that favor the development of a progressive thiol deficiency as a result of drug consumption in a relatively small percentage (3 to 5%) of drug abusers but not the majority, then the facts can be explained. In excessive intravenous exposure to drugs the disposition factors for increased redox sensitivity in cases of relatively low degradation of the reduced glutathione levels could cause a sustained shift in balance to a type 2 cytokine profile as well as a reduced cellular immune response in favor of a greatly increased humoral antibody response. The non-elimination of intracellular agents conditioned by this further increases antibody activity. This process is triggered in predisposed drug abusers, just as in predisposed homosexuals at an early stage of excessive glutathione consuming exposure. The hugely increased numbers of antibodies can be quantitively and qualitatively sufficient to interact with the human cellular test proteins of the "HIV tests" and to induce a positive test result. As drug abusers generally have had a drug career before being imprisoned, the predisposed drug abusers are already "HIV positive" on entering prison. The majority of non-predisposed drug abusers with the same or higher exposure have constantly been "HIV negative" on entry and remain so despite continued exposure to contaminated needles. However, unwittingly, imprisoned "HIV positive" and "HIV negative" drug abusers makes for the most wide-ranging exposure and disposition study that has taken place in Western countries in the last 15 years. 20,000 drug abusers, under state-run supervision, could be observed day to day in Germany alone. There were analogous findings in all other Western countries. The 1988 prognosis, predicted by the author of this book in his capacity as medical director of the largest social therapeutic rehabilitation clinic for delinquent drug addicts in Germany from 1981-1988, was completely confirmed; the alternative prognosis of HIV/AIDS medicine was completely disproved. *These findings clearly demonstrate that toxic exposure and individual disposition are the real causes of pre-AIDS and AIDS.*

The dependency upon disposition for the occurrence of Type-I overregulation and the following Type-II counterregulation is reflected in both the total population and the risk groups, as a Gaussian (bell-shaped) distribution curve with the vast majority of exposed individuals having a variable immune balance and flexible cytokine pattern; however with chemotherapeutic exposure a generalized weakness of intra—and extracellular immunity emerges

Disposition factors can be epidemiologically justified. They also explain why the pathogenetic distribution patterns manifest in a Gaussian distribution curve, equally for excessive expositions as in collective populations and differing risk groups. While the majority of the exposed individuals will maintain a variable redox balance with flexible cytokine patterns, a minor percentage will develop a distinct Type-I overreaction or a distinct Type-II counterreaction. To presume a fatal mass-infection transmissible to everybody, ending in inevitable death was *a priori* a medical construction beyond the biological-evolutionary reality.

In the case of the "HIV-induced" AIDS, it seemed particularly questionable to presume that the humoral (antibody-supported) immunity was operating successfully (Mildvan 1982) while the cellular immunity of the T4 helper cells against intracellular germs failed, so opportunistic infections could develop. Once patients were treated with AZT chemotherapy massive bacterial infections happened as a consequence of maturation inhibition of bone marrow cells (Rosenthal 1994, Marco 1998, Cox 1998). Because the evolutionary and biologically programmed coaction of exposition and disposition factors had not been sufficiently understood, HIV/AIDS medicine provoked the appearance of combined acquired cellular and humoral immune deficiency SCID (severe combined immunodeficiency). The untoward result was the prescription of chemotherapeutics on the basis of the objectively incorrect theory that "HIV causes AIDS."

The clinical and epidemiologic results demonstrate the deficits of modern medicine with abundant clarity. Modern medicine, in its submission to the monied interests of pharmaceutical companies, and the media oversimplification of lobbied politicians, let alone its own information overload and stubborn arrogance, has woefully underestimated the toxic and pharmacotoxic stressors that were its own prescription. The one-sided fixation on outdated 19th century infection theories combined with sophisticated 20th century biotechnological methods has made for a deadly combination.

The actual number of reported AIDS cases in Africa is "surprisingly" low, in sharp contrast to the propagandistic numbers of the media and international organizations; disposition factors have not been closely investigated in relation to this population's generally increased exposure to multiple stressors, since these factors are not recorded during African "HIV" testing practices

The HIV and AIDS establishment's massive projection of a supposed pandemia (mortal infection spreading on whole populations) reveals that even in the case of doubtless increased collective charging with immune stressors (endemic multi-infectiosity, contaminated drinking water, undernourishment, adverse living conditions et al.), special disposition factors must supervene when triggering acquired immunodeficiency.

Professor Duesberg, retrovirus cancer scientist and molecular biologist at Berkeley, California, one of the most severe critics of the "HIV causes AIDS" theory, considers the "HI virus" to be a "passenger virus." He too regards toxic reasons such as excessive consumption of illegal drugs, nitrite inhalation as sexual doping agent, medical chemotherapy and also the injection of highly contaminated clotting protein factors against hemophilia to be the real causes of AIDS in Western countries (Duesberg 1996). On the occasion of the Pretoria specialists' conference, summoned by President Mbeki before the XIII World AIDS Conference in July 2000 (see chapter XII), he stated:

"In the light of this hypothesis the new epidemic of HIV-antibodies would simply reflect a new epidemic of HIV-antibody testing, introduced and inspired by new American biotechnology. This technology was developed during the last 20 years for basic research to detect the equivalents of biological needles in a haystack, but not to "detect" the massive invasions of viruses that are necessary to cause ALL conventional viral diseases (Duesberg 1992 a, Duesberg 1992 b, 1996, 1998, Mullis, 1996, 1998). But this technology is now faithfully but inappropriately used by thousands of AIDS virus researchers and activists to detect latent, i.e. biochemically and biologically inactive HIV or even just antibodies against it (Duesberg 1996 a)! The same technology also provides job security for other virologists and doctors searching for latent, and thus biologically inactive, viruses as their preferred causes of Kaposi's sarcoma, cervical cancer, leukemia, liver cancer, and rare neurological diseases—without ever producing any public health benefits (Duesberg 1992 a) . . . To all of us who have been subjected to the American AIDS rhetoric, and indeed the rhetoric of our first meeting in Pretoria last May, about the 'catastrophic dimensions' of African AIDS (Washington Post, April 30, 2000), the healthy African growth rates come as a big surprise. Take as an example of this rhetoric President Clinton's recent designation of AIDS as a 'threat to US national security' . . . . spurred by US intelligence reports that looked at the pandemic's broadest consequences, ... particularly Africa . . . . [and] projected that a quarter of southern Africa's population is likely to die of AIDS . . . . (Washington Post, April 30, 2000).

The alarming tone of WHO's joint United Nations Program on HIV/AIDS, 'AIDS epidemic update: December 1999' (UNAIDS December 1999), announcing that Africa had gained 23 million 'living with HIV/AIDS,' because they are "estimated" carriers of antibodies against HIV, since the "early 1980s" (WHO, Weekly Epidemiological Record 73, 373-380, 1998) is equally surprising in view of information available to the agency. Neither the WHO nor the United Nations point out that Africa had gained 147 million people during the same time in which the continent was said to suffer from a new

AIDS epidemic. Likewise, South Africa has grown from 17 million to 37 million in 1990 (United Nations Environment Programme, June 15, 2000), and to 44 million now ("HIV/AIDS in the Developing World," U.S. Agency for International Development & U.S. Census Bureau, May 1999). In the last decade South Africa has also gained 4 million HIV-positive people (A. Kinghorn and M. Steinberg, South African Department of Health, undated document probably from 1998, provided at the Pretoria meeting). Thus South Africa has gained 4 million HIV-positives during the same decade in which it grew by 7 million people. Moreover, although the 23 million 'estimated' HIV-antibody positives are said to be 'living with HIV/AIDS' by the WHO, the agency does not offer any evidence for morbidity or mortality exceeding the modest numbers, i.e. about 75,000 cases annually, reported by the it's Weekly Epidemiological Records (0.012% of Africa's whole population) (WHO Weekly Epidemiological Records 73, 373-380, 1998). The agency's estimates of HIV-positives are indeed just 'estimates' because, according to the 1985-Bangui definition of African AIDS as well as to the current 'Anonymous AIDS Notification' forms of the South African Department of Health, no HIV tests are required for an AIDS diagnosis (Widy-Wirski et al., 1988; Fiala, 1998).

In addition, the WHO promotes the impression of a microbial AIDS epidemic by reporting African AIDS cases cumulatively rather than annually (WHO's Weekly Epidemiological Records since the beginning of the epidemic). This practice creates the deceptive impression of an ever growing, almost exponential epidemic, even if the annual incidence declines (Fiala, 1998). It would follow that the estimated increases in African HIV antibody (!)-positives do not correlate with decreases in any African population. On the contrary, they correlate with unprecedented simultaneous increases in the country's populations—hardly the 'catastrophe' imagined by the Washington Post and propagated by the WHO and the American AIDS establishment. But this deceptive AIDS propaganda biases a scientific analysis of African AIDS by all those who are not aware of the facts" (Duesberg 2000).

In other words, the actual figures recorded in the WHO epidemiological reports on total morbidity and death rates in African states are hardly higher than in Western countries. Namely 0.012% of Africa's total population fall ill and die of AIDS per year (WHO Weekly Epidemiological reports since 1991), compared to 0.001 to 0.002% of total populations in Western countries (CDC 1999, Robert Koch Institute 1999). The absurd propagandistic claims insisting on a "African pandemic" distributed to the international media by the WHO are based on arbitrary extrapolation of small random samples received by abusing the "American biotechnology" that uses the "anti HIV antibody test" (Duesberg 2000).

Based on the not very reliable acquisition of pathogen data, compared to Western countries and because of the small fund of medical research results in developing countries, it is much less obvious to draw conclusions on the exposition and disposition interaction for morbidity and mortality in causal connection with systemic diseases of Type-II cell dyssymbiosis. However the population explosion data in African countries shows comparability with demographic processes in Western countries 150 years ago. With gradual improvement in living conditions and medical and social standards, infectious disease rates will decline and toxic stress will increase. Increased collective charge, irrespective of gender, with variegated immunostressors with simultaneously "surprising" (Duesberg 2000) low AIDS incidence (WHO Weekly Epidemiological Records since 1991) when compared to Western countries and the parallel population explosion in Africa give reason to presume that disposition factors must play a role. The consequences for developing countries as for Western countries are the same: protection from the abuse of "American biotechnology" (Duesberg 2000) and the "blessings" of Western chemotherapy and chemoantibiotics while promoting knowledge on evolutionary biologically programmed redox protection.

Over the course of evolution it was favorable to have the individual disposition for an exceptionally redox-sensitive Th2 immune response against invasive extracellular agents, yet in contemporary times it is now a disadvantage; the toxic and pharmacotoxic immune stressors prevalent in modern civilization trigger exactly the same redox-sensitive immune response, and after exhaustion of the redox control system can provoke a persistent Type-II cellular dyssymbiosis (AIDS, cancer and other systemic illnesses) in such predisposed individuals

Disposition factors act via the peroxidation control system (creation of hydrogen peroxides, H_2O_2 and lipid oxides) and nitrosylation of transcription proteins (bonding NO and NO derivatives with hydrogen sulphide groups of proteins containing cysteine, RSNO). In the case of too high glutathione consumption this control system initially raises, as a sensor, the activity of antioxidative genes and the metabolization of H_2O_2, lipidperoxidation and RSNO (Hausladen 1996). After depletion of the neosynthesis of glutathione and other antioxidative enzymes (catalase, superoxide dismutase, selenium dependent glutathione peroxidase, glutathione transferases, NADPH-dependent glutathione reductase), the hypoxic/pseudohypoxic emergency routine is switched on. From an evolutionary biological point of view, the early and sustained switch of the cytokine balance to humoral and antibody-supported immune response was advantageous, because the bacterial threat predominant in the course of the evolution could be efficiently averted. Bacteria proliferate faster than opportunistic pathogens. They can be inhibited and destroyed efficiently through the defense mechanisms of non cell-related humoral immunity, complement formation, opsonization (coating of bacteria membranes by special target molecules for antibodies) and by the antibodies themselves, which are formed by B-cells matured in the bone marrow. The larger fungal and parasitic pathogens, equipped with mitochondria, and mycobacteria with a special cell membrane are stopped most efficiently by interaction between the non-specific and specific immune cell networks. If not inhibited in time by the gas attack, many parasites can invalidate the NO gas synthesis via special surface molecules (glyco-inositol phospholipids).

Multicellular (extracellular) parasites can emit specialized enzymes, which attack tissues (proteinases), and trigger a type 2 cytokine response (Th2 immune response) as a suitable form of reaction, since combating worms, for example, would require too large quantities of NO gas which would in turn damage the body's own tissue cells. Metastatic cancer cells also utilize the biochemical supply of proteinases for pervading tissue and thereby deactivate the NO gas production in neighboring cells. Cancer cells are characterized by low NO gas synthesis (Ignarro 2000) and greatly affected by high NO gas levels (Xie 1996, Chinje 1997). All in all, a one-sided Th2 (cytokine 2) immune response is a disadvantageous disposition for blocking intracellular pathogens (fungi, parasites, mycobacteria, some virus species) and the inhibition of metastatic cancer cells (Zvibel 1993, Liew 1994, 1995 a, 1995b, Mosmann 1996, Abbas 1996, Lucey 1996, Xie 1996). Immune defense depends on an appropriate and flexible combination of defense and regulation strategies.

On balance, the importance of the evolutionary advantage of a redox-sensitive sustained type 2 cytokine immune response has changed through advances in civilization and the developments in modern medicine, especially on introduction of vaccination programs and antibiotics over the last 50 years, while toxic and pharmacotoxic effects of the impact of civilization have gained in importance as a threat to cellular symbiosis.

People with a particularly redox-sensitive disposition are now at a disadvantage because they respond to toxic influences faster and with a more sustained Type-II counterregulation that would be better suited to the inhibition of extracellular bacteria or multicellular parasites.

Thus, the immune system chooses the evolutionary biologically programmed, but "wrong" strategy, because it is mislead by toxic stressors, which did not exist as part of natural evolution. This development is reflected in the steady rise of cancer and other systemic diseases over the last 100 years in the industrialized countries. Today, the main sources of toxic exposition which favor the development of cancer and other systemic diseases in the industrialized countries are: toxin residues in nutrition, in the environment and at working places, and the use of tobacco (Loeppky 1994, Walker 1998, Waite 1998, North 1998) as well as pharmacotoxic medication and toxic pharmaceutical decomposition products (Kalow 1993). The individually predisposed efficiency of redox-dependent detoxification capacity is the critical disease factor for the actual incidence of Type-II cell dyssymbiosis through toxic and pharmacotoxic nitrosation and peroxidation.

Indicative of an individual disposition for redox-efficiency and the detoxification capacity of the cellular symbiosis, patients with manifest systemic illness depend most urgently on replenishment of the cysteine/glutathione systems

Long after Warburg made his historic declaration at the conference of Nobel laureates held in Lindau on Lake Constance in 1967—that there is no disease whose prime cause is better known than cancer (Warburg 1967)—an expanding field of research has been established which examines in humans the effect of individual metabolic disposition on the detoxification of pharmaceuticals. This field of research was very quickly expanded to include the direct and indirect effects of toxic substances on cancer genesis (overview Kalow 1993, Daly 1994). These studies concentrate, corresponding to the molecular genetic mainstream of cancer research, on the variability of genetic expression for biosynthesis of xenobiotic-metabolizing enzymes (genetic enzyme polymorphism):

"The paradigm for mechanism of action of chemical carcinogens has been well established in model cell culture and animal systems, and studies in humans appear to support the possibility that most cancers are initiated by chemical/dietary exposures and proceed through various stages of preneoplastic lesions consisting of partially transformed cells to full metastatic cancers (Vogelstein 1993). In rodent models, the progression stage can be enhanced by treatment with tumor promoters, which themselves do not necessarily exhibit the properties of carcinogens (Hennings 1993). These chemicals are thought to mediate cell proliferations that fix the mutation in the genome. Another class of chemicals called nongenotoxic carcinogens has been described in rodent model systems (Jackson 1993, Barret 1995, Costa 1995). These agents are not metabolically activated to genotoxic derivatives but presumably alter cell-cycle control. Many nongenotoxic carcinogens are also tumor promoters. However, their mechanisms of action are not presently known.

It is widely held that humans differ in their susceptibilities to cancer. Certain individuals may be more susceptible, whereas others are more resistant to cancer. This may be due to a number of factors including health, nutritional status, and gender. From what is known about the mechanism of action of carcinogens, it is thought that genetic background could play a significant role. The responsible genes are probably those encoding the xenobiotic-metabolizing enzymes (XMEs) that activate or inactivate carcinogens (Gonzalez 1995, Nerbert 1996). Variable levels of expression of these enzymes could result in increased or decreased carcinogen activation. In fact, it is well established that genetic differences occur in expression of XMEs" (Hirvonen 1999).

In other words, genes are effectors in complex, self-organized networks, which under the influence of redox-dependent sensors encourage or discourage the biosynthesis of enzymes. If the enzyme systems are individually more strongly predisposed to activating carcinogens rather than deactivating them, then there are more demands on the antioxidative capacity. The thiol pool and other activities could become exhausted more rapidly from protecting the respiratory chain, the macromolecules and lipids. The result is that in the long-term the redox milieu changes and the dominant cytokine profiles switch, earlier and in a more sustained manner, to type 2 cytokines. The production of nitrogen and oxygen oxides are choked and the highly fluid micro-Gaia milieu transforms permanently to a less fluid milieu.

Dependent on time, re-fetalized tumor cells could form (Type-II counterregulation of cell dyssymbiosis). If in this situation prooxidative chemotherapeutics are in use, the desired apoptosis/necrosis can be selectively forced in a part of the cells (Type-I overregulation of cell symbiosis), but by the same token this can also accelerate a fully developed transformation into metastatic cancer cells inside other cells. Basically, all phases of still-to-be-compensated cellular dyssymbiosis, primarily in tumor tissues but also secondarily in differentiated tissues, can switch over unpredictably to a decompensated cellular dyssymbiosis phase. It is a characteristic of the principle of chemotherapeutic treatment that patients with a particularly redox-sensitive disposition, who become ill because of this genetic and supragenetic predisposed redox sensitivity, will not only have cellular dyssymbiosis in manifest tumor tissues but also in other tissue types and that tumor cells will respond to the targeted attack of chemotherapeutics in manifestly decompensated tissues in a diversity of ways in the various phases. Therefore, there can only be a conditional homogenous responsiveness of tumor cells to chemotherapeutics, and the results of therapy schemata cannot be sufficiently calculated individually. Consequently, for patients with a systemic disease, the distinctive genetic polymorphism of carcinogen-activating detoxification enzymes become manifest in the course of the disease. Redox-sensitive variability of the xenobiotic-metabolizing enzymes applies mainly to cytochrome P450-dependent and flavin-containing monoxygenases, epoxide hydrolases, glutathione transferases, N-acetyl transferases, NAD(P)H-ubiquinone oxidoreductases, myeloperoxidases etc. (overview Wilkinson 1997, Hirvonen 1999). Such patients most urgently require a balancing of the thiol pool and redox state. Chemotherapeutical treatment and the consequent extreme prooxidative stress must inevitably have had a counterproductive effect on patients with systemic diseases because such therapy is normally done without compensating for the depletion of the thiol pool, the dysregulation of amino acids and the cysteine balance; and it is done without moderating the Type-II counterregulations. Chemotherapy triggers the desired destructive cell effects as well as individually non-calculable cell dyssymbiotic counterregulations, causing among other things systemic wasting syndrome.

Genetic tests of questionable value were developed to determine the individually predisposed variability of the isoforms of detoxification enzymes. In the USA, for example, prophylactic mastectomies were performed to avoid breast-cancer on the basis of such genetic tests. Such deterministic prognostics by means of genetic tests are to be viewed most critically for a number of reasons. If they have any significance at all, then at the most as an inducement for purposefully influencing the individual balance and regulation therapies in the interplay between exposition and disposition through nutritional measures.

The deterministic forecast of an individual's disposition based on genetic testing of detoxification-enzyme synthesis is to be criticized for many reasons; in reality, the expression of every single gene is redox-dependent, resting primarily on the relative condition of the bioenergetic redox system

"It is anticipated that rapid advances will be made in methodology to determine potential metabolic at-risk genotypes. These advances may include less invasive collection methods for test samples (e.g., buccal cell and urinary cell samples), automated DNA extraction combined with robotic sample handling, and high-density oligonucleotide array-based genetic test methods. At present, many research laboratories are conducting association studies and contradictory reports are emerging in specialist literature. Several sources of potential bias exist that partly account for these divergent findings, usually an initial small study showing a positive association. This raises the important issue of power calculations in planning subsequent studies. High profile reporting to the public of results of studies that may ultimately turn out to be erroneous is also problematic in this context. Also, there recently has been debate about publication bias—selective publishing of only positive associations. If the potential biases mentioned above are carefully controlled, genetic screening studies may in the near future help us identify susceptible individuals and subgroups in environmentally exposed populations. Companies offer gene tests to individuals and employers. As long as this testing is not scientifically and ethically above reproach, it can benefit only companies selling the tests. There is an urgency to address several important ethical questions with regard to societal and public health" (Hirvonen 1999).

This gene-technological development of tests demonstrates the predominant tendency to overemphasize structural gene aberrations instead of considering the bioenergetic conditions for genetic expression for the biosyntheses of enzyme proteins and studying exposure risks and compensating individual dispositions by non-aggressive prevention.

The guiding criteria for diagnosis among those testing "HIV positive"

All available experimental, clinical and epidemiological data result in the main principles of diagnostics, prophylaxis and therapy of systemic diseases in clinical practices. Pre-AIDS and AIDS, because of the relative straightforwardness of the cause and effect relationship between exposure and predisposing factors, present a good model of the overregulation and counterregulation of the cellular symbiotic interactions in immune and non-immune cells and the consequential systemic processes.

There is no reason for panic should a patient find himself stigmatized as "HIV positive" as a result of the "HIV test."

Death prognoses are an expression of limited medical knowledge rather than justified in biological fact. The period of incubation from the "HIV seroconversion" to manifest symptoms averages 12-15 years. In the USA, where patients are treated aggressively and early with prooxidative chemotherapeutics and chemoantibiotics about 5% of patients stigmatized as HIV positive become ill. Consequently, under these conditions, it would take

20 years for all "HIV positives" to actually become manifestly ill. However the actual incidence depends on the persistence of primary exposure risks, on the secondary exposure risk through the aggressive therapy schedule and on the omission of targeted compensatory and regulatory therapies, if they are necessary in the first place.

A careful anamnesis of the patient is necessary; it is not enough just to state that he belongs to a risk group. Allergy predisposition or atopic skin diseases, asthma etc. can be important indicators for a patient's disposition to type 2 cytokine reactions and increased antibody production. The absence of typical bacterial children's diseases can, with other indicators, also be a sign of a type 2-disposition. As more than 70 symptomatic conditions can result in a positive HIV test reaction and even the HIV/AIDS researchers categorize *a priori* 5% of all confirmed positive "HIV tests" as insignificant diagnostic findings, medical actions cannot and must not be guided by the positive result of the "HIV test," irrespective of the non-isolation of an actual immune weakening "HI virus."

The determination of the immune cell status and antibody status are obligatory. The number of differentiated cells measured within the immune cell network and the immunoglobulin classes cannot alone be considered reliable indicators for the actual existence of an immune cell deficiency in symptom-free patients as, within any healthy population, roughly 5% have T4 cell values below 500 per microliter in their blood stream. For HIV/AIDS medicine this T4 cell count is already interpreted as a reason for chemotherapeutic and chemoantibiotic intervention in patients testing HIV positive. In healthy people the T4 cell counts can even drop below 200 per microliter without a serious loss of cellular immunity functions. Without seriously limiting their functionality, the number of T-helper immune cells in the blood stream depends on multiple influences. Valid information can be obtained through the DTH recall antigen test (antigen recall test of the skin, delayed-type hypersensitivity). A strong DTH test reaction is considered a reliable indicator of the actual functionality of type 1 cytokines, activating a cytotoxic NO defense gas against the intracellular pathogens after antigen stimulation (Christou 1986, 1995, Mosmann 1989, Hässig 1998 b).

(Note: Four weeks after the first publication of this book (in November 2001), the DTH test was withdrawn from circulation worldwide by its producer, the pharmaceutical industrial group, Aventis-Mérieux (which includes the subsidiary Mérieux-Pasteur). As Aventis-Mérieux (now merged with French pharmaceutical group Sanofi) holds the patented monopoly of the DTH test, there is no alternative diagnostic instrument. Biosyn, the German DTH test vendor, pointed out in a written statement that Aventis-Mérieux had for no apparent reason abruptly stopped delivering the DTH test. They, Biosyn, had been trying to get a license for the production of the DTH test, but Aventis-Mérieux prevented their attempt. This strange behavior can only be understood by considering the medical political background. Aventis-Mérieux had at that time (November 2001), been involved in studies using so-called naked DNA as an "anti HIV vaccine" on human experimental subjects in Uganda and Thailand. Such a vaccination was considered to promise billions of dollars in sales. An easy-to-handle DTH test could be detrimental to this purpose. In African countries, for example, the "anti-HIV-antibody test" frequently reacts positive for people previously infected with tuberculosis or malaria pathogens, which have endemic proportions there. In addition, conventional scientists deny any connections of this reaction to an "HIV infection." In such cases, the use of DTH skin reaction tests would show a sufficient Th1 immune cell reaction, if subjects of the test didn't manifest chronically present TB or malaria exposure of clinical relevance. A routine use of a DTH test before a mass-vaccination with naked DNA would consequently have been able to unmask the global "HIV infection" as a scientific campaign of disinformation. In the meantime, experiments with naked DNA against "HIV infection" have been suspended. Only after leukaemia appeared in infants, treated with genetically upgraded stem cells, to fight a serious immune deficiency, has a global moratorium on human trials on gene therapy been declared.)

The acute danger of intracellular opportunistic infections is not only due to the positive result of an "HIV test." A weak or anergic (ineffective) DTH skin test reaction indicates the probability of a prevalent shift to type 2 cytokine status and the danger of opportunistic infections. (Note: Nowadays the cellular immunity can be measured using the lymphocyte transformation test (LTT). This test uses comparable antigens to the no-longer-available DTH skin test but the costs are higher. Alternatively it can be measured by cytokine 1-cytokine 2 profiles for determination of a possible Th1-Th2 switch).

Measurement of the values of reduced glutathione in the plasma, in the lung mucosa and intracellularly in the T4 lymph cells of the blood stream is essential (on the laboratory process, see Buhl 1989, Herzenberg 1997, Nuttall 1998). At the same time, the cyst(e)ine level in the plasma must be determined. Major deviations from the non-protein thiol norms must be treated, even in symptom-free patients.

Preventing and treating systemic illnesses with glutathione/cysteine compensation

The organism's need for thiol is often underestimated or neglected. After the predominant scenarios in the "thioester-iron world" one of the essential conditions for the origin of life in the prebiotic world before the creation of cellular organisms, was the capacity of sulfur to generate bonds and exchanges between protons of the sulfhydryl groups through "weak interactions" (De Duve 1991). Saltwater contains a naturally elevated sulfur concentration, but for terrestrial life forms there is a consistent danger of latent deficiencies of non-protein thiols and sulfates. Both are indispensable because they are responsible for the regulation of the redox milieu, the functioning of cell symbiosis in immune and non-immune cells and innumerable biosyntheses and biochemical reactions (Wrong 1993, Hässig 1999).

The pathognomic symptom of cellular immune deficiency (AIDS) and other systemic diseases is lack of cysteine and glutathione. (Herzenberg 1997, Dröge 1997 b, Peterson 1998, Hässig 1998 d, Kremer 1999). In symptom-free and symptomatic patients lack of thiol must be permanently compensated with individually adjusted doses. The "semiconductor thresholds" of redox-sensitive gene expression must be modulated in a sustainable and enduring manner by the negative redox potential, which depends on the glutathione system, in order to retune the enzyme activities necessary for intact cellular symbiosis.

Since the stimulation of the neosynthesis of glutathione, due to the redox-dependent enzyme syntheses, is not guaranteed, at least 2 grams of glutathione and simultaneously 5 to 10 grams of N-acetyl cysteine must be orally administered per day for 2 to 4 weeks at the beginning of compensation therapy. As protection against opportunistic pathogens the glutathione concentrations, especially in the mucous membranes, are considerably higher than in the blood plasma (for example, pulmonary mucosal fluids contain about 150 to 200 micromoles of glutathione, blood plasma less than 5 micromoles). Lack of glutathione in the lung secretion layer is an important conditioning factor for cellular immune deficiency against the *Pneumocystis carinii* fungi, the pathogens of the most common AIDS-indicating disease, PCP of the lungs.

In cases of distinctive resorption dysfunction caused by infectious and non-infectious changes in the intestinal mucosa, corresponding doses of reduced glutathione and N-acetyl cysteine can be administered intraveneously. After balancing the intracellular and the plasma levels of the thiol pool and the glutathione concentrations in the lung and the intestinal mucosal liquids, cysteine treatment should be continued for another six months with a daily dosage of 5 to 10 grams of N-acetyl cysteine. In addition, cysteine and methionine, the latter converted in the liver to cysteine, can be taken as part of the daily nutritional regime and can be found in low fat curds and other native organic dairy products (Bounous 1993).

Additional glutamine and arginine compensation to prevent or treat wasting syndrome (cachexia)

Due to the deficit of convertible protons, thiol deficiency causes a glutamine decrease with exaggerated protein reduction in the skeletal muscles (loss of body weight, wasting syndrome). The oral intake of up to 40 grams per day of glutamine can be used to retune the synergic effect between glutamine and cysteine levels for T-helper cell maturation (Shabert 1999).

Simultaneously this effect improves the regeneration of intestinal and lung mucous membranes, energy metabolism of cell symbiosis and acid-base balancing. The glutamine facilitates detoxification activity in the liver via the glutathione system and slows down the urea production by reducing the arginine splitting to urea and ornithine.

If there is a clear-cut arginine deficit and the linked lack of NO gas production the cellular immune performance (T-4 cells, natural killer cells, neutrophile granulocytes) can be significantly improved by supplementing the thiol and glutamine balance in pre-AIDS and AIDS with doses of up to 30 grams of arginine per day and up to 2% of the caloric intake respectively (Barbul 1990, Bower 1990). Synergistic adjustment of the dysregulation of amino acids cysteine, glutamine and arginine can be achieved in the case of massive immune cell deficiency, forced aerobic glycolysis, malignant cell transformation and cell degeneration as well as a pronounced wasting syndrome, by using small intestinal probes or, if necessary, by parenteral infusion solutions. In critical cases of disease, glutathione can be administered intravenously.

Highly dosed compensation for thiol deficiency and amino acid dysregulation must be seen as the basic therapy of the redox environment and for detoxification. These are providing the organism with much needed and natural survival resources to facilitate its self-regulation. The success of therapy must be continuously supervised by laboratory checks adapted to individual requirements, as the intake of N-acetyl cysteine simultaneously raises the glutamine and arginine levels in plasma (Dröge 1997 a).

Rigorously administered compensatory therapy, in cases of pre-AIDS or AIDS, during a well-monitored treatment phase produces better and more cost effective results than the counterproductive prescription of chemotherapeutic agents (AZT etc., "cocktail therapy," HAART) and permanent prophylaxis with chemoantibiotics (Bactrim etc.) which may bring short-term results, but have been proven to aggravate symptoms. If chemoantibiotics such as Bactrim etc. have to be prescribed for a short time because of acute opportunistic infections, then it is vital to administer a strictly metered compensation of the thiol deficiency.

Obligatory compensation therapy can be effectively supported by a set of specific regulatory measures during the symptom-free phase of acquired immune deficiency as well as in the phase of systemic secondary diseases.

Additional liver protection, in particular with acute/chronic hepatitis B or autoimmune hepatitis (nutritive isothiocyanate, polyphenols, glucuronic acid)

Hepatitis is often evident in members of pre-AIDS and AIDS risk groups—promiscuous homosexuals, intravenous drug users and recipients of highly contaminated blood products (Hässig 1996 b, 1998 e)—and calls for additional liver protection to bring relief to the glutathione system and phase-II detoxification enzymes (Wilkinson 1997). In contrast to the phase-I enzymes, which generate reactive electrophiles (electron-consuming substances) and activate carcinogens, phase-II enzymes inhibit electrophile bonds and turn them into water-soluble excretable substances. "Oltipraz" is a synthetic agent that has proved highly effective. It was originally designed as an anthelminthic against *Schistosoma*, which trigger type 2 cytokine dominance (Lucey 1996) analogous to the earlier stages of acquired immune deficiency. "Oltipraz" is a sulfur-containing dithiolthione and primarily activates the enzyme family of glutathione S-transferases. It exerts a protective function in the liver and in many other cell systems, especially the intestinal mucous membrane. Besides the protective effects against opportunistic germs and endoparasites, the agent has been shown to have antiviral and anticarcinogenic effects (overview Wilkinson 1997). These findings are significant especially after prior prooxidative damage of mitochondrial cell symbiosis caused by AZT etc. and permanent prophylaxis with "Bactrim." "Oltipraz" is equally efficient in the activation of the detoxification enzymes in the T-helper cells (Gupta 1995). A prescription of 125 to 250 milligrams/m2 twice a week for 12 weeks is an adequate dosage, as "Oltipraz" causes a sustainable triggering of the phase-II detoxification enzymes and has very few side-effects. (Note:

dithiolthione, trade name Oltipraz, up until now is only available for clinical studies. There has been no approval by the FDA, only publications about cancer treatment with Oltipraz in clinical research).

Among the natural substances, sulfur-containing isothiocyanates provide effective protection by triggering the variegated phase-II detoxification enzymes (overview Hecht 1995). These thiocyanates are inherent in vegetables like garlic, onions, as well as in broccoli and several other cabbage species.

The other important family of natural liver-protecting agents are polyphenols. Animal and human organisms are not able to synthesize aromatic bonds with benzene rings from preliminary stages. Polyphenols must be taken in from the outside, for example by ingesting algae or plants and are thus similar to vitamins (Hässig 1997 c). The redox cycling between the glutathione system and the polyphenolic substances is crucial for the balancing of the redox milieu and the detoxification done by the polyphenols, as well as for triggering the phase-II detoxification enzymes or, as the case may be, the inhibition of the phase-I enzymes.

Above all, polyphenols assist enzymes in cooperating with reduced and oxidized glutathione, glutathione peroxidase, glutathione reductase, glutathione S-transferases, catalase, NAD(P)H, quinone oxidase; and they inhibit the enzymes of the cytochrome P450 family (overview Wilkinson 1997).

Antioxidative protection of cell symbioses of liver cells and other cell systems including the immune cells, by polyphenols, is of particular importance in the highly acute AIDS state, if intracellular opportunists can proliferate without inhibition, due to the failure of the cytotoxic NO-gas producing Th1 helper cells. In this precarious situation, type 2 cytokine production is amplified on the one hand, but on the other hand the non-specific immune reaction of the phagocytes (macrophages) and the microglia cells in the brain are hyperactivated by the modulation of pro-inflammatory cytokines (interleukin-12, interleukin-1, tumor necrosis factor alpha and others, inflammation mediators and nitrogenic and oxidative radicals).

The elevated quantity of neopterine (as a folic acid metabolism product) and the beta-2 protein in the circulating blood are indirect markers for hyperactivation of the proinflammatory cytokine activity of the unspecific immune cells with a simultaneous suppression of the cytotoxic NO-gas production of the specific immune cells (full-blown AIDS) (Mauri 1990, Odeh 1990, Fuchs 1990, Harrison 1990, Matsuyama 1991, Krown 1991, Hässig 1993, Valdez 1997).

Consequently, well-balanced cell-protecting counterregulations fail and the simultaneous cytotoxic overregulations (prevalence of interleukin-12 compared to type 2 cytokine interleukin-10) incapacitate the feedback functions. In cases of a thiol deficiency and an overconsumption of other antioxidants, the redox balance collapses in the cytokine chaos (Cossarizza 1995).

The clinical studies concerning polyphenols over the last years have mainly concentrated on ellagic acid, the polyphenols in green tea, curcumin, silymarin etc. (overview Stoner 1995, Conney 1997, Wilkinson 1997, Zhao 1999, Plummer 1999).

Another possibility is the Galenic combination of glutathione with polyphenolic anthocyans (Recancostat, Ohlenschläger 1994) or with the ginkgo biloba polyphenol (S-acetyle glutathione, SAG). The polyphenolic complex phytotherapeutic "Padma 28," produced in Switzerland from a traditional recipe of Tibetan medicine, containing 20 herbal flavonoids and tannins, has proved its worth in protecting the liver in chronic cases of hepatitis B (Brzosko 1992, Liang 1992, Hässig 1997 c).

Additionally, reinforcing the supply of glucuronic acid can relieve liver cell symbiosis. Glucuronic acid plays an equally important role as a phase-II regulator of prooxidative and carcinogen-activating foreign agents in the liver by transforming toxins into secretable substances. Kombucha, the organic product from China, containing a symbiosis of fungi and specific bacteria, is a natural source of glucuronic acid that contains, besides high concentrations of glucuronic acid, vitamin B compounds and antibiotic substances. Kombucha can be made at home (Frank 1992).

Prostaglandin (PGE2) modulation (essential fatty acids: omega-3/omega-6; COX2 inhibitors)

The characteristic progression of prostaglandin synthesis, especially PGE 2, under the influence of type 2 cytokine dominance in pre-AIDS or AIDS, as part of the Type-II counterregulation, can also be countermodulated therapeutically or preventively. Elevated quantities of PGE2 inhibit, like the type 2 cytokines, the synthesis of the cytotoxic NO gas and thus enhance opportunistic infections. The prostaglandins are products of the arachidonic acid, an essential fatty acid. Arachidonic acid is enzymatically metabolized into prostaglandin within the cell's plasma membrane by the enzyme cyclooxygenase (COX). In AIDS, cancer and other systemic diseases, the

COX-2 isoform appears elevated. COX-2 increases PGE2 production and also raises the type 2 cytokines interleukin-6 production, which can trigger wasting syndrome (Hack 1996). Symptomatic for all systemic diseases like AIDS and cancer, wasting syndrome can be influenced by the selective inhibition of the COX-2 (O'Hara 1998). PGE2 is enzymatically generated by COX-2. In the same sense as growth factor TGF-ß, it activates the generation of polyamines from the arginine product ornithine. Therefore, the blockade of COX-2 through medication also inhibits tumor growth, reduces wasting syndrome and improves the Th1-Th2 balance of cellular immunity (Subbaramaiah 1997, Huang 1998, Jones 1999, Lipsky 1999 a, 1999 b, Sawaoka 1999, Golden 1999, Masferrer 2000, Kune 2000, Prescott 2000, Reddy 2000, Higashi 2000, Stolina 2000).

However, in symptom-free patients with a weak or an anergic Th1 immune cell population, prostaglandin modulation through essential fatty acids is a better option for treatment. In animal testing the Th1 immune cell population's stimulability in the DTH skin reaction test was inhibited, when 15% of the intake of calories consisted of linolenic acid, but not with the same quantity of fish oil with its high content of omega-3 fatty acid (Alexander 1990). Just as cold water fish can supply their needs of essential fatty acids by eating sea microalgae, patients can cover their requirement of essential fatty acids for prostaglandin modulation by the nutritional intake of contamination-free microalgae in powder or in tablet form (e.g. chlorella vulgaris). Admittedly it is necessary to ingest a couple of grams per day for several weeks in order to stimulate immune cell reaction and inhibit tumor formation. The effect of the mitochondrial cell symbiosis protection is improved by simultaneous substitution with cysteine, glutamine, arginine and RNA (Bower 1990, Cossarizza 1995, Chuntrasakul 1998, Gianotti 1999).

The low or high fluidity of the micro-Gaian milieu of cell symbiosis and the fluidity of the cell membranes reflect the type and the composition of the multi-unsaturated fatty acids (Bower 1990, Fernandes 1998, Simopoulos 1999, Zelenuich-Jaquotte 2000). The interaction between the synthesis of NO and its derivates and the prostaglandin PGE2, which is synthesized from the arachidon essential fatty acid, is equidirectional in small amounts but antagonistic in larger amounts (overview Lincoln 1997, Minghetti 1998). This interaction is of vital importance for the prevention and therapy of Type-II counterregulations of cell dyssymbiosis (systemic diseases) including the type 1 to type 2 cytokine switch (cellular Th1 immune deficiency, pre-AIDS) combined with pro-inflammatory macrophage hyperactivation (opportunistic infections, full-blown AIDS). It is possible to effectively counterregulate massive regressions of the cell symbiosis with omega-3 multi-unsaturated fatty acid and its derivatives (Veierod 1997, Imoberdorf 1997, Gogos 1998, Albert 1998, Ogilvie 1998, De Lorgeril 1998, Tashiro 1998, Rose 1999, Bougnoux 1999, Burns 1999, Bartsch 1999, Biasco 1999).

Individually customized micronutrient compensation (vitamins, minerals, trace elements)

The use of micronutrients (vitamins, minerals and trace elements) must be considered in a differentiated way regarding compensation and regulation therapies for the prevention of pre-AIDS and AIDS as well as for other systemic diseases.

"Nowadays the intake of vitamin E, in combination with vitamin C and ß-carotene, is worldwide the standard antioxidative treatment. *In The Antioxidant Supplement Myth*, Herbert critically analyzes this process (Herbert 1994). He conclusively demonstrates that this process is afflicted with serious disadvantages as pharmacological doses of a single polyphenol, like for example vitamin E in combination with vitamin C and ß-carotene, have some positive, but often damaging effects, depending on the receptor's iron balance. As redox compounds have both prooxidative and antioxidative effects the treatment can be summed up by the sentence: supplementation (of micronutrients) can help some consumers, harm others, but for most people they have no effect whatsoever. Thus, it was demonstrated that vitamin C (ascorbic acid), in the presence of redox-active transition metal ions, like iron (Fe^{3+}) or copper (Cu^{2+}), can act as a prooxidant and indirectly, by the so-called Fenton reaction, help to develop highly reactive hydroxyl radicals (HO) (Fenton 1894, Halliwell 1993, Cottier 1995). The synthesis of hydrogen peroxide (H_2O_2) occurs through a slow pH-dependent dismutation of superoxide radicals: $2O_2{-}\bullet + 2H^+ \rightarrow O_2 + H_2O_2$. Incidentally, as chelators of free metals, tannins can contribute useful services in this situation. Kim et al., who in studies on 14,407 Americans could find no life-prolonging effects in the use of isolated and unbalanced vitamins and mineral nutrition supplements, have extensively affirmed Herbert's critical statement. They identified the annual expenditure of $3.3 billion for nutrition supplements as a virtually useless augmentation of the health care costs (Kim 1993). In conclusion, we would like to state that a sufficient nutritive supply of a natural mixture of tannins and flavonoids is indispensable for a reliable and side-effect free antioxidative effect" (Hässig 1997 c).

Vitamin E and vitamin C generate radical chain reactions as intermediate states, which must be compensated for by the glutathione system (Ohlenschläger 1994), therefore a given thiol deficiency can be further aggravated by the intake of high dosages of these vitamins. Micronutrient requirements, in pre-AIDS and AIDS, should be evaluated in the context of a fine tuning of strict compensation and regulation therapy because deficits of individual micronutrients depend on the redox status, the mitochondrial activity, the cytokine balance, the existence of wasting syndrome, any given resorption dysfunction, severe diarrhea, toxic and infectious stressors, alloantigen overcharge, chemotherapeutic agents, chemoantibiotics, antiparasitics, fungistatics, virustatics etc, excessive alcohol, drug or cigarettes usage and many other factors. Uncontrolled self-medication does not make much sense and can in some cases even be dangerous.

A profiling study of ambulatory pre-AIDS and AIDS patients in relatively good health without a clinically definable wasting syndrome or heavy diarrhea quantified:

- Vitamin A and total carotenes, vitamins C, E, B6, B12, folate, thiamin, niacin, biotin, riboflavin, pantothenic acid, free and total choline and carnitine, biopterin, inositol, copper, zinc, selenium, magnesium and glutathione.

The results of the study confirm a reduction in the circulating concentrations of glutathione and relatively common lower serum concentrations of magnesium, total carotene and total choline plus increased niacin levels. The remaining values were within normal ranges or lower in a minority of the test subjects partly through self-medication with vitamins and minerals (Skurnick 1996).

Today's HIV/AIDS clinical research concerning micronutrients as influencing factors for acquired immune deficiency states (pre-AIDS and AIDS) confirmed the individual dependency on deficiencies in a holistic context of dysfunctional cell symbiosis.

"Deficiencies of single micronutrients are known to adversely affect the immune system by depression of cellular and humoral immunity and the impairment of phagocytosis (Beisel 1982, Klurfeld 1993). Individuals infected with the human immunodeficiency virus type 1 (HIV-1) may be particularly vulnerable to nutritional deficiencies that impair already compromised immune function. In a previous study of HIV-1 infected patients, we found that carotenes and ascorbate were below normal in 27% of the subjects, and vitamins E and A were low in 12% (Bogden 1990). Serum levels of micronutrients in HIV-1 patients have been associated with markers of immune function and stage of disease (Fordyce-Baum 1990, Baum 1991, 1992, Semba 1993). Studies have shown that abnormalities in nutriture both accompany and predict HIV disease progression (Semba 1993, Coodley 1993, Tang 1993, Abrams 1993). These investigations assessed dietary intake or serum concentrations of one or a few micronutrients in selected cohorts" (Skurnick 1996).

The primary influence of micronutrients on the prevention and therapy of cancer was also put into perspective in comparison to the importance of the redox status, NO—and prostaglandin syntheses, the cytokine balance and cell symbiosis activity (World Cancer Research Fund 1997).

An additional measuring of the serum ferritine level must be considered essential, which in pre-AIDS or AIDS patients as in all pro-inflammatory stages of macrophage hyperactivation is evidently elevated (Gupta 1986) and plays an important role in all Type-II counterregulations (Gherardi 1991, Weinberg 1992, Herbert 1992, Gelman 1992, Lacroix 1992, Kiefer 1993). In addition to compensation therapy of the redox status, the reinforcement of the matrix has an important function in regard to the regulation of the iron balance (Pippard 1989, Hässig 1993).

Stabilization of the extracellular matrix (polyanions)

The basic extracellular matrix, which embeds all tissues and organs, functions as filter for all the bioenergetic, substantial, hormonal and sensory inputs and outputs of cellular symbiosis. Among other things, the matrix is composed of a complex network of sulfate-rich protein molecules (glycosaminoglycans, proteoglycans), which are necessary for the negative redox potential. Re-fetalization of the extracellular matrix into sulfate-free hyaline acid, as present in early embryonic tissue, is characteristic for many carcinomas (Heine 1997).

For prevention and therapy, the extracellular matrix can be reinforced by a regular supply of polyanions, chondroitin sulfates in the form of cartilage preparations or shark cartilages, of macroalgae, of agar-agars or by eating macroalgae (Hässig 1992). The balance of the redox potential of the matrix synergistically supports the glutathione system and relieves cell symbioses in states of prooxidative and systemic stress (Hässig 1992, 1997 a, 1998 b).

Direct activation of the mitochondrial respiration chain (coenzyme Q10; L-carnitine; possibly lipoic acid and thiamine)

Direct activation of the mitochondrial cell symbiosis can be stimulated by coenzyme Q10 (Folkers 1986) and L-carnitine (Bremer 1990).

Coenzyme Q10 plays an important role in the electron transfer in the mitochondrial respiratory chain. In symptom-free "HIV positives,", Q10 deficit is already apparent and progressively increases in pre-AIDS and AIDS. Toxic stressors and prooxidative medication (AZT etc., Bactrim etc.) are decisive factors that lead to dysfunction in the mitochondrial respiratory chain and secondary defects in the mitochondrial DNA. Q10 improves the cell symbiosis performance in immune cells and non-immune cells and can be prescribed in a daily dosage of 200 milligrams for a several months without detectable side effects (overview Folkers 1988).

L-carnitine supports the participation of long-chained fatty acids (triglycerides) for the oxidation inside mitochondria. L-carnitine deficits increase glucose metabolism and facilitate a switch to aerobic glycolysis (Warburg Phenomenon). The disturbance in triglyceride transport causes lipid accumulation, which is often observed in treatment with HAART and protease inhibitors (Brinkmann 1999). Pre-AIDS and AIDS have been shown, in the context of a L-carnitine deficit, to be systemic dysfunctions of lipometabolism and of the lipid composition of the T-cells (De Simone 1991). Administrating high doses of L-carnitine, 6 grams per day for two weeks, has improved T-helper cell proliferation, lowered the triglyceride serum levels and decreased the serum values of circulating beta-2 microglobulin and alpha tumor necrosis factor as indicators for hyperactivation of macrophages in HIV positives and AIDS patients. L-carnitine also appears to stabilize the cytokine balance by ameliorating mitochondrial performance (overview De Simone 1993).

Reduced mitochondrial performance as consequence of chemotherapeutics, caused by damage to mitochondrial DNA after the intake of AZT etc. and Bactrim etc., can additionally be compensated by the daily dose of 600 mg lipoic acid (alpha-lipoic acid) plus 300 mg thiamine (vitamin B1) for a month or longer.

Targeted activation of mitochondria is especially significant for "HIV positives" but also for cancer patients, who years after enforced chemotherapy are still under the threat of multiple organ failure (myocardial infarction, sepsis, cerebral infarction, hepatic coma, myopathies etc.) as a result of potentiating mitochondrial DNA defects.

The moderation of hypercortisolism (DHEA-S; glucosaminoglycans; heparin; heparinoids; phytotherapeutic complexes: flavonoids + tannins)

The cytokine balance and the related equilibrium between cell-mediated and antibody-supported immunity are, as all organ systems, closely related to the sensory and hormonally controlled stress systems. The retroactive hormonal stress axis between the hypothalamus, pituitary, and adrenal cortex modulates the cytokine profiles via equilibrium between cortisol and DHEA-S (dehydroepiandrosterone sulfate), both generated in the adrenal cortex. The final cortisol synthesis takes place in the mitochondrial cell symbionts of the adrenal cortex cells (Tyler 1992), so that disturbance and damage of these cells can favor grave psychosomatic stress diseases and systemic diseases like AIDS, cancer and many other symptoms. During states of high stress the synthesis and the release of cortisol increases when compared to the DHEA levels. This causes the inhibition of cytokine synthesis through the interaction of cortisol with transcription factors (Brattsand 1996). Persistent cortisol increase facilitates the antibody-supported immune response and weakens cellular immune reaction. On inhibition of the type 1 cytokine profile, however, under the strong stress stimulation of the macrophages through antigens and toxins, the release of nitrogen and oxygen radicals and of the inflammation mediators interleukin-1 and tumor necrosis factor-alpha can be increased within the macrophages. The neopterin and ferritin levels serve as a direct quantification of the extent of the inflammatory macrophage-activation and as an indirect measurement serve such markers that display the scale of the acute phase reaction, as for example the C-reactive protein (Hennebold 1994, Hässig 1997 d, 1998 b).

Inversely, a shift from a type 1 (Th1) cytokine profile to a type 2 (Th2) cytokine dominance through an increased cortisol/DHEA-S ratio means that a moderation in stress-related hypercortisolism amplifies the effect of DHEA-S on type 1 cytokine synthesis. This means an improvement to the cortisol/DHEA-S ratio in favor of the latter can expand cellular immunity by activating the type 1 cytokine interleukin-2.

There is indeed a direct correlation between the balance of T4 helper immune cells and the increased cortisol level (Th1-Th2 switch) or, as the case may be, the level of DHEA-S, the predominantly synthesized form. The development of acquired cellular immune weakness syndrome is associated with an increasing DHEA-S deficit (Biglieri 1988, Hilton 1988, Raffi 1991, Mulder 1992, Christeff 1996, Ferrando 1999). However, the 24-hour cortisol level seems to be elevated in AIDS patients, (Vilette 1990).

These findings resulted in the hypothesis that DHEA-S substitution (DHEA-S as an anti-cortisol hormone) could enhance cellular immunity for the prevention and therapy of opportunistic infections in cases of pronounced pre-AIDS and AIDS (Frissen 1990, Wisniewski 1993). The DHEA-S level as counterbalance to the ACTH cortisol system is of vital importance not only for the cytokine-controlled functions of cell symbiosis of the immune cells, but also for other cell systems (Parker 1985, Ebeling 1994, Lavallee 1996). DHEA is a precursor molecule for androgenous sexual hormones and the DHEA-S dysregulation is a co-determining factor in tumors in hormone-dependent organs such as the mammary or prostate glands as well as in tumors in other organs (Vermeulen 1986, Heinonen 1987, Barrett-Connor 1990, Stahl 1992, Le Bail 1998, Lissoni 1998, Svec 1998, Eaton 1999).

The moderation of hypercortisolism and the indirect type 1 cytokine stimulation via DHEA-S can in many cases be supported by nutritive measures, including an increase in the extracellular content of glycosaminoglycans (heparin, heparinoids). They reduce the influx of calcium ions into the inner cell and inhibit cortisol bonding on the intracellular receptors. This can be achieved through an intake of cartilage extracts (chondroitin sulfate) or of agar from sea algae (Hässig 1993, 1998 b). Simultaneously, the proinflammatory hyperactivation of macrophages (as counterregulation) in a cortisol-related type 1 to type 2 cytokine shift can be repressed by binding surplus NO and O_2 radicals by intercepting excessive free iron and the increasingly formed catabolic proteases by using complex phytotherapeutics like Padma 28, a Tibetan preparation made of polyphenolic flavonoids and tannins (Liang 1992, Hässig 1993, Gebbers 1995).

The regulation of cytokine chaos in acute full-blown AIDS requires high-dose cysteine/glutathione compensation + DHEA-S + gammaglobulins, in order to curb the antagonism between simultaneous macrophage hyperactivation and the type 1 cytokine inhibition of T-helper immune cells

The moderation of cortisol and the reactivation of DHEA-S in interaction with the inhibition of pro-inflammatory macrophage stimulation are important additionally, as macrophages, because of their phagocytosis-performing capacities, represent a preferred reservoir for intracellular opportunistic pathogens (Rubin 1988, Meltzer 1992). The counteraction to a strong and long-lasting nitrosative, prooxidative and systemic stress effect results in an elevated cortisol/DHEA-S ratio, a weakening of cellular immunity and an inhibition of cytotoxic NO gas defense through a type 2 cytokine switch; it also results simultaneously in a pro-inflammatory mobilization of opportunistic residents in the macrophages (fungi such as *Pneumocystis*, *Candida*, histoplasms, cryptococci, parasites and toxoplasms, bacteria including mycobacteria, *Listeria*, *Legionella* and chlamydia, and many actually-existing viruses, in contrast to the phantom "HI viruses"). These counterregulations must, sooner or later, lead to clinical full-blown AIDS, if the primary stress factors can not be minimized, the proton demand deficiencies are not balanced and the dysregulation of the cell symbiosis is aggravated additionally by the use of "chemo-tactical" weapons.

In full-blown AIDS, there is a crucial antagonism between the behavior of the non-specific immune response of the macrophages, and the specific immune response of T4 helper immune cells: The cortisol brake for the biosynthesis of tumor necrosis factor in the macrophages is suppressed by the activation of interferon-γ under strong or/and long-term stress stimulation (Luedke 1990), and the ratio of cortisol/DHEA-S in the macrophages is regulated in favor of the latter by their inflammatory cytokines (Hennebold 1994). In contrast, the T4 helper cells remain inhibited under the influence of cortisol and synthesize after receiving signals from the glutathione-depleted antigen-presenting dendritic cells, predominantly type 2 cytokines (Peterson 1998). They inhibit cytotoxic NO gas synthesis, contrary to the macrophages (loss of helper Th1 cell functions) and stimulate instead antibody production (overview Mosmann 1996, Lucey 1996, Abbas 1996, Hässig 1996 d, Lincoln 1997). The net result in the T4-immune cells is a change in the ratio of the cortisol to DHEA-S in favor of the former (Wisniewski 1993, Christeff 1996, Ferrando 1999).

The contradictory clinical symptoms of manifest AIDS result from this antagonism of nonspecific inflammatory events, combined with the mobilization of opportunistic pathogens on the one hand and the loss of the specific Th1 gas production against intracellular opportunists on the other hand.

The prooxidative, glutathione-consuming and mitochondriotoxic chemotherapy with AZT etc. and sustained prophylaxis with Bactrim etc. are not able to control the competing cytokine chaos resulting from nonspecific immune hyperactivation within the macrophages (Type-I overregulation of among other things: type 1 cytokine interleukin-12 antagonistic towards type 2 cytokine interleukin-10; tumor necrosis factor alpha increased; type 1 cytokine interferon-γ increased; NO-and oxygen radicals including toxic hydroxyl groups increased) and the deactivation of the specific Th1 immune response (Type-II counterregulation of, among other things: type 2 cytokine interleukin-10 antagonistic towards interleukin-12; in wasting syndrome type 2 cytokine interleukin 6 increased; in tumor cells TGF-ß increased; NO and O_2^- production inhibited). The most effective option is compensating the thiol deficiency, whereby cysteine slows down the cytotoxic effects of tumor necrosis factor within the hyperactivated macrophages and improves glutathione neosynthesis (Cossarizza 1995).

The preventive and therapeutic aim must be to balance the redox milieu, to improve the fluidity of the micro-Gaian milieu, to reconstruct the cytokine balance and simultaneously to moderate the competition between Type-I overregulation of unspecific immunity and Type-II counterregulation of specific immunity. This can only be achieved by a synergistic compensation and regulation therapy.

Overcoming fear and anxiety, and the profound shift in knowledge of healing from chemoantibiosis to nontoxic cellular symbiosis therapy

"Last but not least it is essential to resolutely confront the still widely propagated and officially held belief that every HIV-infected person must sooner or later progress to AIDS and inevitably die (Hässig 1992 b). On the contrary, we should give HIV positives the hope that by adapting their lifestyles to the opportunities given by nature they may be spared from the limitations of AIDS for a long time, maybe forever. To achieve this they have to come to terms with their nutritional problems. In our overview work, "The Rethinking of AIDS," which was published about one year ago, we asked whether this could lead to a general paradigm shift in medicine (Hässig 1992 b). Nowadays, we tend to assume that such a shift will happen. The use of AZT and analogous virucidal medication as recommended by the responsible authorities, is based on the antibiotic paradigm, which means the toxicological extinction of microbial inflammation germs. Man lives, however, in an ongoing symbiosis with a whole range of microorganisms, hence the question is justifiable if it would not be more sensible to support the probiotic, physiological mechanisms of self-healing to support organisms"(Hässig 1993).

The variety of the effective and non-toxic intervention options demonstrates a possible change within medical practice "from antibiosis to symbiosis Therefore, it is the overriding task of physicians to reduce the paralyzing and destructive fear of death and instead encourage people affected by systemic cell dyssymbiosis by reinforcing their natural will to survive by clarification of the actual state of knowledge. The most effective protection against the abuse of "violent medicine" (Albonico 1997) as a modern instrument of terror and fear is the rational knowledge, that every kind of risk for and any targeted attack on the cell symbiosis of immune cells and non-immune cells is answered according to the laws of evolutionary biology.

An imagined "HIV retrovirus," if it were to exist, would be no exception. The actual clinically monitored symptoms in pre-AIDS and AIDS would, if a biologically active "HIV agent" actually were to be the cause of the disease, be conditioned by the disturbance of the redox balance, cell symbiosis damage and by the shifting within the micro-Gaian milieu. The preventive and therapeutic consequences of the deactivation of such a biologically undetected "HIV retrovirus" would be principally the same as for all other prooxidative load factors. Irrespective of the type of exposure, these basic consequences are universally valid whether they are of a toxic, pharmacotoxic, traumatic, inflammatory, infectious, nutritive, radiative, alloantigenic, psychic or any other nature. People with an especially redox-sensitive disposition must all be advised to avoid risks of exposure and orientate their nutrition according to their blood group as a code for the genetically predisposed polymorphism of the enzyme systems (D'Amato 2000).

The lifesaving synergy of a conscientious compensation and regulation therapy is derived from the logic of the natural laws of the co-evolution between microbes and man, the processing of toxins and other bioactive stress factors, including the consequences of undernutrition and malnutrition.

The profound change in "natural" scientific knowledge of the sciences progresses from antibiosis (from the Greek: *anti* = against + *bios* = life) to symbiosis (from the Greek: *sym* = with, together). The foreseeable end of lethal virus hunting and of one-sided aggressive cancer expunging represents, both for those concerned and for medical therapists as well as for general population, a self-critical liberation from the staging of a collective and exploitive terrorism of fear.

Fig. 69) Various factors that damage mitochondria

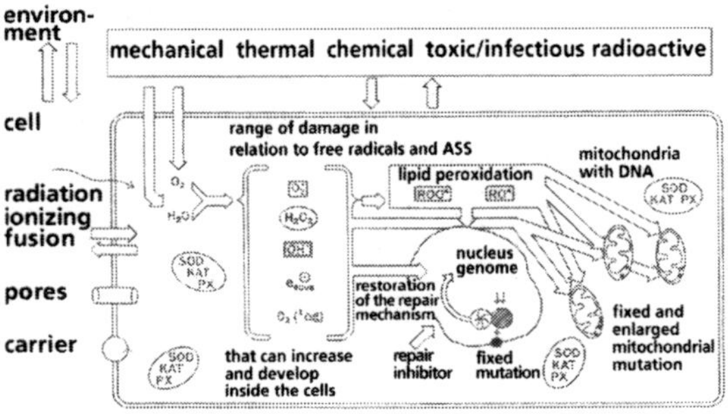
environ-
ment
mechanical thermal chemical toxic/infectious radioactive
cell
radiation
ionizing
fusion
pores
carrier
range of damage in
relation to free radicals and ASS
lipid peroxidation
mitochondria
with DNA
nucleus
genome
restoration
of the repair
mechanism
fixed and
enlarged
mitochondrial
mutation
that can increase
and develop
inside the cells
repair
inhibitor
fixed
mutation
SOD
KAT
PX

Fig.) 70 Glutathione molecule in its reduced (left) and oxidized (right) form.

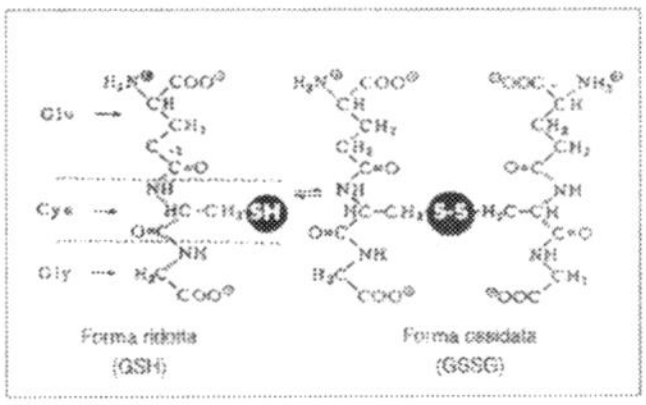
Glu
Cys
Gly
SH
S-S
Forma ridotta
(GSH)
Forma ossidata
(GSSG)

Fig. 71) Glutathione molecule takes part in all the main processes of cellular biology. The relationship between reduced glutathione and oxidized glutathione (about 400:1) has to be continually balanced depending on cell type. Chronic exhaustion of glutathione leads to apoptosis, degeneration or transformation to a tumour cell.

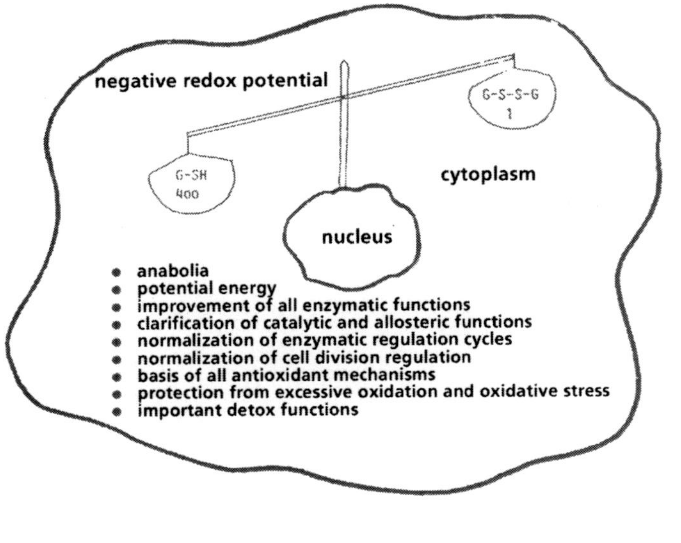
negative redox potential
G-S-S-G
1
G-SH
400
cytoplasm
nucleus
• anabolia
• potential energy
• improvement of all enzymatic functions
• clarification of catalytic and allosteric functions
• normalization of enzymatic regulation cycles
• normalization of cell division regulation
• basis of all antioxidant mechanisms
• protection from excessive oxidation and oxidative stress
• important detox functions

Fig. 72) Diagram of the mechanism of reduced glutathione

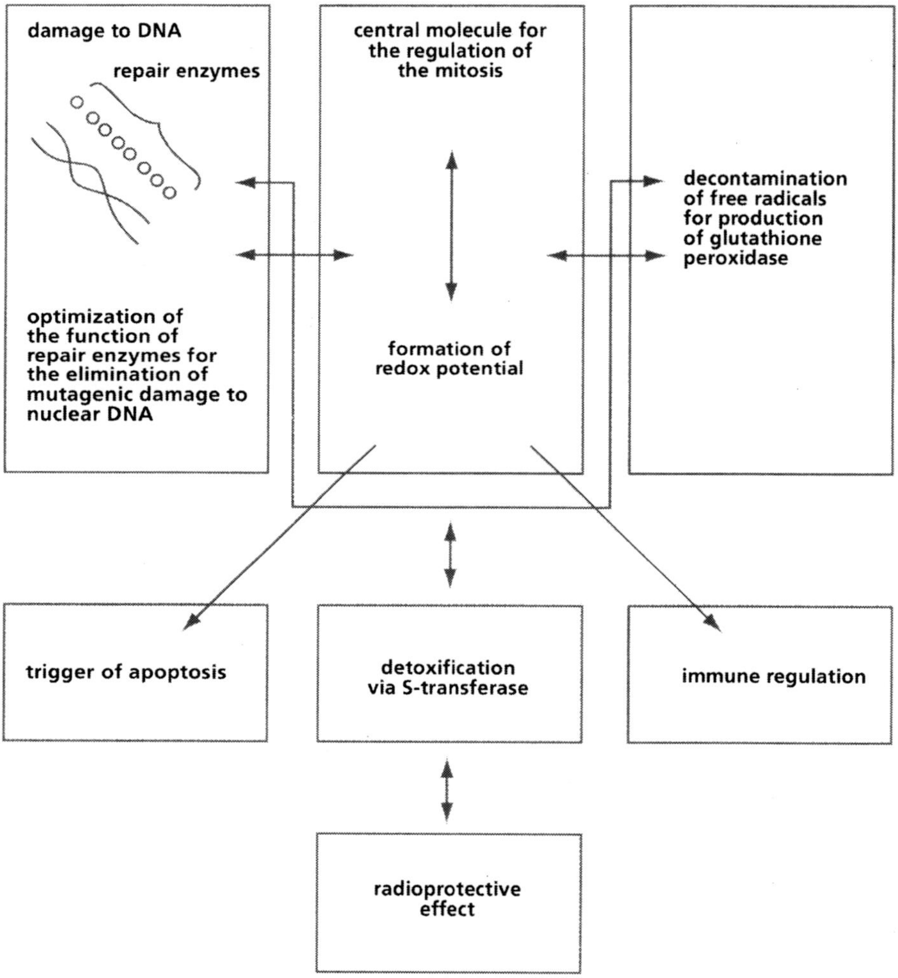
damage to DNA
repair enzymes
optimization of the function of repair enzymes for the elimination of mutagenic damage to nuclear DNA
central molecule for the regulation of the mitosis
formation of redox potential
decontamination of free radicals for production of glutathione peroxidase
trigger of apoptosis
detoxification via S-transferase
immune regulation
radioprotective effect

Fig. 73) Glutathione controls the balance of the immunocytes Th1/Th2 in antigen presenting cells.

An insufficient level of glutathione leads to a permanent switch of the TH1/TH2 balance and promotes the development of AIDS, tumours and many other chronic pathologies. This deficiency must be compensated by therapy.

Proc. Natl. Acad. Sci. USA. Vol 95, pp. 3071-3076. March 1998. Immunology

Fig. 74) Some structural formulas of polyphenols (flavonoids). Flavonoids exchange electrons with glutathione and strengthen its functions. Flavonoids are widespread in plants, however, the human body is not able to synthesise them.

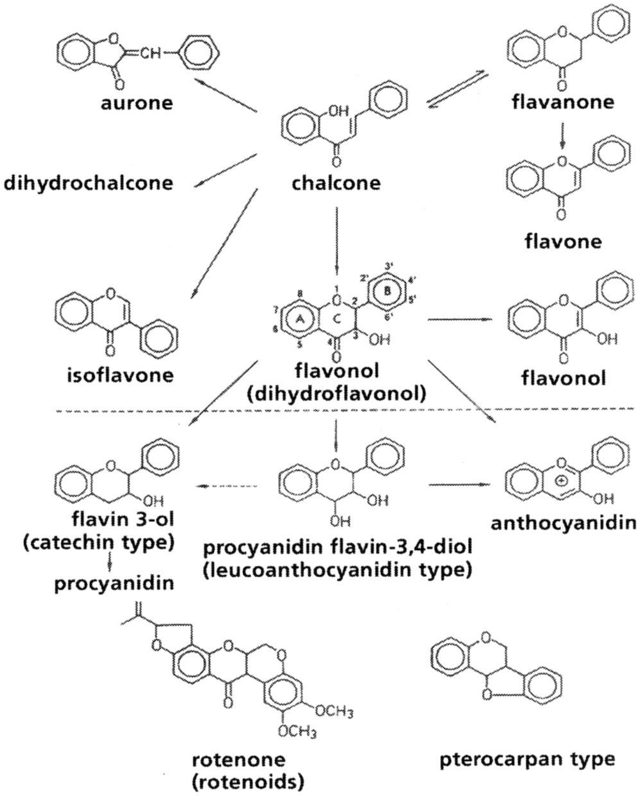

aurone
chalcone
dihydrochalcone
flavanone
flavone
isoflavone
flavonol
(dihydroflavonol)
flavonol
flavin 3-ol
(catechin type)
procyanidin
procyanidin flavin-3,4-diol
(leucoanthocyanidin type)
anthocyanidin
rotenone
(rotenoids)
pterocarpan type

Fig. 75) The anthocyans (flavonoids in flowers and fruit) support the glutathione system in numerous and important functions.

Anthocyans

1. Pelargonidin
2. Peonidin
3. Cyanidin
4. Malvidin
5. Petunidin
6. Delphinidin

- Inhibitors of tumor growth
- Radical captors
- Terminators of the radical chains
- Redox cycling with GSH
- Absorption of UV-light
- Collagenase inhibition
- Stronger antioxidant in hydrophile environments

Fig. 76) An excessive amount of saturated fatty acids in food and obesity promote the formation of toxic acetaldehyde, tumors and other systemic pathologies, chronic and autoimmune as well as metabolic illnesses.

Effects of killer fatty acids on health

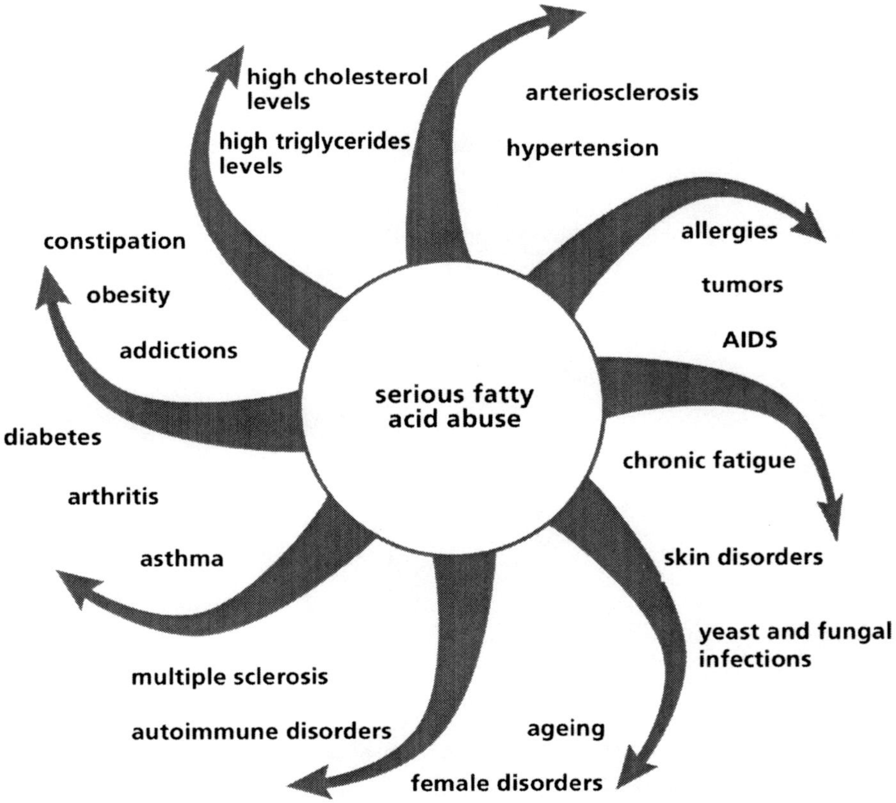

serious fatty acid abuse
high cholesterol levels
high triglycerides levels
arteriosclerosis
hypertension
allergies
tumors
AIDS
chronic fatigue
skin disorders
yeast and fungal infections
ageing
female disorders
multiple sclerosis
autoimmune disorders
asthma
arthritis
diabetes
constipation
obesity
addictions

Fig. 77) Some sources of essential fatty acids (unsaturated)

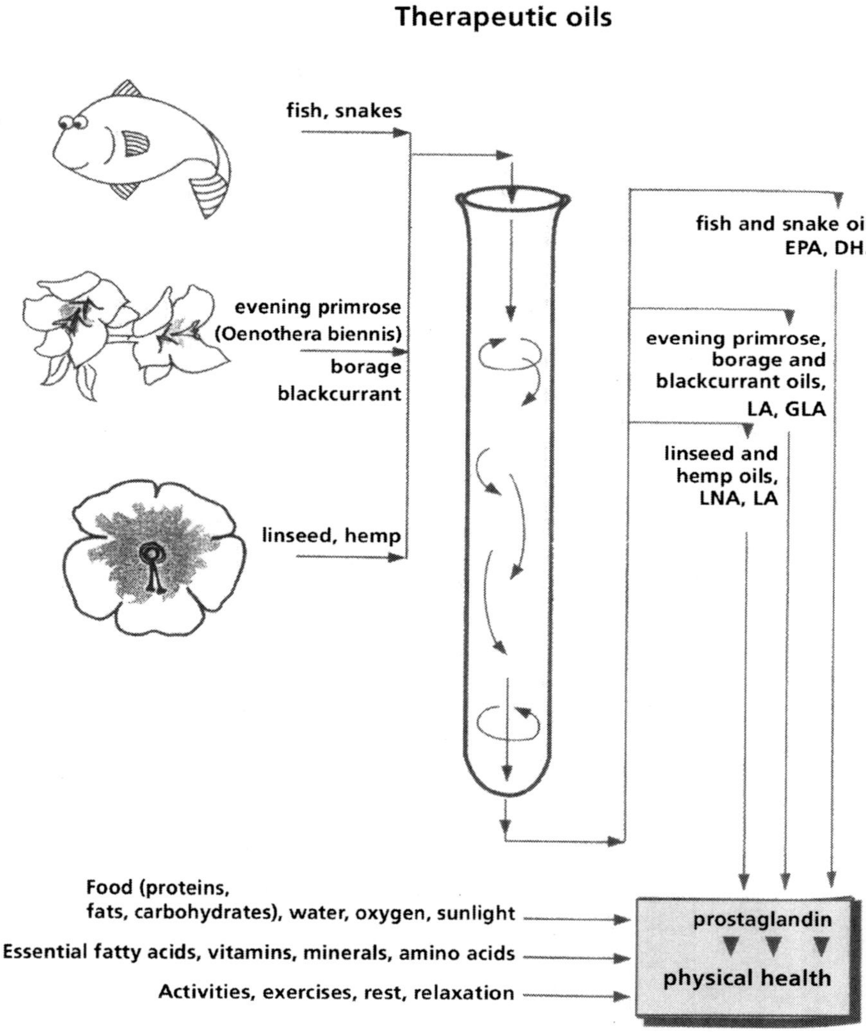
Therapeutic oils
fish, snakes
evening primrose
(Oenothera biennis)
borage
blackcurrant
linseed, hemp
fish and snake oils
EPA, DHA
evening primrose,
borage and
blackcurrant oils,
LA, GLA
linseed and
hemp oils,
LNA, LA
Food (proteins,
fats, carbohydrates), water, oxygen, sunlight
Essential fatty acids, vitamins, minerals, amino acids
Activities, exercises, rest, relaxation
prostaglandin
physical health

Fig. 78) Omega-3 fatty acids promote the production of series 3 prostaglandins and in many clinical trials they have shown a capacity to inhibit tumors. Amongst all the conventional and alternative medicines, only the omega-3 fatty acids, mainly EPA, have so far been shown to be efficacious in the treatment of cachexia in tumor patients.

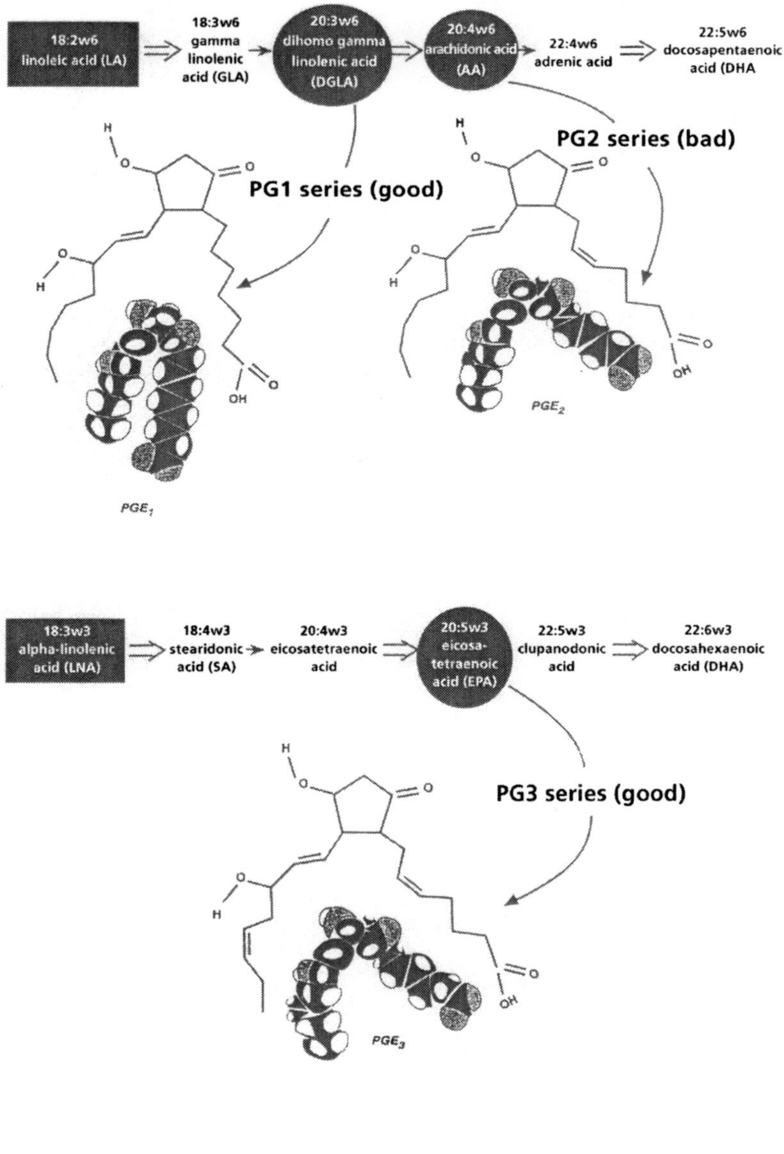

18:2w6 linoleic acid (LA)
18:3w6 gamma linolenic acid (GLA)
20:3w6 dihomo gamma linolenic acid (DGLA)
20:4w6 arachidonic acid (AA)
22:4w6 adrenic acid
22:5w6 docosapentaenoic acid (DHA
PG1 series (good)
PG2 series (bad)
PGE1
PGE2
18:3w3 alpha-linolenic acid (LNA)
18:4w3 stearidonic acid (SA)
20:4w3 eicosatetraenoic acid
20:5w3 eicosa-tetraenoic acid (EPA)
22:5w3 clupanodonic acid
22:6w3 docosahexaenoic acid (DHA)
PG3 series (good)
PGE3

Chapter XII

Resistance Against the Mass Poisoning in Africa

The international initiative of President Mbeki—answers from the South African government's open discussion on the causes of AIDS in the West and developing nations; on the nontoxic prevention and therapy for AIDS; on AZT's true mechanisms and the global terror epidemic spread by physicians and the media—the international HIV cartel's refusal to join the discussion and the disinformation campaign it launched.

On 3 April 2000, three months before the beginning of the World AIDS Conference, the South African President Thabo Mbeki announced in an open letter to the UN General Secretary, Kofi Annan, and other Western leaders, an invitation to open discourse on the toxic effects of AZT and therapeutic alternatives in the treatment of AIDS.

Beforehand, the South African Minister of Health had posed a precisely formulated, written question to the so-called AIDS dissidents:

"Is AZT incorporated in DNA? Can this stop 'HI' viral replication?" (Tshabalala-Msimang 2000).

The background lay in an arrangement between five pharmaceutical companies and the World Health Organization, initiated by the Norwegian physician and former Prime Minister, Brundtland, with the seemingly humanitarian offer of dropping the prices of AZT and other nucleoside substances so that pregnant women and newborns in African and other countries could be supplied with AZT and other nucleoside substances for the prophylaxis and treatment of "HIV infections" and AIDS-indicating illnesses.

But the research data of orthodox medical research presented by the "AIDS dissidents" caused profound shock among those responsible in South Africa and the initiative of the South African president. Mbeki wrote to Kofi Annan and the political leaders of Western countries of his intention of holding an open scientific discourse on the unanswered questions on HIV, AIDS and AZT, and his wish to discuss, among other things, the unanimous condemnation in the international press of his initiative. Mbeki was termed in the international media either "criminal" or "crazy."

"Some elements of this orchestrated campaign of condemnation worry me very deeply. It is suggested, for instance, that there are some scientists who are "dangerous and discredited" with whom nobody, including ourselves, should communicate or interact. In an earlier period in human history, these would be heretics that would be burnt at the stake! Not long ago, in our own country, people were killed, tortured, imprisoned and prohibited from being quoted in private and in public because the established authority believed that their views were dangerous and discredited. We are now being asked to do precisely the same thing that the racist apartheid tyranny we opposed did, because, it is said, there exists a scientific view that is supported by the majority, against which dissent is prohibited. The scientists we are supposed to put into scientific quarantine include Nobel Prize Winners, Members of Academies of Science and Emeritus Professors of various disciplines of medicine!

Scientists, in the name of science, are demanding that we should cooperate with them to freeze scientific discourse on HIV-AIDS at the specific point this discourse had reached in the West in 1984. People who otherwise would fight very hard to defend the critically important rights of freedom of thought and speech occupy, with regard to the HIV-AIDS issue, the frontline in the campaign of intellectual intimidation and terrorism which argues that the only freedom we have is to agree with what they decree to be established scientific truths. Some agitate for these extraordinary propositions with a religious fervour born by a degree of fanaticism, which is truly frightening. The day may not be far off when we will, once again, see books burnt and their authors immolated by fire by those who believe that they have a duty to conduct a holy crusade against the infidels. It is most strange that all of us seem ready to serve the cause of the fanatics by deciding to stand and wait" (Mbeki 2000).

After pressure from the American government, two-thirds of the scientists and physicians at the international specialist conference, held on the 6/7 May

2000 in Pretoria, consisted of people who expressed absolutely no doubt about the theory that "HIV causes AIDS" and who were of the opinion that the toxic effects of AZT and other substances had to be accepted to protect mankind from "lethal HIV infection." In response to the Mbeki initiative the American president Clinton declared that AIDS was a threat to national security. The sponsors in the presidential election campaign, at that time already underway, demanded "business as usual". But many people in the media global village, alerted by the Mbeki initiative, became increasingly bewildered and aware via the internet that the medication used worldwide to combat AIDS and cancer had also been proven to cause AIDS and cancer.

Within the framework of the specialist conference, comprehensive experimental, clinical and epidemiological data, facts and proof were presented by scientists and physicians countering the predominant theory that "HIV causes AIDS," against the use of the "HIV" test and against the highly toxic treatment of "HIV" positive patients with "antiretroviral" chemotherapeutics which cannot be considered life-preserving (Fiala 2000, Papadopulos-Eleopulos 2000 c, Duesberg 2000). The author of this book supplemented and specified this expertise in a written reply to some decisive questions from the South African president and health minister:

Answers to the questions raised by South Africa's President Thabo Mbeki and Health Minister Manto Tshabalala-Msimang, M.D., on the active mechanism of AZT from 23 February 2000 and on HIV/AIDS from 6-7 May 2000.

Q—Is AZT incorporated in DNA?

A—Azidothymidine (AZT) is a nucleoside into which an azido group (=N3) is incorporated, in contrast to the natural nucleoside thymidine. Like all natural and synthetic nucleosides, AZT can only be incorporated into DNA or provirus DNA as a nucleotide in combination with three inorganic phosphorus atoms. Numerous experimental studies have demonstrated that up to 99% of the nucleoside AZT is not metabolized in the nucleotide azidothymidine triphosphate (AZT-TP). Therefore, in theory, 1% of the AZT accepted by the human cells could be incorporated in the DNA nucleus or in some DNA provirus. However, in living human cells, nobody to date has proved the actual incorporation of AZT-TP in the DNA nucleus or in any DNA provirus. Other assertions are completely without foundation.

Q—Can AZT stop replication of the "HIV" viruses?

A—The theoretical possibility of 1% of the AZT absorbed being incorporated in the DNA as AZT-TP means that 5 mg of the prescribed minimum dose of 500 mg or 15 mg of the prescribed maximum dose of 1,500 mg AZT could be incorporated in the DNA nucleus or in some DNA provirus. According to data from the AZT manufacturer Glaxo-Wellcome, the nucleoside analog AZT is accepted after absorption in the alimentary canal in numerous immune cells and non-immune cells. Only a fraction of this low amount of substance from the 5-15 mg of AZT would be available for incorporation in the "HIV" infected Th1 lymphocytes (identical to the T4 or type 1 CD-4 cells). As, according to the 1995 HIV/AIDS theory, the HIV virus is supposed to increase a billion-fold daily, the proportion of the AZT triphosphate allocated to all the HIV-infected Th1 lymph cells in comparison to the amounts of AZT-TP allocated to all the non-infected Th1 lymph cells would be theoretically and actually too low to be able to stop the replication of the "HIV." However, the fixing of the active dose of AZT to inhibit the "HIV" presumes the objectively refuted assertion that ATZ is incorporated as AZT-TP with a high affinity exclusively into the HIV's DNA provirus.

Yet the active mechanism of AZT is another matter. The 99 times higher amount of AZT that cannot be incorporated in DNA, which does not combine with three inorganic phosphoric atoms, actually reacts in a much shorter time with non-DNA molecules in the alleged HIV-infected Th1 lymph cells and in Th1 lymph cells not infected by HIV as well as in other immune cells and non-immune cells. The reactive azido molecule group is used in the experimental mitochondrion research in order to block the cytochrome oxidase enzyme in the mitochondrial respiration chain. The intact mitochondria, former bacterial cell symbionts that appear in all human cells except red blood corpuscles, work with molecular oxygen (0_2) to produce 90% of the adenosine triphosphate (ATP) energy carrier molecules necessary for human life. The blockade of the respiratory enzyme cytochrome oxidase by AZT prevents conversion of electrons into O_2. The immediate result is reduced ATP production and an increased synthesis of toxic oxygen radicals.

The cells suffer from loss of energy. Within a few minutes and at latest within three hours, there is a reaction to the AZT that cannot incorporate in the DNA. Meanwhile, replication of the DNA nucleus or any kind of DNA provirus, which always depends on DNA nucleus replication of active cells, would require 40-72 hours after the theoretical build-up of AZT-TP. The blockade of oxygen respiration and energy production in T-helper cells (T4 cells or CD-4 cells) resulting from AZT medication leads specifically to premature death of immune cells or, under certain conditions in accordance with the law of nature to switching of maturing T-helper immune cells to type 2 T-helper immune cells (Th1-Th2 switch) as part of a Type II counterregulation. Both reaction forms result in immune system weaknesses. The premature dying particularly affects Th1 cells. Their depletion is the principal immunological characteristic of "HIV positive" and AIDS patients. It is the function of Th1 cells to eliminate intracellular pathogens such as parasites, fungi, mycobacteria, and viruses. Since the discovery of nitric oxide (NO) production in human cells (Furchgott and Ignarro, 1987, Nobel Prize, 1998), it has been proven beyond any reasonable doubt that NO gas production in Th1 cells is indispensable for elimination of intracellular pathogens. If the Th1 cells producing NO gas are lacking, opportunistic pathogens may develop (AIDS). The function of the Th2 cells is to prompt antibody formation. Th2 cells produce no NO gas to eliminate intracellular pathogens.

Numerous studies have proven that "HIV positives" have a loss of Th1 cells and a dominance of Th2 cells at the earliest possible stage in "HIV" seroconversion. It is biologically unimaginable that all T-cells should be colonized by "HIV" at this early stage of the "HIV" infection, since the prevailing Th2 cells are intact, and antibody production is even increased. Therefore, according to the laws of logic, the Th1-Th2 switch, which leads to cellular immunity weakness, must have other causes. The active mechanism of NO and AZT (=N3) is identical: inhibition of cytochrome oxidase in complex IV of the mitochondrial respiratory chain is the essential physically and pathophysiologically active factor in human cells through NO and also AZT. Depending on duration and dose of increased NO production as well as medication of AZT, special cell types and disposition of patients, a concurrent rise occurs in cell death (apoptosis, necrosis) and/or Th2 cell dominance (opportunistic infections = AIDS), tumor formation (e.g., Kaposi's sarcoma, lymphoma, carcinoma), or degeneration of the skeleton and heart muscle cells as well as nerve cells). The causes of AIDS in Western countries have been clarified epidemiologically and pathophysiologically without any reasonable doubt in thousands of experimental and clinical studies. Without any doubt, unusual accumulating load factors for exogenously and/or endogenously induced NO over-stimulation have been proved in all so-called risk groups. There is no rational, comprehensible biological reason to assume that the combination of these immune stress factors in Western civilization should have remained completely ineffective and without recognizable disease results. Strong or lasting NO overstimulation leads as a counterreaction to increased cell death and/or in the case of T-helper cells to a Th1-Th2 switch with inhibition of the cellular production of NO and disturbance of the mitochondria's oxygen respiration.

The clinical results (including AIDS) are in no way puzzling but easily understood in terms of biology and evolution. "HIV," the virus that nobody so far has actually isolated according to the standard rules of retrovirology, the virus which was deduced to exist only due to unspecified molecular markers to postulate it hypothetically as cause of disease, is neither sufficient nor necessary. This postulate veils the real cause of AIDS. At the point in time when the "HIV causes AIDS" disease theory was developed, the researchers did not know of NO production in human cells or the existence of two forms of T-helper immune cells with and without NO gas production! Nor were we aware of the dependence of the function of eliminating intracellular pathogens in Th1 cells on their NO gas production nor of the regulation of oxygen respiration in the mitochondria by NO and its derivatives. Failure to consider these research data by HIV/AIDS-researchers can only be construed as lamentable ignorance or unwillingness to learn.

This explanation of AIDS' causes and the active mechanism of AZT is supported by the fact that after introducing clinical medication in malignant forms of lymph cell cancer with substances analogous to nucleosides (that show the same active mechanism as AZT), a massive loss of Th1 cells appeared in the same form among all treated, and so did the inverse ratio of T4/T8 lymph cells and opportunistic infections. Exactly these immunology data and clinical symptoms define the AIDS syndrome. Since presentation of the conclusive data from NO research, cytokine research, mitochondria research, and other experimental and clinical research sectors from the mid-1990s, there are no longer grounds for rational doubt about the actual causes of AIDS in Western countries.

African clinical standards for diagnosing AIDS and test-procedure standards for antibodies against the "HIV" are in no way congruous with those of Western countries. However, regardless of race and country-specific diagnostic practices, all human beings are identical in the response that evolution has programmed into human immune and non-immune cells when affected by nitrosative and prooxidative stress conditions. In Africa it is particularly chronic inflammatory and infectious processes, protein shortages, and malnutrition (nutritional AIDS), contamination of drinking water with nitrifying bacteria, and nitrosamine burdens in nutrients that can lead to clinical symptoms of opportunistic infections (AIDS) as a result of induced Th1-Th2 switches.

Chronic infections stem from mycobacteria, such as chronic tuberculosis or the leprous form of leprosy, spirochete bacteria such as the tertiary form of syphilis, malaria pathogens, trypanosomal, toxoplasmic, and other parasites, fungi pathogens such as pneumocystes, candida forms, histoplasms, Cryptococcus, and many others. These always result from too weak a Th1 immune response and a switch in the Th1-Th2 immune cell balance to Th2 immune state with increased antibody production. Infections such as worm parasites trigger *a priori* a Th2 immune response that can become chronic. If the clinical symptoms of an unspecified sort and duration become chronic, these have been diagnosed in Africa since 1985 as AIDS, based on the Bangui definition, without test evidence of "anti-HIV" antibodies. This pragmatic procedure led to the apparent proof of a suddenly rapid increase in Africa of "HIV"-caused AIDS-indicating diseases.

Arbitrary projections from small random samples of "HIV positive" serum tests and sweeping clinical AIDS diagnoses in Africa still serve the World Health Organization, UNAIDS, the Western countries, and the international news media as basic proof of the HIV pandemic in Africa and derived from this a threat to all humanity. Since children, women, and men can suffer from chronic inflammatory and infectious processes due to general living conditions in developing countries, these AIDS cases can be manipulated at will in terms of sweeping medical statistics as proof of heterosexual transfer and mother-child transfer leading to the "HIV" in Africa.

Since these undoubted facts are logical in view of the high scientific standards of Western medicine and can be understood with little intellectual effort, there is no rational reason to assume that the intended mass poisoning with a mitochondrial inactivator, azidothymidine (AZT), was a tragic scientific error. No HIV-AIDS researcher and no medical specialist to date has been able to answer the inescapable medical-ethics question of why medicinal application of AZT and other substances that trigger the loss of Th1 immune cells, reverse the ratio of T4/T8 lymph cells, and cause opportunistic infections should be indicated to treat patients, preventatively and therapeutically, who are in danger of developing Pre-AIDS and AIDS.

That AZT is effective as inactivator of mitochondria can be derived from the biological fact that azidothymidine was isolated from herring spermatozoa in 1961. The spermatozoa of vertebrates are not allowed to transmit these cellular symbionts to the female ovum, and the mitochondria of the spermatozoa must be inactivated at the time-point of penetration into the ovum. In the case of vertebrates, only the mother's cellular symbionts will be transmitted to descendants. AZT was produced synthetically in 1964 but banned from human trials after tests on mice and rats with leukemia resulted in the development of lymph-cell cancer. AZT was used clinically for AIDS patients from 1986, but without evidence of its actual incorporation in any provirus DNA and without testing for possible mitochondria damage. The question of whether AZT can stop replication of the so-called virus is inseparably linked with the question of evidence of the "HI virus."

The "anti-HIV" antibody test was stocked with stimulated human stress proteins as antigens from lymph cell cultures of manifest AIDS patients and from co-cultivated lymphatic leukemia cells. The test substrates have been calibrated in such a way that a positive test result will appear beyond a certain amount of unspecified antibodies which in the blood serum of test subjects characteristically indicates a long-term Th2 immune-cell response and an increasing antibody reaction. The test reaction level and the number of test antigens in the "anti-HIV" antibody tests have been determined arbitrarily. There are no international obligatory standards for this test reaction level and the required test-antigens. In Africa, for example, a reaction in "HIV" tests is usually rated a positive test result with fewer test antigens than in Western countries. Since no antibodies form in the human immune system that react only with those antigens against which they were originally formed, the statement that "anti-HIV" antibody tests react exclusively with antibodies formed in human organisms against antigens of the "HIV" is already, for this biological reason, objectively false.

"HIV" test antigens, for example, have been shown to react with antibodies against tuberculosis, malaria, and *Pneumocystis* pathogens as well as many other antibodies against microbial and non-microbial antigens. In Western countries too, applied determination of "viral load" with the help of the PCR laboratory technique is, according to the inventor of this DNA-multiplying method, the Nobel Prize winner Kary B. Mullis, completely unsuitable to detect the so-called HIV's RNA. Nobody to date has actually isolated a natural RNA sequence or a provirus DNA sequence of "HIV." All publications on the so-called isolation of "HIV" show nothing other than findings of unspecific molecular markers that are arbitrarily interpreted as "finger prints" of "HIV." Other data of scientific findings can not be expected in view of the pressing epidemiological, immunological, cell-biological, and clinical evidence that Type II counterregulation of human immune and non-immune cells as well as the development of AIDS-indicator diseases are, under certain conditions, evolutionarily programmed. For physiological and pathophysiological understanding of these immunological and clinical phenomena, the assumption of an infection with "HIV" is neither sufficient nor necessary but objectively redundant. It was assumed at the conference of leading HIV-AIDS researchers in 1997 that no disease mechanism of "HIV" could be proved (Balter 1997).

The question is often raised of whether AIDS could be transmitted in another way, sexually, into the bloodstream, via the respiration system or other infection routes if one assumes that the so-called virus is not the cause of AIDS. Many people have mental difficulty in separating certain facts of the immune system, since it is suggested to them that the immune cells of "HIV positives" and AIDS patients react primarily to infectious pathogens that are usually transmitted sexually or from an "HIV positive" mother to her children. However, the biological truth is that human immune cells are influenced by a number of non-microbial immune stressors as well as microbial immune stressors (antigens and toxins). Thus AIDS-indicating diseases must not always be triggered primarily by infections of any kind, as demonstrated by the examples of nutritional AIDS, transplantation AIDS as a result of immunosuppressive therapy, or by AIDS after AZT medication or after medication with other nucleoside analog drugs. A homosexual African, for example, can also become ill with nutritional AIDS, even if he never takes the risks of anal-receptive homosexuals from the West. However, he would be registered in Africa as a heterosexual HIV-AIDS patient. Nor would the apparent mother-child transmission of AIDS have to be caused primarily by infection. Since the immune cells and non-immune cells of the fetus show a dominance of Th2 or type 2 cytokines respectively during pregnancy, the disposition for opportunistic infections after birth (AIDS) depends mainly on whether the mother has transmitted enough intact maternal antibodies and whether a stable Th1-Th2 immune cell balance can be adjusted in the child during the first months of life.

In cases where mothers are lacking nutrition, poorly nourished, or suffering toxic damage before and during pregnancy, the maturing of the infant's T-helper immune cells will be substantially affected. Opportunistic infections (PCP) were already diagnosed during the 1940s among prematurely born children and orphans in Europe. Opportunistic infections also occur among children with congenital thymic aplasia. Why children of nutritionally, infectiously, and toxically damaged mothers in Africa should suddenly be infected by "HI viruses" if they develop opportunistic infections cannot be comprehended rationally, even if the "anti-HIV" antibody test shows a positive result for the reasons mentioned above. Treating such children preventively or therapeutically with AZT or other nucleoside analogues would then be inhumane treatment in the sense of the UN Declaration of Human Rights—even if one works from the assumption that the postulated "HI viruses" exist and could be transmitted from mother to child. The restricted or unrestricted treatment of the not yet matured immune cells of a newborn child by means of substances that demonstrably largely damage the maturity of immune cells fulfills the case for deliberately inflicting bodily harm with fatal results and must be condemned internationally as especially inhumane treatment.

President Mbeki's questions to the conference of experts on May 6-7 2000 in Pretoria show the basic misunderstanding that arises from viewing AIDS as the exclusive result of a sexual infection and taking no account *a priori* of all other immune stressors, whether they are sexually associated or not, infectious, or noninfectious. For example, more than 90% of those older than six in Western countries have antibodies that also react to pneumocystes. But only a few human beings fall ill with *Pneumocystis carinii* pneumonia (PCP), the most frequent AIDS-indicator disease in Western countries. The pathogen is an airborne fungus that is transmitted from person to person. Whether a person becomes diseased from such an opportunistic PCP, depends entirely on whether enough Th1 immune cells are available to produce the cytotoxic NO gas in order to eliminate PCP pathogens after specific signals from antigen-presenting cells and toxin stimulation through pathogens. In cases of the disease, the PCP pathogens benefit from the fact of cellular immunity weaknesses, regardless of whether the preceding Th2 dominance was the result of stressors that were infectious or noninfectious, sexually transmitted or not. Gender and manner of sexual transmission may play a role, but they may just as easily not be factors. Other pathogens that trigger opportunistic infections may gain advantage from previous chronic infections, even though they produce no opportunistic infections themselves.

Such interactions are known in Western countries, for example, among surgical patients after operations and trauma as well as among patients in intensive-care wards. Under the general living conditions in developing countries such interactions of chronic and opportunistic pathogens are frequent and have nothing to do with "HIV," even if the "HIV test" is positive and the T4 cell count is low. On the contrary, such laboratory findings can be given in any cases of marked Th2 immune-cell dominance and existing chronic infections without the presence of any "HIV." However, an AZT medication would even be counter-indicated if the existence of "HIV" were proven, since such "HIV" would only die with the immune cells and because it would kill more immune cells that were not infected with "HIV." But these biological conditions do not mean that AIDS is "transmitted," since AIDS is the clinically resulting syndrome and not the cause of the acquired Th1 immune cell weakness and the inhibition of toxic resistance-gas production. What are transmitted are pathogens that could primarily be involved in developing a Th1 immune weakness or could profit secondarily from an existing Th1 weakness. Yet even among homosexuals, these transmissions in no way result only via the sexual channel but though all possible access channels.

The superficial differentiation between heterosexually and homosexually associated transmissions of "HIV" serves Western HIV/AIDS propaganda as a manipulative suggestion of a fatal "HIV" infection transmittable to anybody through sexual contact. It ignores infectious immune stressors and involvement of non-infectious immune stressors, which have been very effective disease triggers for millions of years without "HIV." However, the predominantly homosexual transmission of "HIV" infections in Western countries and the heterosexual transmission of "HIV" infections in African countries are not explained by HIV/AIDS researchers as being the result of special infectious and non-infectious risks of a minority of homosexual patients and the general living conditions in Africa countries but as a result of the demonstrably special sexual compulsiveness of homosexuals and African men and women. During the past 15 years the international mass media have availed themselves of many a cliché on the fantasized sex lives of African men and women. In order to avert the alleged pandemic for all humanity, it is demanded as if in sheer solicitousness that pregnant women and newborns in Africa be treated with AZT. As start-up help and for seemingly humanitarian reasons, pharmaceutical concerns in cooperation with the WHO and Western countries offered AZT and other nucleoside analogues at dumping prices.

The crucial question in this economic whodunit is no longer whether AZT can stop "HIV" but whether South Africa can serve as the gateway for AZT in developing countries. A problem that first came to public light through the change in knowledge of medical research during the past decades is intensifying for Western countries as well as developing countries: the increasing abuse of chemoantibiotics and mass vaccinations since the end of WWII. Both factors can favor a predisposition for the long-term prevalence of Th2 illnesses such as allergies, ectopic skin diseases, chronic arthritis, certain autoimmune diseases, AIDS, cancer, etc. The reason for this is the lack of training in the ways of Th1 immune cells and the shift in the balance of the Th1-Th2 immune response. An indicator for this two-edged change in the infectious load profile in Western countries is the fact that practically the only patients diagnosed as AIDS patients come from age groups born after WWII. The same applies to patients with organ transplants (without genetic disposition) who have developed transplantation AIDS. This acquired disposition has an even graver impact under the general living conditions in developing countries than in Western countries where the change in disease has already been clearly recognized in the growing number of chronic diseases.

During the ongoing decade, biological laws of co-evolution must be discussed anew in light of medical research's fundamental findings in the 1990s. A future-oriented and rationally based health-care and social policy must be oriented within this context and not in the context of irrational theories that have caused the waste of enormous scientific and economic resources (Kremer 2000 b).

Brief answers to questions raised by South Africa's President Thabo Mbeki at the conference of specialists on HIV/AIDS issues in Pretoria on 6-7 May 2000

Questions:

1. **What evidence is there for the assumption that HIV is the cause of AIDS, and what consequences would result for the emergence of symptoms and their diagnoses?**

This question contains the related questions:

a) **What is the cause of immune deficiencies that lead to AIDS and ultimately to death?**
b) **What are the most efficient options to react to these causes?**
c) **Why is HIV/AIDS transmitted heterosexually in black Africa (south of the Sahara), while it is supposedly transmitted homosexually in the industrialized countries?**

2. **What role can treatment play in developing countries?**

The following related issues should be considered:

What possibilities of treatment are suitable for developing countries?
For AIDS patients?
For HIV-positive patients?

For prevention of mother-child transmission?
In preventing HIV infections through work-related injuries?
In preventing HIV infections after rape?

3. What are the best means of therapeutic prevention of HIV/AIDS?

Discussion should always consider the social and economic context, especially poverty and other frequently occurring diseases as well as the limited infrastructure in developing countries.

(C. Köhnlein and C. Fiala: Report on the 1st meeting at the invitation of South African President Mbeki; C. Fiala: AIDS in Africa, the way forward; Koehnlein-Kiel@t-online.de / christianfiala@aon.at).

Answers:

Furchgott and Ignarro secured evidence for the first time in 1987 (Nobel Prize, 1998) that cell systems of the human organism are controlled by nitric oxide gas. During the following years it was demonstrated that immune cells eliminate microbial disease pathogens within cells by producing nitric oxide (NO) gas. It was found that there are two types of immune cells: those that produce NO gas and its derivatives and those that produce no NO gas but stimulate formation of antibodies to inhibit microbial disease pathogens outside the body cells.

These revolutionary findings have resulted in revising many disease theories held as correct at that time. Immunological disease phenomena that had previously been interpreted as causal results of "HIV," based on prevailing immune-system theories, can now be explained based on the pioneering new research data without contradiction or assumption of an "HIV" infection. These new findings fully justified the critical questions of President Mbeki on HIV/AIDS and have far-reaching consequence for medicine, society, politics, and economics.

There must be a balance between NO gas-producing immune cells and those that do not produce NO gas. This balance in cellular and humoral antibody immunity can be disturbed by non-infectious as well as infectious factors, as either can lead to an acquired cellular immunodeficiency (AIDS). Overstimulation of the immune cells' NO gas production that is either too strong or lasts too long leads to inhibition of NO gas production in the immune cells and increased activation of antibody-producing cells in its place. The result can be an uninhibited rise in intracellular microbes such as fungi, parasites, mycobacteria, and viruses (opportunistic disease pathogens) within the body cells that would normally be eliminated by cytotoxic NO gases without symptoms. This clinical disease diagnosis is defined as AIDS. Oxygen respiration of certain cell systems can be blocked by simultaneous overstimulation of NO gas production and counterregulation of certain cell biology. These cells can switch to energy production independent of oxygen, and this can lead to tumor formation. This process was already known in 1924 (the Warburg Phenomenon). Yet it can only be explained by the NO research findings. Nerve and muscle cells can also suffer degenerative damage by disturbing oxygen respiration for the same reason. AIDS in the defined sense is a rare form of disease in Western countries with an annual incidence amounting to 0.001-0.002% of the entire population.

The largest group of AIDS patients is a minority of anally receptive homosexuals. The causes of NO overstimulation in this risk group are: inhalation of organic nitrogen gases (poppers) as sexual means of doping, abuse of antibiotic chemicals that become metabolized into NO and nitrosamines; acceptance of foreign protein as the result of unprotected anal intercourse that can lead to NO overstimulation analogous to NO overstimulation by microbial antigen protein and antigen toxins in cases of multi-infectiousness if cell detoxification is interrupted.

Intravenous drug addicts are the second largest risk group, and their cellular immune balance is disturbed by drug intoxication itself, by frequent microbial infections resulting from contamination of used needles, toxic additives to the drug substances, low and lack of nutrition related to bodily consumption resulting from drug-dependent lifestyles. Those potentially affected in this risk group amount to about 5% of the total population of intravenous drug users. In relatively rare cases the children of drug-dependent mothers are affected as a result of the mothers' chronic intoxication. The cell respiration disturbance related to it in immune and non-immune cells causes these newborns to suffer maturity damage in cell immunity.

A further risk group are hemophiliacs who have injected commercially obtained but highly contaminated coagulating proteins that result in long-term NO overstimulation (as animal experiments have shown). Multi-transfusion receivers with a serious basic disease are another small risk group in numerical terms. On average they have received 35 storage units of foreign blood. A 10-year clinical study in Canada involving several thousand patients, which was published in 1986, showed that more than 30%

of surgical patients indicated immune anomalies that are viewed today as disturbances in NO gas-producing immune cells and as a preponderance of non-NO gas-producing immune cells. Already during the 1960s it became known that organ transplant patients developed entirely identical diseases after treatment with immunotoxic drugs. These appeared from the late 1970s among homosexual patients. Onward from 1982, they were classified as AIDS. The same AIDS-indicator diseases, inhibition of NO gas production in immune cells, and predominant maturation of non-NO gas-producing immune cells as well as opportunistic infections (AIDS) developed in the same form among patients with blood-cell cancer who were treated with pharmaceutical substances from the substance class to which the AIDS medicine AZT and related substances belong. Immune cells responded to entirely different types of triggers with NO gas production as well and in cases of overstimulation with inhibition of NO gas production. These can be toxic and pharmacotoxic substances, malnutrition or lack of nutrition, foreign protein intake, infections, inflammations, lack of hormone regulation, emotional stress, and many others.

Chronic infectious and inflammatory processes, malnutrition or lack of nutrition, as well as contaminated drinking water play the most vital role in developing countries. The reasons for this lie in general living conditions for which Western countries bear a historically shared responsibility. Under the conditions given, a much higher exposure to microbial disease pathogens exists in developing countries for embryos in the mother's womb, newborns, children, women, and men than in developed industrialized countries. Microbes outside the body cells are inhibited or eliminated by antibodies and other endogenous mechanisms as well as by a variety of cells in the immune-cell network. If they manage to get inside the body cells, according to new findings, they can only be inhibited effectively or eliminated by a functioning NO gas resistance. This applies especially for fungi, parasites, mycobacteria, and a number of viruses. Chronic infections develop if cytotoxic NO gas no longer suffices. This means a constant irritation of the NO gas stimulation. The cells must be protected from potential damage and accelerated death by endogenous gas production. Sulfurous protein, vitamins, and enzymes (antioxidants) fulfill these tasks. These must be accepted or synthesized from nutritional components. The antioxidants are called this because they constantly have to neutralize nitrogen oxide (NO) and its derivatives as well as reactive oxygen species (ROS). If the antioxidants are exhausted, because nutritional intake of antioxidants and/or components to synthesize antioxidants is lacking or one-sided and/or chronic infections and inflammatory processes cause too high use of antioxidants, NO gas production and formation of reactive oxygen molecules can no longer be neutralized sufficiently. Increased cell deterioration and/or cell-biology counterreactions occurs in immune cells and non-immune cells that lead to secondary inhibition of NO gas production. As a result opportunistic infections can occur under these conditions. This vicious circle of a high exposure to for chronic infections and inflammations, anti-oxidative undernourishment and malnutrition, as well as disposition for opportunistic infections is well known as nutritional AIDS in developing countries. (Beisel 1992, 1996). The primary causes of this form of AIDS in developing countries, regardless of gender, concern unborn babies in their mothers' wombs, newborns, children, women, and men. These primary causes usually differ basically from the primary causes of most AIDS-indicating diseases in the risk groups of Western countries.

AIDS in Africa is no more a result of transmitting a so-called AIDS pathogen sexually in Africa than it is in Western countries. There is no such AIDS pathogen. Nor would it be either sufficient or necessary to understand the disease processes. The assumption of such an AIDS pathogen stems from a not too distant time in the history of medicine when the fundamental processes in immune cells and non-immune cells simply had not yet been understood. Even in AIDS cases where primarily infectious processes are a co-deciding cause for failure of NO gas resistance in the immune cells, sexually transmitted infections play no exclusive role. The sexual channel is only one of the possible means of access for infections. Most chronic infections are not transmitted sexually (for example, lung tuberculosis, miliar tuberculosis, malaria, worm infections, and numerous other tropical infections). This also applies for secondary opportunistic pathogens, mainly fungi, parasites, mycobacteria, and cytomegaloviruses, as well as other herpes viruses. The most common AIDS-indicating disease, PC lung infection, demonstrates this point. It is triggered by an airborne fungus pathogen.

The scientific reduction of thought to homosexual or heterosexual transmission of a so-called AIDS pathogen has veiled the actual causes of developing opportunistic infections. All are caused by inhibiting NO gas production in immune cells and non-immune cells as well as by blockading the oxygen respiration of certain cells. HIV/ AIDS medicine has not been able to explain to date why the identical diseases of pharmacotoxic AIDS and nutritional AIDS develop entirely independently of any "HIV" pathogen, while other people, despite analogous excessive toxic, pharmacotoxic, infectious, and nutritive immune stressors or massive administration of immunotoxic foreign protein, are only supposed to develop identical AIDS-indicating diseases when a so-called AIDS pathogen has been transmitted sexually or via the bloodstream. Numerous experimental and clinical studies have established that the antioxidant and sulfurous detoxifying proteins in the immune cells are sharply reduced, and that the immune cells which predominate, produce no more NO gas, but that antibody production is increased among "HIV-positives" at the earliest possible moment of "HIV" seroconversion, when the "HIV test" shows a positive result. This fact proves that the immune cells of these patients cannot be disturbed by a so-called AIDS pathogen, as claimed by HIV/AIDS theory, but that the immune cells have inhibited NO gas production due to a shortage or total lack of antioxidant detoxifying molecules. The Th2-immune cells not producing NO gas are moving mainly outside the bloodstream, where they can take over the stimulation of B-cells for antibody production.

However, the reduced number of immune cells, as alleged proof for destruction by "HIV" viruses, is only measured in flowing blood. This AIDS definition applies in the USA even if no clinical symptoms are at hand but only the number of T4 immune cells in the blood stream has fallen below a certain level and the "HIV" test shows a positive reaction. This obscure diagnostic procedure (AIDS without the clinical syndrome or "AID" without "S") has raised the officially recorded count of "AIDS cases" in the USA since 1 January 1993 by more than 100%. This AIDS definition has not been accepted in Europe, and the numbers of AIDS cases are dropping accordingly. Just as questionable as these definitions is the diagnosis of AIDS diseases in Africa. The Bangui AIDS definition of 1985, which is in use today with variations, enables AIDS diagnosis by appearance based on unspecified symptoms such as coughing, fever, diarrhea, etc., if they last longer than one month. Such symptoms are frequent in developing countries in cases of chronic inflammatory and infectious processes. These cases, recorded as AIDS without diagnostic standards, are reported to the World Health Organization in Geneva. Based on the summary judgment of the assumed "spread dynamics of HIV in Africa," the HIV/AIDS cases are projected, and the data gained is offered to the world press as the current status of the "HIV/AIDS pandemic" in Africa. Given this completely arcane HIV/AIDS data, the international mass media paint a picture of the "dying continent of Africa" without referring to the slipshod method of data gathering. These practices have led to the manipulated world opinion that 90% of all HIV/AIDS infections occur in Africa.

Thus in the USA, Europe, and Africa there are differing factual bases treated in public opinion as HIV/AIDS. To this extent, in view of "the limited infrastructure in developing countries," it only makes sense to raise questions about the cause, therapy, and prevention of AIDS if the real biomedical core of the problem is cleanly separated from manipulated propaganda of HIV/AIDS medicine and their profiteers.

As to the question about the "consequences resulting from the emergence of symptoms and their diagnoses," knowledge of the real background facts in Africa means that the actual causes of patients' diseases are diagnosed incorrectly or not at all. It also means that patients and their family members are placed in mortal fear, excluded, and submitted to hopelessness. There is no proof to support the "HIV causes AIDS" disease theory, but there is an overwhelming abundance of evidence against it. Nobody has actually isolated the "HIV," and the existence of such a virus was concluded by unspecified molecular markers after manipulation of immune cells from the blood of homosexual AIDS patients. These immune cells were stimulated with highly oxidized substances that, as one knows today, trigger reactive NO gas production. Since the cells were greatly decreased by detoxifying molecules containing sulfur, a portion of the cells perishes. This phenomenon then interpreted as destruction by the hypothetical HIV. Another portion of the cells reacted with cell-biology counterregulations. These include formation of regenerative protein and export of oxidized stress protein from the cells. Both molecular markers were seen as exclusive proof of the presence of "HIV" although the same molecular markers could be provoked in numerous other cells under the same laboratory conditions.

All cell experiments that have supposedly detected isolation of the "HIV" are based on evidence of such unspecific markers after stimulation with such highly oxidizing substances in cell cultures. Nobody has been able to demonstrate cell-free HIV in the blood serum of "HIV positives" or AIDS patients without such biochemical manipulations, although they are supposed to multiply a billion-fold according to the HIV/AIDS theory prevailing since 1995. According to the findings of NO research, HIV researchers have confused cause and effect. This knowledge is supported by the fact that the discoverer of the patented "HIV" test of 1984, Dr. Gallo, manipulated cell cultures of AIDS patients with hydrocortisone. The hormone hydrocortisone blocks cell splitting including reproduction of viruses potentially existing that can only reproduce with host cells in synchronized manner. Hydrocortisone also inhibits NO gas production but promotes formation of regenerative protein.

Two of Dr. Gallo's external colleagues, who had worked with him on cell experiments, published in 1987 that the "HIV" sought in AIDS patients' immune cells based on molecular markers (regenerative protein, export of stress protein from the cells in the form of so-called virus-like cell particles) had been demonstrated especially well after adding hydrocortisone to the cell culture. These data referred to experiments in Dr. Gallo's laboratory during 1984 when setting up the "HIV" test. Yet Dr. Gallo, who had deliberately kept this hydrocortisone effect a secret in his publications, had to admit the fact after a reproach at the 1998 press conference of the international World AIDS Congress in Geneva. Dr. Gallo has been unable to explain to this day why the splitting of host cells is blocked after adding hydrocortisone, as every physician knows from the clinical application of hydrocortisone, but the "HIV" reproduced especially well with hydrocortisone present. NO research provides this explanation: unspecific molecular markers, allegedly proof of "HIV" existence, are nothing other than regenerative proteins and cellular waste exported from cells under oxidative stress from cells in virus-like cell particles as the by-product of cellular biological counterregulation. Thus, these markers have nothing to do with "HIV."

Dr. Gallo misinterpreted the protein released after oxidizing stimulation from the immune cells of AIDS patients that were cultivated jointly with human leukemia cells. He identified it as "HIV" protein. Using this human cell protein, Dr. Gallo equipped the test substrate for his patented "anti-HIV" antibody test. This test substrate, which had been adjusted to especially high antibody amounts, reacted with antibodies in blood serum of people whose immune cells form a particularly high level of antibodies.

This is true above all for people whose immune cells no longer produce NO resistance gas but increasingly stimulate synthesis of antibodies instead. *An "HIV positive" test result means nothing more than the proband has particularly high amounts of antibodies in his blood, and these react accordingly with foreign human test protein.* Since there are no antibodies in human blood that react only with the protein against which they were originally formed, the "HIV" test demonstrably reacts to many different antibodies. In Africa, antibodies in the blood serum of test subjects react positively in the HIV test, though the antibodies formed originally against antigen protein from tuberculosis, malaria, and PCP fungi pathogens as well as many other pathogens.

There are, therefore, no "HIV" infections either by sexual transmission or via the bloodstream. *So-called mother-child transmissions are transmissions of maternal antibodies to the child and/or toxic damage to the child's immature immune-cell formation in the mother's womb and/or immune-cell anomalies after birth by toxic medication treatment.* They can also be the result of the mother having a chronic infection that was transmitted to the child. So-called professionally caused "HIV" transmissions or transmission by rape are anecdotal reports. There is no validated proof case of this in all the HIV/AIDS literature. These horror stories are based on the pseudo-logic of the HIV/AIDS theory and serve as alleged confirmation of the "HIV" infection for the general public. Consequently there is also no treatment or prevention against the putatively real "HIV" as the alleged cause of AIDS.

Yet there are effective prevention and treatment possibilities for pre-AIDS and AIDS. Besides compensating for undernourishment and malnutrition as well as the treatment sought for infectious and noninfectious causes of disease and avoidance of specific risks, a suitably dosed antioxidant compensatory therapy is indicated. This calls for proteins containing sulfur and other additives as well as amino acids (glutathione, cysteine, homocysteine, arginine, etc.), vitamins, minerals, trace elements, plant polyphenols, natural protease inhibitors such as polyanions based on sea algae and cartilage preparations, prostaglandin modulators made of fish oils (omega-3 fatty acid) or, in difficult cases, selective cyclooxygenase-2 inhibitors, if necessary difluoromethylornithine as a polyamine inhibitor, and gamma globulin (Hässig 1998 b) in case of opportunistic infections. Non-toxic therapeutics recognizes many possibilities of balancing a disturbance of cellular immunobalance without blocking cellular respiration by AZT and related substances. In recent years orthodox HIV/AIDS medicine too has begun to rediscover the possibilities of consistent antioxidant protection and liver protection for patients with acquired cellular immunodeficiencies. In this sphere, developing countries have an abundance of potential options by using sea products as food supplements, building up a license-free plantation economy for phytotherapeutics, and recollection of ethnomedical experience.

Since 1984, an incredible waste of resources has occurred in Western countries regarding the largest capital investment in medical history based on the objectively false disease theory "HIV causes AIDS." Poor countries can hardly afford the luxury of crippling the will of their people to survive through irrational sex and death fantasies instead of investing their meager resources in improving general living conditions. This also includes comprehensive further education of medical staff to the state of medical knowledge in 2000 instead of 1984. The history of Western medicine has demonstrated that the prevalence of chronic inflammatory and infectious processes was reduced drastically and continuously up until the middle of the previous century prior to introduction of chemotherapeutics, antibiotics, and mass immunization (Sagan 1987). Meanwhile, fundamental findings of Western medical research into NO, cell symbiosis, and other areas have gained significance in other important spheres of preventive and therapeutic medicine outside official

HIV/AIDS medicine. Sooner or later these findings will also prevail in the broadest sense in AIDS prevention and therapy. Scientists, physicians, and others involved, particularly in the news media, have benefited for 16 years from the massive capital flow to research to combat "HIV"/AIDS. They have been outraged by the South African government's critical questions about the cause, treatment and prevention of AIDS, reacting out of ignorance, irrational conformist rhetoric against "conspiracy theories" and, in general, an indolent unwillingness to learn.

However, discriminating against physicians and scientists as AIDS dissidents, who have only drawn rational conclusions from validated medical-research findings based on the best available knowledge, their consciences, and their sense of duty, is an unacceptable violation of general human rights, especially for the patients involved. What would happen if the South African government were to maintain the "HIV causes AIDS" disease theory that, in the meantime, has become scientifically obsolete and approve recommended mass poisoning with AZT and related toxic pharmaceuticals? It would actually trigger the catastrophe suggested to the Africans by interested physicians, mass media, politicians, and drug concerns as well as the large army of profiteers and the stream of capital would flow to exploit the self-staged archaic fear of a plague. After having overcome the racist mania of Apartheid, it must become the historic mission of the South African government to resist the HIV plague mania and to develop its own African way to improve general living standards and standards for prevention and therapy.

Such "HIV positives" have survived in Western countries by resisting mass fear hysteria, recognizing risks of disease, and using a broad range of natural food-supplement resources and antioxidant medicine. Meanwhile, the "HIV positives" who trusted the highly toxic "antiviral" pharmaceutical substances and chemotherapeutics have fallen victims to HIV/AIDS medicine. According to official government statistics published by the German public-health authorities in 1985, for example, each German with "HIV" must have been infected by 1995 and died of AIDS by 2000. These figures, projected by the semi-logarithmic Weibull statistical method, have never been corrected. Instead, the country's mass media have bought these and many other absurd claims as medical facts. The same health-care authorities officially stated in 1999 that 0.0015% of the population was newly registered as "HIV"/AIDS cases, and that it still concerned people from the same risk groups. The same leading news media failed miserably to report on this clear counterargument to the hysterical news a "fatal sex epidemic transmittable to anybody." Instead it promptly reported at the World AIDS Congress on 9 July 2000 in South

Africa that "Almost half of all young women are HIV-positive at age 20, and 58% of them are by the time they are 25. Among men, the infection rate reached its apex at age 32, since 45% had the fatal virus in the blood" (*Der Spiegel*, 3 July 2000). A similar numbers game, the same horror stories about epidemic, sex, and sensation spread in the USA and Europe during the past two decades is being projected at the moment in South Africa, the country that is supposed to serve as a strategic beachhead for the pharmaceutical firms to access all other developing countries.

The director of the Epidemiology Research Unit in Johannesburg, Dr. Williams, is quoted as the only verifiable source of the assertion on the alleged epidemic nature of HIV/AIDS in South Africa: "The sudden increase in tuberculosis cases among gold miners attracted the attention of epidemiologist Williams to Carletonville. Within 10 years the number of tuberculosis patients had almost quadrupled; TB frequency was 100 times greater than in Western industrial nations. The researcher knew that lung disease often comes as the result of a HIV infection. Tests confirmed his suspicion. Every third miner was already infected with HIV, as were 37% of all adult women." (*Der Spiegel*, "Fluch der Jungen," 3 July 2000). What Europe's largest news magazine with the advertising slogan "Spiegel readers know more" failed to tell its readers was that orthodox HIV/AIDS researchers at America's Harvard University had established in a comprehensive 1994 study that "HIV-1," ELISA and WB results should be interpreted with caution when screening individuals infected with *M. tuberculosis* or other mycobacterial species.

So, too, ELISA and WB may not be sufficient for a HIV diagnosis in AIDS-endemic areas of Central Africa where the prevalence of mycobacterial disease is quite high. There is a very high rate of false-positive ELISA and WB results in "HIV tests" (Kashala 1994). Like many other leading media, *Der Spiegel*, has been informed several times in writing, with submissions from scientific publications, of the untenable nature of the HIV/AIDS claim in Africa. But it has not changed its deliberately false coverage. Even in 1985 the ELISA test had only been accepted as an "HIV" diagnostic test by Western countries due to the "90% false-positive HIV results." According to Western testing guidelines, a second positive ELISA test result must be confirmed by a positive test result in the so-called WB test. In Africa, as a rule, only the ELISA test is carried out, if any, on cost grounds, and then using two test antigen proteins. Such HIV-positive test results do not count as confirmed positive results in Western countries. Since 1992 the WB confirmation test has not been allowed as an "HIV" confirmation test in Great Britain as it was considered too unreliable. There are no binding international standards for "HIV" tests. However, the biomedical truth is that any "HIV" test is false-positive, and none of these tests can show antibody bond against "HIV," since nobody has provided proof that the test substrate of the "HIV" test contains "HIV" protein. On the other hand, any informed person knows the specific causes for tuberculosis and other infections among itinerant workers in African gold-mines are related to the labor conditions and living conditions in the residential camps. To understand these diseases, as recent medical research has sufficiently explained, there needs to be no "HIV" infection or "HIV positive" test results among people in Africa who have come into contact with the endemic tuberculosis pathogen.

Does the South African government really want to expose the South African people to the arcane practitioners of international epidemic speculators and the "brutality typical of concerns in the pharmaceutical sector" (*Der Spiegel*, 26 June 2000)? Years of experience in Western countries has taught that preventive and therapeutic recommendations were not understood and could not have been implemented to target groups properly during recent decades without basic communication of medical research's changing knowledge.

Medicine and health-care policy are always part of a tacit system knowledge dominance that must be counterchecked by transparency. However, during the past two decades counterchecking by institutionalized medicine and leaders of medical opinion speaking in trade journals has failed in the case of HIV/AIDS medicine, since the self-styled "HIV-retrovirus" researchers were the initiators of the epidemic hysteria and at same time chief consultants deciding on release of immense amounts of research money as well as publishing on HIV/AIDS in the specialized media (Lang 1998). The South African government will have to find a more than rhetorical response to the extremely dangerous challenge of the World AIDS Congress in its own country that is known to have been sponsored by the international pharmaceutical concerns. The degree of the unscrupulous mixture of deliberate medical perjury, distortion of scholarly based counter-analyses, malicious personal discrimination and discrediting of a sovereign government's members can hardly increase in the service of "brutal" economic interests.

"Shortly before the13th World AIDS Conference that took place in the harbor city of Durban 9-14 July," reported *Der Spiegel*, "Chief of State Thabo Mbeki also caused annoyance and confusion. He sought to speak to scientists who championed the long refuted thesis that AIDS is not the result of an HIV infection but the consequence of drug and alcohol abuse, poverty, and underdevelopment. As the Boers' racist regime was forced to abdicate in 1994, the country still had a chance to stem the epidemic. Yet the national

AIDS plan broke down due to an authority free-for-all, mistrust for white experts, and a lack of political will to lead. In his five-year term in office, the country's first black president, the globally respected Mandela dedicated less public time to the South African AIDS topic than he did to a PR meeting with the Spice Girls, Naomi Campbell, and Michael Jackson. Prominent black pop stars had indeed already warned in 1990 that AIDS could 'ruin the fulfillment of our dreams,' indeed a health-card paper written by the then still exiled African National Congress (ANC) had conceded that almost 60,000 freedom fighters could be infected, yet none of the returnees were tested. And only once, at the end of 1998 at an economic forum in Switzerland, did Mandela make AIDS the topic of a detailed speech. Every fifth new South African mother was already HIV-positive at the time.

Meanwhile 22.4% of all newborns countrywide are infected. The epidemic rate among women under 30 even lies at almost 26%. Nonetheless, in no year since the ANC's takeover of power has the national AIDS budget even been fully spent. At the same time the health minister refuses AZT "on cost grounds," though it would reduce the probability of HIV transmission to the newborn by half" (*Der Spiegel*, 3 July 2000).

Even though thoroughly informed, the editorial board of *Der Spiegel*, which prides itself on having the most serious journalistic reputation, suppresses the following important fact in its coverage: *Highly toxic AZT blocks maturation of antibody-producing immune cells in bone marrow* (Rosenthal 1994).

The newborn will be protected against extracellular disease pathogens during the first months of life by antibodies transmitted from the mother. Newborn antibodies measured by the "HIV" test are therefore antibodies of the mother.

About 12% of newborns with "HIV positive" mothers in Western countries react positively in these tests. In the sense of HIV/AIDS theory, this finding means that 88% of newborns are supposed to have received no antibodies in the mother's womb via the common circulatory system, although the mother's "HIV" is supposed to have increased a billion times a day and the mother's antibodies may have had to survive for years against the "HIV" in the blood serum. On the other hand, 12% of newborns are supposed to have accepted the mother's "HIV" antibodies and react positively to the "HIV" test. This assumption means an insoluble contradiction in the sense of HIV/AIDS theory, since any newborn accepts antibodies from the mother and logically, according to HIV/AIDS theory, must also receive the "HIV" allegedly multiplying a billion-fold in the blood serum of the "HIV positive" mother. In this logical difficulty, one treats all "HIV positive" pregnant mothers with AZT, although one knows that pregnant mothers in Africa even within the framework of HIV/AIDS theory could show a "very high rate of false-positive results in ELISA and WB HIV tests" (Kashala 1994). If the newborn is negative in the "HIV" test after birth, one claims that the "HIV" infection has been prevented through AZT. On the other hand, if the newborn is positive in the "HIV" test, the newborn will continue to be treated with AZT.

Nobody really knows with which antibodies the mother and newborn have reacted positively to the test. Since the sensitivity threshold of the "HIV" test is adjusted to a certain amount of antibodies, the "positive HIV" test means only that the mother and newborn indicate a sufficiently high amount of antibodies to react positively to the "HIV" test's protein. A "negative HIV" test for a newborn of an "HIV positive" mother merely indicates that the newborn has not accepted enough antibodies from the mother or has already formed them itself to register a positive result in the "HIV" test. Yet the "HIV" could still have been transmitted from the mother to the newborn if one assumes that the "HIV" exists in the mother's bloodstream, as demonstrated by the "HIV" test, with which all kinds of antibodies can react. Since AZT, due to its biochemical properties, suppresses immune cells producing newly maturing antibodies among pregnant women treated with AZT the probability increases that the newborn accepts fewer antibodies than would be required for a positive result in the "HIV" test. The claim that "use of AZT reduces the probability of HIV transmission to the newborn by half" (*Der Spiegel*, 3 July 2000) is based on this effect.

In reality, neither an "HIV positive" nor an "HIV negative" result for the newborn would express anything about transmission of the "HIV" after an "HIV positive" pregnant woman has been treated with AZT, even if one assumes that she were actually infected by the "HIV." Even in this (fictitious) case, the "HIV" test result would provide only information that more or less of the mother's antibodies were transmitted to the child without being able to know if they were antibodies against (fictitious) "HIV" or antibodies against other antigens.

However, the biological truth is that AZT, due to its biochemical properties, could not inhibit "HIV," since the substance is not integrated in any DNA or any provirus DNA of an "HIV." Rather it blocks the cell respiration of immune and non-immune cells and causes secondary DNA damage to these cells. Thus the logical consequence would be that HIV would not be inhibited if prescribed to all pregnant women in South Africa with positive "HIV tests" (allegedly 22.4% of all pregnant women) as a prophylaxis against transmission of the "HIV" to the newborn. AZT does not do what it allegedly should do but demonstrably does what the substance should supposedly prevent, namely promote acquired immunodeficiency. AZT has caused in newborns serious birth defects and other maturity disturbances (Kumar 1994, Moye 1996). Administration of AZT is strictly contraindicated for all "HIV positives" and AIDS patients, pregnant women, newborns, children, women, and men including those patients diagnosed as "HIV-positives" without a "positive HIV" test finding according to the Bangui definition of AIDS cases. *"A critical analysis of presently available data which claim that AZT has anti-HIV effects shows there is neither theoretical nor experimental evidence which proves that AZT, used either alone or in combination with other drugs, has any such effect"* (Papadopulos-Eleopulos 1999).

The real active mechanism of AZT is clearly known. AZT inhibits certain enzymes in cell respiration of immune and non-immune cells. The result is development of opportunistic infections (AIDS), certain tumors, and degeneration of muscle and nerve cells. Even the manufacturer warns: "Retrovir (Zidovudine = AZT) may be associated with severe hematologic toxicity including granulocytopenia and severe anemia . . . . Prolonged use of Retrovir has also been associated with symptomatic myopathy . . ." (Glaxo Wellcome, 1998).

The fact that AZT also inhibits enzymes in microbes has been misinterpreted as inhibiting "HIV" replication. Since opportunistic pathogens can adapt better to the inhibiting effect than the cell systems of patients whose immune systems have already been weakened, AZT medication, sooner or later, will favor uninhibited development of opportunistic pathogens (AIDS). Due to their similar action, AZT and over-stimulation of NO gas have identical effects: accelerated cell deterioration and/or cell-biology counterregulations. However, fixation on "HIV" infection veils this causal relationship. The AZT manufacturer admits "similar pathological changes such as those produced by HIV illness have been associated with long-term medication of AZT" (Glaxo Wellcome, 1998). However, symptoms of "HIV" illness (anomalies of cellular immunity, positive "HIV" test, and opportunistic infections) can be explained free of contradiction by NO research findings and without assuming the existence of "HIV." The test findings of Dr. Brian Williams ignore the fact that this causal relationship can be demonstrated as follows:

"The ELISA and WB test results should be interpreted with caution when screening individuals infected with *M. tuberculosis* or other mycobacterial species . . . The ELISA and WB HIV test cannot be sufficient for HIV diagnosis in AIDS-endemic areas of Central Africa where the prevalence of mycobacterial diseases is very high" (Kashala, 1994).

The lack of a well-informed medical base has had disastrous effects for South Africa and other developing countries. The World Health Organization (WHO) based much of its prognosis on positive "HIV test" findings by the director of the Epidemiology Research Unit in Johannesburg, Dr. Williams, working with cases of tuberculosis infections in Carletonville and other areas in South Africa.

"Every other South African youth will die of AIDS, a WHO study predicted," reported *Der Spiegel*. "Every hour another 70 South Africans are infected with the fatal virus. And nowhere, believes epidemiologist Brian Williams, 55, is the situation as bad as in the mining city of Carletonville. Because gold mining offers the ideal breeding grounds for a virus transmitted by sexual acts. Some 70,000 lonesome men live in the barracks of the mining companies around the small town and its black townships. This is the result of a job-creation policy introduced during Apartheid. Gold lies several thousand meters below ground in Carletonville. Not much more than a gram is gained from every ton of boulders extracted. If the mining is to pay, itinerant workers must be shipped to the mining sites. To this day they only see their families every two to three months. The rest of the year they live crammed together, 14 men to every 45 square meters" (*Der Spiegel*, 3 July 2000).

Every experienced industrial physician knows that the working and living conditions described are ideal breeding grounds for tuberculosis and other microbial infections in view of the low medical standards in African countries. The "sudden increase in tuberculosis cases among gold miners made epidemiologist Williams aware of Carletonville," *Der Spiegel* continued. "Within 10 years the number of tuberculosis patients almost quadrupled. TB incidence was 100 times greater than in Western industrialized countries. The researcher knew that lung disease often comes after an HIV infection. Tests confirmed his suspicion: HIV had already infected every third miner. Another 37% of all adult women were also infected. Completely unprepared, the researcher concluded the extent to which the epidemic had infected Khutsong's young people. Among girls the HIV infection rate rose with a leap at age 15; at age 20 almost half of all young women were HIV-positive;

at age 25 some 58% had been infected. Among men the epidemic rate reached its apex at age 32, since 45% had the fatal virus in their blood" (*Der Spiegel*, 3 July 2000).

These claims on the alleged epidemic rates in South Africa were diagnosed with so-called ELISA HIV diagnostic tests that even in orthodox HIV/AIDS medicine, from the outset, recorded 90% false-positives. Moreover, the test result depends on the blood's viscosity, and this is higher in tropical countries than in Western countries. Testing preparation and testing technique in African countries do not qualify as meaningful in Western HIV/AIDS medical circles, so that people who test "HIV-positive" in Africa regularly show "HIV-negative" test results in repeat tests in Western countries. Despite this, these "HIV-positive" test results were bought by the WHO, Western HIV/AIDS physicians, and the international news media as biological facts in order to exert political and economic pressure on developing countries. Yet from the viewpoint of scientifically based medicine with a minimum claim to seriousness, it is crucial to know for reasons of interpretation what these antibody reaction tests in case of serial tests in Africa could tell us, if anything at all. That is:

- Whether "HIV" tests react positively to antibodies in the blood stream of test subjects that were supposed only to have been formed against "HIV" after sexual transmission of "HIV" to people with a healthy immune system.

- Or whether the test subjects in "HIV" tests react positively to antibodies that have formed in their bloodstream after primarily latent or manifest infection with mycobacteria (*M. tuberculosis, M. leprosy, M. avium*), fungal microbes (*Pneumocystis carinii, Candida, Cryptococcus, Coccidioides, Histoplasma*, etc.) or other microbes entirely without a hypothetical infection with "HIV."

The answer to these crucial diagnostic questions can be demonstrated by comparisons with assertions of HIV/AIDS theory and the data from NO research as well as findings actually validated scientifically (see end of this chapter).

The research data show clearly that "HIV" tests react positively to antibodies formed against mycobacteria and fungus microbes. The assertion of HIV/AIDS medicine that "positive HIV" test results in Africa should be given equal diagnostic weight with a fatal "HIV" infection is not scientifically viable. The assertion of Dr. Williams that development of tuberculosis among

Africans is the result of an "HIV" infection is without medical foundation. The biological truth is rather that a mycobacterial tuberculosis infection leads to antibody formation that could react positively to test protein in the "HIV" test. The mycobacterial infection precedes a positive result in the "HIV" test and not vice versa. If a positive result in the "HIV" test actually indicates a still active mycobacterial or fungal infection or another infection it cannot be decided on the basis of an "HIV" test. Specific diagnostic processes must be used for such a statement. The antibody reaction in the "HIV" test could involve existing antibodies stemming from an earlier infection, and this test fails to show which infection it has identified. To this extent, use of an "HIV" test is senseless, misleading, and highly unethical.

Scientific and deliberately false assertions on lethal "HIV" infections in South Africa make perfidious use of pseudo-evidence of "positive HIV" tests to allot political guilt to the South African government and to spread irrational death fears out of vested political and economic interest.

"Half of the young people will die of the epidemic because the state has failed to act." warned *Der Spiegel.* "The major death toll has just begun . . . A catastrophe of unimaginable extent looms in countries such as Zimbabwe, Zambia, Botswana, and South Africa. The land at the Cape was the last to register the pandemic. At first the disease seemed to affect above all white homosexuals. That was in the late 1980s when the Boers still ruled. They regarded the epidemic as divine punishment for sexual perversion. Health-care policy measures were not taken. Then the radical change occurred. A civil war raged in the country's most populated state, Kwazulu-Natal. Right-wing white militants threatened a coup as the blacks celebrated the release of their hero, Nelson Mandela, after 27 years of imprisonment. The virus was forgotten. Ten years later it has inflicted more than one tenth of the population. And almost all victims are black. Yet the political leadership still reacts helplessly to the epidemic. Indeed a health-care paper written by the African National Congress (ANC) had conceded while still in exile that nearly 60,000 freedom fighters could be infected. Yet none of the returnees were tested" (*Der Spiegel,* 3 July 2000).

Thus it gave the impression that 60,000 freedom fighters potentially infected with the lethal "HIV" had dragged the "HIV" epidemic into the country upon their return, and the ANC government had looked on idly at "the death of half of the young people." Yet the same news magazine had already declared Africa to be the "dying continent" in 1991 (*Der Spiegel,* 17 June 1991). Since then, according to data from the United Nations, the population in Africa has increased by more than 100 million people. If the South African government, under pressure from the international epidemic speculators, were to adopt the medically and scientifically untenable HIV/AIDS theory as national doctrine and approve the mass poisoning with AZT and other toxic AIDS medicines, this would in fact be "criminal betrayal of responsibility to one's own people" (Mbeki: Letter to world leaders on AIDS in Africa, 3 April 2000).

The World AIDS Congress hops from continent to continent every two years, invading another country like a plague of locusts. The horror story of the homosexual scene as the breeding grounds of the "death virus," transmittable to anybody through sex, has lost its impact among the Western public. For example, according to the official 1999 medical statistics from Germany, a total of about 800 "HIV" stigmatized people died of AIDS. All of these victims were treated pharmacotoxically. In contrast to the non-event of the mass epidemic predicted for years, some 11,000 stars and their supporting cast staged the HIV/AIDS travelling circus during the millennium year. The doctors, scientists, health-care officials, media reporters, and epidemic activists had been lured to South Africa with sponsoring funds from the drugs firms. There they would tell the gruesome epidemic saga of the 60,000 demilitarized bush warriors who had returned to their country untested for the death germ they were prepared to sow among every other youth. In return, shareholders wanted to see the turnover of pharmacotoxic products increased with "the brutality typical of the sector" (*Der Spiegel*, 26 June 2000).

The turnover figures in developing countries would pay off in view of stagnating sales in Western countries, even at the rock bottom prices offered by the World Health Organization and the Western pharmaceutical firms. Millions of poisoned corpses should pay the price for the grotesque epidemic. The opening strategy should focus on treatment of "HIV positive" pregnant women with "antiviral" AIDS medicines that inhibit maturing of antibody-producing bone-marrow cells and in this way fake inhibition of "HIV" in newborn babies.

South Africa, *quo vadis*? Will the freedom fighters of the ANC stop the virus hunt? Or will epidemic Apartheid replace racial Apartheid?

"Not long ago in our own country," President Mbeki wrote to world leaders concerning AIDS, "people were killed, tortured, imprisoned, and inhibited from being quoted in private and in public, because the established authority believed that their views were dangerous and discredited. We are now being asked to do precisely the same thing that the racist apartheid tyranny we opposed did, because it is said, there exists a scientific view that is supported by the majority, against which dissent is prohibited." (Mbeki: Letter to world leaders on AIDS in Africa, 3 April 2000).

Yet today the issue is no longer scientific dissent. It is hard medical facts suppressed by vested interests. This specifically concerns the "clean torture" of millions of defenseless people who have been placed in deathly fear and are supposed to be treated with demonstrably toxic pharmaceutical substances. These form the diagnostic basis of antibody reaction tests that demonstrably indicate anything else than an infection with a fatal "HIV." And it specifically concerns medical and social standards in developing countries to improve the state of knowledge in the year 2000 in order to hinder the actual causes of AIDS (in the most narrow and broadest senses) preventively and therapeutically. This task of the century will also demand use of all powers and resources in an intelligent manner and without the obsession of HIV/AIDS medicine, which simplifies and compounds in a terrifying fashion the problem facing us.

The speech of President Mbeki at the opening of the 13th World AIDS Congress in Durban on 9 July 2000 was the right signal for all independent scientists if the practice of future health-care policy is not to be determined by organized disinformation but by sober factual analysis.

"According to predictions presented in Durban by two American officials, the Bureau of Statistics and the Agency for International Development (AID), life expectancy in Botswana is 29 years, in South Africa, Swaziland, and Namibia 30 years—the most pessimistic prediction on the catastrophic development so far. On the other hand, Mbeki said at the opening of the congress that poverty is the greatest cause of death in the world and the most important reason for disease and suffering. At least indirectly he expressed doubt on the extent of the AIDS catastrophe in South Africa. In Botswana every third person in the sexually active population is infected, the highest percentage in the world. In South Africa 4.2 million people carry the virus—every fifth adult—more than in any other country in the world. From 2003 on, according to new American studies, the population in South Africa and Botswana will shrink. Some 70% of the 34 million HIV victims and almost all of the 11 million AIDS orphans of the world live in sub-Sahara Africa. In Mbeki's opening speech to the congress, where more than 11,000 doctors, scientists, and AIDS activists met for more than six days, he even disappointed hopes of those from his area that he would change his controversial position on the cause and combating of AIDS. He said one could not simply place all the blame on a virus but avoided comments on the link between HIV and AIDS.

In contrast to the overwhelming opinion of the scientists, he obviously did not consider this link crucial. In a letter to the South African opposition leader Leon, Mbeki repeated his doubts on the effectiveness of AIDS medicine, which unsettled scientists all the more. The South African health minister, Dr. Manto Tschambalala-Msimang, also expressed this doubt. She said on the second day of the congress that the effect and possible danger of the drug Nevirapine must be checked carefully before it could be used in South Africa. The German pharmaceutical enterprise Boehringer Ingelheim, manufacturer of Nevirapine, that could greatly reduce transmission of AIDS from mothers to their unborn children or after the birth through mother milk, had offered to supply the drug to South Africa and other developing countries without cost for five years." (*Frankfurter Allgemeine Zeitung*: Weitere Kontroversen auf dem AIDS-Gipfel in Durban 11 July 2000).

Nevirapine is a so-called non-nucleoside analog substance used as an "HIV" replication inhibitor. Analogous to AZT, the substance inhibits the maturing of antibodies producing bone-marrow cells and can cause an "HIV-negative" result in the "HIV" test for newborns. A critical analysis of currently available data shows that Nevirapine exercises just as little "anti-HIV" effect as AZT (Papadopoulos-Eleopulos 1999).

Anyone who looks at the pseudo-logic of the HIV/AIDS theory rationally does not need "careful study of the effect and possible danger of the Nevirapine resource," because there is just as little indication for use of this immunotoxic substance as for AZT. On the contrary there are only strict contraindications. Anyone who has not understood the pseudo-logic of the HIV/AIDS theory must keep in mind that AZT, Nevirapine, and other "antiviral" AIDS medicines could not inhibit "HIV" even if somebody had validated the existence of the "HIV."

Even in this case, there is no indication for "careful study on the effect and possible danger of the Nevirapine resource," but there are clear contraindications.

Anyone who considers the pseudo-logic of the HIV/AIDS theory to be correct because the vast majority of physicians present it as correct for rational reasons will be forced, not only, theoretically and experimentally to make a "careful study of the effect and possible danger of the Nevirapine resource." Additionally, one will be forced to study carefully, under pressure from the rationally incomprehensible public assertion that every second young person must die from the fatal "HIV" infection, therapeutical use of

Nevirapine and other "antiviral" AIDS medicines in treating pregnant women, newborns, children, young people, other women, and men. The tragedy of the HIV/AIDS medicine in Western countries during the past 14 years has sufficiently established this predictable fact.

The result of giving "careful study" to prescribing Nevirapine, AZT, etc. to "HIV positive" pregnant women and their newborns in South Africa and other developing countries would be programmed from the outset. The effects of Nevirapine, etc., would only prove that unspecified antibodies could be manipulated toxically. According to random statistical distribution of the substance by pharmacokinetics and pharmacodynamics, a portion of newborn children of mothers testing "HIV-positive" during pregnancy would react "HIV positive" to the unsuitable, because it is unspecific, test while another portion would test "HIV negative." This pseudo-proof of inhibiting the "HIV" at the cost of serious immunotoxic damage that has been found to appear biologically after brief medication with so-called AIDS medication would justify regular use of Nevirapine or its competitors by millions of pregnant women and newborns. The immunotoxic damage appearing would be blamed on the "HIV." Nobody would any longer be prepared to discuss the verifiable fact that the HIV/AIDS medicine specialists, despite knowing better, had confused cause and effect. And the cell-biology counterregulations constantly resulting from immune-system stress would be explained as proof of the "lethal HIV."

The free offer for "basic study" of Nevirapine, for example, was presented in context of competition with other pharmaceutical firms and their toxic products. The payback for the manufacturer would multiply after five years. In the long term the South African government would be hopelessly handed over to a dictatorship by the pharmaceutical concerns and practitioners of "HIV" laboratory medicine through this refined marketing ploy.

Indeed, the manipulated world citizenry would honor the South African government's immunotoxic mass poisoning of its own people, and the accusation of "lack of will in political leadership" (*Der Spiegel*, 3 July 2000) would no longer be heard!

If the fundamental findings of NO gas research and other biomedical research sectors during the early 1980s had already been known, nobody would have needed an explanation concerning development of opportunistic infections (AIDS) by "HIV." Nobody would have considered it necessary for laboratories to act in designing an "HIV" test. And nobody would have been able to justify thorough research on the effect and possible dangers of immunotoxic substances paradoxically to treat people with acquired immunodeficiencies.

One would have established and verified the antioxidant state of endangered and diseased people, that the antioxidant deficits and NO gas inhibition of immune cells are present long before the manifest appearance of opportunistic infections. One would have recognized the specific risks of endangered and diseased immunodeficient patients in Western countries and developing countries. And would have tried to avoid this through preventive medicine and to restore the immunobalance through targeted compensatory therapy and inhibition of cell-biology counterregulation. This is not the first time in medical history that serious vitamin-deficiency diseases, for instance, have been confused with viral infections.

As an answer, the "HIV" propaganda headquarters of the United Nations (UNAIDS) has pointed accusingly to the conduct of President Mbeki:

"If things continue in this manner, all efforts invested in development aid will have been for nothing, which would naturally have an impact on the world economy. In the worst case, anarchy threatens." (*Der Spiegel*: "Zeitbombe vor der Haustür," July 10 2000). The veiled political blackmail could hardly have been expressed more clearly.

However, the propaganda noise of paranoiacs serving the pharmaceutical industry could not entirely cover up the fact that even medical advocates of the organized mass poisoning supported the critical position of the South African government.

"The problem for most of those affected today is still the side effects of therapy," *Der Spiegel* reported. "Experts even consider it possible that in 10 years this will result in widespread coronaries among those infected with HIV. And even cancerous diseases could become the problem then due to weakened immune systems as a result of the 'side effects' of therapy" (*Der Spiegel*, "Zukunft der Todgeweihten," 10 July 2000).

It could hardly be more absurd: The same toxic mixers who assert that immunotoxic "antiviral" AIDS medicines would prevent immune-cell weaknesses now predict as experts that the same immunotoxically treated patients would develop widespread coronaries and also cancerous diseases "due to immune systems weakened by the side effects of therapy."

The biological truth is that, viewed objectively, all "antiviral" AIDS medicines can cause immune deficiencies, heart muscle weakness, and transformations of cells into cancer cells due to inhibition of cell respiration. This is especially true among people whose immune systems are already weakened. But AIDS medication cannot inhibit any "HIV," even if the actual existence of "HIV" were to be detected by somebody.

The course of discussion at the 13th World AIDS Congress had confirmed the view of the Wall Street Journal in 1996 that "HIV-positives" and AIDS patients treated with "antiviral" AIDS medicines "are practically the guinea pigs of drug research in one of the largest and most expensive medical experiments of our time."

The South African government has been the first in the world to counter the uninhibited running amok of "HIV"/AIDS medicine and its profiteers with rational and humanitarian standards. The consequence must again be to recognize fundamental findings on the ancient laws of co-evolution between humans and microbes in healthcare and social policies. The AIDS problem demonstrates civilization's vulnerability if the manipulative potential of modern medicine is abused to exploit humanity worldwide by staging irrational fear of epidemics without effective and rational countercontrols. The deceptive strategies of the virus hunters and their propagandists and profiteers are more insidious than the old colonialism, since the human right to life and freedom from bodily harm is being annulled under the mask of humanitarian aid instead of the scientifically validated real causes of AIDS being treated with the nontoxic resources available.

HIV/AIDS medicine has produced monstrous problems, but it has not solved a single problem. The expiry dates of the promised healings become ever shorter, the means of disinformation ever more incredible, and medical ethics have long been forgotten. For 16 years the prospect has been held out of developing sera against the "HIV" during the next 2-10 years. This occurred for the first time in April 1984 when the American government announced the national doctrine "HIV is the most probably cause of AIDS." (It remains a mystery today how they wanted to develop a serum against a "probable" cause.) Since then the trickery has been repeated regularly by promising an "anti-HIV" serum before and during every World AIDS Congress. These are the simple methods applied at the stock market to maintain the capital flow for new research money. Yet the feeling of being threatened must be raised each time, by means of propaganda at the cost of people in developing countries. The congenital defect of HIV/AIDS medicine was the patent office registration by the discoverer of the "HIV" test before submitting it to any scientific publication. The premature commercialization corrupted HIV/AIDS medicine from the very start.

In contrast, the findings of NO research, cytokine research, and cell symbiosis research are available to anybody free of patent for preventive and therapeutic use.

Comparison of Predictions between HIV/AIDS Theory and NO Research on Cause and Incidence of Tuberculosis and Other Opportunistic Infections and Real Scientific Findings

A. Predictions of HIV/AIDS Theory

1. Exposure and disposition:
    - Transmission of "HIV" by sexual exposure
    - Sexual transmission possible to anyone without special disposition
    - Transmission from mother to child, women to men, men to women, men to men

2. Immune system anomalies:
    - Sharp reduction in number of T-helper immune cells in blood serum (Th cells) resulting from destruction of Th cells by "HIV."
    - Positive "HIV" test: reaction to test protein with antibodies in blood serum that should only occur again "HIV" protein.
    - Molecular "HIV" markers: characteristic only for "HIV."

3. Opportunistic infections (AIDS):
    - Immune system deficiencies in combating tuberculosis, fungal, and parasite pathogens resulting from destruction of Th cells by "HIV."

4. Prevention and therapy:
    - Inhibited reproduction of "HIV" by "antiviral AIDS" medicines.
    - Anti-microbial treatment with chemical antibiotics.

B. Predictions of NO Research

1. Exposure and disposition:
    - Increased exposure to *M. tuberculosis* and other mycobacteria, fungal, and parasite pathogens resulting from higher epidemic rates in

the total population. Too few preventive check-ups, low medical standards, lack of hygiene, and other factors.
- Increased disposition due to undernourishment and malnutrition, burdening work, housing, and living conditions, more frequent burdens from other chronic infections.

2. Immune system anomalies
   - Functional change in Th cells after intensive and/or long-lasting NO over-stimulation.
   - Maturation arrest and accelerating death of NO gas-producing Th1 cells as result of exhaustion and/or low acceptance or synthesis of antioxidants for detoxification.
   - Dominance and emigration of non-NO gas-producing Th2 cells from the blood serum (Th1-Th2 switch).
   - Increased antibody production influenced by type 2 cytokines of Th2 cells.
   - Positive "HIV" test: unspecified reaction of test proteins with antibodies that would form against antigens of tuberculosis and other mycobacterial pathogens as well as fungal and parasitic pathogens.
   - Molecular "HIV" markers: characteristic cell products resulting from cell biology counterregulations, primarily by NO over-stimulation and secondarily by NO inhibition due to insufficiently eliminated intracellular infection with mycobacteria as well as fungal and parasitic microbes.

2. Opportunistic infections (AIDS):
   - Poor elimination of intracellular tuberculosis and other mycobacterial pathogens as well as fungal and parasitic pathogens including after Th1-Th2 switch with surviving Th2 dominance.
   - Characteristic with inhibited NO gas production by Th1 cells after previously intensive and/or long-lasting NO gas over-stimulation.
   - Exhaustion of antioxidant detoxification and/or lack of antioxidants (reduced synthesis and/or reduced nutrient supply).

3. Prevention and therapy:
   - Antioxidant compensation therapy and inhibition of cell-biology counterregulation to restore the balance of immune cells and other cell systems.
   - Nontoxic anti-microbial treatment.

C. Current Scientific and Medical Findings

1. Exposure and disposition:
   - Continuous decline in the prevalence and incidence of tuberculosis and other infections in Western countries during the 1840-1940 period to a very low level by improving working, housing, and living conditions, hygiene, nutrition, and medical standards before the introduction of chemotherapy, BCG, and other immunizations (Sagan 1997).

2. Immune system anomalies:
   - Th1-Th2 switch and surviving Th2 dominance as well as inhibition of NO gas production in Th1 cells in the case of all chronic mycobacteria as well as fungal, parasitic, and worm infections among others
   - Increased antibody production influenced by dominant type 2 cytokine patterns of Th2 cells with all chronic mycobacterial, fungal, parasitic, and worm infections among others.
   - Positive "HIV" test: very high rates of false-positive ELISA and WB "HIV" test results with mycobacterial infections (*M. tuberculosis, M. leprae, M. avium intracellulare*) and fungal infections (including *Pneumocystis carinii, Candida, Cryptococcus, Coccidoides, Histoplasma*).
   - Molecular "HIV" markers as a result of intensive or long-lasting nitrosative and prooxidative stress ubiquitous in human cell systems as characteristic regeneration enzymes, regenerative cytokines, and stress protein. (Lincoln 1997, Lucey 1996, Kashala 1994, Papadopulos-Eleopulos 1997 c, Temin 1985, Teng 1997, Brattsand 1996, Del Prete 1998).

3. Opportunistic infections (AIDS):
   - Characteristic in case of Th2 dominance (Lucey 1996, Abbas 1996, Mosmann 1996).
   - Characteristic in case of NO gas-production inhibition (Lincoln 1997).
   - Characteristic systemic exhaustion of antioxidant detoxification among symptom-free HIV-positives and AIDS patients (Buhl 1989, Greenspan 1993).
   - Characteristic nutrient antioxidant shortage (Beisel 1996, Bower 1990).

4. Prevention and therapy:
   - Dramatic increase of Th1 cells and stable balance of Th1-Th2 immune cell production after high doses of compensatory therapy with antioxidants (Herzenberg 1997, Greenspan 1993).
   - Successful treatment of lethal parasitic and fungal infections as well as transformed tumor cells by inhibiting cell biology counterregulations (polyamine and prostaglandin inhibition) (Sjoerdsma 1984, Subbaramaiah 1997, Stoner 1995)

(End of the brief answers to the questions raised by President Mbeki on 6-7 May 2000) (Kremer 2000 c).

Between the first and second sessions of the specialist conference that was summoned by President Mbeki on 7/8 May 2000 in Pretoria for an open discussion about the contradictions of the HIV/AIDS theory and alternatives to the treatment of "HIV positive" and AIDS patients with AZT (see above), one of the contributors, Dr. Montagnier from the Pasteur Institute in Paris, supposedly the first person to discover "HI viruses," organized the collecting of signatures of around 5,000 physicians and scientists in defense of the HIV/AIDS theory. This was then published in the leading scientific journal *Nature* after he was confronted at the specialist conference by a few independent physicians and scientists about the objective inconsistencies of the disease theory "HIV causes AIDS." It was officially agreed to present the arguments for and against the HIV/AIDS theory in a concerned way during the second session of the specialist conference, a few days before the World AIDS conference in Durban. The fear that the world at large would learn for the first time of scientific counterarguments, bypassing the perfectly functioning media monopoly up until that time, was so great that dogmatism succeeded over open discourse.

The South African government had planned to film the second session and to publish the course of the discussion.

Unfortunately for open scientific discourse, Dr. Montagnier is not only a researcher, but also an entrepreneur in his own right, receiving 1% in patent fees for every "HIV" test used worldwide in the same way as the American researcher Dr. Gallo's objectivity and communications are impaired by his financial interests.

Additionally, Montagnier is president of the World AIDS Foundation, which receives the rest of the patent fees for every "HIV" test and whose express mission is the propagation and maintenance of the HIV/AIDS theory. It is to the credit of all independent physicians, scientists and journalists that everyone who is interested can inform themselves about the medical and scientific counter arguments on the internet and through participation in open discourse can form their own opinions. Informed opinion-making is the first step in overcoming mortal fear and through self-help to counteract the fate of a medically programmed death by poisoning. In recent years many sufferers have used this chance of survival. The dictatorial behavior of the opinion-makers of HIV/AIDS medicine have shown that the actors know that the business of fear, as in all dictatorships, can only be maintained if freedom of expression and information are suppressed. This suppression is bought by the targeted control of the flow of capital for research funds, such as, for example, the World AIDS Foundation's funding of research laboratories and clinics.

The sources of finance of the "HIV" tests and profits from sales of chemotherapeutics simmer away only as long as the staged mortal fear can maintain the willingness of the general public to finance the host of specialists. The end of virus hunting began long ago as simple, plausible truths, which can be physically felt, reveal their own dynamics, and are stronger than the "invisible hand of the market."

(Information at: *www.ummafrapp.de, www.aliveandwell.org, www.virusmyth.org, www.theperthgroup.com, www.robertogiraldo.com, www.tig.org; www.altheal.org)*

In the meantime, the relatively small group of directors of this deadly drama and their governors in individual countries know exactly that the evolutionary biological and medical advances in knowledge and the consequences of the planned mass poisoning that can no longer be negated, have left the actors of HIV/AIDS medicine exposed and hard pressed to explain. The international mass media, up until now knowingly complicit in the "most brutal spreading of information," could change course. As the South African president summoned the international specialists conference on May 6-7 in Pretoria, in the run-up to the World AIDS Conference, for an open forum on the special problems of AIDS in Africa and the possible preventative and therapeutic alternatives to the administration of pharmacotoxins, an initiative was started by the two-thirds orthodox majority of the participants, including the patent-holder of the "HIV" test Dr. Montagnier, in which the disputed "contradictions and open questions regarding HIV/AIDS, particularly with reference to Africa" were supposed to be defined "by means of a majority vote" for a clarification on the official line.

As this was "the first open and official discussion on disagreements that are in part very disparate, since the appearance of AIDS" and "that even in the preliminary stage the initiative was characterized by attempts of political control by the USA and Europe" (Köhnlein 2000) this process confirms in an exemplary manner at which level medical insights as biological truths in that medical insights would be dictated by biological truth and are released by the world media. On the second day of the specialist conference the majority endorsed "those who fundamentally agree with the existing convictions." In the minority group were "those who had criticized major points of the procedural methods over the last 15 years." The majority in the "first open and official discussion since the appearance of AIDS" were obviously not prepared to even acknowledge the argumentation of the minority let alone discuss it openly and parted with the following agreement:

"Over the next two months the participants should try to objectively discuss the open questions point for point on the internet. The findings then being consolidated in a second meeting at the beginning of July 2000" (Köhnlein 2000).

This agreement was boycotted by the majority. Dr. Montagnier, in his capacity as president of the World AIDS Foundation, organized a collection of signatures from the 5,000 scientists and physicians for the defense of the HIV/AIDS theory and published the claims that have been known for 16 years in the leading scientific journal *Nature*, without allowing the scientists and physicians from the critical minority group the opportunity to comment (Papadopulos-Eleopulos 2000 c). A few days before the World AIDS Conference in South Africa the world at large must have had the impression that there was no alternative to the HIV/AIDS disease theory.

This development in the "first open and official discussion since the appearance of AIDS" spotlights the depths to which medical research has sunk at the cost of millions of affected patients. President Mbeki had previously stated:

"We will not, ourselves, condemn our own people to death by giving up the search for specific and targeted responses to the specifically African incidence of HIV-AIDS. I make these comments because our search for these specific and targeted responses is being stridently condemned by some in our country and the rest of the world as constituting a criminal abandonment of the fight against HIV-AIDS. Some elements of this orchestrated campaign of condemnation worry me very deeply" (Mbeki 2000).

Mbeki in his letter to the world leaders alludes to the fate of Galileo a number of centuries ago, who would have ended being burnt at the stake had he not astutely renounced his theory that the Earth revolves around the sun and not vice versa. The famous scientist in the playwright Bertolt Brecht's play *The Life of Galileo,* says: "I tell you: A person who does not know the truth is just a fool, but a person who knows the truth and calls it a lie, he is a criminal!" Foolishness is out of the question with the protagonists of the of HIV/ AIDS medicine run amok; rather it is a question of a collective scientific mental block, but with the rigorous will to commercially exploit its own medical malpractice at the cost of life to the affected patients.

The Secret of Cancer: "Short-Circuit" in the Photon Switch.

Change in the medical world-view of tumorology—The rational Cell Symbiosis Therapy concept

In Western countries, every third person suffers from some form of cancer, and every fourth person dies of it. The prognoses of the WHO state that by the year 2050 half of all mortalities will be due to a cancerous disease.

According to the prevailing cancer theories chance defects (mutations) in the DNA in the nucleus, which are regarded as irreparable, are considered to be the primary cause of the disease. Standard therapy in oncology (operations, chemotherapy and/or radiation therapy) is based on this assumption. The cure rates of cancer (minimum of 5 years survival after diagnosis) are given as being 45% (22% surgical treatment, 12% radiation therapy, 5% chemotherapy, 6% combined standard therapies). 60-70% of patients with incurable cancer are palliatively treated with radiation therapy, 50% with chemotherapy and less than 1% of the patients are treated surgically (EU data, 2003). In the USA, for instance 20% of the overall health budget is spent annually on chemotherapy for cancer patients.

The Nobel Prize winner Professor Watson, who together with Crick discovered the double helix of DNA in the nucleus, the most prominent promoter of the 1971 "War on Cancer" succinctly declared in 2003: "First we have to understand cancer before we can cure it."

The background to this sobering thought after decades of most intensive research efforts and a massive capital injection is the fact that the classic mutation theory of oncogenesis has been forever shaken by newer research. Under the mutation theory a tumor colony develops from a single "degenerated" body cell that through uncontrolled division is thought to pass on identical DNA defects to all daughter cells. However, it has become apparent that each individual cancer cell, even within the same tumor of a patient, features genetically varies.

The internationally respected cancer researchers Professor Weinberg from the MIT in Cambridge, USA and Professor Hahn from the Dana Farber Cancer Research Center in Boston, both supporters of the classic mutation theory, published in 2002 an overview of the ostensibly still puzzling six insiduous "acquired capabilities" of cancer cells. These attributes include the ability to:

1. resist exogenous growth-inhibitory signals
2. generate their own mitogenic signals
3. bypass apoptosis
4. acquire vasculature
5. gain potential immortality
6. invade and metastasize

The "Cell Dyssmybiosis Concept" (Kremer 2001) explained for the first time the six "acquired capabilities" of cancer cells as an evolutionary-biologically programmed natural (albeit overregulated) protective switch of the divisionally active human cells during permanent chronic cell stress. The origin of this concept was the evolutionary-biological discovery that humans owe their biological existence, like all nucleated single—or multi-cellular creatures (eukaryotes), to a unique act of integration deep in the history of evolution. Roughly 2 billion years ago two unicellular organisms without nuclei from the archaea and bacteria domains fused to form a new single cell type that is now termed protista. Comprehensive comparative sequence analyses regarding the genetic make-up and specific proteins of archaea, bacteria, and a multitude of eukaryotic organisms (including humans), produced an astonishing result: about 60% of the genes in a human nucleus originate from the primeval archaea (A genome) the remaining genes having a bacterial origin (B genome), which in particular in the nucleus are delegated by the bacterial endosymbionts that have survived up until today in all human cells as mitochondria (on average 1,500 per cell).

There is a controlled division of labor between the A and B genomes: the A genome dominates the late cell division phases, while the B genome drives the early cell division phase and the functions of the various differentiated cell types.

From these fundamental cellular biological facts, and integrating a large number of new experimental and clinical research data, the cell symbiosis concept leads to the following conclusions about oncogenesis and cancer therapy:

1. There is a controlled toggle-switch between the mitochondria and both nuclear subgenomes.

2. Transformation to cancer cells is a functional (not structural) failure of this toggle-switch, after the divisional phase cells are no longer sufficiently able to switch back to the differentiated cell performance phases
3. The cause of this permanent functional failure is the gradual deficiency of one of the central functions of mitochondria, namely to supply ca. 90% of the "universal energy-storing and energy-transporting molecule" adenosine triphosphate (ATP) for practically all biosyntheses and metabolic processes. Under normal circumstances roughly one's body weight of ATP has to be synthesized and then broken up every day. ATP cannot be stored and the actual stock in human beings is enough for only 5 seconds. When the mitochondrial functions are disturbed, cancer cells intermittently or permanently revert to the archaic form of ATP synthesis in the cytoplasm (glycolysis) with, potentially, up to a 20-fold increase in the glucose turnover at the cost of the organism as a whole (cachexia resulting from the forced degradation, especially of muscle proteins for the benefit of carbon intermediary products for glycolysis, is one of the most frequent causes of death in cancer patients).
4. Hitherto perceptions about the synthesis and function of ATP molecules, the basis of all cellular biological medical theories, are, however, objectively false. ATP has 3 molecule groups: 1 base adenine ring molecule that absorbs the light quanta at near-ultraviolet levels of 270 nm, 1 sugar molecule with 5 carbon atoms as well as a—molecule string with 3 phosphate groups. The current dogma, based on a theory formed more than 60 years ago by the later Nobel Prize winner Lippmann, is that electron energy is transferred in the respiratory chains of mitochondria (of which there are literally thousands in every mitochondrion as shown by EM photographs) on discharge of "energy-rich" electrons from nutrients via a kind of electrochemical battery, to protons which for their part drive ATP synthesis energetically and store their surplus energy in the phosphate bonds of ATP. These "energy-rich" phosphate bonds of ATP transported into the cytoplasm then release this stored energy via hydrolysis mainly to maintain the energetic processes of cell metabolism. Biochemical experiments have clearly shown, however, that the phosphate bonds of ATP are not especially rich in energy and that, upon hydrolysis, only heat energy is released that can at the most be used for heat production by isotherm cells (constant cell temperature). The fundamental question of the actual mechanism for the acquisition of cell energy remains unanswered. This fact explains the predominant failure of cancer prevention and therapy up until now.
5. Biochemistry and medical science have failed to this day to explain the function of the adenine groups of ATP, as no biochemical reaction with

this adenine ring molecule is shown. However, an understanding can be gained, within the framework of the cell symbiosis concept, from the biophysical attributes of light absorption of the adenine group. All essential components of mitochondrial cell respiration are light-absorbing molecules with characteristic "frequency windows" of absorption maxima from near the UV spectrum to the longer wave yellow/orange spectral range of visible light up to ca. 600nm. Yet the source of the electromagnetic energy is not sunlight. In fact a low frequency pulsating electromagnetic field is induced by the constant flow of uncoupled, paramagnetically aligned electrons in the respiratory organelles. The electromotive power generated by this process is catalytically enormously strengthened by the enzyme complexes of the respiratory chain (acceleration factor of 10^{17}). This effects an interaction between the electrons and the protons likewise aligned parallel to the induced magnetic field dependent on the strength of the magnetic field between the antiparallelly aligned electrons and protons. This process produces a quantum dynamic transfer of information via photonic energy exchange. The ultimate source of photons are fluctuations of resonance frequencies of the physical vacuum (zero-point energy field). The transferred information is stored in the spin of the protons that proceed to the ATP synthesis complex via proton gradients. There, the resonance information is transferred by a unique rotation system to the adenine group of ATP whose electrons can move freely in the alternating double bonds of the ring molecules. The ATP serves as an "molecular antenna" for the reception and relaying of resonance information from the "morphogenetic field." Human symbiosis is consequently not a heat power machine but a light frequency-modulated information-transforming medium. All the time this cell symbiosis is resonance coupled with the lowest, not-yet-materialized energy status (the physical vacuum as an inexhaustible "global information pool").

6. In oncogenesis, for a diversity of reasons, there is a functional disturbance especially to the 4th enzyme complex of the respiratory chain. The task of this complex, according to conventional opinions, is to transfer the inflowing electrons to molecular oxygen at the end of the respiratory chain and thus reduce it to water. In the cell symbiosis concept, however, the crucial factor is that, in reducing O_2 to water, completed electron couplings induce an antimagnetic impulse, and the electromagnetic alternating field for resonance information transfer switches on and off at an extremely fast periodic time interval (in picoseconds). If the electron flows to O_2, however, are permanently disturbed then a failure in the modulation of ATP occurs and increasing numbers of oxygen and other radicals form that can attack and damage the macromolecules (nucleic acids, proteins,

lipids, carbohydrates). In order to prevent this danger the key enzyme hemoxygenase upregulates. This enzyme uses O_2 as cofactor for the production of carbon monoxide (CO). In cases of long-term surplus production CO gas has crucial effects on cancer cell transformation:

- CO gas effects a characteristic phase shifting of the absorption of visible light from components of the respiratory chain and as a result "short-circuits" the photon switch for the modulation of the information transfer to the mitochondrial ATP.
- CO gas activates in the cytoplasm certain regulator proteins for the stimulation of the cell division cycle also without external growth signals (see above: 1st "acquired capability").
- CO gas effects via enzymatic overactivation of the important secondary messenger substance cyclic guanosine monophosphate (cGMP) the inhibition or blockade of communication between neighboring cells (2nd "acquired capability" of cancer cells).
- CO gas blocks programmed cell death by bonding onto the bivalent iron in important key enzymes (3rd "acquired capability" of cancer cells).

The result is a polar program reversal: The transformed cancer cells remain trapped, dependent on the degree of malignancy, in a continuous cell division cycle and can not switch back to the differentiated cell performances of the respective cell types without biological compensatory aid. According to recent clinical knowledge the cancer cells become especially malignant and massively disperse metastatic cells when the O_2 supply to tumor cells via capillary blood vessels is impeded. In these cases chemotherapy and radiation treatment are no longer effective as without the presence of molecular oxygen programmed cell death of the cancer cells can no longer be induced. In this situation cancer patients are considered incurable by oncologists using standard cancer therapy.

- The cell symbiosis concept postulates that when the cofactor O_2 is deficient, then the even more effective cyanide gas (HCN) is formed instead of CO. HCN is in humans the strongest mitochondrial respiratory poison and produces an even stronger phase switching of the absorption of visible light, probably by the well known inhibition of the reduction of trivalent irons to bivalent irons of certain hemocytochromes of the respiratory chain. This hypothesis can support the evolutionary-biological views of the cell symbiosis concept as cancer cells regress *de facto* to unicellular organisms (as a result of the loss of cell-to-cell communication with neighboring tissue cells) and that is why they behave like "parasitic cells" (4th, 5th, and 6th "acquired capability" of cancer cells). In this sense, cancer cells represent a regression to the early eukaryotic stage of a colony of protist cells, and so use the conserved archive of evolution in human nuclear genomes as a strategy of survival, depending on the actual given milieu conditions of the individual cancer cells (for the individual genetic variations, see above).

7. In 2003, American cancer researchers confirmed a functional disruption of cancer cells in the 4th complex of the respiratory chain despite simultaneously intact messenger RNA and intact mitochondrial DNA, without being able to explain this phenomenon. However, at the end of 2002 a cancer research group from Helsinki University, after many years of animal experiments and clinical studies, were able to exactly document for the first time—using electron microscopes and mass spectrometers—that the transformation to cancer cells is actually caused by the loss of control of the cell division cycle of the mitochondria.

The clinical research team could demonstrate that the tumor cells after a relatively short time had re-programmed to intact, normal differentiated cells without signs of programmed cell death by using a particular experimentally mediated bioimmunological compensation therapy on various human cancer diseases. These patients under conventional tumor therapy had a survival status of on average less than 12 months. In 2003 researchers from the Anderson Cancer Research Center of the University of Texas in Houston published the first wide-ranging overview about the hundreds of animal experiments on the effects of curcumin, the active ingredient of turmeric (*Curcuma longa*, from the ginger family, biochemically, curcumin I from the molecular family of polyphenols, also termed bioflavonoids, synthesized from plants) on cancer cells and metastases. *The researchers were amazed to discover that curcumin effectively inhibited nearly all signal paths in tumor cells and metastases.*

The researchers were unable to provide an explanation of this wide-ranging effect. The actions of curcumin can, however, be explained if you know that curcumin in the violet spectral range of visible light absorbs with nearly the same wavelength—415 nm—as the electron-transferring molecule cytochrome *c* that is more rapidly broken up by the protective enzyme hemoxygenase in cancer cells. In cancer cells curcumin, so to say, bridges the III and IV complex photon switch "short-circuit" of the respiratory chain in mitochondria and thus normalizes the information transfer for maintaining modulation of ATP.

The quoted research data show that (in opposition to the prevailing cancer theories of supposedly irreparable gene defects in the nucleus) the demonstrated functional disruptions of the transfer of information in cell symbionts can be re-normalized by means of an adequate biological compensation therapy. The concept of cell symbiosis therapy (Kremer 2001) derived from knowledge gained from cell symbiosis research has in the meantime led to some spectacular therapeutic successes (in individual cases even in cancer diseases that had been declared incurable). There is a broad spectrum of classes of substances responding to natural light available and the potential is by no means exhausted. What is desperately needed, however, is a comprehensive overhaul of the current state of research with the aim of developing optimized therapeutic formulations and to make them available for clinical and therapeutic practice. Admittedly, achieving this purpose through an interdisciplinary research group within the established health system is not to be expected in the foreseeable future, as conventional medical science has largely remained stuck in the one-sided thermodynamic energy concepts of the 19th Century.

(First published in Townsend Letter Aug. /Sept. 2007)

The Concept of Cell Symbiosis Therapy

The Way Out of the Therapeutic Dead End

In July 2003, "the roof of the genetic world caved in" as one researcher commented. What had happened? At an international genetics congress in Melbourne, genetic researchers from all over the world declared the "the end of the beginning" and "the beginning of the new era" in genomics research. Prior to this, the conclusive findings of one of the most ambitious research projects in modern medicine had been published; since the end of the 1980s, an alliance of international research groups had catalogued all the genes of the human nuclei, comprising over 3 billion sequences in total, using computer-assisted automatic sequencing machines. The expectation was that the human genome contained at least 120,000 genes—special sections in DNA with a coded sequence of the DNA building blocks: the four classic nucleic bases adenine (A), guanine (G), cytosine (C) and thymine (T). This assumption was based on the fact that there are over 100,000 proteins in human cells, which require a genetic blueprint for their synthesis outside the nucleus. On top of this, there are the some 20,000 regulating genes that are necessary to guide the genetic expression—the total process of the transcription of genes from messenger RNA transcripts to completed protein. In a parallel research program, genetic researchers sequenced the genes of DNA molecules in the nuclei of murine (mouse) cells. The findings were alarming: the murine nuclear genome had about 24,000 genes, nearly the same as the human nuclear genome of approximately 25,000 genes. Today, genetic researchers speak of only 21,000 human nuclear genes. This is hardly more than the number found in the tiny threadworm used in genetic research, which is only a few millimetres in length with exactly 969 cells. In comparison, humans have roughly 50 billion cells. In contrast, simple plants such as *Arabidopsis thaliana (thale cress)* feature proportionally more nuclear genes than human nuclei.

The Nobel prize laureate David Baltimore, one of the most respected leaders of opinion on genetic determinism of human existence at the time, observed in an almost desperate commentary on the preliminary findings of the Human Genome Project published in 2001:

"Unless the human genome contains a lot of genes that are opaque to our computers, it is clear that we do not gain our undoubted complexity over worms and plants by using many more genes. Understanding what does give us our complexity . . . remains a challenge for the future" (Baltimore, D. 2001 Our Genome Unveiled. *Nature* 409:814-816).

What Baltimore and the vast majority of his colleagues do not state, after the collapse of the genetic worldview, is the fact that all fundamental theories of modern gene technology focussed medicine on cell energy, cell information and cell-to-cell communication are in need of comprehensive revision.

This author, on the basis of analysis of a great diversity of evolutionary biological research data, postulated (in contrast to the perceptions of contemporary evolutionary researchers) that the human nucleus in actuality has a double genome: an evolutionary biologic legacy, borne from the integration of two primeval akaryotic unicellular micro-organisms, which simultaneously formed the nucleus,. This postulate of the "hermaphroditic" nature of human cell systems has proven to be most fruitful in therapeutic practice, for the understanding of health and illness, ageing and death.

In the early 1970s, previously unknown procaryonts were brought up from the depths of the ocean where absolutely no sunlight penetrates by remotely operated vehicles (ROV). For a long time, these organisms were classified as a new form of bacteria. Later, however, comprehensive sequence comparisons of the nucleic acids and proteins of these micro-organisms showed fundamental differences to bacteria, so that evolutionary biologists reclassified the 5 kingdoms of life to three domains: Archaea, single-celled organisms lacking nuclei; Bacteria, which also lack nuclei; and Eukarya, organisms *with* nuclei (single-celled protists, single—and multi-celled algae, single—and multi-celled fungi, plants, animals and humans).

The revolutionary realization—that all Eukarya, including humans, owe their existence to a unique act of fusion in the history of evolution, namely the colonization of a voluminous type of Archaea as host/stem cell by single-cellular organisms from the bacterial domain—was decisive. This formation of an intracellular symbiosis from members of two different domains, and the integration of the two inherently incompatible alien genome cultures into a common nucleus, termed "cell symbiosis" by the author, took place 2.1 billion years ago at a very striking point of time in the Earth's history.

The first of three periods when the earth was completely covered by ice occurred some 2.4 billion years earlier. Geologists have shown that before this Ice Age, the Earth's atmosphere was free of molecular oxygen (O_2), but dominated by carbon dioxide (CO_2) and methane gas (CH_4). The CO_2 was a result of volcanic activities in the Earth's crust, whereas the methane gas (CH_4) was produced by the ubiquitous Archaea which convert CO_2 into CH_4.

After the melting of the global ice sheet, the O_2 concentrations of the atmosphere rose exponentially, while methane concentrations fell exponentially. Cell symbiosis took place at exactly the point in time that these two atmospheric gas curves intersected.

To date, evolutionary biologists still have not answered the question as to how the strictly anaerobic Archaea (as they are still now termed in textbooks) for which minimal amounts of O_2 are highly toxic and their bacterial symbionts which had already developed an O_2-dependant respiratory chain could encounter each other in the same milieu. The puzzle can be immediately resolved once you know that a certain type of Archaea, under gradually increasing threat to existence by O_2 gas pressure, in the ocean and in the earth's atmosphere, evolved to facultative aerobics and learned to metabolize CH_4 with the aid of O_2in a moderately O_2-enriched milieu and to obtain electrons and protons for the essential supply of adenosine triphosphate (ATP). This ATP metabolism has been demonstrated by microbiologists in methane-producing archaea and bacteria. In oxygen-free milieus, however, the same archaea can survive by switching ATP production to the oldest metabolic pathway in all organisms—glucose degradation (glycolysis). This action of facultative aerobic archaea was the decisive condition for cell symbiosis with the bacterial symbionts which had already developed an O_2-dependent respiratory chain.

Until the end of the 1990s, evolution researchers were able to secure and publish important findings about human cell symbiosis: roughly 60% of the genes in the human genome are derived from the genes of stem cells of facultative aerobic archaea (termed as A-genome by the author). The A-genome is dominant during the cell division cycle from the S-phase (the DNA replication phase). The remaining genes (termed as B-genome by the author) come predominantly from the genes ascribed to the bacterial symbionts in the mutual nucleus. The B-genome is dominant during the phases of differentiated cell activities depending on the respective cell types.

On the basis of the scenario sketched here, the author was able to reinterpret the process of cancer. In the 1920s, the biochemist and later Nobel prize winner, Otto Warburg, first described the phenomenon that cancer cells, despite the presence of O_2, seemed to undertake ATP production mainly via glycolysis in the cytoplasm. This "Warburg Phenomenon" is to this day still controversially discussed as the progeny of these bacterial symbionts, which evolved to the highly complex performers in all cell types—termed mitochondria—and have been shown to have a not inconsiderable O_2 consumption, also in cancer cells.

In 2002, Australian cancer researchers published the findings of a precise measurement of the actual O_2 consumption in the MCF-7 breast cancer cell line, commonly used for such analyses, over a five-day period using the latest oxygen electrodes. At the same time, the researchers criticized measurements of this type as being too short-term. The puzzling result was that the O_2 consumption in these cancer cells was not much below that of many intact differentiated cells and glycolysis not much higher. But the researchers could not identify 65% of the metabolic substrate for the production of electrons and protons needed for O_2-dependent ATP production. (Guppy et al. Contribution to different fuels and metabolic pathways to the total ATP turnover of proliferating MCF-7 breast cancer cells. Biochem J. (2002). May 15; 364 (pt1): 309-15).

These findings demonstrate that the "hermaphroditic" nature of the human cell system is to this day still not understood by clinical cancer researchers. In order to resolve this dilemma the author has adopted the well-founded assumption that the cancer process reflects—like a rear view mirror—the development phases of evolution: the functional disturbance on the regulatory level of aerobic O_2 utilization for ATP production by means of the enzymatic oxidase system in mitochondria, forces a protective switching at the regulatory level of facultative aerobic O_2 utilization for ATP production by means of the enzymatic oxygenase system in the cytoplasm. Such an evolutionary-biologically programmed protective switching can for the first time explain the up until now non-identified substrate portion for the O_2-dependent production of electrons and protons in tumor cell colonies and also the Warburg Phenomenon.

Warburg had postulated an either/or situation as he had assumed a structural defect in the cytochrome oxidase complex of the respiratory chain of mitochondria: Either O_2 respiration in the intact differentiated cells in mitochondria, or glycolysis without utilization of O_2 despite the presence of O_2 in the cytoplasm. However, to the postulated model of the double genome a system of doubled O_2 utilization has to be assigned. Under long term chronic cell stress of a diverse nature the cells active in division can regress to the evolutionary biological older intermediate stage of ATP production—both

ATP production with O_2 utilization in mitochondria and in the cytoplasm with varying proportions and also ATP production through glycolysis without O_2 utilization in the cytoplasm, the latter proportionally dependent on the state of regression of the forming cancer cells. The B-genome gradually is losing control over the differentiated cells performance in favour of an increasing dominance of the A-genome as an archaic programmed strategy of survival.

In this context it can also be explained why since the declaration of "War against Cancer" in the USA in 1971 the expectation of survival in the most common solid carcinomas has not been markedly improved. Aggressive therapy with pharmaceutical toxins and ionizing radiation is still based on the objectively false theory of chance genetic mutation as the cause of cancer. This form of therapy can only inhibit or destroy more or less differentiated cells which are found in the regulations phase of the facultative aerobic ATP production. Simultaneously, however, there is still the danger that surviving cancer cells through the production of oxygen and nitrogen radicals associated to the therapy are forced into the strictly anaerobic phase or find themselves already in this phase. These cancer cells, resistant to conventional therapy, metastasize and dictate the fate of cancer patients.

Proof that this is the case is supplied by the recent discovery of tumor stem cells in solid carcinomas, firstly breast cell carcinomas in 2003 and since then in many other cancer cell types. These tumor stem cells are today regarded as the really dangerous cancer cells against whose uninhibited division tendency there are still no treatment methods in conventional cancer therapy (Clarke, M.F., Fuller, M. Stem Cells and Cancer: two Faces of Eve. Cell (2006), 126, 1111. Huntley, B.J.P., Gilliland, D.G. Leukaemia Stem Cells and the Evolution of Cancer Stem-cell Research, Nature Reviews Cancer (2005 Apr.) 5:4,311).

In contrast, forms of therapy derived from the concept of cell symbiosis have yielded impressive success in treatment (Lowenfels, D. The Dual Strategy of the Immune Response. A Review of Heinrich Kremer's Research on the Pathophysiology of AIDS, Cancer and Other Chronic Immune Imbalances. Townsend Letter, June 2006, 68-75 (USA). This is true not only for "over-therapied" patients, but also for other tumor sufferers in all stages, patients with cellular and humoral immune deficiencies, inflammatory illnesses, autoimmune diseases, cardiac diseases, atherosclerosis, diabetes (also therapy resistant forms), osteoporosis, burn-out syndrome, CFS, fibromyalgia, neurodegenerative diseases including Alzheimer's disease and other forms of dementia, Parkinson's disease, depression, psychoses and many more symptomatic states and deficiencies in performance which can be classified primarily as mitochondriopathies.

The realization of the author that, in short, contrary to the then-current theories, the respiratory chain of mitochondria operates as a light quantum—(photon-) processor was decisive for the development of recipes for the Cell Symbiosis Therapy® (Kremer, H. The Secret of Cancer: Short-Circuit in the Photon Switch, Townsend Letter. Aug/Sept 2007, pp.121-124).

The multidimensional modulated information generated by this is transferred to the delocalized electrons of the double bonds in the adenine molecule of adenosine triphosphate. This explains why ATP, directly or indirectly 'activating' or rather 'informing', has to be involved in practically all metabolic processes. Thus, for example, the complex modulated ATP nucleobases,inform' the necessary nucleobase building blocks before every neosynthesis of a DNA or RNA sequence, conveying a coded oscillating energy to them.

The geneticist Baltimore's question quoted above on "what gives us our complexity" can in principal be answered as follows: information is a non-material size that is communicated from a space/time independent matrix of potential information to our 'antennae molecules' like ATP as 'creative information' via quantum dynamic series. So, cells are not simply thermal generators but information transforming media. But not all ATP is the same: ATP information modulated in human mitochondria is certainly more complexly modulated than ATP information modulated in mice. Similarly, ATP modulated under facultative aerobic conditions is certainly less complexly modulated than mitochondrial ATP from intact differentiated cells, or conversely, ATP modulated under glycolytic anaerobic conditions is certainly the least complexly modulated. Cancer researchers speak of the latter as 'dedifferentiated' cells.

Baltimore should have asked himself why, after copying a protein coded DNA sequence to a messenger RNA sequence and after the processing of this sequence, a poly A tail has to be attached to the 'mature' messenger RNA as otherwise protein synthesis would not work. The instructions for this process cannot be found in the genes. So, how do the cells know what they have to do? The answer is that the 270-odd adenine molecules of the poly A tail, which originate from modulated ATP, are resonance coupled to the non-material information field. If you imagine these poly A tails to be variable light quantum modulated adenine elements, then this results in a coded light quantum profile and anyone can understand the total organism as a highly complex 'informed' light quantum field. (For a quantum dynamic model concept see the publication of the Nobel price laureate David Bohm (1990) A New Theory of the Relationship of Mind and Matter. Philosophical Psychology: Vol. 3 N. 2.271-86).

This is why in Cell Symbiosis Therapy®, natural substances are deployed which absorb and emit photons above certain wavelengths in the near UV range and in the visible spectrum. The therapeutic potential of such natural substances has been confirmed in recent research publications (Middlestone, E., Jr, et al (2000) The Effects of Plant Flavonoids on Mammalian Cells: Implications for Inflammation, Heart Disease, and Cancer. Pharmacol. Res. 52,673-751; Aggarwal B.B. et al. (2003) Anticancer Potential of Curcumin: Preclinical and Clinical Studies. Anticancer Res. Jan-Feb: 23(1A):363-98).

The concept of Cell Symbiosis Therapy® has been supported particularly by the fascinating new findings of experimental and clinical research into ageing processes. In conjunction with the discovery of the new enzyme class, sirtuin (silent information regulators) that mute certain genes and molecules by removing an activating molecular group—astonishing effects have been detected in all eukarya. Thus, for instance, the sirtuin enzymes of mice which are particularly predisposed for cancer and diabetes, are activated by particular natural substances from the large family of vegetable polyphenols. In comparison to normal control mice, the predisposed mice lived considerably longer and developed strikingly fewer cancer, diabetic or neurodegenerative diseases.

These research data prove that there is a superordinated regulatory system, also in humans, as sirtuin enzymes have also been detected in the nuclei, the cytoplasm and the mitochondria of humans. As a result, photon-absorbing vegetable polyphenols activate the O_2-dependent mitochondrial activity via multiple networked regulatory cycles. The long held scientific bias that the ageing process and the typical diseases connected to it, like cancer, diabetes, cardiovascular diseases and neurodegenerative disease types are unavoidable natural deterioration processes can now be challenged (Wood, J.G. et al. (2004), Sirtuin Activators Mimic Caloric Restriction and Delay Aging in Metazoans. Nature, 430, 686-89. Porcu, M., Chiarugi, A. (2005) Sirtuin interacting Drugs: From Cell Death to Lifespan Extension. Trends in Pharmacological Sciences, 26 N. Sinclair, D.A. (2005) Towards a Unified Theory of Caloric Restriction and Longevity Regulation, Mechanisms of Aging and Development, 126:9,987.

Structurally analogous, photon-modulating vegetable polyphenols (free from chemical residues, heavy metals and contaminants) are an essential part of dispensing of the Cell Symbiosis Therapy® both in combined and special galenic preparation forms. Polyphenols cannot be synthesised by mammals, which is why for humans they have the characteristics of vitamins. They are essential for intact mitochondrial function and for this reason vegetable polyphenols in an appropriate combination with other natural products are indicated for the prevention and treatment of serious defects in mitochondrial performance, systemic diseases and premature ageing. They are prescribed as nutritional supplements therapeutically by doctors and alternative practitioners in an individual preventative or treatment concept.

Note:

Information about certified education seminars on the principles and practice of Cell Symbiosis Therapy® for doctors and therapists, about laboratory documented treatment reports and participation in medically supervised research in a multi-centre practice study on applied Cell Symbiosis Therapy® can be found at www.cellsymbiosis-netzwerk.de

(First published in Townsend Letter Aug./Sept. 2008)

The Dual Strategy of the Immune Response

A Review of Heinrich Kremer's Research on the Pathophysiology of AIDS, Cancer, and Other Chronic Immune Imbalances

By David Lowenfels

[First published in Townsend Letter #275 6/2006, Revised 4/2008]

In 1984, Bob Gallo and Margaret Heckler held a press conference in which they attributed AIDS to infection with the allegedly exogenous retrovirus, HIV. This pronouncement bypassed the scientific peer-review process and jumped straight into the hands of the media and the minds of the masses. To understand the context of this event, it is important to remember the politics of Nixon's Retrovirus-Cancer research, Bob Gallo's misleading laboratory deceptions in his thirst for fame and fortune, and the gross medical oversight of the challenges of the "fast-lane" gay lifestyle ofthe 1970's, which have boon elaborated previously [Duesberg 1996, Crewdson 2002, Roberts 2006, Root-Bernstein 1993, de Harven 2003, Kremer 1996, 2001, 2003]

Since the time of Gallo's media announcement, many so-called "AIDS dissidents" have vociferously disputed the HIV theory of AIDS causality (Duesberg and Rasnick, The Perth Group, Root-Bernstein, Giraldo, to name but a few), but a coherent model for the pathophysiology of immune dysfunction and a corresponding nontoxic clinical therapy for disease reversal has been lacking. Mainstream HIV-centric AIDS therapies have focused on chemotoxic eradication, which at best is a stop-gap measure with ultimately grave consequences. HIV theorists continually invent convoluted explanations for how a phantom virus that can hardly be found *in vivo* (and only then by surrogate markers) could cause a total collapse of the immune system.

Most non-HIV theories of treatment revolve around drug abstinence, good nutrition, and avoidance of infections and other oxidative strcssors. While these measures are supportive to prevention and health maintenance, they have not been very useful in the actual reversal of AIDS and pre-AIDS, due to a lack ofbiochemical understanding of the actual disease mechanisms.

The one exception that this author has encountered is the work of German doctor Heinrich Kremer MD, which is deeply grounded in modern biochemistry, immunology, and cell physiology.

This article is a summary of the pathophysiological model of chronic immune dysfunction, as elaborated by Dr. Kremer in his 2001 book, *A Quiet Revolution in Cancer and AIDS Medicine (Die Stille Revolution der Krebs und AIDS-Medizin)*. An Italian version was published in 2003, and the translation of this monumental work into English is currently underway.

An understanding of Kremer's model is based on three fundamental concepts, which are introduced here and will subsequently be elaborated:

- the function of nitrogen oxides and thiols (antioxidative sulfur compounds) as bioregulators of redox metabolism in cellular life forms and, particularly, the importance of nitric oxide (NO) in humans;
- the generalized functional dichotomy of the immune system and its cytokines (immunoregulatory messaging proteins), between the cell-mediated and humoral immunity, and its evolutionary interplay with NO; and
- the symbiotic nature of multicellular organisms, particularly regarding the mitochondrion, which is an endosymbiotic proteobacterium and is regulated by the intracellular redox balance.

Some of the finer points cannot be covered in this short format, nor can some of the more recent insights. However, what will be elaborated is a solid overview of the biological mechanisms and treatment of the chronic immune imbalance known as AIDS.

The Discovery of Nitric Oxide as an Endogenous Bodily Regulator

Research on the effect of nitrogen oxides in humans began in the late 1800s, when amyl nitrate and nitroglycerine were used as vasodilators in the treatment of cardiac disorders such as angina pectoralis [Brunton 1867, Fye 1986, Berlin 1987]. Over a century would pass until light was shed on the biochemical mechanism of these drugs. Research beginning in the late 1970s by the teams of Furchgott, Ignarro, and Murad led to the eventual discover of NO as an endogenous (self-made) signaling chemical used not only in the vascular system. but also throughout the body; for this those researchers were awarded the 1998 Nobel Prize in Physiology and Medicine.

NO is a highly reactive, but short-lived, paramagnetic radical. Due to its electrical neutrality, tiny size, and gaseous nature, NO can diffuse freely through cell membranes to foster cell-to-cell communication without need for specialized receptors—a phenomenon that was never before seen in biology. For decades, this mechanism was overlooked, as scientists were adamant that animal cells could not synthesize such a primitive molecule.

Today, we know that NO is crucial to a massive variety of processes in the animal organism and is not just limited to the regulation of blood pressure. The body has several different enzymes used to produce NO, of the family called NO synthase (NOS). Nearly all human cell systems produce (dependent on the level of intracellular calcium) small amounts of NO from L-arginine as part of normal and pathological processes [Moncada 1991]. A sampling of such systems includes neural, mucosal, splee, cardiac, bone, cartilage, liver, and skin cells [Lincoln 1997]. Of particular importance to immunological discussions is the calcium-independent enzyme called inducible NOS (iNOS), which can manufacture NO in large amounts over an extended period of time.

Redox Potentials Direct Cellular Processes

From the perspective of evolutionary biology, reactive nitrogen species (RNS)—i.e., nitrogen oxides—and other reactive oxygen species (ROS) are ancient but universal methods of intracellular and cell-to-neighbor communication, which operate via manipulation of biological redox potentials [Kremer 2001]. Redox potential describes the quality of a system as electron-rich (reduced) or electron-poor (oxidized), usually measured in millivolts.

Changes in the cellular redox status in turn affect the activation of genes and transcription of proteins [Sen and Racker 1996, Marshall 2000]. In an analogous manner, the intracellular redox status influences the production of cytokines by the immune cells, which then regulates immune function [Peterson 1997, Marshall 2000].

The primary biological counterpart to oxidation by RNS and ROS is reduction (ie., antioxidation) by thiols, also known as mercaptans. These sulfur-containing molecules are strongly nucleophilic and can donate an electron in order to quench a free radical, themselves becoming oxidized in the process. These oxidized thiols are then either excreted or recycled by other antioxidants. The ocean is the primary source of biological sulfur, and land-based life forms face continual risk for latent sulfur deficiency [Hässig and Kremer 1999]. It is therefore necessary to maintain a sufficient sulfur reservoir, or "thiol pool," in the organism to counterbalance normal regulatory and pathological oxidative processes. For example, healthy mitochondria are one of the primary sources of ROS in the human organism, and thus their maintenance is dependent on cellular antioxidants that scavenge these byproduct radicals from oxidative phosphorylation [Cardoso 1999, Sastre 2003].

Aside from the aforementioned changes in genetic transcription, alterations in the cell redox status can also manifest as alterations of sulfur-iron groups in the mitochondrial respiration chain, or as cystine (S-S) cross-linking in enzymes and proteins that contain the amino acids cysteine or methionine [Moncada 1991]. Cysteine and methionine share the feature of a sulfhydryl (S-H) group, which is a potent antioxidant. The primary intracellular antioxidant is glutathione (GSH), which is a tripeptide synthesized from cysteine, glutamate, and glycine. (Figure 2) The balance between oxidized and reduced glutathione (GSH and GSSG respectively) can guide many important cellular processes [Sen and Racker 1996].

The Dual Strategy of the Immune Defense

An additional scientific prerequisite to Kremer's model involves an understanding of the functional dichotomy of the immune system and its cytokines. between the cell-mediated defense and the humoral defense. Cytokines (formerly known as lymphokines) are messaging proteins secreted by various immune cells. Patterns of cytokine expression form a complex and interrelated feedback network, which regulates the functioning of the immune system. (See Figure 1)

In 1986, the research group of Mosmann and Coffman demonstrated that CD4+ T-cells could be differentiated into two distinct functional patterns, which they named Th1 and Th2 (T-helper Type-1 and Type-2, respectively) [review in Mossmann 1989]. T-cells are lymphocytes that, when matured and activated, can perform as effector cells to assist the immune system in carrying out its tasks. The letter T stands for thymus, which is where these cells are trained and matured after their birth in the bone marrow. There are several kinds of T-cells, including helper, suppressor, and cytotoxic types. The term "helper" was originally coined before the discovery of Th1 cells to explain how Th2 cells assist B-cells in antibody production. Mosmann and Coffman's groundbreaking Th1/Th2 discoveries opened up a whole new paradigm in immunology, in which scientists attempted to classify diseases based on the pattern of cytokine responses [overview with Kidd 2003). Many other types of regulatory and suppressor T-cells have been discovered since [Mosmann 1996], but the CD4+ Thl/Th2 dichotomy will suffice for this simplified introduction. The Type-1 cytokines are associated with the cell-mediated immunity (CMI), while the Type-2 cytokines are associated with the humoral immunity. Both types of cytokines have a tendency to counteract each other (i.e., reciprocal inhibition by negative feedback.) (Figure 1)

The CMI is the front-line defense of the immune system, which responds against intracellular parasites (e.g., fungi, virii, and myoobacteria). The macrophages, natural killer (NK) cells, and Th1 cells primarily carry out this function, which is regulated by Type-1 cytokines. The CMI is also involved in cancer defense, delayed-type hypersensitivity (DTH) reactions, and homeostatic cellular "housekeeping" of dead or damaged cells.

The humoral immunity is the second-line of defense, which blocks extracellular parasites (e.g., bacteria and worms) from entering cells, via antibodies. The B-cells (B for maturation in the bone marrow) and Th2 cells primarily carry out this function, which is regulated by Type-2 cytokines. The humoral arm of the immune system is responsible for the manufacture of antibodies, as well as allergic and autoimmune reactions.

Th1 Cells Can Synthesize Large Amounts of NO Gas, While Th2 Cells Cannot

While the body has several enzymes for producing NO under different circumstances and in different cell systems, the inducible form (iNOS) is of crucial importance to the immune system. Inducible nitric oxide synthase (iNOS) is used by the cell-mediated immunity (CMI) to create clouds of cytotoxic (cell-killing) NO gas. The humoral Th2 cells do not have this ability to manufacture large amounts of NO gas. The cytotoxic NO gas spray is an integral weapon in the defense against intracellular pathogens (e.g., fungi, viruses, and mycobacteria). (Table 1) Macrophages, NK, and Thl cells use this gas to disrupt and/or kill intracellular microbes, via inhibitory binding to their metalloenzymes and thiopeptides crucial for metabolism [Kröncke 1995]. In the process, the infected cells are also destroyed and, depending on the severity of the assault, sometimes innocent "bystander" cells are as well.

Figure 1: Diagram of Cytokine Regulation and Feedback Pathways.

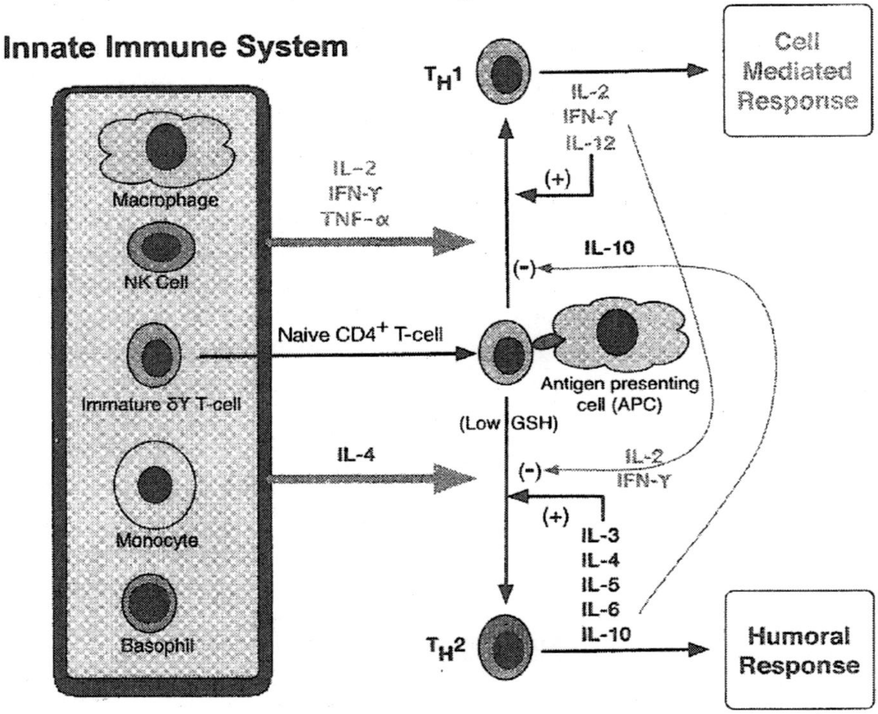

Innate Immune System
Macrophage
NK Cell
Immature δY T-cell
Monocyte
Basophil
IL-2
IFN-γ
TNF-α
Naive CD4+ T-cell
IL-4
TH1
TH2
Cell Mediated Response
Humoral Response
IL-2
IFN-γ
IL-12
(+)
IL-10
(-)
Antigen presenting cell (APC)
(Low GSH)
(-)
IL-2
IFN-γ
(+)
IL-3
IL-4
IL-5
IL-6
IL-10

IL = Interleukin
IFN = Interferon
TNF = Tumor Necrosis Factor
NK cell = Natural Killer cell

Table 1: Pathogens and Cellular Targets of NO

Viruses
Herpes simplex virus (a,d)
Coxsackie virus (a)
Vaccinia virus (d)
Ectomelia virus (d)

Bacteria
Francisella tularensis (a)
Mycobacterium tuberculosis (a,e)
Mycobacterium bovis (f)
Mycobacterium leprae (a,b)
Mycobacterium avium (e)
Listeria monocytogenes (a)
Chlamydia trachomatis (a)

Fungi
Cryptococcus neoformans (a,b)
Histoplasma capsulatum (g)

Parasites
Leishmania species (a,b,c)
Trypanosoma cruzi, musculi and *brucei* (a,c)
Plasmodium falciparum (a,c), *chabaudi* (h)
Toxoplasma gondii (b,c)
Schistosoma mansoni (b,c)
Entamoeba histolytica (a,i)

Mammalian cells
Tumour cells (a)

Pathogens that have been shown to induce the expression of type II NOS either *in vitro* or *in vivo* and are subject to the toxic effects of NO. Selected references are indicated in parentheses.

(a) Lowenstein, Dinerman & Snyder, 1994;
(b) Langrehr *et al.*, 1993;
(c) James, 1995;
(d) Nathan, 1995;
(e) Greenberg *et al.*, 1995a;
(f) Yang *et al.*, 1995;
(g) Zhou *et al.*, 1995;
(h) Jacobs, Radzioch & Stevenson, 1995;
(i) Lin *et al.*, 1995.

Excerpted from: Burnstock G, Hoyle C, Lincoln G. *Nitric Oxide in Health and Disease: Biological Research Topics 1.* London: Cambridge Univ. Press, 1997.

The Thiol Depletion Sensor Regulates the Cytokine Synthesis

The question remains: how does the immune system know whether to activate Type-1 or Type-2 cytokines? The answer remained a mystery until a major discovery at Stanford in 1998, when researchers there found that the level of GSH in antigen-presenting cells (APCs)—i.e., macrophages, dendritic cells, and B-lymphocytes—controls the switching between synthesis of Type-1 or Type-2 cytokines [Peterson 1998, Murata 2002].

In other words, a decline in the GSH:GSSG ratio signals the APCs to manufacture Type-2 cytokines, which then instruct naïve Th0-cells to mature into the Th2 type. The abundance of Type-2 cytokines causes reciprocal downregulation of Type-1 cytokines, which in turn inhibits any further synthesis of NO. (Figure 1) This event is called the Thl-to-Th2 switch, or a shift towards Type-2 cytokine dominance. The outcome is the hyperactivation of antibody production at the expense of inhibited CMI. In most cases, this shift is temporary. However, if a long-lasting shift occurs, the weakness of the CMI can invite intracellular opportunistic infections (OIs, the hallmark of "HIV"/AIDS). (Table 2) A simple and reliable measurement for Th2 dominance with Type-1 cytokine inhibition is the DTH skin test (originally used in sepsis research): an anergic result is an indicator for strong risk of OI due to insufficient Interleukin-2 (IL-2) [overviews with Christou 1995 and Kremer 2001].

Self-Protection from Oxidative Damage

The reason for the inhibitory switching of NO lies in an ancient evolutionary program for self-protection from oxidative damage. GSH can be seen as the "gas mask" for the Type-1 immune cells used to protect them from oxidative damage by NO [Kremer 2001]. However, reduced thiols are only available in a finite supply, dependent on the nutritional intake of cysteine/methionine and other antioxidants. The unfortunate side effect of using NO is that the immune cells themselves can become severely oxidized. If the initial CMI response is not effective against an invader, the immune system is in danger of harming itself with the double-edged sword of NO gas. This can also happen if the CMI response is excessive (perhaps due to multiple co-infections) or long-lasting (due to chronic infection). In fact, any of the myriad forms of oxidative and/or nitrosative stress can contribute to the Th2 shift by systemic antioxidant depletion. These prooxidative factors can be any combination of infectious, traumatic, psychoemotional, chemotoxic, or nutritional stressors [Hässig 1997].

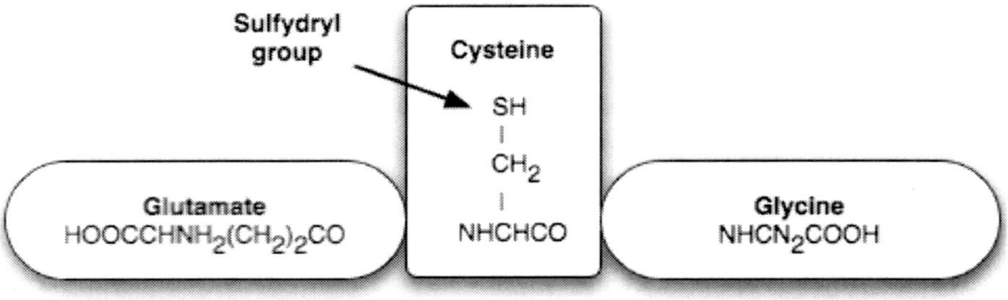
Sulfydryl group
Cysteine
SH
CH2
NHCHCO
Glutamate
HOOCCHNH2(CH2)2CO
Glycine
NHCN2COOH

The Molecular Structure of Glutathione (GSH)

A "Fire Alarm" for Extreme Prooxidative Threat

The Th1-to-Th2 switch evolved as a "fire alarm" for extreme prooxidative threat. From an evolutionary biological perspective, the Th1 cell is first seen in simple invertebrates such as sponges. The Th2 cell appears later during the early evolution of vertebrates such as amphibians and the bony fish [Roitt 1985]. Evidence suggests that the development of Th2 cells and antibodies was an evolutionary solution to parasitic colonization by other invertebrate organisms. Bony fish have a complex circulatory system, which makes them susceptible to invasion by multicellular parasites such as worms. Imagine the tiny Thl cells attacking a large worm that would be like using firecrackers to attack a giant monster. In that case, an excessive Th1 response using NO gas would not defeat the worm, but would instead cause harm to the fish via extreme tissue oxidation and inflammation. A backup system is needed for this emergency, and over time, Mother Nature equipped the more complex animals with such a solution: the Type-2 cytokine switch [Kremer 2001]. A Th2 dominance is generally an effective defense against prevention and healing of worm infections [Mosmann 1996].

In pre-Industrial times, humans with an aggressive Type-2 switch had a survival advantage, because they could successfully fight off worms and bacteria. Humans in those times also were not exposed to the oxidative stressors in the environment, food, and medicine now present in modern civilization. (See Sidebar.) In addition, the modern practice of vaccination also leads to more aggressive Type-2 switching. Today, these additional stress burdens flip the Type-2 switch too easily. The net result is a population-wide increase in chronic immunological diseases such as allergies, atopic skin disorders, asthma, autoimmune conditions, and cancer [Kremer 2001].

Table 2: Clinical Pictures of Th1 vs Th2 Response

Th1 (NO gas)	Mixed Th1/Th2	Th2 (antibody)
Tuberculosis (localized)		Tuberculosis (systemic)*
Leprosy (tissue-destroying tuberculoid form)		Systemic Lepromatosis
Primary Syphilis	Secondary Syphilis	Tertiary Syphilis (malignant)
(N/A)		Worm Infection
Leishmaniasis (self-limiting)		Leishmaniasis (Kalaazar)
Candidiasis (localized)		Candidiasis (systemic)*
Toxoplasmosis (self-limiting)		Toxoplasmosis (brain and lymph)*
Salmonella (self-limiting)		Salmonella sepsis*
Pneumocysts w/o illness (ubiquitous in inhaled air)		Pneumocystis pneumonia*
Infertility/Miscarriage		Successful Pregnancy

(*clinical AIDS)

AIDS Patients and Type-2 Cytokine Dominance

Immunological observations of AIDS patients demonstrate a Type-2 cytokine dominance. The initial findings of AIDS clinics noted DTH anergy, reduced T-cell proliferation after stimulation, increased B-cell activity, and specific antibody production, all of which glaringly point towards the shift to Type-2 cytokine dominance (a.k.a. Type-2 counter-regulation) [Gottlieb 1981, Masur 1981, Mildvan 1982].

The immunological response of AIDS patients is not new, as the Th2 switch has existed in animals for millennia. Rather, the unprecedented collective exposure to oxidative stressors precipitated the relabeling of the symptoms of the counterregulatory Th2 switch as "AIDS." Among other tbings, the primary prooxidative factors involved in gay men include combinations of nitrite inhalation ("poppers"), consumption of immunotoxic medicines and recreational drugs (including Septra/Bactrim, AZT, and more recently, Viagra), and exposure to antigens and endotoxins via repeated infections. All of these factors induce the synthesis of NO gas, ultimately leading to exhaustion of the thiol pool. Protein malnutrition seen in the Third World can also lead to a long-term functional inhibition of NO synthesis [Kremer 2001].

Results from research on seropositive patients showed Th1 cell impairment even in asymptomatic individuals with normal T-cell counts [Giorgio 1987. Miedema 1988, Clerici 1989 a, 1989 b]. In 1989, it was observed that asymptomatic "HIV"-seropositive individuals are systemically deficient in glutathione [Buhl 1989]. In 1993, Clerici and Shearer were the first to hypothesize about Th2 dominance in A1DS patients. which remained a tantalizing but controversial topic for many years until the Peterson group's 1998 breakthrough [Clerici, 1994, M06smann 1994, Fakoya 1997, Klein 1997].

In 2000, Breitkreutz et al. reported that asymptomatic seropositive patients showed a "massive loss" of approximately 10g of sulfur compounds via daily urination, leading to an "alarming negative balance of approximately 2 kg of cysteine per year" [Breitkreutz 2000]. Such a cumulative loss of thiols would obviously lead to chronic Type-2 counterregulation, the consequences of which include rising levels of antibodies (hypergammaglobulinemia) over time, leading to allergic and autoimmune complications, as well as a progressive diminishment in the CMI response, creating susceptibility to intracellular "opportunistic" infections. These sequelae are characteristic of the progression to AIDS and are the direct result of the inhibition of NO gas synthesis due to thiol depletion.

It has been reported that hypergammaglobulinemia precedes "HIV"-antibody seroconversion in hemophiliacs [Brenner 1991]. The Perth Group also has pointed out that "studies conducted in drug users show that the decrease in T4 cells precedes a positive antibody test" [Papadopolous 2004]. Further evidence for acquired immunodeficiencies (AIDS) of the CMI, without the manifest syndrome of OIs, in both "HIV+" and "HIV-" individuals from risk groups, is discussed in Root-Bernstein's 1993 book. The entirety of evidence convincingly suggests that the shift towards Th2 dominance begins long before seroconversion.

Glutathione

Glutathione (GSH) is a tripeptide made of cysteine, glutamate. and glycine. GSH plays important roles in cell and liver detoxification, mineral metabolism, antioxidant quenching of free radicals, and regulation of mitochondrial symbiosis. Due to its large size, GSH usually must be synthesized from components inside the cell, with cysteine and its antioxidant sulfhydryl group (sulfur-hydrogen bond) being the rate-limiting factor. One of the safest ways to boost systemic glutathione is oral N-acetylcysteine (NAC). Modern stressors which consume reduced gluathione (GSH) include the following:

4. All manners of oxidative stress
5. Chemical poisoning, via environment or via food/water
6. Carcinogens
7. Synthetic pharmaceuticals
8. UV and X-rays (ionizing radiation)
9. Electro-smog (non-ionizing radiation)
10. Oxygen, under—and oversupply
11. Infections
12. Overexertion from sports
13. Questionable nourishment
14. Heavy metal intoxication
15. Free-radical reactions
16. Chronic illnesses

Oxidized GSSG is reduced back to GSH by the enzyme glutathione reductase and the coenzyme NADPH. However, this reduction depends on a well-functioning status of the enzyme glutathione reductase and sufficient coenzyme NADPH. Both enzyme and coenzyme are damaged via electrophillc bonding with toxins. With a burden of frequent detoxification, they can no longer perform their task: too much oxidized glutathione (GSSG) remains, and the vital balance of (GSH):(GSSG) becomes disturbed from its approx. 400:1 ratio. Thereby, the redox regulation so dependent on this balance is interrupted.

(Original German by Dr. Gerhard Ohlenschlaeger, 2003)

"HIV" Cellular Characteristics and the Depletion of Reduced Thiols

Many researchers have argued that the immune weaknesses in risk groups simply leads to greater susceptibility to putative "HIV infection." According to Kremer, this is a gross confusion of cause and effect. The characteristics attributed to HIV in cell cultures, namely reverse transcription, "virus-like" particles, and catabolic cellular debris, are part of the evolutionary response against prooxidation.

Reverse transcription is a well-known factor in the repair of oxidatively damaged nuclear DNA [Kremer 2001]. Cell cultures of HIV are necessarily subjected to unusual oxidative and mitogenic stressors (including hydrocortisone), in order to express the "HIV proteins" [Barre-Sinnousi 1983, Popovic 1984, Gallo 1984]. The genetic expression of pathological proteins (e.g., HIV1 TAT) by dysfunctional cells is just another symptom of intracellular/systemic imbalance. Because it is the epigenetic oxidative mechanisms which result in unusual gene transcription, HIV researchers are confusing cause and effect.

The inflammatory Th1 cytokines, interferon-gamma and tumor necrosis factors, activate the production of oxygen radicals that can lead to increased cell death by both apoptosis (programmed cell death) and necrosis (unprogrammed cell death). Necrosis exposes intracellular proteins to the extracellular matrix, which activates autoimmune reactions in both Thl and Th2 cells [Kremer 2001].

A fact widely overlooked by AIDS researchers is that everyone has "HIV proteins" in minute amounts; those stigmatized as "HIV+" simply have higher amounts than the arbitrary threshold of the "HIV [auto]antibody" ELISA test kit, which calls for unusually high serum dilution (Giraldo 1998. Kremer 1998, 2002, 2003]. Therefore, an "HIV+" test result is pathognomonic (a distinctive indicator) for reduced thiol insufficiency (i.e., cysteine deficiency) and resultant cellular catabolism.

Mitochondrial Symbiosis Depends on Reduced Thiols and NO

The final nail in the coffin for the HIV theory is that the cell types used to derive "HIV proteins" (Gallo used cancer cells, and Montagnier used embryonic cells) all have altered mitochondrial bioenergetics that predispose them for Type-2 counterregulation [Barre-Sinnousi 1983, Gallo 1984, Kremer 2002].

Fueled by oxygen, mitochondria are the energy powerhouses that generate nearly all the ATP used for cellular processes. Currently accepted theory maintains that the mitochondria are endosymbiotic bacteria, long ago incorporated into eukaryotic cells [Margulis 1981]. The overwhelming evidence for this is that mitochondria have their own genome (mtDNA). Because the mitochondria are themselves relatives of bacterial organisms, they are also susceptible to suffocation by nitrogen oxides when present in cytotoxic concentrations [Kremer 2001].

Mitochondria are responsible for regulating cellular metabolism, including the initiation of apoptosis [Green 1998, Desagher 2000]. Laboratory research is currently lacking on the exact mechanisms that maintain the mitochondrial symbiosis. As mentioned earlier, normal mitochondrial respiration is the leading source of oxidative radicals in the cell. For this reason, a continual supply of antioxidants are needed to mop up these radicals, the primary one being glutathione peroxidase (GSH-Px), which contains both selenium and GSH. AIDS researchers in the past decade have noted deficiencies in selenium, which was erroneously postulated as excess transcription of GSH-Px by HIV [Look 1997, Taylor 1997, Foster 2000]. The GSH deficiencies that cause the inhibition of NO synthesis also lead to the dissolution of the mitochondrial symbiosis (a.k.a. "Warburg Phenomenon") [Kremer 2001].

Not surprisingly, disturbances of the mitochondria are evident even in asymptomatic seropositive individuals [Cote 2002]. This problem is made worse by the administration of nucleoside analogues such as AZT, which suffocate mitochondrial respiration enzymes and interfere with the synthesis of mtDNA via inhibition of polymerase-gamma [Cherry 2003]. Other

AIDS drugs can deplete systemic GSH by liver toxicity. It is imperative to focus on restoring the mitochondrial symbiosis as a primary goal of AIDS therapy [Kremer 2001, 2003], and current research in China substantiates this paradigm [Miao 2005].

Mitochondrial dysfunction is also tied to cancer, as demonstrated by Nobel Laureate Otto Warburg, who showed that a breakdown of oxidative cell respiration and increase of lactic acid fermentation was a precursor to cancer [Warburg 1966, Kremer 2003]. Stimulated by Kremer, cutting-edge cancer research in Germany and Spain is currently corroborating Warburg's theories [Isidore 2005, Schulz 2006].

The Case of the Missing T-Cells

A paradox overlooked by the initial AIDS researchers was that an "unknown agent" was supposedly killing the T-helper cells, yet the antibody production of the B-cells and antibodies remained intact. Another paradox is that AIDS researchers could only find the nonspecific laboratory artifacts that indirectly implicated a retrovirus amongst Th2 cell clones, but not Th1 clones [Maggi 1994, Chehimi 1995, Abbas 1996, Lucey 1996]. "How can a killer be responsible for murder if it was never even at the scene of the crime?" [Kremer 2001]

Although HIV-theorists have come up with many imaginative explanations for this conundrum, the obvious logical solution is that the decline of T-cells seen in the peripheral blood is not due to any postulated "HIV-mediated cell killing," but rather is just another consequence of the thiol-mediated cytokine shift.

A predominance of Type-2 cytokines leads to the production of Th2 cells, which reside primarily in the bone marrow (where they can contact the B-cells) and out of view from peripheral blood counts. To cite an analogy given by Kremer, the "police officers" of the bloodstream are missing from the streets, not because gangsters have killed them, but instead because they have taken desk jobs [Kremer 2001].

The bone marrow disruption that occurs with highly active antiretroviral therapy (HAART) is responsible for damage to the maturation of B-cells. As a result, the Th2 cells cannot make contact with mature B-cells and so return to circulation in the peripheral bloodstream. This toxic disruption explains the transient increase of CD4+ blood counts seen with nucleoside inhibitors

[Kremer 2001, 2003]. The cell-count increase is misleading because Th2 cells cannot produce cytotoxic NO gas and are therefore lame against preventing Ols. Because Th1 and Th2 cells cannot be differentiated by their surface proteins, the only way to get reliable information on immune function is by cytokine profiling or DTH skin testing.

Antioxidants Improve Immune Function

It must be underscored that there is a direct connection between the uptake of antioxiants from food or supplements and the levels of GSH in the immune cells. Therefore, there are two general ways in which antioxidant depletion and the corresponding immune imbalances can occur. The first way is through a lack of antioxidant intake, in other words. malnutrition or starvation. The second way is through redox overload due to prooxidative stressors (toxic, infectious, psychoemotional, etc.) which, alone or in combination, exceed the capacity of cellular antioxidant supply. The end result of both these situations is a systemic starvation for freely available electrons, corresponding with deficiencies of thiols and other reducing substances, which ultimately triggers the biologically evolved program of Type-2 counterregulation.

A extensive range of antioxidants have been claimed to inhibit "HIV infection" *in vitro* [Schreck 1992, Jaruga 2002]. In fact, many of the newer AIDS drugs have potent antioxidant capacity [ScienceBlogs 2006], either directly via their metabolites or indirectly via inhibition of enzymes, like cytochrome P450. Over the long term, the enzymatic inhibition that these drugs cause is quite toxic, particularly due to the disruption of mitochondrial replication and repair [ScienceBlogs 2006, Cherry 2003]. As early as 1989, a lack of cysteine was noticed in AIDS patients. This lack could have suggested a non-toxic supplemental therapy, if researchers were not blinded by the glamour of virus-hunting [Dröge 1989]. The replenishment of thiols in AIDS prevention by the GSH pro-drug, n-acetylcysteine (NAC), was first suggested by Dröge in 1993 [overview with Kelly 1998]. Clinical trials in subsequent years proved astounding results, and NAC is universally recommended for seropositive patients [Dröge 1997, De Rosa 1997, Herzenberg 1997, Breitkreuitz 2000]. Given the knowledge of this enormous benefit, it is troubling that doctors are not prescribing NAC to their patients; presumably its lack of popularity is due to the lack of patentability (i.e., profitability) of an endogenous (bodily made) substance derived from a simple amino acid. Mainstream AIDS-drug "cocktail" therapy cannot possibly address this massive cysteine deficiency. In fact, the Herzenberg study showed that individuals taking HAART therapy generally had the worst levels of intracellular GSH and thus benefited most from NAC supplementation.

Kremer's Approach to Healing Immune Dysfunction

This article bas provided an outline of Kremer's theory of pathophysiology behind the immune dysfunction seen in AIDS, as explained by the shift to Th2 dominance. It has only briefly touched on the therapy, which is still being researched and has been outlined elsewhere [Kremer 2001 b, de Fries 2005]. There is no "magic bullet" solution to this disorder, since there is no actual HI-Virus to be eradicated. Even if HIV were to actually exist, the laws of evolutionary biological immunology would still call for an identical thiol-replenishing treatment rationale. The process of reversing Th2 dominance is complex and highly individual; it requires time, patience, and the help of a truly knowledgeable physician. Excerpted from Kremer's book, here is the general strategy for healing the Thl/Th2 imbalance:

- Minimization of prooxidative stress
- Replenishment of thiol deficiency
- Balancing of amino acid dysregulation
- Liver protection to lighten the burden of systemic thiol deficiency
- Modulation of Type-2 counterregulation
- Micronutrient replenishment
- Fortification of the extracellular matrix
- Mitochondrial revitalization
- Attenuation of stress hormones
- Fear reduction and psychological assistance (i.e., de-hexing) [Kremer 2001].

This author hopes you share his excitement for the English publication of Kremer's book, which is the result of a monumental effort of love by a dedicated team. There is still much to be discovered regarding the healing powers of orthomolecular cell-symbiosis compensation therapy for AIDS. However, the scientific basis of pathophysiology is solid, and clinical applications in such regard continue to demonstrate immense benefit. My deepest gratitude goes out to Dr. Kremer and his devoted German-speaking colleagues [Felix de Fries, Oliver Langkopf, Alfred Hässig (deceased)], who have gifted us greatly in our understanding of health and disease.

References

Abbas AK, Murphy KM, Sher A. Functional diversity of helper T-Iymphocytes. *Nature.* 1996;383: 787-793.

Barre-Sinoussi F, Chermann JC, et al. [Montagnier]. Isolation of a T-lymphotrophic retrovirus from a patient at risk for acquired immune deficiency syndrome (AIDS). *Science.* 1983;220:868-871.

Breitkreutz R, Pittack N, et al. Improvement ofimmune functions in HIV infection by sulfur supplementation: two randomized trials. *Journal of Molecular Medicine.* 2000;78(1): 55-62.

Breitkreutz R, Holm S, et al. Massive loss of sulfur in HIV infection. *AIDS Res Hum Retroviruses.* 2000;16: 203-209.

Brenner B, Schwartz S, et al. The prevalence and interaction of human immunodeficiency virus and hepatitis B virus infections in Israeli hemophiliacs. *Isr J Med Sci.* 1991 Oct; 27(10):557-6l.

Brunton TL. On the use of nitrite of amyl in angina pectoris. *The Lancet.* 1967;2: 97-98.

Berlin R (1987) Historical aspects of nitrate therapy. *Drugs.* 1987;33(Suppl4): 1-4.

Buhl, et al. Systemic glutathione deficiency in symptom free HIV-seropositive individuals. *The Lancet.* Dec 21989;1294-1297.

Chehimi J, Frank I, Ma X, Trinchieri G. Differential regulation of IL-1O and role of T-helper cells. In:Abstr. 408. Second National Conference on Human Retroviruses, Infectious Diseases Society of America. Alexandria, VA, 1995.

Cherry CL, Wesselingh SL. Nucleoside analogues and HIV: the combined cost to mitochondria. *J Antimicrobial Chemotherapy. 2003;51:1091-1093.*

Christou NY, Meakins JL, Gordon J et al. The delayed hypersensitivity response and host resistance in surgical patients. 20 years later. *Ann Surg.* 1995;222 (4): 534-546.

Clementi E, Nisoli E. Nitric oxide and mitochondrial biogenesis: a key to long-term regulation of cellular metabolism. *Comp Biochem Physiol A Mol Integr Physiol.2005;142(2):102-10.*

Clerici M, Shearer GM. A THl-7TH2 switch is a critical step in the etiology of HIV infection. *Immunology Today.* 1993;14(3):107-111.

Clerici M, Shearer GM. The Thl-Th2 hypothesis ofHIV infection: new insights. *Immunology Thday. 1994* Dec; 15(2):575-81.

C1erici M, Stocks NI, Zajak RA et al. (1989 a) Interleukin-2 production used to detect antigenic peptide recognition by T-helper lymphocytes from asymptomatic HIV-seropositive individuals. *Nature. 1989;339:383-385*

Clerici M, Stocks NI, Zajak RA et al. Detection of three distinct patterns of T-helper cell dysfunction in asymptomatic human immunodeficiency virusseropositive patients: independence of CD4 cell number and clinical staging. *J Clin Invest. 1989;84:* 1892-1899.

Cote HC, Brumme ZL et al. Changes in mitochondrial DNA as marker of nucleoside toxicity in HIVinfected patients. *N Engl J Med. 2002;346:811-20.*

Crewdson, J. *Science Fictions:* a *Scientific Mystery,* a *Massive Cover-Up, and the Dark Legacy of Robert Gallo.* Boston: Little, Brown & Co., 2002, ISBN 0316-13476-7. *[http://www.sciencefictions.net]*

de Fries F, Lowenfels D. (2005) AIDS-defining illnesses: their causes and treatment. [http://aliveandwellsf.org/therapy].

de Harven, E. Problems with Isolating HIV. European Parliament, Brussels, Dec 08, 2003. http://www.altheal.org/isolationlisolhiv.htm

De Rosa SC, Zaretsky MD, et al. N-acetylcysteine replenishes glutathione in HIV infection. *Eur J Clin Invest.* 2000;30: 915-929.

Desagher S & Martinou JC. Mitochondria as the central control point of apoptosis. *Trends Cell Bioi.* 2000;10(9):369-77.

Dröge W, Breitkreutz R. Glutathione and immune function. *Proc Nutr Soc.* 2000 Nov; 59(4):595-600.

Dröge W, Holm E. Role of cysteine and glutathione in HIV infection and other diseases associated with muscle wasting and immunological dysfunction. *FASEB J.* 1997 Nov; 11(13):1077-89.

Dröge W, Gross A, Hack V et al. Role of cysteine and glutathione in HIV infection and cancer cachexia: Therapeutic intervention with N-acetyl-cysteine (NAC). *Adv Pharmacol.* 1997; 38:581-600.

Dröge W. Cysteine and glutathione deficiency in AIDS patients: A rationale for the treatment with Nacetylcysteine. *Pharmacol.* 1993; 46:61-65.

Dröge W. Metabolische Storungen bei HIV-lnfektion. *Project News.* 1989;2:4-5. AIDS-Zentrum des Bundesgesundheitsamtes Berlin.

Duesberg, P. *Inventing the AIDS Virus.* Regnery USA, 1996, ISBN 0-89526-470-6.

Elfering S, Sarkela T, Giulivi C. Biochemistry of mitochondrial nitric-oxide synthase. *J Biol Chem.* Oct 11 2002.

Fakoya A, Matear PM et al. HIV infection alters the production of both type 1 and 2 cytokines but does not induce a polarized type 1 or 2 state. *AIDS.* 1997; 11:1445-1452.

Foster, H.D. AIDS and the "selenium-CD4-T cell tailspin": The geography of a pandemic. *Townsend Letter for Doctors and Patients.* 2000;209, 94-99.

Fye WE T. Lauder Brunton and amyl nitrite: a Victorian vasodilator. *Circulation. 1986;74:222-229.*

Gallo RC, Salahuddin SZ, Popovic M, et al. Frequent Detection and Isolation of Cytopathic Retroviruses *(HTLV-III)* from Patients with AIDS and at Risk for AIDS. *Science. 1984;224:500-502.*

Giorgio JV, Fahey JL, Smith DC et al. Early effects of HlV on CD4 lymphocytes *in vivo. J Immunol.* 1987;138: 3725-3730.

Giraldo, R. Everyone tests positive. *Continuum.* Winter 1998/1999.

Gottlieb MS, Schroff R, Howard M et aI. Pneumocystis carinii pneumonia and mucosal candidiasis in previously healthy homosexual men. evidence of a new acquired cellular immunodeficiency. *NEJM.* 1981;305:1425-1431.

Gow AJ, StamlerJS. Reactions between nitric oxide and haemoglobin under physiological conditions. *Nature. 1998;391:169-173.*

Green DR & Reed JC. Mitochondria and apoptosis. *Science. 1998;281(5381):1309-12.*

Hässig, A. On politics, risks and therapies: interview with Prof. Alfred Hassig. *Continuum.* June/July 1997;4 (6).

Hässig A, Kremer H, Liang W-X et al. Seriously seeking sulphur: sulphur tames oxygen and converts it from foe to friend. *Continuum.* 1999;5 (5): 54-55. [http://garynull.com/Documents/Continuum/SeriouslySeekingSulphur.html].

Herzenberg LA, De Rosa SC, Dubs JG, et al. Glutathione deficiency is associated with impaired survival in HIV disease. *Proc Nat Acad Sci USA.* 1997 ;94(5):1967-1972.

Jaruga P, Jaruga B, Gackowski D, Olczak A, Halota W, Pawlowska M, and Olinski R Supplementation with antioxidant vitamins prevents oxidative modification of DNA in lymphocytes ofHIV-infected patients. *Free Radic Biol Med. 2002;32:414-420.*

Kelly GS. Clinical applications of n-acetylcysteine. *Alt Med Rev. 1998;3(2):114-127.*

Kidd, P. Th1/Th2 balance: the hypothesis, its limitations, and implications for health and disease. *Alternative Medicine Review.* Aug. 2003.

Klein SA, J,rgen MD et al. Demonstration of the Thl to Th2 cytokine shift during the course of HIV-l infection using cytoplasmic cytokine detection on single cell level by flow cytometry. *AIDS. 1997;* 11:1111-1118.

Kremer, H. Acquired iatrogenic death syndrome: pneumonias & lung diseases. *Continuum.* Nov./Dec. 1996. [http://www.virusmyth.net/aids/data/hkpneumo.html].

Kremer, H. Did Dr. Gallo and His Colleagues Manipulate the "AIDS-Test" to Order? *Continuum.* Summer 1998.

Kremer, H. (2001) Die Stille Revolution der Krebs—und AlDS-Medizin. Neue fundamentale Erkenntnisse über die tatsachlichen Krankheits—und Todesursachen bestatigen die Wirksamkeit der biologischen Ausgleichstherapie. (The quiet revolution in cancer and AIDS medicine: new and fundamental cognition about the actual causes of illness and death, prove the effectiveness of the biological balancing therapy). *Ehlers Verlag,* Wolfratshausen 2nd ed, 2002.

Kremer, H. The perversions of AIDS medicine. raum+zeit 121, 50-64; Jan./Feb. 2003. [http://*www.altheal.org/overview/pervmed.html].*

Kremer, H. (2001 b) The Lifesaving Knowledge on Healing, draft translation excerpt from Chapter XI of Die Stille Revolution. Available at http://aliveandwellsf.org/kremer/.

Kröncke K-D, Fehsel K, Kolb-Bachofen V. Inducible nitric oxide synthase and its product nitric oxide, a small molecule with complex biological activities. *Biol Chemistry Hoppe-Seyler.* 1995;376: 327-343.

Lincoln J, Hoyle CHV, Burnstock G (ed.) *Nitric Oxide in Health and Disease.* Cambridge, England: Cambridge University Press, 1997.

Look MP, et al. Serum selenium, plasma glutathione (GSH) and erythrocyte glutathione peroxidase (GSH-PxHevels in asymptomatic versus symptomatic human immunodeficiency virus-l (HIV-l) infection. *EurJ of Clin Nutr.* 1997; 51: 266272.

Maggi E, Mazzetti M, et al. Ability of HIV to promote a Thl to ThO shift and to replicate preferentially in Th2 and ThO cells. *Science.* 1994 Jul 8; 265(5169):244-8.

Margulis, L. *Symbiosis in Cell Evolution.* (2nd Edition 1993). New York: Freeman, 1981.

Marshall HE, Merchant K, Stamler J. Nitrosation and oxidation in the regulation of gene expression. *FASEB.2000;14:1889-1900.*

Masur H, Michelis MA, Green JB et al. An outbreak of community-acquired pneumocystis carinii pneumonia. *N Engl J Med. 1981;305:1431-1438.*

Miao B, Li J, et al. Sulfated polymannuroguluronate, a novel anti-AIDS drug inhibits T-cell apoptosis by combating oxidative damage of mitochondria. *Mol Pharmacol. 2005;68(6):1716-27.*

Miedema F, Petit AJC, Terpstra FG et al. Immunological abnonnalities in human immunodeficiency virus (HIV)-infected asymptomatic homosexual men. HIV affects the immune system before CD4+ T-helper cell depletion occurs. *J Clin Invest. 1988;82:* 1908-1914.

Mildvan D, Mathur RW, Enlow PL et al. Opportunistic infections and immune deficiency in homosexual men. *Ann Intern Med.* 1982; 96: 700-704.

Moncada S, Palmer RMJ, Higgs EA. Nitric oxide: physiology, pathophysiology, and pharmacology. *Pharmacol Rev.* 1991;43: 109-142.

Mosmann TR. Cytokine patterns during the progression to AIDS. *Science.* 1994 Jul 8;265(5169):193-4.

Mosmann TR, Cherwinski H, Bond MW et al. Two types of murine helper T cell clone: 1. Definition according to profiles of Iymphokine activities and secrete proteins. *J Immunol.* 1986;136: 2348-2357.

Mosmann TR, Coffman RL. THI and TH2 cells: different patterns of lymphokine secretion lead to different functional properties. *Annual Review of Immunology.* 1989,7:145-173.

Mosmann TR, Sad S. The expanding universe of T cell subsets: TH1, TH2 and more. *Immunol Today.* 1996;17 (3): 138-146.

Murata, Y et al. The polarization ofThl/Th2 balance is dependent on the intracellular thiol redox status of macrophages due to the distinctive cytokine production. *International Immunology.* 2002; 14(2): 201-212.

Papadopulos-Eleopulos E et al. A critique of the Montagnier evidence for the HIV/AIDS hypothesis. *Med Hypotheses. 2004;63(4):597-601.*

Parcell, S. Sulfur in human nutrition and applications in medicine (review). *Alternative Med. Rev.* Feb. 2002.

Peterson JD, Herzenberg LA, Vasquez K, Waltenbaugh C. Glutathione levels in antigen-presenting cells modulate Thl versus Th2 response patterns. *Proc Nat Acad Sci USA.* 1998; 95:3071-3076.

Popovic M, Sarangadharan, M, et al [Gallo]. Detection, isolation, and continuous production of cytopathic retroviruses (HTLV-III) from Patients with AIDS and Pre-AIDS. *Science.* 1984; 224:497-500.

Roberts, J. HIVgate (2006). available at http://sparks-of-light.org

Roitt JM, Brostoff J, Male DK. *Immunology.* London: Gower Medical Publishing, 1985.

Root-Bernstein R. *Rethinking AIDS; The Tragic Cost of Premature Consensus.* New York: The Free Press/ Macmillan USA, 1993, 527 pages, ISBN 0-02926905-9.

Schreck R, Albermann K, and Baeuerle PA (1992) Nuclear factor kappa B: an oxidative stressresponsive transcription factor of eukaryotic cells. *Free Radic Res Commun. 17:221-237.*

Schulz T. J. Thierbach R. Voigt A. Drewes G. Mietzner B. Steinberg P. Pfeiffer A.F.H. Ristow M. Induction of oxidative metabolism by mitochondrial frataxin inhibits cancer growth: Otto Warburg revisited *J. Biol. Chem. Vol. 281, Issue 2, 977-981 2006 January 13*

ScienceBiogs (2006). Comments by "jean" published at [http://scienceblogs.com/aetiology/2006/02/discussion_of_the_padian_paper.php].

Sen CK, Packer L. Antioxidant and redox regulation of gene transcription. *FASEB J.* 1996 May;10(7): 709-20.
Snyder SH, Bredt DS. Biological roles of nitric oxide. *Scientific American.* 1992;266: 28-35.
Taylor, E.W. Selenium and viral diseases: facts and hypotheses. *Journal of Orthomolecular Medicine.* 1997;12(4):227-239.

About the author:

David Lowenfels is a scientist, engineer, and musician, with Master's degrees from MIT and Stanford. He began questioning the "HIV=AIDS" model in 1999 and encountered Dr. Kremer's work in 2003. He is greatly excited by the emerging paradigm of future medicine: moving beyond the current strategy of eradication and suppression, beyond "complementary alternative" therapy, and into new realms of biological understanding which yield methods for guiding and, balancing the body's innate healing processes. He is currently a student of Dr. Yurkovsky's Field Control Therapy (FCT).

Bibliography

A

Abbas AK, Murphy KM, Sher A (1996)
Functional diversity of helper T-lymphocytes
Nature 383: 787-793.

Abel U (1990)
Die zytostatische Chemotherapie fortgeschrittener epithelialer Tumoren
Hippokrates Verlag, Stuttgart

Abrams B, Duncan D, Hertz-Picciotto I (1993)
A prospective study of dietary intake and acquired immune deficiency syndrome in HIV-seropositive homosexual men
J Acquir Imm Def Syndr Hum Retrovir 6: 949-958

ACTUP New York (1993)
Conference on oxidative stress in HIV / AIDS
A potential for new therapies. Nov 8-10, 1993
Oxidative Stress 11: 8-10

Adams J (1989)
AIDS. The HIV myth
St. Martin's Press, New York

Ader R (1980)
Psychoneuroimmunology
Academic Press, New York

Akaike T, Suga M, Maeda H (1998)
Free radicals in viral pathogenesis: Molecular mechanisms involving superoxide and NO
Proc Soc Exp Biol Med 217 (1): 64-73

Akerlund B, Jarstrand C, Lindeke B et al. (1996)
Effect of N-Acetylcysteine (NAC) treatment on HIV-1 infection: A doubleblind placebo-controlled trial
Eur J Clin Pharmacol 50: 457-461

Albert CM, Hennekens CH, O'Donnell CJ (1998)
Fish consumption and risk of sudden cardiac death
JAMA 279 (1): 23-28

Albonico HU (1997)
Gewaltige Medizin
Verlag Paul Haupt, Bern-Stuttgart-Wien

Alexander JW, Peck MD (1990)
Future prospects for adjunctive therapy: pharmacologic and

nutritional approaches to immune system modulation
Crit Care Med 18: S1 59-64

Alexander J, Scharton-Kersten TM, Yap G, Roberts CW, Liew FY, Sher A (1997)
Mechanisms of innate resistance to Toxoplasmose gondii infection
Philos Trans R Soc Lond B Biol Sci 29: 352 (1359): 1355-1359

Alexander JW, Meakins JL (1972)
A physiological basis for the development of opportunistic infections in man
Ann Surg 176: 273-287

Altmann R (1894)
Die Elementarorganismen und ihre Beziehung zu den Zellen
Veit, Leipzig

Amin AR, Abramson SB (1998)
The role of nitric oxide in articular cartilage breakdown in osteoarthritis
Curr Opin Rheumatol 10 (3): 263-268

Ammich O (1938)
Über die nichtsyphilitische interstitielle Pneumonie des ersten Kindesalters
Virchows Arch Path Anat 302: 539-554

Anderson R, Grabow G, Oosthuizen R et al. (1980)
Effects of sulfamethoxazole and trimethoprim on human neutrophil and lymphocyte functions in vitro: In vivo effects of co-trimoxazole
Antimicrob Agents Chem 17: 322-327

Angier N (1988)
Natural obsession: the search for oncogenes
In: Epstein S (1998)
Winning the war against cancer? .... Are they even fighting it?
The Ecologist 28 (2): 69-80

Aoki T, Muller WA, Cahill GF (1972)
Hormonal regulation of glutamine metabolism in fasting man
Adv Enzyme Regul 10: 145-151

Aoki T, Miyakoshi H, Usuda Y, Herberman RB (1993) Low NK syndrome and its relationship to chronic fatigue syndrome
Clin Immunol Immunopathol 69: 253-265

Appelton L, Tomlinson A, Willoughby DA (1996)
Induction of cyclooxygenase and nitric oxide-synthase in inflammation
Adv Pharmacol 35: 27-78

Ardawi MS, Newsholme EA (1982)
Maximum activities of some enzymes of glycolysis, the tricarboxylic acid cycle and ketone-body and glutamine utilization pathways in lymphocytes of the rat
Biochem J 208: 743-748

Argiles JM, Lopez-Soriano FJ (1990)
Why do cancer cells have such a high glycolytic rate?
Med Hypotheses 32: 151-155

Armengol CE (1995)
A historical review of Pneumocystis Carinii JAMA 273 (9): 247-251

Arnaudo E, Dalakas MC, Shanshe et al. (1991)
Depletion of muscle mitochondrial DNA in AIDS-patients with zidovudine induced myopathy
Lancet 337: 508-510

Arzuaga J, Moreno S, Miralles P et al. (1994)
Lower respiration tract-infections in HIV-infected patients 10th Inti Conf AIDS, Yokohama, Japan

Auerbach DM, Bennett Jv, Brachmann PS et al. (1982)
Epidemiologic aspects of the current outbreak of Kaposi's sarcoma and opportunistic infections
N Engl J Med 306: 248-252

Azano Y, Hoder RJ (1983)
T-cell regulation of B-cell activation: Antigen-specific and antigen-nonspecific suppressor pathways are mediated by distinct T-cell subpopulations
J Immunol 130 (3): 1061-1065

B

Bacellar H, Munoz A, Miller EN et al. (1994)
Temporal trends in the incidence of HIV-1-related neurologic diseases: Multicenter AIDS Cohort Study (MACS) 1985-1992
Neurology 44: 1892-1900

Bach MC (1989)
Failure of zidovudine to maintain remission in patients with AIDS
N Engl J Med 320: 594-595

Bachrach D, Heimer YM (eds.) (1989)
The physiology of polyamines
CRC Press Inc, Florida. VoLl

Bader JP (1975)
Reproduction of RNA tumor viruses
In: Fraenkel-Conrat H, Wagner RR (ed.) Comprehensive Virology
Plenum Press, New York

Bagetto GL (1992)
Deviant energetic metabolism of glycolytic cancer cells
Biochimie 74: 959-974

Bagetto GL (1997)
Biochemical, genetic and metabolic adaptations of tumor cells that express the typical multidrug-resistance phenotype.
Reversion by new therapies
J Bioenerget Biomembr 29 (4): 401-413
Baker DH, Wood RI (1992)
Cellular antioxidant status and HIV replication Nutrition Reviews 501: 15-18

Balter M (1997)
How does HIV overcome the body's T-cell body guards?
11th Colloquium of the Cent-Gardes Marnes-la-Coquette, France, 27 to 29 October 1997
Science 287: 1399-1400

Baltimore D (1985)
Retroviruses and retrotransposons: The role of reverse transcription in shaping the eucaryotic genome
Cell 40: 481-482

Bani D, Marini E, Bello MG et al. (1995)
Relaxin activates the L-arginine-nitric oxide pathway in human breast cancer cells
Cancer Research 55: 5272-5275

Bannasch P, Klimek F, Mayer D (1997)
Early bioenergetic changes in hepatocarcinogenesis: Preneoplastic phenotypes mimic responses to insulin and thyroid hormone
J Bioenergetics Biomembr 29 (4): 303-312

Barbul A, Wasserkrug HL, Seitter E et al. (1980)
Immunostimulatory effects of arginine in normal and injured rats
J Surg Res 29: 228-235

Barbul A, Sisto DA, Wasserkrug HL et al. (1981)
Arginine stimulates lymphocyte immune response in healthy human beings
Surgery 90: 244-251

Barbul A, Fishel RS, Shimazu S et al. (1985)
Intravenous hyperalimentation with high arginine levels improves wound healing and immune function
J Surg Res 38: 328-334

Barbul A (1986)
Arginine: Biochemistry, physiology and therapeutic implications
J Parenteral Enteral Nutr 10: 227-238

Barbul A (1990)
Arginine and immune function
Nutrition 6: 53-62

Barcellini W, Rizzardi Gp, Borghi MO (1994)
TH1 and TH2 cytokine production by peripheral blood mononuclear cells from HIV-infected persons
AIDS 8: 757-762

Barnalba V, Francs M, Paroli R (1994)
Selective expansion of cytotoxic T lymphocytes with a CD4+ CD56+ surface phenotype and a T helper type 1 profile of cytokine secretion in the liver of patients chronically infected with hepatitis B virus
J Immunol 152: 3074-3087

Barnes JM, Magee PN (1954)
Some toxic properties of dimethylnitrosamine
Brit J and Mad 11: 167-174

Barnes PI. Liew FY (1995)
Nitric oxide and asthmatic inflammation
Immunol Today 16: 128-130

Barré-Sinoussi F, Chermann JC, Rey F (1983)
Isolation of a T-lymphotropic retrovirus from a patient at risk for

acquired immunodeficiency syndrome (AIDS)
Science 220: 868-871

Barré-Sinoussi F (1996)
HIV as the cause of AIDS
Lancet 348: 31-35

Barret IC (1995)
Mechanisms for species differences in receptor—mediated carcinogenesis
Mut Res 333: 189-202

Barrett-Connor E, Friedlander NI. Khaw KT (1990)
Dehydroepiandrosterone sulfate and breast cancer risk Cancer Res 50 (20): 6571-6574

Bartlett I. Fauci AS, Goosby E et al. (1997)
HHS Guidelines for the treatment of HIV infection in aduts and adolescents
The Federal Register 1997

Barton LL (1983)
Energy coupling to nitrite respiration in the sulfate-reducing bacterium Desulfovibrio gigas
J Bacteriol 153: 867

Bartsch H, O'Neill JK, Schulte-Herrmann R (ed.) (1987)
Relevance of N-Nitroso compounds to human cancer
Exposures and mechanisms
IARG Scientific publications no. 84. International Agency for Research on Cancer, Lyon

Bartsch H, Nair J, Owen RW (1999)
Dietary polyunsatured fatty acids and cancers of the breast and colorectum: Emerging evidence for their role as risk modifiers
Carcinogenesis 20 (12): 2209-2218

Bauer MKA, Lieb K, Schulze-Osthoff K et al. (1997)
Expression and regulation of cyclooxygenase-2 in rat microglia
Eur J Biochem 243: 726-731

Baum MK, Mantero-Atienza E, Shor-Posner et al. (1991)
Association of vitamin B6 status with parameters of immune function in early HIV-infection
J Acquir Imm Def Syndr Hum Retrovir 4: 1122-1132

Baum MK, Shor—Posner G, Bonvehi P et al. (1992)
Influence of HIV infection on vitamin status and requirements
Ann NY Acad Sci 669: 165-173

Bauss F, Droge W, Mannel DN (1987)
Tumor necrosis factor mediates endotoxic effects in mice Infect Immun 55: 1622-1625

Becker-Wegerich P, Steuber M. Olbrisch R et al. (1998)
Defects of mitochondrial respiratory chain in multiple symmetric lipomatosis
Arch Dermatol Res 290: 652-655

Beisel WR (1982)
Single nutrients and immunity Am J Clin Nutr 35: 417-468

Beisel WR (1992)
History of nutritional immunology: Introduction and overview
J Nutr 122: 591-596

Beisel WR (1996)
Nutrition and immune function: Overview J Nutr 126: 2611 S—2615 S

Beizhuizen A, Werners I, Haanen C (1998)
Endogenous mediators in sepsis and septic shock Adv Clin Chem 33: 55-131

Benbrik E, Chariot P, Bonavaud S et al. (1997)
Cellular and mitochondrial toxicity of zidovudine (AZT), didanosine (ddl), and zalcitabine (ddC) on cultured human muscle cells
J Neurol Sci 149: 19-25

Bendich A, Borenfreund E, Sternberg SS (1974 a)
Penetration of somatic mammalian cells by sperm Science 183: 857

Bendich A, Borenfreund E, Beju D (1974 b)
Alteration of mammalian somatic cells following uptake of spermatozoa Acta Cytol 18: 544

Benecke E (1938)
Eigenartige Bronchiolenerkrankung im ersten Lebensjahr
Verh Dtsch Ges Path 31: 402-406

Beral V, Peterman TA, Berkelman RL et al. (1990)
Kaposi's sarcoma persons with AIDS: A sexually transmitted infection?
Lancet 335: 123-127

Berdnikoff G (1959)
Fourteen cases of Pneumocystis carinii pneumonia Canad Med J 80: 1-5

Bergsma D,Good RA (ed.) (1968)
Immunologic deficiency disease in man The National Foundation, New York

Bergström J, Fürst P, Holmstrom BU et al. (1981)
Influence of injury and nutrition, water and electrolytes
Ann Surg 193: 810-816

Berkovic SF, Andermann F, Shoubridge EA et al. (1991)
Mitochondrial dysfunction in multiple symmetricallipomatosis
Ann Neurol 29: 566-569

Berlin R (1987)
Historical aspects of nitrate therapy
Drugs 33 (Suppl 4): 1-4

Bernhard W, Leplus R (1964)
In: Fine structure of the normal and malignant human lymph node
Pergamon Press, Oxford

Berridge V, Strong P (eds.) (1993)
AIDS and contemporary history
Cambridge University Press, Cambridge U.K.

Berzofsky JA, Berkower n, Epstein SL (1993)
Antigen-antibody interactions and monoclonal antibodies
In: Paul WE (ed.)
Fundamental Immunology. 3rd ed. Raven, New York (pp. 421-465)

Bess JW, Gorelick RIo Bosche WJ et al. (1997)
Microvesicles are a source of contaminating cellular proteins found in purified HIV-1 preparations
Virol 230: 134-144

Bessen LJ, Greene JB, Louie E et al. (1988)
Severe polymyositis-like syndrome associated with zidovudine therapy of AIDS and ARC
NEJM 318: 708

Betz M, FOX BS (1991)
Prostaglandin E2 inhibits lymphokines
J Immunol 146: 108-113

Beutler E, Gelbart T (1985)
Plasma glutathione in health and in patients with malignant disease
J Lab Clin Med 105: 581-584

Biasco G, Paganelli GM (1999)
European trials on dietary supplementation for cancer prevention
Ann NY Acad Sci 889: 152-156

Bierer BE, Hollander G, Fruman D, Burakoff SJ (1993)
Cyclosporin A and FK506: Molecular mechanisms of immunosuppression and probes for transplantation biology
Curr Opin Immunol 5: 763-773

Biglieri EG (1988)
Adrenal function in the acquired immunodeficiency syndrome (AIDS)
West J Med 148: 70-73

Birkmayer JGD, Vrecko C, Vole D, Birkmayer W (1993)
Nicotinamide adenine dinucleotide (NADH)—a new therapeutic approach to parkinson's disease. Comparison of oral and parenteral application
Acta Neurol Scand 87: Suppl 146: 32-35

Birks EJ, Yacoub MH (1997)
The role of nitric oxide and cytokines in heart failure Coron Artery Dis 8: 389-402

Blattner WA (1989)
Retroviruses
In: Evans A (ed.)
Viral Infections in Humans
Plenum Medical Book Company, New York. 3rd edn.

Blazar BA, Rodrick ML, O'Mahony JB et al. (1986)
Suppression of natural killer cell function in humans following thermal and traumatic injury
J Clin Immunol 6: 26-36

Bloom BR (1993)
The power of negative thinking
J Clin Invest: 1265-1266

Blumenfeld W, Wagar E, Handley WK (1984)
Use of the trans bronchial biopsy for opportunistic pulmonary infections

in the acquired immunodeficiency syndrome (AIDS)
Am J Clin Pathol 81: 1-5

Bodey GP (1966)
Fungal infections complicating acute leukemia
J Chron Dis 19: 667-673

Boeke JD (1996)
DNA repair. A little help for my ends
Nature 383: 579-581

BogdenJD,BakerH,FrankOetal.(1990)
Micronutrient status and human immuno-deficiency virus (HIV) infection
Ann NY Acad Sci 587: 189-195

Bogovski P, Bogovski S (1981)
Animal species in which N-nitroso compounds induce cancer
Int J Cancer 27: 471-474

Boice J, Greene MH, Killen IV et al. (1983)
Leukemia and preleukernia after adjuvant treatment of gastrointestinal cancer with Gemustine (methyl CCNU)
NEJM 309: 1079-1084

Bolanos JIP' Almeida A, Stewart Vet al. (1997)
Nitric oxide—mediated mitrochondrial damage in the brain: mechanisms and implications for neurodegerterative diseases
J Neurochem 68: 2227-2240

Bonuous G, Baruchel S, Falutz I. Gold P (1993)
Whey proteins as a food supplement in HIV-seropositive individuals
Clin Invest Med 16: 204-209

Bougnoux P (1999) n-3 polyunsatured fatty acids and cancer
Opin Clin Nutr Metabol Care 2 (2): 121-126
Bower RH (1990)
Nutrition and immune function
Nutrition in Clinical Practice 3: 189-193

Bowman A, Gillespie JS, Pollork D (1982)
Oxyhaemoglobin blocks non-adrenergic non-cholinergic inhibition in the bovine retractor penis muscle
Europ J Pharmacol 85: 221-224

Brambilla G (1985)
Genotoxic effects of drug-nitrite interaction products: Evidence for the need of risk assessment
Pharmacol Res Commun 17 M: 307-321

Brand K, Leilbold W, Luppa P et al. (1986)
Metabolic alterations associated with proliferation of mitogenic-activated lymphocytes and of lymphoblastoid cell lines: Evaluation of glucose and glutamine metabolism
Immunobiology 173: 23-34

Brand K, Hermfisse U (1997 a)
Aerobic glycolysis by proliferating cells: A protective strategy against reactive oxygen species
FASEB J 11: 388-395

Brand K (1997 b)
Aerobic glycolysis by proliferating cells: Protection against oxidative stress at the expense of energy yield
J Bioenergefics Biomernbr 29 (4): 355-364

Brattsand R, Linden M (1996)
Cytokine modulation by glucocorticoids: mechanisms and actions in cellular studies discussion
Aliment Pharmacol Ther 10 Suppl 2: 81-90; discussion 9192

Bredt IDS, Snyder SH (1990)
Isolation of a nitirc oxide synthetase, a calmodulin-requiring enzym
Proc Nate Acad Sci (USA) 87: 682-685

Bredt IDS, Snyder SH (1992)
Nitric oxide, a novel neuronal messenger Neuron 8: 3-11

Bremer J (1990)
The role of carnitine in intracellular metabolism J Clin Chem Clin Biochem 28: 297-301

Brennan MF (1977)
Uncomplicated starvation versus cancer-cachexia Cancer Res 37: 2359-2364

Brinkman K, ter Hofstedter HJM, Burger DM (1998)
Adverse effects of reverse transcriptase inhibitors: Mitochondrial toxicity as common pathway
AIDS 12:1735-1744

Brinkman K, Smeitink JA, Romijn A, Reiss P (1999)
Mitochondrial toxicity induced by nucleoside-analogue reverse transcriptase inhibitors is a key factor in the pathogenesis of antiviral-therapy-related lipodystrophy Lancet 354: 1112-1115

British HIV Association (1997)
Guidelines for antiretroviral treatment of HIV seropositive individuals
Lancet 349: 1086-1092

Brittenden J, Heys SD, Ross J, Eremin O (1996)
Natural killer cells and cancer
Cancer 77: 1226-i243

Broaddus C, Dake MID, Stuibarg MS et al. (1985)
Bronchoaiveolar lavage of pulmonary infections in the acquired immunodeficiency syndrome
Ann Intern Med 102: 747-752

Brock TD, Madigan MT, Martinko JM, Parker J (1994)
Biology of microorganisms
Prentice Hall International Editions

Brosman JT (1987)
The role of the kidney in amino acid metabolism and nutrition
Can J Physiol Pharmacol 65: 2335-2343

Brouckaert P, Spriggs DR, Demetri G (1989)
Circulating interleukin-6 during a continuous infusion of tumor necrosis factor and interferon-gamma
J Exp Med 169: 2257-2262

Brüne B, Dimmler S, Molina y Vedia L, Lapetina EG (1994)
Nitric oxide: A signal for ADP-ribosylation of proteins
Life Sciences 54: 61-70

Brüne B, Mohr S, Messmer UK (1996)
Protein thiol modification and apoptotic cell death as cGMP-independent nitric oxide (NO) signaling pathways
Rev in Physiol Biochem and Pharmacol 127: 1-30

Brüne B, Sandau K, von Knethen A (1998)
Apoptotic cell death and nitric oxide: Activating and antagonistic transducing pathways
Biochemistry 63 (7): 817-825

Brunton TL (1967)
On the use of nitrite of amyl in angina pectoris
Lancet 2: 97-98

Brun-Vezinet F, Rouzioux C, Barré-Sinoussi F et ai. (1984)
Detection of IgG antibodies to lymphadenopathy-associated virus in patients with AIDS of lymphadenopathy syndrome
Lancet i: 1253-1256

Brzosko WJ, Jankowski A (1992)
PADMA 28 bei chronischer Hepatitis.
Klinische und immunologische Wirkungen Schweiz Zschr Ganzheits Med 4 (Suppl 1): 13-14

Buchbinder Sp, Katz MH, Hessol NA et ai. (1994)
Long-term HIV-1 infection without immunologic progression
AIDS 8: 1123-1128

Buhl R, Jaffe JA, Holroyd K, Mastrangeli A et ai. (1989)
Systemic glutathione deficiency in symptom free HIV seropositive individuals
Lancet 2: 1294-1297

Buimovici-Klein E, Lange M, Ong KR et al. (1988)
Virus isolation and immune srudies in a cohort of homosexual men
J Med Virol 25: 371-385

Burk D, Woods M, Hunter J (1967)
On the significance of glycolysis for cancer growth, with a special' reference to Morris rat hepatoma
J Natl Cancer Instit 38: 839-863

Burns Cp, Halabi S, Clamon GH et ai. (1999)
Phase I clinical study of fish oil fatty acid capsules for patients with cancer cachexia: Cancer and leukemia group B study 9473
Clin Cancer Res 5 (12): 3942-3947

Burton HR, Bush LP (1994)
Accumulation of tobacco-specific nitrosamines during curing and aging of tobacco
In: Loeppky RN, Michejda CJ (ed.) op.cit.

Busch HFM, Jennellens FGI, Scholte HR (eds.) (1981)
Mitochondria and Muscular Diseases
Mefar, b.v. Beesterzwaag, The Netherlands

Bushby SRM, Hitchings (1968)
Trimetoprim, a sulphonamide potentiator
Br J Pharmacol Chemother 33: 72-90

Buttke TM, Sandstrom PA (1994)
Oxidative stress as a mediator of apoptosis
Immunol Today 15: 7-10

C

Calabrese LH (1989)
The rheumatic mainfestations of infection with the human immunodeficiency virus

Calder PC (1994)
Glutamine and the immune system
Clin Nutr 13: 2-6

Callen M (1990)
Surviving AIDS
Harper Collins, New York

Calvano SE (1986)
Hormonal mediation of immune dysfunction following thermal and traumatic injury
In: Gallin JI, Fauci AS (ed.)
Advances in Host Defence Mechanisms. Vol. 6
Raven Press, New York

Campos Y, Martin MA, Navarro C et al. (1996)
Single large-scale mitochondrial DNA depletion in a patient with mitochondrial myopathy associated with multiple symmetric lipomatosis
Neurology 47: 1012-1014

Cantwell A (1984)
AIDS. The Mystery and the Solution.
Aries Rising Press, New York

Cao Y, Qin L, Zhang L et al. (1995)
Virologic and immunologic characterization of long-term survivors of human immunodeficiency virus type 1 infection
N Engl J Med 332: 201-208

Capron M, Capron A (1994)
Immunoglobulin E and effector cells in schistosomiasis
Science 264: 1876-1877

Capuano F, Guerrieri F, Papa S (1997)
Oxydative phosphorylation enzymes in normal and neoplastic cell growth
J Bioenerget Biomembr 29 (4): 379-384

Carpenter CC, Fischl MA, Hammer SM et al. (1996)
Antiretroviral therapy for HIV—infection in 1996. Recommendations of an international panel International AIDS Society—USA
JAMA 276: 146-154

Carpenter CC et al. (1997)
Antiretroviral therapy for HIV—infection in 1997: Updated recommendations of the international AIDS Society—USA panel
JAMA 277: 1962-1969

Carr A, Samaras K, Burton S et al. (1998 a)
A syndrome of peripheral lipodystrophy, hyperlipidaemia and insulin resistance in patients receiving HIV protease inhibitors
AIDS 12: F51-58

Carr A, Samaras K, Chisholm DJ, Cooper DA (1998 b)
Pathogenesis of HIV-1 protease-inhibitor-associated peripheral lipodystrophy, hyperlipidaemia, and insulin resistance
Lancet 351: 1881-1883

Carr A, Samaras K, Thorisdottir A et al. (1999)
Diagnosis, prediction, and natural course of HIV-1 protease-inhibitor-associated lipodystrophy, hyperlipidaemia, and diabetes mellitus: A cohort study
Lancet 353: 2093-2099

Carter LL, Mang X, Dubey C et al. (1998)
Regulation of T cell subsets from naive to memory
J Immunother 21 (3): 181-187

CDC (1981 a)
Pneumocystis Pneumonia—Los Angeles
MMWR 30: 250-252

CDC (1981 b)
Kaposi's Sarcoma and Pneumocystis Pneumonia among homosexual men—New York City and California
MMWR 30: 3-5

CDC (1987)
Revision of the CDC surveillance case definition for acquired immunodeficiency syndrome
MMWR 36 (Suppl 1 S): 3S-15S

CDC (1993 a)
HIV / AIDS surveillance report
Atlanta, USA. February 1993: 16

CDC (1993 b)
Centers for Disease Control Faxback document # 320320,
January 1993

CDC (1998)
Report of the NIH panel to define principles of therapy of HIV and guidelines for the use of antiretroviral agents in adults and adolescents
Morb Mort Weekly Report 47: 1-83

CDC (1999)
U.S. HIV and AIDS cases reported through June 1999
HIV/AIDS Surveillance Report II (1): 1-37

CDC (2000)
Nur bei jedem zweiten wird HIV-Vermehrung durch Kombitherapie unterdrückt. Therapie lässt noch zu wünschen übrig.
Bericht uber HMRT-Studie der CDC (Holmberg S), vorgetragen auf dem Welt-AIDS-Kongress in Durban / Sudafrika 9.-14. Juli 2000
Ärztezeitung 13. Juli 2000

Ceppi ED, Smith FS, Titheradge MA (1997)
Nitric oxide, sepsis and liver metabolism
Biochem Soc Trans 25: 925-934

Cerami A (1992)
Inflammatory cytokines
Clin Immunol Immunopathol 62: 3-10

Chase MW (1945)
Cellular transfer of cutaneous hypersensitivity to tuberculin
Proc Soc Exp Biol Med 59: 134-137

Chassagne J, Verelle P, Fonck Y et al. (1986)
Detection of lymphadenopathy-associated virus p18 in cells of patients with lymphoid diseases using a monoclonal antibody
Ann Institut Pateur / Immunol 137 D: 403-408

Chehimi J, Frank I, Ma X, Trinchieri G (1995)
Differential regulation of IL-10 and role of T-helper cells
In: Abstr. 408. Second National Conference on Human Retroviruses Infectious Diseases Society of America. Alexandria. Va

Cherfas J (1989)
AZT still on trial
Science 246: 882
Chemov HI (1986)
Review and evaluation of pharmacology and toxicologic data, NDA 19-655.
FDA document under the Freedom of Information Act
In: Lauritsen J (1990)
Poison by Prescription. The AZT Story. Asklepios, New York

Cheson BC (1997)
Toxicities associated with purine analog therapy
In: Cheson BC, Keating MJ, Plunkett W (ed.)
Nucleoside analogs in cancer therapy
Marcel Dekker, New York

Chinje EC, Stratford IJ (1997)
Role of nitric oxide in growth of solid tumours: A balancing act
Essays Biochem 32: 61-72

Chiu DT, Duesberg PH (1995)
The toxicity of azidothymidine (AZT) on human and animal cells in culture at concentrations used for antiviral therapy
Genetica 95 (1-3): 103-109

Chlebrowski RT, Beall G, Grosbenor M et al. (1993)
Long-term effects of early nutritional support with new enterotropic peptide basal formula vs. standard enteral formula in HIV-infected patients: Randomized prospective trial
Nutrition 9: 507-514

Christeff N, Lortholary O, Casassus P. et al. (1996)
Relationship between sex steroid hormone levels and CD4 lymphocytes in HIV infected men
Experim Clin Endocrinol Diabetes 104 (2): 130-136

Christie H (1997)
>From hype to hesitation
Continuum 4 (5): 11-12

Christou NY, Meakins JL, Gordon J et al. (1979)
Delayed hypersensitivity: a mechanism for anergy in surgical patients
Surgery 86: 78-82

Christou NV (1986)
Delayed hypersensitivity in the surgical patient In: Gallin n, Fauci AS (ed.)
Advances in host defence mechanisms. Vol. 6
Raven Press, New York

Christou NY, Meakins JL, Gordon J et al. (1995)
The delayed hypersensitivity response and host resistance in surgical patients. 20 years later.
Ann Surg 222 (4): 534-546
Chuntrasakul C, Siltharm S, Sarasombath S et al. (1998)
Metabolic and immune effects of dietary arginine, gluta. mine and omega.3 fatty acids supplementation in immu. nocompromised patients
J Med Assoc Thail 81 (5): 334-343
Clark JA, Rockett KA (1996)
Nitric oxide and parasitic diseases.
Adv Parasitol 37: 1-56

Clark JA, al Yaman FM, Jacobson LS (1997)
The biological basis of malarial disease
Int J Parasitol 27: 1237-1249

Claude A (1947,1948)
Studies on cells: Morphology, chemical constitution, and distribution of biochemical functions
The Harvey Lectures, Series XLIII, pp.121-164

Clayton J (1990)
Bronchitis drug may help AIDS sufferers
New Scientist 16 June 1990, p.13
Clerici M, Stocks NI, Zajak RA et al. (1989 a)
Interleukin-2 production used to detect antigenic peptide recognition by T-helper lymphocytes from asymptomatic HIV-seropositive individuals
Nature 339: 383-385

Clerici M, Stocks NI, Zajak RA et al. (1989 b)
Detection of three distinct patterns of T—helper cell dysfunction

in asymptomatic human immunodeficiency virus-seropositive patients: independence of CD4 cell number and clinical staging
J Clin Invest 84: 1892-1899

Clerici M, Shearer GM (1993 a)
A TH1-TH2 switch is a critical step in the etiology of HIV infection.
Immunol Today 14: 107-111

Clerici M, Lucey DR, Pinto JA et al. (1993 b)
Restoration of HIV-specific cell mediated immune responses by interleukin-12 in vitro
Science 262: 1721-1724

Clerici M, Shearer GM (1994)
The TH1 / TH2 hypothesis of HIV infection: new insights
Immunol Today 15: 575-581

Clerici M, Shearer GM, Clerici E (1998)
Cytokine dysregulation in invasive cervical carcinoma and other human neoplasias: Time to consider the TH1/TH2 paradigm
J Natl Cancer Institute 90 (4): 261-263

Clipstone NE, Crabtree GR (1992)
Identification of calcineurin as a key signaling enzyme in T lymphocyte activation
Nature 357: 695

Cobbold S, Waldmann H (1998)
Infectious tolerance
Curr Opin Immunol 10 (5): 518-524

Coffey RG, Hadden JW (1985)
Neurotransmitters, hormones, and cyclic nucleoticles in lymphocyte regulation
Fed Proc 44: 112-117

Coffman RL, Carty J (1986)
A T cell activity that enhances polyclonal Ig E production and its inhibition by interferon-gamma
J Immunol 136: 949-954

Coffman RL, Mocei S, O'Garra A (1999)
The stability and reversibility of TH1 and TH2 population
Curr Top Microbiol Immunol 238: 1-12

Cohen J (1997)
The media's love affair with AIDS research: Hope vs. hype
Science 275: 298.-299

Cohen RD, lies RA, Barnett D et al. (1971)
The effect of changes in lactate uptake on the intracellular pH of perfused rat liver
Cli Sci (London) 41: 159-170

Cohen SS (1987)
Antiretroviral therapy for AIDS
NEJM 317: 629

Colosanti M, Persidini T, Menegazzi M (1995)
Induction of nitric oxide synthase in RNA expression
J Biel Chem 270: 26731-26733

Committee on the Safety of Medicines (1985)
Deaths associated with cotrimoxazole, ampicillin and trimethoprim
Curr Prob 15: 1

Committee on the Safety of Medicines (1995)
Revised indications for co-trimoxazole (Septrin, Bactrim, various generic preparations)
Curr Prob Pharmacovigil 21: 6

Concorde Coordinating Committee (1994)
Concorde: MRC/ANRS randomised double-blind controlled trial of immediate and deferred zidovudine in symptom—free HIV—infection
Lancet 343: 871-881

Conney AH, Lou Y-R, Xie J-G et al. (1997)
Some perspectives on dietary inhibition of carcinogenesis: Studies with curcumin and tea
P.S.E.M.B. 216: 234-244

Coodley CO, Coodley MK, Nelson HO, Loveless MO (1993)
Micronutrient concentrations in the HIV wasting syndrome
AIDS 7: 1595-1600

Cooper DA, Emery S (1999)
Latent reservoirs of HIV infection: Flushing with IL-2?
Nature Medicine 5: 611-612
Cooper SW, Kimbrough RD (1980)
Acute dimethylnitrosamine poisoning outbreak
J Forensic; Sci 25: 874-882

Cossarizza A, Franceschi C, Monti D et al. (1995)
Protective effect of N-Acetylcysteine in tumornecrosis factor-alpha-induced apoptosis in U 937 cells: The role of mitochondria
Exp Cell Res 220(1): 232-240

Costa M (1995)
Model for the epigenetic mechanism of action of nongenotoxic carcinogens
Am J Clin Nutr 61: 666S-669S

Cotelle N, Bernier J-L, Catteau J-P et al. (1996)
Antioxidants properties of hydroxy—flavones
Free Rad Biol Med 20: 35-43

Cottier H, Hodler I, Kraft R (1995)
Oxidative stress: Pathogenetic mechanisms

Forsch Komplementärmed 2: 233-239

Cotton P (1990)
Controversy continues as experts ponder zidovudine's role in early HIV infection
JAMA 263: 1605

Cowdry EV (1918)
The mitochondrial constituents of protoplasm
Contrib Embryol 8: 39-160

Cox S, Cadman I. Dietz P et al. (1998)
The antiviral report.
A critical review of new antiretroviral drugs and treatment strategies
Treatment Action Group (TAG), New York
Crabtree HG (1929)

Observations on the carbohydrate metabolism of tumours
Biochem J 23: 536-545

Craddock M (1995)
My analysis of the Ho and Shaw papers email: marck@solution.maths.unsw.edu.au

Craddock M (1996 a)
Some mathematical considerations on HIV and AIDS
In: Duesberg PH (ed.)
AIDS: Virus or Drug Induced?
Kluwer Academic Publishers, Dordrecht-Boston-London

Craddock M (1996 b)
HIV: Science by press conference
In: Duesberg PH (ed.)
AIDS: Virus or Drug Induced?
Kluwer Academic Publishers, Dordrecht—Boston London

Craddock M (1997)
Supplementary Notes for HIV: Science by Press Conference
In: Lang S (1997)
HIV and AIDS. Throwing Math and Statistics at People.
Reader from Department of Mathematics, Yale University, New Haven, USA

Cribb AE, Spielberg SP (1990)
Hepatic microsomal metabolism of sulfamethoxazole to the hydroxylamine
Drug Metabol Dispos 18: 748-757

Cribb AE, Spielberg SP (1992)
Sulfamethoxazole is metabolized to the hydroxylamine in humans
Clin Pharmacol Ther 51: 522-526

Cuezva JM, Ostronoff LK, Ricar J et al. (1997)
Mitochondrial biogenesis in the liver during development and oncogenesis
J Bioenerget Biomembr 29 (4): 365-377

Cunningham AL, Dwyer DE, Mills I, Montagnier L (1996)
Structure and function of HIV
Med J Aust 164: 161-173

Cupps TR, Fauci AS (1982)
Corticosteroid-mediated immunregulation in man
Immunol Rev 65: 133-155

D

D'Adamo PJ, Whitney C (1996)
Eat right for your type
G.P. Putnam's Sons, New York
published in German (2000):

Das Kochbuch für ein gesundes Leben.
Piper Verlag, München

D'Elios M, Del Prete G (1998)
Th1/Th2 balance in human disease
Transplant Proc 30 (5): 2373-2377

Dalakas MC, Illaa I, Pezeshkpour GH et al. (1990)
Mitochondrial Myopathy caused by long-term zidovudine toxicity
N Eng J Med 322: 1098-1105

Daly AK, Cholerton S, Armstrong M et al. (1994)
Genotyping for polymorphisms in xenobiotic metabolism as predictor of disease susceptibility
Environ Health Perspect 102: S44-S61

Daly JM, Reynolds JV, Thorn A et al. (1988)
Immune and metabolic effects of arginine in the surgical patient
Ann Surg 208: 512-523

Daly JM, Reynolds JV, Sigal BK (1990)
Effect of dietary protein and amino acids of immune function
Crit Care Med 18: 586-593

Dang CV, Lewis BC, Dolde C et al. (1997)
Oncogenes in tumor metabolism, tumorigenesis, and apoptosis
J Bioenerget Biomembr 29 (4): 345-353

Dangl J (1998)
Plants just say NO to pathogens
Nature 394: 525-527

Dannenberg AM (1991)
Delayed hypersensitivity and cell-mediated immunitiy in the pathogenesis of tuberculosis
Immunol Today 12: 228-232

Davis RE (1986)
Clinical chemistry of folic acid
Advances in Clinical Chemistry 25: 233-294

De Duve Chr (1991)
Blueprint for a cell: the nature and origin of life
Neil Patterson Publishers, Burlington, North Carolina

De Groote MA, Fang FC (1995)
NO inhibitions: Antimicrobial properties of nitric oxide
Clin Infect Dis 21 S 162-S 165

De Harven E (1998 a)
Pioneer deplores "HIV". Maintaining errors is evil
Continuum 5 (2): 24
Available online at: http://www.garynull.com/Documents/Continuum/PioneerDeploresHIV.htm

De Harven E (1998 b)
Retrviruses: The recollections of an electron microscopist
Contribution to 1998 World AIDS Congress in Geneva
Tel. / Fax: (33) 493 60 28 39

Available online at: http://www.virusmyth.net/aids/data/edhrecol.htm

De Harven E (1965)
Remarks on viruses, leukemia and electron microscopy
Methodological Approaches to the Study of Leukemias. pp 147-156
The Wistar Institute Press, Philadelphia

De Harven E (1998 c)
Remarks on methods for retroviral isolation
Continuum 5 (3): 20-21
Available online at: http://www.garynull.com/Documents/Continuum/RemarksRetroviralIsolation.htm

De Lorgeril M, Salen P. Martin JL et al. (1998)
Mediterranean dietary pattern in a randomized trial: Prolonged survival and possible reduced cancer rate
Arch Intern Med 158 (11): 1181-1187

De Rosa SC, Zaretsky MD, Dubs JG et al. (2000)
N-acetylcysteine replenishes glutathione in HIV infection
Eur J Clin Invest 30 (10) : 915-929

De Simone C, Tzantzoglou S, Famularo G et al. (1993)
High dose L-carnitine improves immunologic and metabolic parameters in AIDS patients
Immunopharmacol Immunotoxicol 15 (1): 1-12

De Simone C, Tzantzoglou S, Jirillo E et al. (1991)
L-Carnitine deficiency in AIDS patients
AIDS 6: 203-205

De Waal Malefyt R (1997)
The role of type 1 interferons in the differentiation and function of Th1 and Th2 cells
Semin Oncol 24 (3 suppl 9): S9-94-S9-98

De Wys WD, Begg C, Lavin PT et al. (1980)
Prognostic effect of weight loss prior to chemotherapy in cancer patients
Am J Med 69: 491-497

De Wys WD, Curran I, Henle W et al. (1982)
Workshop on Kaposi-Sarcoma: Meeting report
Cancer Treatment Reports 66 (6): 1387-1390

Deamer WC, Zollinger HU (1953)
Intersitial "plasma cell" pneumonia of premature and young infants
Pediatrics 12: 11-22

Dean JH, Luster MI, Mungon AE, Kimber T (eds.) (1994)
Immunotoxicology and immunopharmacology
Raven Press, New York. 2nd edn.

Decker O, Schöndorf M, Bidlingmaier F et al. (1996)
Surgical stress induces a shift in the type-1/type-2 T-helper cell

balance, suggesting down-regulation of cell-mediated and up-regulation of antibody mediated immunity commensurate to the trauma
Surgery 119: 316-325

Dei Prete G (1998)
The concept of type-1 and type-2 helper T cells and their cytokines in humans
Int Rev Immunol 16 (3-4): 427-455

Delespesse G, Yang LP, Ohshima Y et al. (1998)
Maturation of human neonatal CD4+ and CD8+ T lymphocytes into Th1 / Th2 effectors
Vaccine 16 (14-15): 1415-1419

Delledonne M, Xia Y, Diton RA, Lamb C (1998)
Nitic oxide functions as a signal in plant disease resistance
Nature 394: 585-588

Des Jarlais DC, Friedman SR, Marmor M et al. (1987)
Development of AIDS, HIV seroconversion, and potential cofactors for T4 cell loss in a cohort of intravenous drug abusers
AIDS 1: 105-111

Des Prez RM, Heim CR (1990)
Mycobycterium tuberculosis
In: Mendell GL, Douglas RG, Bennett JE, 8th ed.
Principles and practices of infectious diseases 3rd ed. Churchill Livingstone, New York

Descotes J (1988)
Immunotoxicology of drugs and chemicals
Elsevier, Amsterdam-New York-Oxford, 2nd edn.

Detels R, English p, Vischer BR et al. (1989)
Seroconversion, sexual activity and condom use among 2915 seronegative men followed for up to 2 years
J Acquir Immun Def Syndr 2: 77-83

Deutscher Bundestag (1994)
Zweite Beschlussempfehlung und Schlussbericht des 3. Untersuchungsausschusses nach Artikel 44 des Grundgesetzes
Drucksache 12/8591 vom 25.10.1994

Dewanjee MK (1997)
Molecular biology of nitric oxide synthases. Reduction of complications of cardiopulmonary bypass from platelets and neutrophils by nitric oxide generation from arginine and nitric oxide donors
ASAIO J 43: 151-159

Di George AM (1968)
Congenital absence of the thymus and its immunologic consequences: Concurrence with congenital hypoparathyroidism
In: Bergsma O, Good RA (ed.)
Immunologic Deficiency Disease in man
The National Foundation, New York

Diamond I. Blisard KS (1976)
Effects of stimulant and relaxant drugs on tension and cyclic nucleotide levels in canine femoral artery
Molecular Pharmacol 12: 688-692

Djordjevic MV, Fan I. Krzeminski J (1984)
Characterisation of N-nitrosamino acids in'Tobacco In: Loeppky RN, Michejcla CJ (ed.) op. cit.

Dona G, Frasca O (1997)
Genes, immunity, and senescence: looking for a link
Immunol Rev 160:159-170

Dorward A, Sweet S, Moorehead R, Singh G (1997)
Mitochondrial contributions to cancer cell physiology: Redox balance, cell cycle and drug resistance
J Bionerget Biomembr 29 (4): 385-390

Dourmashkin RR, O'Toole CM, Bucher O, Oxford JS (1991)
The presence of budding virus-like particles in human lymphoid cells used for HIV cultivation
VIII. International Conference on AIDS. Florence 1991: 122

Doyle Mp, Terpstra JW, Pickering RA et al. (1983)
Hydrolysis, nitrosyl exchange, and synthesis of alkyl nitrites
J Org Chem 48: 3379-3382

Drabick JJ, Magill AI. Smith KJ et al. (1994)
Hypereosinophilia syndrom associated with HIV infection
South Med J 87: 525-529

Dröge W (1989)
Metabolische Störungen bei HIV-Infektion
In: Project News Nr.2, pp.4-5
AIDS-Zentrum des Bundesgesundheitsamtes Berlin

Dröge W (1993)
Cysteine and glutathione deficiency in AIDS patients: A rationale for the treatment with N-acetylcysteine
Pharmacol 46: 61-65

Dröge W, Eck H-P, Mihm S (1992)
HIV—induced cysteine deficiency and T cell dysfunction: A rationale for treatment with N-acetylcysteine
Immunol Today 13: 211-214

Droge W, Eck Hp, Näher H et al. (1988)
Abnormal amino acid concentration in the blood of patients with acquired immune deficiency syndrome (AIDS) may contribute to the immunological defect
Biol Chem Hoppe-Seyler 369: 143-148

Droge W, Gross A, Hack V et al. (1997 a)
Role of cysteine and glutathione in HIV infection and cancer cachexia. Therapeutic intervention with N-acetyl-cysteine (NAC)
Adv Pharmacol 38: 581-600

Droge W, Holm E (1997 b)
Role of cysteine and glutathione in HIV infection and other diseases associated with muscle wasting and immunological dysfunction
FASEB J 11: 1077-1089

Dröge W, Mihm S, Bockstette M, Roth S (1994)
Effect of reactive oxygen internediates and antioxidants on proliferation and function of T-Iymphocytes
Methods Enzymol 234: 135-151

Dröge W, Roth S, Altmann A, Mihm S (1987)
Regulation of T-cell functions by L-Iactate
Cell Immunol 108: 405-416

DTB (1969)
Septrin and Bactrim: A combination of trimethoprim and sulfamethoxazole
Drugs and Therapeutics Bulletin 7: 13-15

DTB (1995)
Co-trimoxazole use restricted
Drugs and Therapeutics Bulletin 33: 92-93

Dubozy A, Husz S, Hunyadi J et al. (1973)
Immune deficiencies and Kaposi's sarcoma
Lancet 2: 265-269

Duesberg PH (1987)
Retroviruses as carcinogenes and pathogens: Expectation and reality
Cancer Res 47: 1199-1220

Duesberg PH (1992 a)
AIDS acquired by drug consumption and other noncontagious risk factors
Pharmacol Therap 55: 201-277

Duesberg PH (1995)
Foreign-protein-mediated immunodeficiency in hemophiliacs with and without HIV
Genetica 95 (1-3): 51-70

Duesberg PH (1996)
Inventing the AIDS virus
Regnery Publishing Inc., Washington DC

Duesberg PH (2000)
The african AIDS epidemic—new and contagious—or—old under a new name?
Presentation Presidential AIDS Advisory
Panel Meeting on May /July 2000 in Pretoria
Net: www.virusmyth.com (front news)

Duesberg PH, Bialy H (1996 a)
Duesberg and the right of reply according to Maddox-Nature
In: Duesberg PH (ed.)
AIDS: Virus or drug induced?
Kluwer Academic Publishers, Dordrecht-Boston-London

Duesberg PH, Rasmick O (1998)
The AIDS dilemma: Drug diseases blamed on a passenger virus
Genetica 104: 85-132

Duesberg PH, Schwartz JR (1992 b)
Latent viruses and mutated oncogenes: No evidence for pathogenicity
Proc Nucleic Acid Res Mol Biol 43: 135-204

Durack DT (1981)
Opportunistic infections and Kaposi's sarcoma in homosexual men
NEJM 305: 1465-1467

Duthie SJ, Johnson W, Dobson VL (1997)
The effect of dietary flavonoids on DNA damage (Strand breaks and oxidised pyrimidines) and growth in human cells
Mutation Res 390: 141-151

Dutz W (1970)
Pneumocystis Carinii Pneumonia
Pathol Ann 3: 309-340

Dvorak HF, Mihm MC, Dvorak AM (1979)
Morphology of delayed-type patients
Ann Surg 190: 557-564

Dworikin BM, Rosenthal WS (1986)
Selenium deficiency in AIDS
J PEN 10: 405-407

E

Eaton NE, Reeves GK, Appleby PN, Key TJ (1999)
Endogenous sex hormones and prostate cancer: a quantitative review of prospective studies
Br J Cancer 80 (7): 930-934

Ebeling P, Koivisto VA (1994)
Physiological importance of dehydroepiandrosterone
Lancet 343 (8911): 1479-1481

Eck HP, Gmünder H, Hartmann M et al. (1989)
Low concentrations of acid globule thiol (cysteine) in the blood plasma of HIV-1 infected patients
Biol Chem Hoppe-Seyler 370: 101-108

Eigenbrodt E, Giossmann H (1980)
One of the keys to cancer?
Trends Pharmacol Sci 1: 240-245

Ellekany S, Whiteside TL (1987)
Analysis of intestinal lymphocyte subpopulation in patients with AIDS and ARC
Am J Clin Pathol 87: 356-364

Ender F, Havre G, Helgebostad A et al. (1964)
Isolation and identification of a hepatotoxic factor in herring meal produced from sodium nitrite preseved herring
Naturwissenschaften 51: 637-638

Epstein S (1996)
Impure Science.
AIDS, activism, and the politics of knowledge
University of California Press, Berkeley-Los Angeles-London

Epstein S (1998)
Winning the war against cancer? Are they even fighting it?
The Ecologist 28 (2): 69-80

Ericson LS (1983)
Splanchnic exchange of glucose, amino acids and free fatty acids in

patients with chronic inflammatory
disease
Gut 24: 1161-1168

Ernster L, Schatz G (1981)
Mitochondria: A historical review
J Cell Biol 91: 227 S—255 S

Esterly JE (1967)
Pneumocystis carinii in lungs of
adults at autopsy
Am Rev Resp Dis 97: 935-939

Evetett GM (1975)
Amyl nitrite ("poppers") as an
aphrodisiacum
In: Sandler M, Gessa GL (ed.)
Sexual Behavior: Pharmacology
and Biochemistry
Raven Press, New York

Eyster ME, Nau ME (1978)
Particulate material in
antihemopbiliac factor (AHF)
concentrates
Transfusion 9/10: 576-581

Ezekowitz RA, Williams OJ, Koziel
H et al. (1991)
Uptake of Pneumocystis carinii
mediated by the macrophage
mannose receptor
Nature 351: 155-158

F

Farber C (1989)
Sins of omission: The AZT scandal
Spin Magazine, Nov 1989

Fauci AS (2000)
Neue Strategien sind bei der
Bekämpfung der HIV-Infektion
nötig
Bericht über HAART-Studie der
NIAID (Fauci AS), vorgetragen
auf dem Welt-AIDS-Kongress in
Durban / Südafrika 9.-14.Juli 2000
Ärztezeitung 14. Juli 2000

Wird HIV trotz Therapie-Pausen
gebändigt? op. cit.
Ärztezeitung 13.07.2000
Net: www.aids2000.com

Fauci AS, Dale DC (1974)
The effect of in vivo hydrocortisone
on subpopulations of human
lymphocytes
J Clin lnvest 53: 240-246

Fauci AS, Dale DC (1975)
The effect of hydrocortisone on
the kinetics of normal human
lymphocytes
Blood 46: 235-243

Fauci AS, Lane HC (1994)
Human immunodificiency (HlV)
disease, AIDS and related disorders
In: Issellbacher KJ, Braunwald Em
Wilson JD et al. (ed.)
Harrisons Principals of Internal
Medicine. 13th ed.
McGraw-Hill Inc., New York
(pp. 1566-1618)

Fauci AS, Pratt Kr (1976 b)
Activation of human B lymphocytes.

I. Direct plaque-forming cell assay for the measurement of polyclonal activation and antigenic stimulation of human B lymphocytes
J Exp Med 144: 674-684

Fauci AS, Pratt KR, Whalen G (1976 a)
Activation of human B lymphocytes. II. Cellular interactions in the PFC response of human tonsillar and peripheral blood B lymphocytes to polyclonal activation by pokeweed mitogen
J Immunol 117: 2100-2104

Fauci AS, Haynes BF (1977)
Activation of human B lymphocytes. III. Concanavalin A—induced generation of suppressor cells of the plague-forming cell response of normal human B ???
J Immunol 118: 2281-2287

Fauci AS, Pratt KR, Whalen G (1977)
Activation of human B lymphocytes. IV. Regulatory effects of corti co steroids on the triggering signal in the plaque-forming cell response of human peripheral blood B lymphocytes to polyclonal activation
J Immunol 119: 598-603

Fearon DT, Locksley RM (1996)
The instructive role of innate immunity in the acquired immune response
Science 272: 50-54

Fedyk ER, Brown OM, Phipps RP (1997)
PGE2 regulation of B lymphocytes and T helper 1 and T helper 2 cells: induction of inflammatory versus allergic responses
Adv Exp Med BioI 407: 237-242

Fein R, KeIsen Dp, Geller N (1985)
Adenocarcinomas of the oesophagus and gastroesophageal junction: Prognostic factors and results of therapy
Cancer 25: 12-18

Felig P, Owen OE, Wahren J, Cahill GF (1969)
Amino acid metabolism during prolonged starvation
J Clin Invest 48: 584-594

Fenton HJH (1884)
Oxidation of tartaric acid in presence of iron
J Chem Soc 65: 899-910

Fernandes G, Troyer DA, lolly CA (1998)
The effects of dietary lipids ongene expression and apoptosis
Proceedings Nutr Soc 57 (4): 543-550

Fernandez de Allbornoz IL, Ostreicher R (1984)
Foreword. Vorträge auf dem Kongress "AIDS—the epidemic of Kaposi's Sarcoma and opportunistic infections" March 1983, New York University Medical Center

In: Friedman-Kien AE, Laubenstein LJ (ed.) op. Cit.

Ferrando SJ, Rabkin JG, Poretsky L (1999)
Dehydroepiandrosterone sulfat (DHEAS) and testosterone: Relation to HIV illness stage and progression over one year
J Acquir Imm Def Syndr 22 (2): 146-154

Fiala C (1998)
AIDS in Africa: Dirty tricks
New African, pp. 36-38

Fiala C (2000)
Seit 20 Jahren leben wir mit HIV / AIDS.
Aufruf zu einer offenen Diskussion der widersprüchlichen Fakten.
Präsentation zur Spezialisten-Konferenz auf Initiative des Südafrikanischen Präsidenten Mbeki Mai/Juli 2000 in Pretoria eMail: christianfiala@aon.at
Fax: +43-1-5973190

Fiala C (1997)
Lieben wir gefährlich? Ein Arzt auf der Suche nach den Fakten und Hintergründen von AIDS
Franz Deuticke Verlagsgesellschaft, Wien-München

Fischl MA, Richman DO, Hansen N et al. (1990)
The safety and efficacy of Zidovudine (AZT) in the treatment of subjects with mildly symptomatic human immunodeficiency virus type 1 (HlV) infection
Ann Intern Med 112: 727-737
Fletcher BS, Kujubu DA, Perrin OM, Herschman H (1992)
Structure of the nitrogen-inducible TIS 10 gene and demonstration that the TIS10-encoded protein is a functional prostaglandin G/H synthase
J Biol Chem 267: 4338-4344

Folkers K, Langsjoen P, Nara Yet al. (1988)
Biochemical deficiencies of Coenzyme Q 10 in HlV-infection and exploratory treatment
Biochem Biophysic Res Communic 153 (2): 888-896

Folkers K, Yamamura Y (eds.) (1986)
Biomedical and clinical aspects of coenzyme Q 10
Elsevier, New York
Fong LYY, Bevill RF, Thurson JC, Magee PN (1992)
DNA adduct dosimetry and DNA repair in rats and pigs given repeated doses of procarbazine under conditions of carcinogenicity and human cancer chemotherapy respectively
Carcinogenesis 13: 2153-2159

Fontana L, Sitianni MC, De Sanctis G et al. (1986)
Deficiency of natural killer activity, but not a natural killer binding, in patients with lymphadenopathy syn~me positive for antibodies to HTLV-III
Immunobiology 171: 425-435

Fordyce-Baum MK, Montero-Atienza E, Morgan R et al. (1990)
Toxic levels of dietary supplementation in HlV-1 infected patients
Arch AIDS Res 4: 149-157

Franchini A, Conte A, Ottaviani E (1995)
Nitric oxide: An ancestral immunocyte of effector molecule
Adv Neuroimmunol 5 (4): 463-478

Frank GW (1992)
Kombucha. Das Teepilz-Getrank. Praxisgerechte Anleitung für die Zubereitung und AnWendung
Verlag W. Ennsthaler, A-4402 Steyer

Fraziano M, Montesano C, Lombardi VR et al. (1996) Epitope specificity of anti-HlV antibodies in human and murine autoimmune diseases
AIDS Res Human Retroviruses 12: 491-496

Frenkel JK, Gwod JT, Schultz JA (1966)
Latent Pneumocystis infection of rats: relapse and chemotherapy
Lab Invest 15: 1559

Freund HA (1937)
Clinical manifestations and studies in parenchymatous hepatitis
Ann Internal Med 10: 1144-1155

Friedland GH (1990)
Early treatment for HIV: the time has come (editorial)
N Engl J Med 322: 1000-1002

Friedman PI (1987)
Is wasting itself lethal? A case-control prospective study
Nutr Res 7: 707-717

Friedman-Kien AE, Laubenstein LJ (ed.) (1984)
AIDS: The epidemic of Kaposi's sarcoma and opportunistic infections
Masson Publishing, New York

Friedman-Kien AE, Ostreicher R (1984 a)
Overview of classical and epidemic Kaposi's sarcoma
In: Friedman-Kien AE, Laubenstein LJ (ed.), op. cit.

Friedman-Kien AE, Saltzman BR, Cao Y et al. (1990)
Kaposi's sarcoma in HIV negative homosexual men
Lancet 1: 168
Frissen PHJ, Mulder JW, Masterson JG, Lange JMA (1990)
DHEA administration in HIV infection
European AIDS Conference, Denmark March 1990

Fry TC (1989)
The Great AIDS Hoax
Life Science Institute, Austin, Texas

Fuchs O, Jager H, Popescu M et al. (1990)
Immune activation markers to predict AIDS and survival in HIV—I seropositives Immunology Letters 26: 75

Fumento M (1989)
The Myth of Heterosexual AIDS
Regnery Gateway, Washington DC

Furchgott RF, Zawadzki JV (1980)
The obligatory role of endothelial cells in the relaxation of arterial smooth muscle by acetylcholine
Nature 288: 373-376

Furchgott RF, Vanhoutte PM (1989)
Endothelium-derived relaxing and contracting factors
FASEB J 3: 2007-2018

Furio MM, Wordell CJ (1985)
Treatment of infectious complications of acquired immunodeficiency syndrome
Am Pharmacol 4: 539-554

Furman PA, Fyfe JA, St. Clair M, Weinhold K, Rideout JL, Freeman GA, Nusinoff-Lehrman S, Bolognesi Dp, Broder S, Mitsuya H, Barry OW (1986)
Phosphorylation of 3'-azido-3'-deoxythymidine and selective interaction of the 5'-triphosphate with human immunodeficiency virus reverse transcriptase
Proc Natl Acad Sci USA 83: 8333-8337

Fye WB (1986)
T. Lauder Brunton and amyl nitrite: A Victorian vasodilator
Circulation 74: 222-229

G

Gabrielsen AE, Good RA (1967)
Chemical suppression of adaptive immunity
Adv Immunol 6: 91-2229

Gajdusek O (1957)
Pneumocystis Carinii—etiologic agent of interstitial plasma cell pneumonia of premature and young infants
Pediatrics 19: 543-565

Galli M, Ridolfo AL, Gervasoni C et al. (1999)
Incidence of fat tissue abnormalities in protease inhibitor-naive patients treated with NRTI combination
Antiviral Ther 4 (Suppl 2): 29

Gallo RC (1986)
The first human retrovirus
Scientific American 235 (6): 88-98

Gallo RC (1991)
Virus Hunting
Basic Books, New York

Gallo RC (1999)
Acceptance speech upon receiving the Paul Ehrlich and Ludwig Darmstaedter award, on 14.03.1999
Paul-Ehrlich-Gesellschaft, Frankfurt a. Main

Gallo RC, Mann O, Broder S et al. (1982)
Human T-cell leukemia-lymphoma virus (HTLV) is in T—but not

B-Iymphocyte from a patient with cutaneous Ted?? lymphoma
Proc Natl Acad Sci USA 79: 5680-5683

Gallo RC, Salahuddin SZ, Popovic M et al. (1984)
Frequent detection and isolation of cytopathic retrovirus (HTLV-III) from patients with AIDS and at risk for AIDS
Science 224: 500-503

Garbuglia AR, Salvi R, Di Caro A et al. (1996)
In vitro activation of HlV RNA expression in peripheral blood lymphocytes as a marker to predict the stability of non-progressive status in Iongterm survivors
AIDS 10: 17-21

Garthwaite I. Charles SL, Chess-Williams R (1988)
Endothelium-derived relaxing factor release on activation of NMDA receptor suggests role as intercellular messenger in the brain
Nature 336: 385-388

Garthwaite I. Garthwaite G, Ralmer RM, Moncada S (1989)
NMDA receptor activation induces nitric oxide synthesis from arginine in rat brain slices
Europ J Pharmacol 172: 413-416

Gatti RA, Good RA (1971)
Occurence of malignancy in immunodeficiency diseases
Cancer 28: 89-98

Gaylarde PM, Sarkany I (1972)
Suppression of thymidine of human leukocytes by cotrimoxazole
Brit Med J 3: 144-149

Gebbers JO (1995)
Antioxidantien in der Ernährung
Forsch Komplementärmed 2: 232-288

Gelmann EP, Popovic M, Lomonilo A et al. (1984)
Evidence for HTLV-infection in two patients with AIDS
In: Friedman-Kien AE, Laubenstein LJ (ed.), op. cit.

Gelman BB, Rodriguez-Wolf MG, Wen J et al. (1992)
Siderotic cerebral macrophages in the acquired immunodeficiency syndrome
Arch PathoI Lab Med 116: 509

George AJT, Ritter MA (1996)
Thymic involution with aging: Obsolescence or good housekeeping?
Immunol Today 17: 267-272

Gervasoni C, Ridolfo AL, Trifir`o G et al. (1999)
Redistribution of body fat in HIV-infected women undergoing combined antiretroviral therapy
AIDS 13: 465-471

Gherardi RK, Mhiri C, Baudrimont M et aI. (1991)
Iron pigment deposits, small vessel vasculitis and erythrophagocytosis in the muscle of human immmunodeficiency virus-infected patients
Human Pathol 22: 1187

Ghilchick MW, Morris AS, Reeves OS (1970)
Immunosuppressive powers of the antibacterial agent trimethoprim
Nature 227: 393-394

Gianotti L, Braga M, Fortis C et aI. (1999)
A prospective randomized trial on preoperative feeding with an arginine-, omega 3 fatty acid-, and RNA-enriched enteral diet: Effect on host response and nutritional status
JPEN J Parenter Enter utrition 23 (6): 314-320

Gill PS, Parick M, Byrnes RK et aI. (1987)
Azidothymidine associated with bone marrow failure in the acquired immunodeficiency syndrome (AIDS)
Ann Intern Med 107: 502-505

Gillespie JS, Liu XR, Martin W (1989)
The effects of L-arginine and N-monomethyl L-arginine on the response of the rat anococcygeus muscle to NANC nerve stimulation
Br J PharmacoI 98: 1080-1082

Gilli RM, Sari JC, Lopez CL et aI. (1990)
ComparatiVe thermodynamic study of the interaction of some antifoIates with dihydrofolate reductase
Biochemica et Biophysica Acta 1040: 245-250

Gillin JS, Shike M, Alcock N et al. (1985)
Malabsorption and mucosal abnormalities of the small intestine in AIDS
Ann Intern Med 102: 619-622

Gillis S, Crabtree GR, Smith KA (1979 a) Glucocorticoid-induced inhibition of T cell growth factor production. I. The effect on mitogen-induced lymphocyte proliferation
J Immunol 123: 1624-1630

Gillis S, Crabtree GR, Smith KA (1979 b)
Glucocorticoid—induced inhibition of T cell growth factor production. II. The effect on the in vitro generation of cytolytic T cells
J Immunol 123: 1632-1638

Giorgio JV, Fahey JL, Smith DC et al. (1987)
Early effects of HlV on CD4 lymphocytes in vivo
J Immunol 138: 3725-3730

Giraldo RA (1999 a)
Everybody reacts positive on the ELISA test for HlV
Continuum 5 (5): 8-10

Net: http://www.robertogiraldo.com/eng/papers/EveryoneTestsPositive.html

Giraldo RA, Ellner M, Farber C et al. (1999 b)
Is it rational to treat or prevent AIDS with toxic antiretroviral drugs in pregnant women, infants, children and anybody else? The answer is negative
Continuum 5 (6): 39-52
Net: http://www.robertogiraldo.com/eng/papers/IsItRational.html

Glaxo Wellcome (1998)
Retrovir (Zidovudine)
In: Physician's Desk Reference. pp. 1167-1175
Medical Economic Co., Monvale, NJ. 1998

Gluschankof P, Monclor I, Gelderblom HR et al. (1997)
Cell membrane vesicles are a major contaminant of gradient-enriched human immunodeficiency virus type-1 preparations
Virol 230: 125-133

Gmünder H, Dröge W (1991)
Differential effects of glutathione depletion on T-cell subsets
Cell Immunol 138: 229-237

Godfried JP, van Griensven G, Tielman R et al. (1987)
Risk factors and prevalence of HIV antibodies in homosexual men in the Netherlands
Am J Epidemiol 125: 1048

Goedert JJ, Neuland CY, Wallen WG et al. (1982)
Amyl nitrite may alter T Lymphcytes in homosexual men
Lancet 1: 412-416

Goedert JJ, Sarngadharen MG, Biggar RJ et al. (1984)
Determinants of retrovirus (HTLV-III) antibody and immunodeficiency conditions in homosexual men
Lancet 2: 711-716

Golz J, Mayr C, Bauer G (1995)
HIV und AIDS.
Behandlung, Beratung, Betreuung.
Urban und Schwarzenberg, München-Wien-Baltimore. 2. Aufl.

Gogos CA, Clinopoulos P, Salsa B et al. (1998)
Dietary Omega-3 polyunsaturated fatty acids plus vitamin E restore immunodeficiency and prolong survival for severely ill patients with generalized malignancy: A randomized control trial
Cancer 82 (2): 395-402

Gold KN, Weyand CM, Gorozny JJ (1994)
Modulation of helper T cell function by prostaglandins
Arthritis Rheum 37: 925-933

Golden BD, Abranson SB (1999)
Selective Cyclooxygenase-2 inhibitors
Rheum Dis Clin North America 25: 359-378

Goldsmith Z (1998)
Cancer: A disease of industrialization
The Ecologist 28 (2): 93-105

GoIshani—Hebroni SG, Bessman SP (1997)
Hexokinase binding to mitochondria: a basis for proliferative energy metabolism
J Bioenerget Biomembr 29 (4): 331-338

Gonzalez FJ (1995)
Genetic polymorphism and cancer susceptibility: Fourteenth Sapporo Cancer Seminar
Cancer Res 55: 710-715

GonzaIez-Quintial R, Baccala R, AIzari PM et aI. (1990)
Poly (GIu60Ala30Tyr10) (GAT)-induced IgG monoclonal antibodies cross-react with various self and non-self antigens through the complementary determining regions. Comparison with IgM monoclonal poIyreactive natural antibodies
Euro J Immunol 20: 2383-2387

Good SS, Durack DT, Miranda P (1986)
Biotransformation in various species and in humans of 3-azido-3-deoxythymidine, a potential agent for the treatment of AIDS
Fed Proc 45: 444, abstract

Goppelt-Struebe M (1995)
Regulation of prostaglandin endoperoxide (cyclo-oxygenase) isoenzyme expression
Prostaglandins Leukot Essent Fattyacids 52: 213-222

Gorard DA, Guilodd RJ (1988)
Necrotizing myopathy and Zidovudine
Lancet i: 1050

Gottlieb MS, Schroff R, Howard M et aI. (1981)
Pneumocystis carinii pneumonia and mucosal candidiasis in previously healthy homosexual men.
Evidence of a new acquired cellular immunodeficiency
NEJM 305: 1425-1431

Gray MW, Burger G, Lang BF (1999)
Mitochondrial Evolution
Science 283: 1476-1481

Green LC, Ruiz de la Luzuriaga K, Wagner DA (1981)
Nitrate biosynthesis in man
Proc Natl Acad Science USA 78: 7764-7768

Green SJ, Scheller LF, Marletta MA et aI. (1994)
Nitric oxide: Cytokine regulation of nitric oxide in host resistance to intracellular pathogens
Immunol Lett 43 (1-2): 87-94

Greenspan HC (1993)
The role of reactive oxigen species, antioxidants and phytopharmaceuticals in human immunodeficiency virus activity
Medical Hypotheses 40: 85-92

Gregory SH, Wing EJ, Hoffman RA, Simmons RL (1993)
Reactive nitrogen intermediates suppress the primary immunologic response to Listeria
J Immunol 150: 2901-2909

Greider CW, Blackburn EH (1996)
Telomeres, telomerase and cancer
Sci Am 274 (2): 80-85

Grey O, Hamilton-Miller JMT (1977)
Trimethoprim-resistant bacteria: Cross-resistance patterns
Microbios 19: 45-54

Grieko MH (1989)
Immunoglobulins and hypersensitivity in human immunodeficiency (HIV) infection
J Allergy Clin Immunol 84: 1-4

Griffin DE, Ward BJ (1993)
Differential CD4 T cell activation in measles
J Infect Dis 168: 275-281

Grünfeld C, Feingold KR (1992)
Metabolic disturbances and wasting in the acquired immunodeficiency syndrome
N Engl J Med 327: 329-332

Gruetter CA, Barry BK, McNamara DB et al. (1979)

Relaxation of bovine coronary artery and activation of coronary guanylate cyclase by nitric oxide, nitroprusside and a carcinogenic nitrosamine
J Cycl Nucleotide Res 5: 211-224

Grupta S, Imam A, Licorish K (1986)
Serum ferritin in acquired immune deficiency syndrome
J Clin Lab Immunol 20: 11-13

Guilbert B, Fellous M, Avrameas S (1986)
HLA-DR-specific monoclonal antibodies crossreact with several self and non-self non-MHC molecules
Immunogenetics 24: 118-121

Guilbert B, Mahana W, Gilbert Met al. (1985)
Presence of natural autoantibodies in hyperimmunized mice
Immunol 56: 401-408

Guiliano F, Rampin O, Benoit G, Jardin A (1997)
The peripheral pharmacology of erection
Progr Krol 7: 24-33

Gupta E, Olopade OJ, Ratain MJ et al. (1995)
Pharmokinetics and pharmacodynamics of Olipraz as a chemopreventive agent
Clin Cancer Res 1: 1133-1138

Guslandi M (1998)
Nitric oxide and inflammatory bowel diseases (review)
Eur J Clin Invest 28: 904-907

Gysling E (1995)
Cotrimoxazol. Sulfamethoxazol / Trimethoprim
Pharma-Kritik 17 (21): 81-86

H

Haanen JBAG, de Waal Malefijt R, Res PCM et al. (1991)
Selection of a human T helper type-l like T cell subset by mycobacteria
J Exp Med 174: 583-592

Habib FM, Springall DR, Davies GJ et al. (1996)
Tumor necrosis factor and inducible nitric oxide synthase in dilated cardiopathy
The Lancet 347: 1151-1155

Hachtel W (1998)
Pflanzen wehren sich mit Stickoxid
Spektrum der Wissenschaft 11 (Nov.): 39-42

Hack V, Gross A, Kinscherf R et al. (1996)
Abnormal glutathione and sulfate levels after interleukin-6 treatment and in tumor-induced cachexia
FASEB J 10: 1219-1226

Hack V, Schmid O, Breitkreuz R (1997)
Cystine levels, cystine flux, and protein catabolism in cancer cachexia, HIV / SlV infection, and senescence
FASEB J 11: 84-92

Hadden JW (1977)
Cyclic nucleotides in lymphocyte proliferation and differentiation.
In: Hadden JW, Coffey RG, Spreafico F (ed.)
Immunopharmacology
Plenum Medical. New York and London

Hässig A, Hodler I. Liang W-X, Stampfli (1992 a)
Neuere nutritive und phytotherapeutische Behandlungsmöglichkeiten
Schweiz Zschr Ganzheits Med 4 (Suppl 1): 5

Hässig A (1992 b)
Umdenken bei AIDS
Schweiz Zschr Ganzheits Med 4: 171

Hässig A, Jolter P, Liang W-X, Stampfli K (1993)
Hinweise zur Prophylaxe von AIDS bei Hl—Virusträgern. Auf der Grundlage eines plausiblen pathogenesemodells dieser Erkrankung
Schweiz Zschr Ganzheitsmed 4: 188-192

Hässig A, Lang W-X, Stampfli K (1994 a)
Lässt sich die HIV-AIDS-Kontroverse lösen?
1st AIDS die Folge von andauernden übermäßigen Stressbelastungen des Organismus?
Schweiz Zschr Ganzheitsmed 6: 304-308

Hässig A, Liang W-X, Stampfli K (1994 b)
Azidothymidin (AZT) und AIDS. Offene Fragen beim Einsatz von AZT zur Prävention und Behandlung von AIDS
Schweiz Zschr Ganzheitsmed 5: 280-283

Hässig A, Kremer H, Liang W-X, Stampfli K (1996 a)
Offene Fragen zur Spezifizitat der Anti-HIV-Antikörper
Schweiz Zschr Ganzheitsmed 8 (6): 294-298

Hässig A, Kremer H, Liang W-X, Stampfli K (1996 b)
Parenteral übertragene Hepatitis-Viren und AIDS
Schweiz Zschr Ganzheitsmed 8 (7/8): 325-330

Hässig A, Liang W-X, Stampfli K, Kremer H (1996 c)
HIV—can you be more specific?
Continuum 4 (2): 10-12

Hässig A, Liang W-X, Stampfli K (1996 d)
Can we find a solution to the human immunodeficiency virus / aquired immune deficiency syndrome controversy? Is acquired immune deficiency syndrome the consequence of continuous excessive stressing of the body?
Medicai Hypotheses 46: 388-392

Hässig A, Kremer H, Liang W-X, Stampfli K (1997 a)
Hyperkatabole Krankheiten
Schweiz Zschr Ganzheitsmed 9 (2): 79-85

Hässig A, Kremer H, LiangW-X, Stampfli K (1997 b)
AIDS und Autoimmunität
Schweiz Zschr Ganzheitsmed 9 (5): 219-221

Hässig A, Liang W-X, Schwabi H, Stampfli K (1997 c)
Flavonoide und Tannine: Pflanzliche Antioxidanzien mit Vitamincharakter
Schweiz Zschr Ganzheits Medizin 4/97

Hässig A, Liang W-X, Stampfli K (1997 d)
Neuroendokrine Steuerung der Immunreaktionen
Die Blaue Liste Schweiz 1997: 22-24

Hässig A, Kremer H, Lanka S, Liang W—X, Stampfli K (1998 a)
15 jahre AIDS.
Eine kritische Stellungnahme zur Situation
Schweiz Zschr GanzheitsMed 10 (4), Mai 1998

Hässig A, Kremer H, Liang W-X, Stampfli K (1998 b)
The role of the Th-l to Th-2 shift of the cytokine profiles of CD4 helper cells in pathogenesis of autoimmune and hypercatabolic diseases
Medical Hypotheses 51: 59-63

Hässig A, Kremer H, Lanka S, LiangW-X, Stampfli K (1998 c)
15 years of AIDS
Continuum 5 (3): 32-37

Hässig A, Kremer H, LiangW-X, Stampfli K (1998 d)
Errors in views on pathogenesis, prevention and treatment of AIDS. A persistent glutathione deficiency is the key of the understanding of this disease
Continuum 5 (4): 28-29

Hässig A, Kremer H, Lanka S, Liang W-X, Stampfli K (1998 e)
AIDS und Hepatitis.
Beruht ein positiver Anti-HIV-Test auf stressinduzierten Aktivierungen von chronischen Hepatitiden?
Schweiz Zschr Ganzheits Med 10 (1), Febr 1998

Hässig A, Kremer H, Liang W-X et al. (1999)
Seriously seeking sulphur.
Sulphur fames oxygen and converts it from foe to friend. Its importance in the formation of proteoglycans and cysteine-containing antioxidants
Continuum 5 (5): 54-55

Haussinger O (1989)
Glutamine metabolism in the liver: Overview and current concepts
Metabolism 38: 14-20

Hagen-Mann K, Mann W (1994)
Quantitative PCR
In: Wink M, Werle H (1994)
PCR im medizinischen und biologischen Labor. GIT, Darmstadt

Haguenau F (1959)
Le cancer du sein chez la femme. Etude comparative au microscope optique
Bull Assoc Franc Etude du Cancer 46: 177-211

Haley TJ (1980)
Review of the physiological effects of amyl, butyl and isobutyl nitrites
Clin Toxicol 16: 317-329

Halliwell B, Chirico S (1993)
Lipid peroxidation: Its mechanism, measurement, and significance
Am J Clin Nutr 57 (Suppl): 715S-724S (discussion)

Halliwell B, Cross CE (1991)
Reactive oxygen species, antioxidants, and AIDS
Arch Intern Med 151: 29-31

Halliwell B, Gutteridge JMC (1990)
The antioxidants of human extracellular fluids
Arch Biochem Biophys 280: 1-8

Halliwell B, Gutteridge JMC (1992)
Free radicals in biology and medicine
Clarendon Press, Oxford. 3rd ed.

Hamlin WE (1968)
Pneumocystis carinii
JAMA 204: 173-177

Hammarqvist F, Wernerman J, Ali R et al. (1989)
Addition of glutamine to total parenteral nutrition after elective abdominal surgery spares free glutamin in muscle, counteracts the fall in muscle protein synthesis, and improves nitrogen balance. Ann Surg 209: 455-463

Hamouda O, Voß L, Siedler A, Iselborn M (1997)
AIDS / HIV 1997.
Bericht zur epidemiologischen Situation in der Bun-desrepublik Deutschland zum 31.12.1996
Robert-Koch-Institut, Berlin

Han J, Stamler JS, Li H-L, Griffith O (1995)
Inhibition of gamma-glutamyicysteine synthetase by S-nitrosylation
In: Biology of nitric oxide (IV) Stamler JS, Gross S, Moncada S, Higgs A (eds.) Portland Press, London

Harakeh S, Jariwalla RJ (1991)
Comparative study of the anti-HIV activities of ascorbate and thiol-containing agents in chronically HIV-Infected cells
Am J Clin Nutr 54: 1231 S—1235 S

Harrison A, Skidmore SJ (1990)
Neopterin and Beta-2 Microglobulin levels in asymptomatic HIV-infection. The predictive value of combining markers
J Med Vir 32: 128

Harver T, Harrer E, Kalams SA et al. (1996)
Strong cytotoxic T cell and weak neutralizing antibody responses in a subset of persons with stable nonprogressing HIV type 1 infection
AIDS Res Human Retroviruses 12: 585-592

Harwood AR, Osoba O, Hofstader SL et al. (1979)
Kaposi's sarcoma in recipients of renal transplants
Am J Med 67: 759-765

Harwood AR, Osoba O, Hofstader SL et al. (1984)
Kaposi's sarcoma in renal transplantant patients
In: Friedman-Kien AE, Laubenstein LJ (ed.), op. cit.

Hausladen A, Privalle CT, Keng T et al. (1996)
Nitrosative Stress: Activation of the transcription factor OxyR
Cell 86: 719-729

Haverkos HW, Curran JW (1982)
The current outbreak of Kaposi's sarcoma and opportunistic infections
CA Bulletin of Cancer Progress 32: 330-339

Haverkos HW, Dougherty JA (ed.) (1988)
Health Hazards of Nitrite Inhalants
National Institute on Drug Abuse, Rockville U.S.

Haverkos HW, Friedman-Kien AE, Drotman P et al. (1990)
The changing incidence of Kaposi's sarcoma among patients with AIDS
J Am Acad Dermatol 22: 1250 f.

Hayakawa M, Ogawa T, Sugiyama S et al. (1991)
Massive conversion of guanosine to 8-hydroxyguanosine in mouse liver mitochondrial DNA by administration of azidothymidine
Bichem Biophys Res Commun 176: 87-93

Haynes BE, Fauci AS (1977)
Activation of human B lymphocytes. III. Concanavalin A—induced generation of suppressor cells of

the plaque-forming cell response of normal human B lymphocytes
J Immunol 118: 2281-2287

Haynes BE, Fauci AS (1978)
The differential effect of in vivo hydrocortisone on the kinetics of subpopulations of human peripheral blood thymus-derived lymphocytes
J Clin lnvest 61: 703-707

Hedht SS (1995)
Chemoprevention by isothiocyanates
J CeIl Biochem 22 (S): 195-209

Heme H (1997)
Lehrbuch der biologischen Medizin. Grundregulation und extrazellulare und Systematik
Hippokrates Verlag, Stuttgart, 2. Aufl. Matrix-Grundlagen

Heinonen PK, Kivula T, Pystynen P (1987)
Decreased serum level of dehydroepiandrosterone sulfate in postmenopausal women with ovarian cancer
GynecoI Obstetric Invest 23 (4): 271-274

Helbert M, Fletcher T, Peddle B et al. (1988)
Zidovudine-associated myopathy
Lancet ii: 689-690

Hengel RL. Watts NB, Lennox JL (1997)
Benign symmetric lipomatosis associated with protease inhibitors
Lancet 350: 1596

Hennebold JD, Daynes RA (1994)
Regulation of macrophage dehydroepiandrosterone sulfat metabolism by inflammatory cytokins
Endocrinology 135: 67

Hennings H, Glick AB, Greenhalgh DA et al. (1993)
Critical aspects of initiation, promotion and progression in multistage epidermal carcinogenesis
Proc Soc Exp Biol Med 202: 1-8

Henry J. Kaiser Family Foundation and HIV/AIDS Treatment Information Service (1997)
Recommendations for antiretroviral therapy
Net: www.cdcnac.org

Henry Y, Lepoivre M, Drapier JC (1993)
EPR characterisation of molecular targets for NO in mammalian cells and organelles
FASEB J 7:1124-1134

Herbert V (1992)
Everybody should be tested for iron disorders
J Am Diet Assoc 92: 1502-1510

Herbert V (1994)
The antioxidant supplement myth
Am J Clin Nutr 60: 157-158

Hernandez-Pando R, Rook GA (1994)
The role of TNF-alpha in T-cell mediated inflammation depends on the Th1/Th2 cytokine balance
Immunology 82: 591-595

Herron DC, Ahank RC (1980)
Methylated purines in human liver DNA after probable dimethylamine poisoning
Cancer Res 40: 3116-3117

Herschman HR (1996) Prostaglandin synthase 2
Biochem Biophys Acta 1299: 125-140

Hersh EM, Reubin JM, Bogerd H et al. (1983)
Effect of the recreational agent isobutyl nitrite in human peripheral blood lymphocytes and in vitro interferon production
Cancer Res 43: 1365-1371

Hertog GL, Hollman PCH, Katan MB (1992)
Content of potentially anticancerogenic flavonoids of 28 vegetables and 9 fruits commonly consumed in the Netherlands
J Agric Food Chem 40: 2379-2383

Herzenberg LA, De Rosa SC, Dubos JG et al. (1997) glutathione deficiency is associated with impaired survival in HIV disease
Proc Natl Acad Sci USA 94: 1967-1972

Heurtier AH, Boitard C (1997)
T-cell regulation in murine and human autoimmune diabetes: The role of TH1 and TH2 cells
Diabetes Metabol 23 (5): 377-385

Heymsfield SB, Mc Manus CB (1985)
Tissue components of weight loss in cancer patients
Cancer 55: 238-249

Hibbs JBJ, Taintor RR, Vavrin Z (1987)
Macrophage cytotoxicity: Role for L-arginine deiminase and imino nitrogen oxidation to nitrite
Science 235: 473-476

Hibbs JB, Westenfelder C, Taintor R et al. (1992)
Evidence for cytokine-inducible nitric oxide synthesis from L-arginine in patients receiving interleukin-2 therapy
J Clin Invest 89: 867-877

Higashi Y, Hawcroft G, Hull MA (2000)
The effect of non-steroidal anti-inflammatory drugs on human colorectal cancer cells: Evidence of different mechanisms of action
Europ J Cancer 36 (5): 664-674

Hilkens CMU, Vermeulen H, van Neerven RJJ et al. (1995)
Differential modulation of T helper type 1 (Th1) and T helper type 2 (Th2) cytokine secretion by prostaglandin E2 critically depends on interleukin-2
Eur J Immunol 25: 59-63

Hill RB, Rowlands DT, Riflkind D (1964)
Infectious pulmonary disease in patients receiving immunosuppressive therapy for organ transplantation
NEJM 271:1021-1025

Hilton CW, Harrington PT, Prasad C, Svec F (1988)
Adrenal insufficiency in the acquired immunodeficiency syndrome
South Med J 81: 1493-1495

Hirvonen A (1999)
Polymorphisms of xenobiotic-metabolizing enzymes and susceptibility to cancer
Environ Health Perspect 107: S37-S47

Hitchings GH (1989)
Nobel lecture in Physiology or Medicine—1988 Selective inhibitors of dihydrofolate reductase
In Vitro Cellular Development Biol 25 (4): 303-310

Ho DD (1995 b)
Time to hit HIV, early and hard
NEJM 333: 450-451

Ho DD (2000)
New strategies are necessary to fight HIV infection
Report on HIV/AIDS research results
Speech during World AIDS Congress in Durban, South Africa 09-14.07.2000
Ärztezeitung 14.07.2000

Ho DD, Neumann AU, Perelson AS et al. (1995 a)
Rapid turmover of plasma virons and CD4 lymphocytes in HIV-1 infection
Nature 373: 123-126

Hobbs GA, Keilbaugh SA, Rief PM, Simpson MV (1995)
Cellular targets of 3-azido-3-deoxythimidine: An early (non-delayed) effect on oxidative phosphorylation
Biochem Pharmacol 50: 381-390

Hodgkinson N (1996)
AIDS: The failure of contemporary science
How a virus that never was deceived the world
Fourth Estate, London

Hoel DG, Davis DL, Miller AB et al. (1992)
Trends in cancer mortality in 15 industrialized countries. 1969-1986
J Natl Cancer Inst 84: 313-320

Hogervorst E, Jurriaans S, Wolf F et al. (1995)
Predictors for non-and slow progression in human immunodeficiency virus (HIV) type 1 infection: Low viral RNA copy numbers in serum and maintenance of HIV-1 p24-specific but not V3-specific antibody levels
J Infect Dis 171: 811-821

Holland SM, Eisenstein EM, Kuhns DB et al. (1994)
Treatment of refractory non-tuberculous mycobacterial infection with interferon gamma
N Engl J Med 330: 1348-1355

Holt PG, Macaubas C, Cooper D et al. (1997)
Th-1 / Th-2 switch regulation in immune responses to inhaled antigens.
Role of dentritic cells in the aetiology of allergic respiratory disease
Adv Exp Med Biol 417: 301-306

Hong RW, Rounds JD, Helton WS et al. (1992)
Glutamine preserves liver glutathione after lethal hepatic injury
Ann Surg 215: 114-118

Hoofman RA, Langrehr JM, Billiar TR et al. (1990)
Alloantigen-induced activation of rat splenocytes is regulated by the oxidative metabolism of L-arginine
J Immunol 145: 2220-2226

Hoover DR, Rinaldo C, He Y et al. (1995)
Long-term survival without clinical AIDS after CD4+ cell counts fall below 200x1O6 /L
AIDS 9: 145-152

Horrobin DF (1990)
Essential fatty acids, lipid peroxidation, and cancer
In: Omega 6 essential fatty acids. Pathophysiology and roles in clinical medicine. pp.351-377 Alan R. Liss Inc., New York

Hortin GL, Landt M, Pokiderly WG (1994)
Changes in plasma amino acid concentrations in response to HIV-infection
Clin Chem 40: 785-789

Horwitz JP, Chua J, Noel M (1964)
Nucleosides.
V. The monomesylates of 1—(2,—deoxy-beta-D-Iyxofuranosyl) thymidine
J Org Chem 29: 2076

Hoshaw RA, Schwartz RA (1980)
Kaposi's sarcoma after immunosuppressive therapy with prednisone
Arch Dermatol 116: 1280-1282

Houdyk APJ, Rijnsburger ER, Jansen J et al. (1998)
Randomized trial of glutamine-enriched enteral nutrition. on infectious morbidity in patients with multiple trauma
Lancet 352: 772

Howarth PH (1998)
Is allergy increasing?—Early life influences
Clin Exp Allergy 28 SuppI 6: 2-7

Huang M, Stolina M, Sharma S et al. (1998)
Non-small cell lung cancer cyclooxygenase-2-dependent regulation of cytokine balance in lymphocytes and macrophages: Up-regulation of interleukin 10 and down-regulation of interleukin 12 production
Cancer Res 58 (6): 1208-1216
Hughes WT, Feldman S, Sanyal SK (1975)

Treatment of pneumocystis carinii pneumonitis with trimethoprim-sufamethoxazole
Can-Med J 112 (Suppl): 47-50

Hurd ER (1977)
Drugs affecting the immune response
In: Hollborrow EG, Reeves WG (ed.) Immunity in Medicine
Academic Press, London
Husstedt JW (Hrsg.) (1998)

HIV—und AIDS.
Fachspezifische Diagnostik und Therapie
[Specialized diagnostics and therapy]
Springer Verlag, Berlin-Heidelberg-New York

Huzzell JGR (1982)
Monoclonal Hybridoma Antibodies: Techniques and Application
CRC Press, New York

I

Ignarro LJ (1992)
Pharmacological, biochemical and chemical evidence that EDRF is NO or a labile nitroso precursor
In: Endothelial regulation of vascular tone
Ryan US, Rubanyi GM (ed.) pp. 37-49
Marcel Dekker Inc., New York

Ignarro LJ (2000)
El óxido nitrico permite inhibir el crecimiento de algunos tumores
[Nitric oxide inhibits the growth of some tumors]
Talk given at Navarra University, May 10th, 2000
Net: www.diariomedico.com/oncologia/n100500.html

Ignarro LJ, Buga GM, Wood KS et al. (1987)
Endothelium-derived relaxing factor produced and released from artery and vein is nitric oxide
Proc Natl Acad Sci (USA) 84: 9265-9269

Ignarro LJ, Lippton H, Edwards JC et al. (1981)
Mechanism of vascular smooth muscle relaxation by organic nitrates, nitrites, nitroprusside and nitric oxide: Evidence for the involvement of S-nitrosothiols as active intermediates
J Pharmacal Experiment Therapeutics 218: 739-749

Imoberdorf R (1997)
Immuno-nutrition: Designer diets in cancer
Supportive Care in Cancer 5 (5): 381-386

Isreal-Biet D, Labrousse F, Tourani J-M et al. (1992)
Elevation of IgE in HIV-infected subjects, a marker of poor prognosis
J Allergy Clin Immunol 89: 68-75

Isrealstarn S, Lambert S, Oki G (1978)
Poppers, a new recreational drug craze
Can J Psychiatry 23: 493-495

Ivady G, Paldy L (1958)
Ein neues Behandlungsverfahren der interstitiellen plasmazelligen Pneumonie Frühgeborener mit fünfwertigen Stilbium und aromatischen Diamidinen
[A new treatment procedure of the interstitial plasma-cellular pneumonia of premature infants with pentavalent Stilbium and aromatic Diamidinen]
MIschr Kinderheilk 106: 10-14

Ivady G, Paldy L, Koltay M et al. (1967)
Pneumocystis carinii pneumonia
Lancet 1: 616-617

J

Jackson CD (1979)
Volatile nitrite
NTP working paper
Office of Scientific Intelligence, National Center for Toxicological Research, pp. 22, U.S.

Jackson MA, Stack HF, Waters MD (1993)
The genetic toxicology of putative nongenotoxic carcinogens
Mut Res 296: 241-277

Jaffe HW, Choi K, Thomas PA et al. (1983)
National case-control study of Kaposi's sarcoma and pneumocystis carinii pneumonia in homosexual men: Part I. Epidemiologic results
Ann Intern Med 99: 145-151

James SL (1995)
Role of nitric oxide in parasitic infections
Microbiol Rev 59 (4): 533-547

Janssen GME, van Kranenburg G, Geurten P (1988)
Gender difference in decline of urea concentration during the first 2-3 days postmarathon
Can J Sport Sci 13: 18P

Jarstrand C, Akerlund B, Lindeke B (1990) glutathione and HIV infection (Letter)
Lancet i: 235

Javier JJ, Fodyce—Baum MK (1990)
Antioxidant micronutrients and immune function in HIV infection
FASEB Proc 4: A940

Jick H, Derby LE (1995)
A large population—based follow-up study of trimethoprim-sulfamethoxazole, trimethoprim and cephalexin for uncommon serious drug toxicity
Pharmacotherapy 15: 428-432

Jochum M, Gippner-Steppert C, Machheidt Wet al. (1994)
The role of phagocyte proteinases and proteinase inhibitors in multiple organ-failure
Am J Respir Grit Care Med 150 (Suppl): 123-130

Johansson KU, Carlberg M (1995)
NO-Synthase: What can research on vertebrates add to what is already known?
Adv Neuroimmunol 5 (4): 431-442

Johns DR (1996)
The other human genome: Mitochondrial DNA and disease. Mutations in mitochondrial genes are increasingly implicated in human disease
Nature medicine 2: 1065-1068

Johnson C (1996)
Viral load and the PCR—why they can't be used to prove HIV infection
Continuum 4 (4): 32-37

Johnston LD, Malley PM, Bachman JG et al. (1986)
Drug abuse among American High School students, College students and other young adults
National trend through 1985
National Institute on Drug Abuse, Rockville U.S.

Jones MK, Wang H, Peskar BM et al (1999)
Inhibition of angiogenesis by nonsteroidal anti-inflammatory drugs: insights into mechanisms and implications for cancer growth and ulcer healing
Nature Medicine 5 (12): 1418-1423

Jun C-D, Choi B-M, Kim H-M, Chung H-T (1995)
Involvement of protein kinase C during taxol-induced activation of murine peritoneal macrophages
J Immunol 154: 6541-6547

K

Kahan D (1984)
Cyclosporine A: Biological activity and clinical applications
Grune and Stratton Inc., New York

Kalow W (1993)
Pharmagenetics: Its biologic roots and the medical challenge
Clin Pharmacol Ther 54: 235-241

Kalyanaraman VS, Sarngadharan MG, Bunn DA et al. (1981 b)
Antibodies in human sera reactive against an internal structural protein (p24) of human T-cell lymphoma virus
Nature 294: 271-273

Kalyanaraman VS, Sarngadharan MG, Poiesz B et al. (1981 a)
Immunological properties of a type C retrovirus isolated from cultured human T-Iymphoma cells and comparison to other mammalian retroviruses
J Virol 38: 906-915

Kayanaraman VS, Sarngadharan MG, Robert-Guroff et al. (1982)
A new subtype of human T-cell leukemia virus (HTLV-II) associated with a T-cell variant of hairy cell leukemia
Science 218: 571-573

Kaposi M (1872)
Idiopathisches multiples Pigmentsarkom der Haut
Arch Dermatol Syphil 4: 265-272

Karp CL, EI-Safi SH, Wym TA et al. (1993)
In vivo cytokine profiles in patients with kalaazar
J Clin Invest 91: 1644-1648

Karupiah G (1998)
Type 1 and type 2 cytokines in antiviral defense
Vet Immunol Immunopathol 63 (1-2): 105-109

Kasakura S (1998)
A role for T helper type 1 and type 2 cytokines in the pathogenesis of various human diseases
Rinsho Byori 46 (9): 915-921

Kashala O, Marlink R, Ilunga M et al. (1994)
Infection with human immunodeficiency virus type-l (HIV-1) and human T celllymphotropic viruses among leprosy patients and contacts: Correlation between HIV-1 cross-reactivity and antibodies to lipoarabinomannan

J Infect Dis 169: 296-304
Katamura K, Shintaku, Yamauchi Y et al. (1995) Prostaglandin E2 at priming of naive CD4+ T cells inhibits acquisition of ability to produce IFN-gamma and IL-2, but not IL-4 and IL-5
J Immunol 155: 4604-4612

Keilin D (1933)
Cytochrome and intracellular respiratory enzymes
Ergebn Enzymforsch 2: 239-271

Kerwin JF, Lancaster JR, Feldman PL (1995)
Nitric oxide: A new paradigm for second messengers
J Med Chem 38: 4343-4362

Kestens L, Melbye M, Biggar RJ et al. (1985)
Endemic African Kaposi's Sarcoma is not associated with immunodeficiency
Int J Cancer 36: 49-54

Ketteler M, Cetto C, Kirdorf M et al. (1998)
Nitric oxide in sepsis-syndrome: Potential treatment of septic shock by nitric oxide synthase antagonists
Kidney Int Suppl 64: S 27-30

Keusch GT, Farthing MJG (1986)
Nutrition and infection
Ann Rev Nutrition 6: 131-154

Khatsenko O (1998)
Interactions between nitric oxide and cytochrom P-450 in the liver
Biochemistry (Moscow) 63: 833-839

Kieffer F (1993)
Wie Eisen und andere Spurenelemente die menschliche Gesundheit beeinflussen
[How iron and other trace elements affect human health]
Mitt. Gebiete Lebensm Hyg: 84-148

Kim I, Williamson DF, Byers T, Koplan JP (1993)
Vitamin und mineral supplement use and mortality in a US cohort
Am J Public Health 83: 546-550

Kim Y-M, Bergonia H, Lancaster JR (1995)
Nitrogen oxide-induced autoprotection in isolated rat hepatocytes
FEBS Lett 374: 228-232

King CL, Hakimi MT, Shata MT, Medhat A (1995)
IL-12 regulation of parasite antigen-driven IgE production in human helminth infections
J Immunol 155: 454-461

King CL, Otteson EA, Nutman TB (1990)
Cytokine regulation of antigen-driven immunoglobulin production in filarial parasite infection in humans
J Clin Invest 85: 1810-1815

Kingsley LA, Kaslow R, Rinaldo CR et al. (1987)
Risk factors for seroconversion to human immunodeficiency virus among male homosexuals
Lancet i: 345-348

Kinlen II (1982)
Immunosuppressive therapy and cancer
Cancer Surv 1: 565

Kinscherf R, Fischbach T, Mihm S et al. (1994)
Effect of glutathione depletion and oral N-acetyl-cysteine treatment on CD4 and CD8 cells
FASEB J 8: 448-451

Kinscharf R, Hack V, Fischbach T et al. (1996)
Low plasma glutamine in combination with glutamate levels indicate risk for loss of body cell mass in healthy individuals: The effect of N—acetylcysteine
J Mol Med 74: 393-400

Kion TA, Hoffman GW (1991)
Anti-HIV—and anti-MHC antibodies in alloimmune and autoimmune mice
Science 253: 1138-1140

Kirk SJ, Regan MC, Barbul A (1990)
Cloned murine T-Iymphocytes synthesize a molecule with the biological characteristics of nitric oxide
Biochem Biophys Res Commun 173: 660-665

Kirkeboen KA, Strand OA (1999)
The role of nitric oxide in sepsis—an overview
Acta Anaesthesol Scand 43 (3): 275-288

Klatzmann D, Barré-Sinoussi F, Nugeyre MT (1984)
Selective tropism of lymphadenopathy associated virus (LAV) for helper-inducer T-Iymphocytes
Science 225: 59-63

Klatzmann D, Montagnier L (1986)
Approaches to AIDS-therapy
Nature 319: 10-11

Klebic T, Kinter A, Poli G et al. (1991)
Suppression of HIV expression in chronically infected monocytes by glutathione, glutathione-esters and N-acetylcysteine
Proc Natl Acad Sci USA 88: 986-990

Klingenstein RJ, Sawarese AM, Dienstag JL et al. (1981)
Immunoregulatory T cell subsets in acute and chronic hepatitis
Hepatology 1: 523-527

Klopstock T, Naumann M, Schalke B et al. (1994)
Multiple symmetric lipomatosis: Abnormalities in complex IV and multiple deletions in mitochondrial DNA
Neurology 44: 862-866

Klurfeid DM (1993)
Nutrition and immunology
Plenum Press, New York

Knowles RG, Moncada S (1994)
Nitric oxide synthases in mammals
Biochem J 298: 249-258

Knox A (1997)
AIDS trial terminated
The Boston Globe, 25th February 1997

Koch ER (1990)
Boses Blut. Die Geschichte eines Medizinskandals
[Bad blood. The history of a medicine scandal]
Hoffmann und Campe, Hamburg

KohnIein C, Fiala C (2000)
AIDS in Africa—the way forward
Expert meeting by invitation of South African president Mbeki
Report on the first meeting (May 6-7) in Pretoria. May 22, 2000

Dr. Claus Köhnlein—eMail: kiel-koehnlein-kiel@t-online.de
Dr. Christian Fiala, Vienna—eMail: christian.fiala@aon.at

Kohlstädt S (2000)
Immer mehr Krebsviren [Even more cancer viruses]
Kongressbericht über "Viren als Ursache von Tumoren",
Deutsches Krebsforschungszentrum Heidelberg
Frankfurter Allgemeine Zeitung 114: N1-N2

Kolb H, Kolb-Bachofen V (1998)
Nitric oxide in autoimmune disease: cytotoxic or regulatory mediator
Immunol Today 19: 556-561

Kosaka T, Miyata A, Ihara Y et al. (1994)
Characterization of the human gene (PTGS2) encoding prostaglandin endoperoxide synthase 2
Eur J Biochem 221: 889-897

Kotler DB Tierney AR, Wang J, Pierson RN (1989)
Magnitude of body cell mass depletion and the timing of death from wasting in AIDS
Am J Clin Nutr 50: 444-450

Kotler DB Tierney AR, Culpepper-Morgan JA et al. (1990)
Effect of home total parenteral nutrition on body composition in patient with acquired immunodeficiency syndrome
JPEN 14: 454-460

Kotler DB Tierney AR, Ferraro R et al. (1991)
Enteral alimentation and repletion of body cell mass in malnourished patients with aquired immunodeficiency syndrome
Am J Cin Nutr 53: 149-155

Kovacs JA (1993)
Diagnosis, treatment, and prevention of Pneumocystis carinii pneumonia in HIV-infected patients
AIDS Updates 6: 1-13

Krebs HA (1972)
The Pasteur effect and the reactions between respiration and fermentation
Essays Biochem 8: 1-34

Kremer H (1990)
Wie seriös ist die Seuchenmedizin? AIDS haben und AIDS machen raum&zeit 47: 12-19

Kremer H (1994)
Weltmythos AIDS emotion 11: 134-147

Kremer H (1996 a)
AIDS—Ein von Arzten forciertes Todessyndrom? raum&zeit 86: 23-32 (Sonerdruck Ehlers Verlag, Wolfratshausen)

Kremer H, Lanka S (1996 b)
Vorsicht AIDS-Medizin: Lebensgefahr! raum&zeit 79: 81-90

Kremer H (1996 c)
Acquired Iatrogenic Death Syndrome (AIDS)
Continuum 4 (4): 8-13

Kremer H (1996 d)
Überlegungen für eine experimentelle Studie zur Wirkung von Folsäure-Inhibitoren auf die Ultrastruktur und Funktion von Mitochondrien in humanen
Lymphozyten und in mikrobiellen Opportunisten des Menschen Unveröffentlichtes Forschungskonzept

Kremer H (1997 a)
Has mankind get out on a path of micro-ecological selfdestruction
Continuum 4 (6):10-11

Kremer H (1997 b)
From abiosis to symbiosis: The role of natural protective substances in chronic diseases, with special emphasis on mitochondria
In: Chronic Disease Processes: Pathogenesis and Treatment.
The Perspective of Phytopharmacology of Multiherbal Compounds International Interdisciplinary Symposium.
University of Roskilde, Denmark, September 28th and 29th, 1997

Kremer H (1998 a)
Has Dr. Gallo manipulated the AIDS-Test in order?
Continuum 5 (4): 10-14

Kremer H (1998 b)
A.E.D.S., not AIDS
Abstract on the XII World AIDS Congress. Geneva 1998

Kremer H (1998 c)
Wird manipuliertes Eiweiß-Gemisch als "AIDS-Test" verkauft?
Das Milliardengeschaft mit der Todesangst—vor einem nicht vorhandenen Virus raum&zeit 95: 41-51

Kremer H (1998 d)
Krebs des Ratsels Lösung?
Weshalb die bioenergetische Krebsforschung aussichtsreicher ist als die Gen-Forschung raum&zeit 94 (Juli/August): 32-36

Kremer H (1999)
Darwins Irrtum und die Krebsmedizin.
Erkenntnisse der Evolutionsbiologie und Bioenergetik eröffnen neue Behandungschancen raum&zeit 99: 5-17

Kremer H (2000 a)
Cancer, SIDA y la silenciosa revolucion de la investigacion sobre la immunidad
Curso de formacion en conocimiento de la vida
Dias 13 y 14 de mayo 2000, Plural-21-Associación para el cuidado de la vida en un planeta vivo
Tel.: +34/934501300, Fax: +34/934564825

Kremer H (2000 b)
Answers to questions on the action of AZT of 23.02.2000, and the Questions on HIV/AIDS of 06./07.05.2000 from the South African health minister, Mrs. Dr. Tshabalala Tshabalala-Msimang, and/or President Mbeki. July 15, 2000
Net: www.AIDS-info.net—www.virusmyth.com

Kremer (2000 c)
Answers to questions, particularly to the cause, prevention and treatment of AIDS, submitted by President the Mbeki to the Specialist Conference on May 6-7, 2000 in Pretoria, regarding the complex problem of HIV/AIDS in developing countries. July 15, 2000
Net: www.AIDS-info.net—www.virusmyth.com

Krenger W, Ferrara JL (1996)
Graft-versus-host disease and the Th1 / Th2 paradigm
Immunol Res 15: 50-73

Krentz AJ, Koster FT, Crist DM et al. (1993)
Anthropometric, metabolic and immunological effects of recombinant human growth factor in AIDS and AIDS-related complex
J Acquir Immune Def Syndr 6: 245-253

Krikorian GG, Anderson JL, Bieber CP et al. (1978)
Malignant neoplasias following cardiac transplantation
JAMA 240: 639-643

Kroemer G, Zamzami N, Susin SA (1997)
Mitochondrial control of apoptosis
Immunol Today 18: 44-51

Kröncke K-D, Fehsel K, Kolb-Bachofen V (1995)
Inducible nitric oxide synthase and its product nitric oxide, a small molecule witb complex biological activities
Biol Chemistry Hoppe-Seyler 376: 327-343

Krown SE, Niedziviecki D, Bhalla RB et al. (1991)
Relationship and prognostic value of endogenous interferon a, ß2-microglobulin, and neopterin serum levels in patients with Kaposi's sarcoma and AIDS
J Acquir Imm Defic Syndr 4: 871-880

Kucera I, Dadak V (1983)
The effect of uncoupler on the distribution of the electron flow between the oxygen and nitrite in the cells of Paracoccus denitrificans
Biochem Biophys Res commun 117: 252

Kulkarni SS, Bhateley DC, Zander AR et al. (1984)
Functional impairment of T-lymphocytes in mouse radiation chimeras by a nucleotide-free diet
Exp Hematol 12: 694-699
Kulkarni AD, Fanslow WC, Drath DB et al. (1986)
Influence of dietary nucleotide restriction on bacterial sepsis and phagocytic cell function in mice
Arch Surg 121: 169-172

Kulkarni AD, Fanslow WC, Rudolph FB et al. (1987)
Modulation of delayed hypersensitivity in mice by dietary nucleotide restriction
Transplantation 44: 847-849

Kumar RM, Hughes PF, Khurranna A (1994)
Zidovudine use in pregnancy: A report of 104 cases and the occurrence of birth defects
J Acquired Immunodeficiency Syndromes 7: 1034-1039

Kune GA (2000)
Colorectal cancer chemoprevention: Aspirin, other NSAID and COX-2 inhibitors
Austral New Zealand J Surg 70 (6): 452-455

Kunz D, Walker G, Eberhardt W, Pfeilschifter J (1996)
Molecular mechanism of dexamethason inhibition of nitric oxide synthase expression in interleukin-1-stimulated mesangial cells: Evidence for the involvement of transcriptional and posttranscriptional regulation
Proceedings of the National Academy of Science USA 93: 255-259

Kwon OJ (1997)
The role of nitric oxide in the immune response of tuberculosis
J Kor Med Sci 12: 481-487

L

L'age-Stehr J, Helm EB (1994)
AIDS und die Vorstadien. Ein Leitfaden für Praxis und Klinik
Springer-Verlag, Berlin-Heidelberg-New York

Lacey RW, Hawkey PM, Devaraj SK et al. (1985)
Co-trimoxazole toxicity
Br Med J 291: 48.1

Lafaille JJ (1998)
The role of helper T cell subsets in autoimmune disease
Cytokine Growth Factor Rev 9 (2): 139-151

Lambie DG, Johnson RH (1985)
Drugs and folate metabolism
Drugs 30: 145-155

Lancaster JR (1992)
Nitric Oxide in cells
Am Scientist 80: 248-259

Lander HM, agister JS, Pearce SF et al. (1995)
Nitric oxide-stimulated guanosine nuclectide exchange on p21ras
J Biol Chem 270: 7017-7020

Landsteiner K, Chase MW (1942)
Experiments on transfer of cutaneous sensitivity to simple chemical components
Proc Soc Exp Biol Med 49: 688-692

Lang S (1998)
Challenges.
The Gallo Case, pp. 361-600.
The Case of HIV and AIDS, pp. 601-714.
Springer Verlag, New York

Lange WR, Dax EM, Haertzen CA et al. (1988)
Nitrite Inhalants: Contemporary patterns of Abuse
In: Haverkos HW, Dougherty JA (ed.) (1988)
Health Hazards of Nitrite Inhalants
National Institute on Drug Abuse, Rockville U.S.

Langton C (1990)
Computation on the Edge of Chaos: Phase transition and emergent computation
Physics 42 D: 12-17

Lanka S (1994)
Fehldiagnose AIDS? Bisher konnte das AIDS-Virus nicht isoliert werden
Wechselwirkung 12 (Dez): 48-53

Lanka S (1995)
HIV—Realitat oder Artefakt?
[HIV—Reality or Artifact?]
raum&zeit 77: 17-26
(Sonerdruck Ehlers Verlag, Wolfratshausen)

Lanka S (1997)
No viral identification—no cloning as proof of isolation
Continuum 4 (5): 31-33

Larhoven L (1990)
A review of the discussion about AZT: Medication or Genocide?
Dossier Alternative AIDS Research 1987-1990
Stichting voor Alternatief AIDS Onderzoek

Larhoven L (1993)
A review of the discussion about the cause of AIDS.
Dossier HIV 1.0 1987-1990
Stichting voor Alternatief AIDS Onderzoek
Net: www.virusmyth.com (front news) (actual information) eMail: info@virusmyth.com
SVA A.O. PO. Box 5241, 5603 BC Eindhoven, The Netherlands

Lascroix C, Said G (1992)
Muscle siderosis in AIDS: a marker for macrophages dysfunction?
J Neurol 239: 4

Laurent-Crawford AG, Krust B, Muller S et al. (1991)
The cytopathic effect of HIV is associated with apoptosis
Virol 185: 829-839

Lauritsen J, Wilson H (1986)
Death rush: poppers and AIDS
Pagan Press, New York

Lauritsen J (1987)
AZT on trial: Did the FDA rush to judgment—and thereby further endanger the lives of thousands of people?
New York Native 19 Oct 1987, 13-17

Lauritsen J (1988 a)
AZT: Iatrogenic genocide
New York Native 28 March 1988,13-17

Lauritsen J (1988 b)
AZT disinformation
New York Native 6 June 1988, 17-18

Lauritsen J (1989 a)
The AZT front: Part one
New York Native 2 Jan 1989, 16-18

Lauritsen J (1989 b)
The AZT front: Part two
New York Native 16 Jan 1989,16-19

Lauritsen J (1989 c)
AZT causes cancer: Burroughs Wellcome issues advisory
New York Native 18 Dec 1989,14-15

Lauritsen J (1990 a)
Poison by Prescription: The AZT Story
Asklepios, New York

Lauritsen J (1990 b)
More science by press conference: FDA committee recommends AZT for healthy people
New York Native 12 Feb 1990, 10

Lauritsen J (1990 c)
A "state of the art" AZT conference, VA doctor finds no benefit from AZT treatment
New York Native 19 March 1990, 17-20

Lauritsen J (1990 d)
AZT watch: New research does not prove efficacy
New York Native 30 April 1990, 17-19

Lauritsen J (1993)
The AIDS War. Propaganda, Profiteering and Genocide from the Medical Industrial Complex
Asklepios, New York

Lauritsen J (1997)
Protease inhibitors in Provincetown
Continuum 4 (5): 8-10

Lavallee B, Provost PR, Roy R et al. (1996)
Dehydroepiandrosterone-fatty acid esters in human plasma formation, transport and delivery to steroid target tissues
J Endocrinol 150 Suppl: S119-124

Lawson DH, Richmond A, Nixon DW et al. (1982)
Metabolic approaches to cancer cachexia
Annu Rev Nutr 2: 277-301

Layne SP, Merges MJ, Dembo M et al. (1992)
Facts underlying sponaneous inactivation and susceptibility

to neutralization of human immunodeficiency virus
Virol 189: 695-714

Le Bail JC, Allen K, Nicolas JC, Habrioux G (1998)
Dehydroepiandrosterone sulfate estrogenic action at its physiological plasma concentration in human,breast cancer cell lines
Anticancer Res 18 (3A): 1683-1688

Le Quoc K, Le Quoc D (1982)
Control of mitochondrial inner membrane permeability by sulfhydryl group
Arch Biochem Biophys 216: 639-651

Lehrer RI (1970)
Defective candidacidal activity of leucocytes from patients with systemic candidiasis
Clin Res 18: 443-449

Lehrer RI, Cline MJ (1971 a)
Leucocyte candidacidal activity and resistance to systemic candidiasis in patients with cancer
Cancer 27: 1211-1218

Lehrer RI (1971 b)
Inhibition by sulfonamides of the candidacidal activity of human neutrophils
J Clin Invest 50: 2498-2505

Leist M, Nicotera P (1998)
Apotosis, exitotoxicity and neuropathology
Exp Cell Res 115: 239: 183-201

Leite-de-Moraes MC, DyM (1997)
Natural killer T cells: A potent cytokine-producing cell population
Eur Cytokine Netw 8 (3): 229-237

Lenton TM (1998)
Gaia and natural selection
Nature 394: 439-447

Levine AS (1982)
The epidemic of acquired Immune Dysfunction in homosexual men and its sequelae-opportunistic infections, Karposi's sarcoma and other malignancies: An update and interpretation
Cancer treatment Reports 66: 1391

Levine AS (1984)
Viruses, immune dysregulation, and Oncogenesis: Inferences Regarding the Cause and Evolution of AIDS
In: Friedman-Kien AE, Laubenstein U (1984), a-a.O.

Levine PH (1985)
The acquired immunodeficiency syndrome in persons with hemophilia
Ann Intern Med 103: 723-726

Lewis W, Dalakas MC (1995)
Mitochondrial toxicity of antiviral drugs
Nature Medicine 1: 417-422

Liang W-X, Stampfli K, Hässig A (1992)
Therapeutische Wirkungsmechanismen Komplexer Phytopharmaka
Schweiz Zschr Ganzheits Med 4 (Suppl 1): 24

Liew FY (1994)
Regulation of nitric oxide synthesis in infections and autoimmune diseases
Immunol Letters 43: 95-98

Liew FY (1995 a)
Nitric oxide in infections and autoimmmune diseases
In: Chadwick D, Cardev G (ed.)
T cell subset in infections and autoimmune diseases
Ciba Foundation Symposium 195. Wiley, Chichester

Liew FY, Wei XQ, Proudfoot L (1995 b
Interactions between cytokines and nitric oxide
Adv Neuroimmunol 5 (2): 201-209

Liew FY, Wei XQ, Proudfoot L (1997)
Cytokines and nitric oxide as effector molecules against parasitic infections
Philos Trans R Soc Lond B Biol Sci 352 (1359): 1311-1315

Lijinsky W (1992)
Chemistry and Biology of N-Nitrosocompounds
University Press, Cambridge

Lijinsky W (1994)
Chemical Structure of Nitrosamines Related to Carcinogenesis
In: Loeppky RN, Micheida CJ (1994 a), op. cit.
Lijinsky W, Taylor HW, Snyder C, Nettersheirn C (1973)
Malignant tumours of liver and lung in rats fed aminopyrin of heptamethyleneimine together with nitrite
Nature 244: 176-178

Lin H, Mosmann TR, Guilbert L et al. (1993)
Synthesis of T helper type-2 cytokines at the maternal-fetal interface
J Immunol 151: 4562-4573

Lincoln J, Hoyle CHV, Burnstock G (ed.) (1997)
Nitric oxide in health and disease
Cambridge University Press, Cambridge U.K.

Lindinger M (2000)
Planckscher Oszillator aus zwei Photonen. Lichtquanten im Resonator.
Frankfurter Allgemeine Zeitung 114: Nl

Lipsky PE (1999 a)
The clinical potential of cyclooxygenase-2-specific inhibitors
Am J Med 106 (5B): 51S-57S

Lipsky PE (1999 b)
Role of cyclooxygenase -1 and -2 in health and disease
Am J Orthoped (Chatham, NJ) 28 (3 Suppl): 8-12

Lischner HW, Huff DS (1975)
T-cell deficiency in Di George syndrome
In: Bergsma D, Good RA, Finstad J, Paul NW (eds.)
Immunodeficiency in man and animals
Sinauer, Sunderland, Mass

Lissoni P, Rovelli F, Giani L et al. (1998)
Dehydroepiandrosterone sulfate (DHEAS) secretion in early and advanced solid neoplasms: Selective deficiency in metastatic disease
Internat J Biological Markers 13 (3): 154-157

Lo JC, Mulligan K, Tai VW et al. (1998)
"Buffalo hump" in men with HIV-1 infection
Lancet 351: 867-870

Loeppky RN (1994 b)
Nitrosamine and N-Nitroso compound. Chemistry and Biochemistry
In: Loeppky RN, Michejda CJ (1994 a)

M

Mallal S, John M, Moore C et al. (1999)
Protease inhibitors and nucleoside analogue reverse transcriptase inhibitors interact to cause subcutaneous fat wasting in patients with HIV-infection
Antiviral Ther 4 (Suppl. 2): 28-29

Mannucci PM, Gringersi A, de Biasi R et al. (1992)
Immune status of asymptomatic HIV-infected hemophiliacs: Randomized, prospective, two year comparison of treatment with a high-purity or an intermediate-purity factor VII! concentrate
Thrombosis and Haemostasis 67: 310-313

Manzari V, Gallo RC, Franchini G et al. (1983)
Abundant transcription of a cellular gene in T-cells infected with human T-cell leukemia-lymphoma virus
Proc Natl Acad Sci USA 80: 12-19

Marchetti P, Decaudin O, Macho A et al. (1997)
Redox-regulation of apoptosis: impact of thiol oxidation status on mitochondrial function
Eur J Immunol 27: 289-296

Marco M, Kass S, Dietz P, et al. (1998)
The OI-Report. A critical review of the treatment and prophylaxis of HIV-related opportunistic infections
Treatment Action Group (TAG), New York

Margosiak SA, Applenan JR, Santi DV, Blakley RL (1993)
Dihydrofolate reductase from the pathogenic fungus Pneumocystis carinii: catalytic properties and interactions with antifolates
Archives of Biochemistry and Biophysics 305: 499-508

Margulis L (1970)
Origin of eukaryotic cells
Yale University Press, New Haven

Margulis L (1988)
Serial endosymbiotic theory (SET). Undulipodia, mitosis and their microtubulic systems preceded mitochondria
Endocytobiosis and Cell Res 5: 133-162

Margulis L, Dolan MF (1997)
Swimming against the current
In: Margulis L, Sagan O (ed.)
Slanted truths. Essay on Gaia, Symbiosis and Evolution
Springer, New York

Marjanovic S Wielburgki A, Nelson BD (1988)
Effect of phorbol myristate acetate and concanavalin A on the glycolytic enzymes of human peripheral lymphocytes
Biochem Bephys Acta 970: 1-6

Marjanovic S, Wollberg ID, Skog S et al. (1993)
The effects of cAMP on the expression of glycolytic enzymes in activating peripheral human T lymphocytes
Arch Biochem Biophys 302: 398-401

Marletta MA (1993)
Nitric oxide synthase structure and mechanism
J Biological Chemistry 268: 12231-12234

Marietta MA, Yoon PS, lyengar R et al. (1988)
Macrophage oxidation of L-arginine to nitrite and nitrate: nitric oxide is an intermediate
Biochemistry 27: 8706-8711

Marmor M, Friedman-KienAE, Laubenstein LJ et al. (1982)
Risk factors for Kaposi's sarcoma in homosexual men: A seroepidemiologic case-control study
Ann Intern Med 100: 809-815

Marmor M, Friedman-Kien AE, Laubenstein LJ et al. (1982)
Risk factors for Kaposi's sarcoma in homosexual men Lancet i: 1083-1087

Marmor M (1984)
Epidemic Kaposi's sarcoma and sexual practices among male homosexuals.
In: Friedman-KienAE, Laubenstein II (eds.)
AIDS: The epidemic of Kaposi's sarcoma and opportunistic infections
Masson Publishing, Chicago 1984

Marquart KH (1986)
AIDS associated Kaposi's sarcoma in Africa
Br Med J 292i 484

Martin W, Smith JA, Lewis MJ, Henderson AH (1988)
Evidence that inhibitory factor extracted from bovine retractor penis is nitrite, whose acid-activated derivative is stabilized nitric oxide
Br Pharmacol 93: 579-585

Marx JL (1983)
Human T-cell virus linked to AIDS
Science 220: 806-809

Marx JL (1989)
Drug resistant strains of AIDS virus found
Science 243: 1551

Masferrer JL, Leahy KM, Koki AT et al. (2000)
Antiangiogenic and antitumor activities of cyclooxygenase-2 inhibitors
Cancer Res 60 (5): 1306-1311

Masur H, Michelis MA, Green JB et al. (1981)
An outbreak of community-acquired pneumocystis carinii pneumonia
N Engl J Med 305:1431-1438

Masur H (1992)
Prevention and treatment of Pneumocystis pneumonia
NEJM 327: 1853-1860

Mathupala Sp, Rempel A, Pedersen PL (1997)
Aberrant glycolytic metabolism ofcancer cells: A remarkable coordination of genetic, transcriptional, post-translational, and mutational events that lead to a critical role for type-II hexokinase
J Bioenerget Biomembr 29 (4): 339-343

Matsiota P, Chamaret S, Montagnier L (1987)
Detection of normal autoantibodies in the serum of anti-HIV positive individuals
Ann Institut Pasteur / Immunol 138: 223-233

Matsumori A (1997)
Molecular and Immune mechanisms in the pathogenesis of cardiomyopathy—role of viruses, cytokines, and nitric oxide
Jpn Circ J 61 (4) : 275-291

Matsuyama T, Kobayaski N, Yamamoto N (1991)
Cytokines and HIV infection: Is AIDS a tumor necrosis factor disease?
AIDS 5: 1405

Matthews DA, Bolin JT, Buridge JM (1985)
Dihydrofolate reductase. The stereochemistry of inhibitor selectivity
J Biol Chemistry 260: 392-399

Matthews R, Smith D, Midgley J et al. (1988)
Candida and AIDS: Evidence for protective antibody
Lancet i: 263-266

Maturana H, Varela FJ (1987)
Der Baum der Erkenntnis
Scherz, München

Matzinger P (1994)
Tolerance, danger and the extended family
Ann Rev Immunol 12: 991-1045

Mauri UJ, Lahdevirta J (1990)
Correlation of serum cytokine levels with haematological abnormalities in human immunodeficiency virus infection
J Int Med 227: 253

Mayer KH (1983)
Medical consequences of the inhalation of volatile nitrites
In: Ostrow DG, Sandholzer TA, Felman YM (ed.)
Sexually transmitted diseases in homosexual men
Plenum Medical Book, New York

Mayers I, Johnston D (1998)
The nonspecific inflammatory response to injury
Can J Anaest 45: 871-879

Mazurek S, Boschek CB, Eigenbrodt E (1997)
The role of phosphometabolites in cell proliferation, energy metabolism and tumour therapy
J Bioenerget Biomembr 29 (4): 315-330

Mbeki, T (2000)
Letter to world leaders on AIDS in Africa. April 3, 2000
Net: www.virusmyth.com/aids/news/lettermbeki.htm

Mc Cann PP, Pegg AE, Sjoerdsma A (eds.) (1987)
Inhibition of polyamine metabolism: Biological significances and basis fo new therapies
Academic Press Inc., Orlando

Mc Cann SM, Kimura M, Karanth S et al. (1998 a)
Role of nitric oxide in the neuroendocrine response of cytokines
Ann NY Acad Sci 1: 174-184

Mc Cann SM, Kimura M, Walczewska A et al. (1998 b)
Hypothalamic control of FSH and LH by FSH—RF, LHRH, cytokines, leptin and nitric oxide
Neuroimmunomodulation 5 (3-4): 193-202

Mc Keehan WL (1982)
Glycolysis, glutaminolysis and cell proliferation, energy metabolism and tumour therapy
J Bioenerget Biomembr 29 (4): 315-330

Mc Leod GX, Hammer SM (1992)
Zidovudine: Five years later
Ann Intern Med 117: 487-501

Mc Quaid KE, Keenan AK (1997)
Endothelial barrier dysfunction and oxidative stress: Rules for nitric oxide?
Exper Physiol 82: 369-370

Meakins JL, Pietsch JB, Bubenick A (1977)
Delayed hypersensitivity: Indicator of acquired failure of host defenses in sepsis and trauma
Ann Surg 186: 241-250

Meister A, Anderson ME (1983)
glutathione
Ann Rev Biochem 52: 711-760

Meister A (1995)
Mitochondrial changes associated with glutathione deficiency
Biochim Biophys Acta 1271: 35-42

Meltzer MS, Gendelman HE (1992)
Mononuclear phagocytes as targets, tissue reservoirs, and immunregulatory cells in human immunodeficiency virus disease
In: Russel SW, Gordon S (eds.)
Macrophage Biology and Activations
Springer-Verlag, Berlin

Meyaard L, Otto SA, Keet JPM et al. (1994)
Changes in Cytokin secretion of CD4+ T cell clones in human immunodeficiency virus infection
Blood 84: 4262-4268

Miedema F, Petit AJC, Terpstra FG et al. (1988)
Immunological abnormalities in human immunodeficiency virus (HIV)-infected asymptomatic homosexual men. HIV affects the immune system before CD4+ T-helper cell depletion occurs
J Clin Invest 82: 1908-1914

Mijasaka N, Hirata Y (1997)
Nitric oxide and inflammatory arthritides
Life Sci 61: 2073-2081

Milano S, Arcoleo F, Dieli M et al. (1995)
Prostaglandin E2 regulates inducible nitric oxide synthase in the murine macrophage cell line J 774
Prostaglandins 49: 1O5-115

Mildvan D, Mathur RW, Enlow PL et al. (1982)
Opportunistic infections and immune deficiency in homosexual men
Ann Intern Med 96: 700-704

Miles AM, Bohle DS, Glasbrenner PA et al. (1996)
Modulation of superoxide-dependent oxidation and hydroxyIation reactions by nitric oxide
J Biol Chemistry 271: 40-47

Miller DJ, Hersen M (1992)
Research fraud in the behavioral and biomedical sciences
John Wiley and Sons, Inc., New York

Miller KD, Jones E, Yanovski JA et al. (1998)
Visceral abdominal-fat accumulation associated with use of indinavir
Lancet 351: 871-875

Minghetti L, Levi G (1998)
Microglia as effector cells in brain damage and repair: Focus on prostanoids and nitric oxide
Progress Neurobiol 54: 99-125

Mirvish SS, Ramen MD, Babcock DM (1988)
Indication from animals and chemical experiments of a carcinogenic role for isobutyl nitrite
In: Haverkos HW, Dougherty JA (ed.) Health Hazards of Nitrite Inhalants
National Institute on Drug Abuse, Rockville U.S.

Mitchell HH, Shoule HA, Grindley HS (1916)
The origin of the nitrates in the urine
J Biol Chem 24: 461-490
Mitsuya H, Weinhold G, Furnman PA. et 0.1. (1985) 3-Azido-3 deoxythimidine (BW A509 U):
An antiviral agent that inhibits the infectivity and cytopathic effect of human

T-lymphotropic virus type III / lymphadenopathy-associated virus in vitro
Proc Natl Acad Sci USA 82: 7096-7100

Miyoshi I, Kubonishi K, Yoshimoto S et al. (1981 a)
Detection of type-C partikels in cord leucocytes and human leukemic T-cells
Nature 294: 770-771

Miyoshi I, Kubonishi K, Yoshimoto S, Shiraishi Y (1981 b)
A T-cell line derived from normal human cord leucocytes by co-culturing with human leukemia T-cells
Gann. 72: 978-981

Modlin RL, Bloom BR (1993)
Immune regulation: Learning from Leprosy
Hosp Pract 28: 71-84

Modolell N, Corraliza 1M, Link F et al. (1995)
Reciprocal regulation of the nitric oxide synthase / arginase balance in mouse bone marrow-derived macrophages by TH1 and TH2 cytokines
Eur J Immunol 25: 1101-1104

Moncada S, Palmer RMJ, Higgs EA (1991)
Nitric oxide: Physiology, pathophysiology, and pharmacology
Pharmacol Rev 43: 109-142

Moncada S, Bagetta G (eds.) (1996)
Nitric oxide and the cell: proliferation, differentiantion and death
Portland, London

Montagnier L (1985)
Lymphadenopathy-associated virus: from molecular biology to pathogenicity
Ann Intern med 103: 689-693

Montefiori DC, Pantaleo G, Fink LM et al. (1996)
Neutralizing and infection-enhancing antibody responses to human immunodeficiency virus type 1 in long-term nonprogressors
J Infect Dis 173: 60-67

Morel PA, Oriss TB (1998)
Crossregulation Thl and Th2 cells
Crit Rev Immunol 18 (4): 275-303

Morré OJ, Wu L-Y, Morré DM (1998)
Response of a cell-surface NADH oxidase to the antitumor sulfonylurea N—(4-methylphenyl-sulfonyl)—N'—(4-chlorophenyl urea) (LYI81984) modulated by redox
Biochimica et Biophysica Acta 1369: 185-192

Mosmann TR (1988)
Helper T cells and their lymphokines
In: Feldmann M, Lamb J, Owen M (ed.)
T cells
Wiley, New York

Mosmann TR, Cherwinski H, Bond MW et al. (1986)
Two types of murine helper T cell clone: I. Definition according to profiles of Iymphokine activities and secrete proteins
J Immunol 136: 2348-2357

Mosmann TR, Coffman RL (1989)
TH 1 and TH 2 cells: Different patterns of lymphokine secretion lead to different functional properties
Ann Rev Immunol 7: 145-173

Mosmann TR, Sad S (1996)
The expanding universe ofT cell subsets: TH1, TH2 andmore
Immunol Today 17 (3): 138-146

Moss AR, Osmond D, Bacchetti P et al. (1987)
Risk factors for AlDS and HIV seropositivity in homosexualmen Am J Epidemiol125: 1035-1047

Mourad FH, Turnvill JL, Farthing MJG (199)
Role of nitric oxide in intestinal water and electrolyte transport
Gut 44: 143-147

Moye J, Rich KC, Kalish LA et al. (1996)
Natural history of somatic growth in infants born to women infected by human immunodeficiency virus
J Pediatrics 128: 58-67

Mrochek JE, Katz S, Christie WH, Dinsmore SR (1974)
Acetaminophen metabolism in man, as determined by high-resolution liquid chromatography
Clin Chem 20: 1086-1096

Müller WEG, Bachmann M, Weiler BE et al. (1991)
Antibodies against defined carbohydrate structures of Candida albicans protect H9 cells against infection with human immunodeficiency virus-l in vitro
J Acquir immun Defic Syndr 4: 694-703

Müller WEG, Schröder HC, Reuter P et al. (1990)
Polyclonal antibodies to mannan from yeast also recognize the carbohydrate structure of gp120 of AlDS virus: An approach to raise neutralizing antibodies to HIV-1 infection in vitro
AIDS 4 : 159-162

Muller JW, Jos Frissen PH, Krijnen P et al. (1992)
Dehydroepiandrosterone as predictor for progression to AIDS in asymptomatic human immunodeficiency virus infected men
J Infect Dis 165: 413-418

Mullis K (1993)
Interview in:
Carroll: The weird way to win a Nobel prize
San Francisco Chronicle, 21 Oct 1993, E9

Mullis K (1996)
Foreword
In: Duesberg PH (1996)
Inventing the AIDS Virus, pp. XI-XIV
Regnery Publishing Inc., Washington DC

Mullis K (1998)
Dancing naked in the minefield
Pantheon Books, New York

Mullis K (2000)
Interview in: Behr A, Reichardt L
Wenn 99 Prozent
allerWissenschaftler einer
Meinung sind. ist sie mit großer
Wahrscheinlichkeit falsch
Süddeutsche Zeitung Magazin, 7.
August 2000, 22-24

Murad F, Mittal CK, Arnold WP et
al. (1978)
Guanylate cyclase: Activation by
azide, nitro compounds, nitric oxide,
and hydroxyl radical and inhibition by
hemoglobin and myoglobin
Advances in Cyclic Nucleotide Res 9:
145-158

Muraille E, Leo O (1998)
Revisiting the Th1/Th2 paradigm
Scand J Immunol 47 (1): 1-9

Murayama T, Nomura Y (1998)
The actions of NO in the central
nervous system and in thymocytes
Jap J Pharmakol 76: 129-139

Murell W (1879)
Nitroglycerin as a remedy for angina
pectoris
Lancet i: 8O-1,113-115,151-
152,225-227

Murphy S, Simmons ML, Agullo L
et al. (1993)
Synthesis of nitric oxide in CNS glial cells
Trends in Neuroscience 16: 323-328

Murphy JT, Mueller GE. Whitman
ST (1997)
Redefining the growth of the
heterosexual HIV / AIDS epidemic
in Chicago
J AIDS Hum Retrovirol 16: 122-126
Murphy JJW, Bistom F, Deepe GS et
al. (1998)
Type 1 and type 2 cytokines: From
basic science to fungal infections
Med Mycol 36 Suppl 1: 1O9-118

Murray MF (1999)
Niacin as a potential AIDS
preventive factor
Medical Hypotheses 53 (5): 375-379

N

Nast-Kolb D, Waydhas Ch, Jochum
M et al. (1992)
Biochemische Faktoren als objektive
Parameter zur Prognoseabschatzung
beim Poly trauma
Unfallchirurg 95: 59-66

Nathan C, Xie Q-W (1994)
Nitric oxide synthases: Roles, tolls,
and controls
Cell 78: 915-918

Navikas V, Link J, Wahren B et al.
(1994)
Increased levels of interferon-gamma
(IFN-gamma), IL-4 and transforming
growth factor (TGF-ß) in RNA
expressing blood mononuclear cells in
human HIV infection
Clin Exp Immunol 6: 59-63

Nebert DW, Mc Kinnon RA, Puga A (1996)
Human drug-metabolizing enzyme polymorphisms: Effects on risk of toxicity and cancer
DNA Cell Biol 15: 273-280

Nelson E, Morioka T (1963)
Kinetics of the metabolism of acetaminophen by humans
J Pharmacol Sci 52: 864-868

Neu J, Riog JC, Meetze WN et al. (1997)
Enteral glutamine supplementation for very low birth weight infants decreases morbidity
J Pediatr 131: 691

Newberne PM (1977)
Effect of folic acid B, choline and methionine on immunocompetence and cell-mediated immunity
In: Suskind RM (ed.) (1977)
Malnutrition and the immune response
Raven Press, New York

Newell GR, Adams SC, Mansell PWA, Hersh EM (1984)
Toxicity, immunosuppressive effects and carcinogenic potential of volatile nitrites—Possible relationships to Kaposi's sarcoma
Pharmacotherapy 4: 284-291

Newell GR, Spitz MR, Wilson MB (1988)
Nitrite Inhalants: Historical Perspective
In: Haverkos HW, Dougherty JA (ed.) (1988)
Health Hazards of Nitrite Inhalants
National Institute on Drug Abuse, Rockville U.S.

Newman GW, Guarnaccia JR, Vance EA et al. (1994)
Interleukin-12 enhances antigen-specific proliferation of peripheral blood mononuclear cells from HIV-positive and negative donors in response to mycobacterium avium
AIDS 8: 1413-1419

Newsholme EA, Parry-Billings M (1990)
Properties of glutamine release from muscle and its importance for the immune system
JPEN 14 (Suppl): 563

Newsholme EA (1996)
The possible role of glutamine in some cells of the immune system and the possible consequence for the whole animal
Experientia 52: 455-459

Nickerson M, Parker JO, Lowry TP, Swenson EW (1979)
Isobutyl Nitrite and related compounds
Pharmex Ltd., San Francisco

Nickolson LB, Kuchroo VK (1996)
Manipulation of the Th1 / Th2 balance in autoimmune disease
Curr Opin Immunol 8 (6): 837-842

North R (1998)
Pesticide use on farm animals: can we regulate it?
The Ecologist 28 (2): 106-109

Null G (1997)
AIDS—a second opinion
In: Video-Film: Interviews with scientific and medical AIDS—Dissidents
New York-London
Available at: Continuum, 172 Foundling Court, Brunswick Centre London WC IN lQE, UK
Tel.: +44(0) 1717137071
Fax: +44(0) 1717137072

Nussbaum B (1990)
Good intentions: How big business, politics, and medicine are corrupting the fight against AIDS
Atlantic Monthly Press, New York

Nussler AK, Billiar TR (1993)
Inflammation, immunoregulation and inducible nitric oxide synthase
J Leukocyte Biol 54: 171-178

Nuttal SL, Martin U, Sinclair AJ, Kendall MJ (1998) glutathione: in sickness and in health
Lancet 351: 645-646

O

O'Garra A, Steinman L, Gijbels K (1997)
CD4+ T-cells subsets in autoimmunity
Curr Opin Immunol 9 (6): 872-883

O'Garra A (1998)
Cytokines induce the developement of functionally heterogenous T helper cells
Immunity 8 (3): 275-283

O'Hara CJ, Groopmen JF, Federman M (1988)
The ultrastructural and immunohistochemical demonstration of viral particles in lymphnodes from human immunodeficiency virus-related lymphadenopathy syndromes
Human Pathol 19: 545-549

O'Harra N, Chang SW (1982)
Kaposi's sarcoma and the HLA-DR5 alloantigen
Ann Intern Med 97: 617-622

O'Riordan DM, Standing JE, Limper AH (1995)
Pneumocystis carinii glycoprotein A binds macrophage mannose receptors
Infect-Immun 63: 779-784

Ochoa JB, Curti B, Peitzman AB et al. (1992)
Increased circulating nitrogen oxides after human tumor immunotherapy: Correlation with toxic hemodynamic changes
J Natl Cancer Institute 84: 864-867

Odeh M (1990)
The role of tumor necrosis factor-alpha in acquired immunodeficiency syndrome
J Int Med 228: 549

Oefner C, D'Arcy A, Winkler FK (1988)
Crystal structure of human dihydrofolate reductase complexed with folate
Eur J Biochem 174: 377-385

Oettle AG (1962)
Geographical and racial differences in the frequency of Kaposi's sarcoma as evidence of environmental or genetic causes
In: Symposium on Kaposi's sarcoma
Unio Internationalis Contra Cancrum. Vol. 18.
Karger, Berlin

Ogilvie GK (1998)
Interventional nutrition for the cancer patient.
Clin Techniques in Small Animal Practice 13 (4): 211-216

Ohara M, Sawa T (1998)
Current topics in the regulation of prostanoids-2. The interactions with cytokines
Masui 17 (12): 1471-1477

Ohlenschlager G (1991)
Das Glutathionsystem.
Ordnungs—und informationserhaltende Grundregulation lebender Systeme
Verlag für Medizin Dr. Ewald Fischer, Heidelberg

Ohlenschlager G (1992)
Die Rolle des Glutathion in der Antikanzerogenese.
Das Glutathionsystem wird zunehmend für die Detoxikation von Schadstoffen aufgebraucht
Natur—und Ganzheitsmedizin 5: 221-228

Ohlenschlager G (1994)
Betrachtungen zur Nichtglechgewichts—Thermodynamik des Glutathionssystems in lebenden Systemen
Praxis-Telegramm Sonderbeilage 1/94: 1-16

Olivier R (1995)
Flow cytometrie technique for assessing effects of N-acetylcysteine on apoptosis and cell viability of human immunodeficiency virus-infected lymphocytes
Methods Enzymol 251: 270-278

Olweny ChL (1984)
Epidemiology and clinical features of Kaposi's sarcoma in tropical Africa
In: Friedman-Kien AE, Laubenstein LJ (ed.), op. cit.

Ono K, Nakane H (1990)
Mechanisms of inhibition of various cellular DNA and RNA polymerases by several flavonoids
J Biochem 108: 608-613

Oppenheim JJ, Cohen S (1983)
Interleukins, Lymphokines and Cytokines Academic Press, London

Orusevic A, Lala PK (1998)
Role of nitric oxide in IL-2 therapy-induced capillary leak syndrome
Cancer Metastasis Rev 17 (1): 127-142

Oshima H, Bartsch H (1994)
Chronic infections and inflammatory processes as cancer risk factors: possible role of nitric oxide in carcinogenesis
Mutation Research 305: 253-264

Osmond DG (1993)
The turnover of B-cell populations
Immunol Today 14 (1): 34-37

Ostrom N (1989)
The poisoning continues. Pregnant women with AIDS to be given AZT
New York Native July 31, 1989, 15

Ostrom N (1996)
Poison makes a comeback
New York Native, 15.07.1996

Ottaviani E, Franceschi C (1998)
A new theory of the common evolutionary origin of natural immunity, inflammation and stress response: The invertebrate phagocytic immunocyte as an eye-witness
Domest Anim Endocrinol 15 (5): 291-296

Owen M, Steward M (1996)
Antigen recognition
In: Raitt I, Brostoff J, Male D (eds.)
Immunology, 4th ed. (7.1-7.12)
Mosby, London

P

Paganelli R, Fanales-Belasio D, Scala E et al. (1991)
Serum eosinophil cationic protein (ECP) in human immunodeficiency virus (HIV) infection
J Allergy Clin Immunol 88: 416-418

Paganelli R, Scala E, Ansotegui IJ et al. (1995)
CD8+ T lymphocytes provide helper activity for IgE synthesis in human immunodeficiency virus-infected patients with hyper IgE
J Exp Med 181: 423-428

Palmer RMJ, Ferrige AG, Moncada S (1987)
Nitric oxide release accounts for the biological activity of endothelium-derived relaxing factor
Nature 327: 524-526

Palmer RMJ, Ashton DS, Moncada S (1988)
Vascular endothelial cells synthesize 'nitric oxide from Larginine
Nature 333: 664-666

Pantaleo G, Menzo S, Vaccarezza M et al. (1995)
Studies in subjects with long-term nonprogressive human immunodeficiency virus inffection
N Engl J Med 332: 209-216

Papadopulos—Eleopulos E (1988)
Reappraisal of AIDS—is the oxidation induced by the risk factors the primary cause?
Medical Hypotheses 25: 151-162

Papadopulos-Eleopulos E, Hedland-Thomas B, Dufty AP (1989)
An alternative explanation for the radiosensitization of AIDS patients
Int J Radiat Oncol Biol Phys 17: 695-696

Papadopulos-Eleopulos E, Turner VF, Papadimitriou JM (1992 a)
Oxidative Stress, HIV and AIDS
Res. Immunol 143: 145-148

Papadopulos-Eleopulos E, Turner VF, Papadimitriou JM (1992 b)
Kaposi's Sarcoma and HIV
Medical Hypotheses 39: 22-29

Papadopulos—Eleopulos E, Turner VF, Papadimitriou JM (1993 a)
Is a positive Western Blot proof of HIV infection?
Bio/Technology 11: 696-702

Papadopulos—Eleopulos E, Turner VF, Papadimitriou JM (1993 b)
Has Gallo proven the role of HIV in AIDS?
Emergency Medicine 5: 71-147

Papadopulos—Eleopulos E, Turner VB Papadimitriou JM et al. (1995 a)
A critical analysis of the HIV—T4-cell-AIDS hypothesis
Genetica 95 (1-3): 5-24

Papadopulos-Eleopulos E, Turner VF, Papadimitriou JM, Causer D (1995 b)
Factor VIII, HIV and AIDS in haemophiliacs: An analysis of their relationship
Genetica 95 (1-3): 25-50

Papadopulos-Eleopulos E, Turner VB Papadimitriou JM, Bialy H (1995 c)
AIDS in Africa: Distiguishing fact and fiction
World J Microbiol Biotechnol 11: 135-143

Papadopulos-Eleopulos E, Turner VB, Papadimitriou JM, Causer O (1996)
The isolation of HIV: Has it really been achieved?
Continuum 4: 1s—24s

Papadopulos—Eleopulos E (1997 a)
Why no whole virus?
Continuum 4 (5): 27-30

Papadopulos-Eleopulos E, Turner VB, Papadimitriou JM, Causer D (1997 b)
A critical analysis of the evidence for isolation of HIV
Net: www.virusmyth.com/aids/data/epapraisal.htm

Papadopulos-Eleopulos E, Turner VB, Papadimitriou JM et al. (1997 c)
HIV antibodies: Further questions and a plea for clarification
Curr Med Res Opinion 13 (10): 627-633

Papadopulos-Eleopulos E et al. (1998 a)
Between the lines. A critical analysis of Luc Montagnier's interview answers to Djamel Tahi
Continuum 5 (2): 35-45

Papadopulos-Eleopulos E, Turner VB, Papadimitriou JM (1998 b)
A brief history of retroviruses
Continuum 5 (2): 25-29

Papadopulos-Eleopulos E, Turner VB, Papadimitriou JM (1999)
A critical analysis of the pharmacology of AZT and its use in AIDS
Curr Med Res Opinion 15 S1-S45

Papadopulos-Eleopulos E, Turner VF, Papadimitriou JM et al. (2000 a)
The last debate.
March 2000
Net: www.virusmyth.com/aids/data/epdebate.htm

Papadopulos-Eleopulos E, Turner VB Papadimitriou JM et al. (2000 b)
Perth Group responds to Rasnick
Net: www.virusmyth.com/aids/data/epreprasnick.htm

Papadopulos-Eleopulos E, Turner VF (2000 c)
HIV testing and surveillance.
Presentation Presidential AIDS Advisory Panel Meeting on May/July 2000 in Pretoria
Net: www.virusmyth.com (front news)

Park KGM, Hayes PD, Garlick PJ et al. (1991)
Stimulation of lymphocyte natural cytotoxicity by L-arginine
Lancet 337: 645-646

Parker LN, Levin ER, Lifrak ET (1985)
Evidence for adrenocortical adaptation to severe illness
J Clin Endocrinol Metabol 60: 947-952

Parker WE, Cheng YC (1994)
Mitochondrial toxicity of antiviral nucleoside analogs
The J of NIH Research 6: 57-61

Parkin JM, Eales U, Galazka AR, Pinching AJ (1987)
Atopic manifestations in the acquired immune deficiency syndrom: Response to recombinant interferon gamma
Br Med J 294: 1185-1186

Parkinson JF, Mitrovic B, Marrill JE (1997)
The role of nitric oxide in multiple sclerosis
J Met Med 75:174-186

Paronchi P, Maggi E, Romagnani S (1999)
Redirecting Th2 responses in allergy
Curr Top Microbiol Immunol 238: 27-56

Parravicini CL, Klatzmann D, Jaffray P et al. (1988) Monoclonal antibodies to the human immuno-deficiency virus p18 protein cross-react with normal human tissues AIDS 2: 171-177

Parry-Billings M, Blomstrand E, Mc Andrew N, Newsholme EA (1990)
A communicational link between skeletal muscle, brain and the cells of the immune system
Int J Sports Med 11, Suppl 2: S122-S128

Pasteur L (1876)
Etudes sur la biere Gauthier-Villars, Paris

Paul-Ehrlich-Stiftung (1998)
Schreiben des Prasidentender Paul-Ehrlich-Stiftung vom 02.12.1998

Pearlman JT, Adams GL (1970)
Amyl nitrite inhalation fad
JAMA 212:160

Pearson CJ, Mc Devitt HO (1999)
Redirecting Th1 and Th2 responses in autoimmune disease
Curr Top Microbiol Immunnol 238: 79,122

Pedersen BK, Kappel M, Klokker M et al. (1994)
The immune system during exposure to extreme physiologic conditions
Int J Sports Med 15: S116-S121

Pedersen PL (ed.) (1997)
Bioenergetics of cancer cells
J Bioenergetics Biomembranes 29 (4): 299-413

Penn I (1979)
Kaposi's sarcoma in organ transplantant recipients
Transplantation 27: 8-11

Penn I (1981)
Malignant lymphoma in organ transplant recipients
Transplantation 31: 738-738

Penn I (1991)
Principles of tumor immunity. immunocompetence and cancer
In: De Vita V, Heltmann V, Rosenberg S (eds.)
Lippinscott, Philadelphia

Perelson AS (1997)
Decay characteristics of HIV-1 infected compartments during combination therapy
Nature 387: 188-191

Perrier A, Rask-Madsen J (1999)
Review article: The potential role of nitric oxide in chronic inflammatory bowel disorders
Aliment Pharmacol Ther 13: 135-144

Peterhans E (1997)
Reactive oxygen radical and nitric oxide in viral diseases
Biol Trace Elem Res 56 (1): 107-116

Peterson JD, Herzenberg LA, Vasquez K, Waltenbaugh C (1998)

Glutathione levels in antigen-presenting cells modulate Th1 versus Th2 response patterns
Proc Natl Acad Sci USA 95: 3071-3076

Petros A, Lamb G, Leone A et al. (1994)
Effects of a nitric oxide synthase inhibitor in humans with septic shock
Cardiovascular Res 28: 34-39

Petrovsky N, Harrison LC (1998)
The chronobiology of human cytokine production
Int Rev Immunol 16 (5-6): 635-649

Phillips AN, Smith GD (1997)
Viral load and combination therapy for human immunpodeficiency virus
NEJM 336: 958-959; 960 discussion

Philpott P (1997)
The isolation question.
How an Australian biophysicist and her simple observations have taken center stage among AIDS reappraisers
Reappraising AIDS 5 (6): 1-12
(Group for the reappraisal of the HIV/AIDS-hypothesis, 7514 Girard Ave. 1-331
La Jolla, CA 92037 eMail: philpott@wwnet.com
Tel.: (810) 772-9926 (Detroit)
Fax: (619) 272-1621 (San Diego)

Philpott P, Johnson C (1996)
Viral Load of Crap
Reappraising AIDS 4 (Oct. 1996)

Piatak M, Saag MS, Clark SJ et al. (1993)
High levels of HIV-l in plasma during all stages of infection determined by competitive PCR
Science 259: 1749-1754

Pifer LL, Hughes W~T, Stagno S et al. (1978)
Pneumocystis Carinii infection: Evidence for high prevalence in normal and immuno-suppressed children
Pediatrics 61: 35-41

Pifer LL, Wang YF et al. (1987)
Borderline immunodeficiency in male homosexuals: Is lifestyle contributory?
South Med J 80: 687-697

Pinto L, Sullivan J, Berzofsky et al. (1995)
ENV-specific cytotoxic T lymphocyte responses in HIV seronegative health care workers occupationally exposed to HIV-contaminated body fluids
J Clin Invest 96: 867-873

Pippard MJ (1989)
Clinical use of iron chelation
In: de Sousa M, Brock JH (eds.)
Iron in immunity, cancer and inflammation
J. Wiley and Sons Ltd., Chichester, USA

Pizzo, PA et al. (1988)
Effect of continuous intravenous infusion of zidovudine (AZT) in children with symptomatic HIV infection
NEJM 319: 889-896

Platt JL, Grant BW, Eddy AA, Michael AF (1982)
Immune cell populations in cutaneous delayed-type hypersensitivity

J Exp Med 158: 1227-1242
Pluda JM, Yarchoan R, Jaffe ES et al. (1990)
Development of non-Hodgkin lymphoma in a cohort of patients with severe human immunodeficiency virus (HIV) infection on long-term antiretroviral therapy
Ann Intern Med 113: 276-282

Poiesz BJ, Ruscetti FW, Gazdar AF et al. (1980)
Detection and isolation of type C retrovirus particles from fresh and cultured lymphocytes of a patient with cutaneous T-cell lymphoma
Proc Natl Acad Sci 77: 7415-7419

Poli G, Introna M, Zanaboni F et al. (1985)
Natural Killer cells in intravenous drug abusers with lymphadenopathy syndrome

Clin Ex Immunol 62: 128-135
Pollock JS, Förstermann U, Mitchell JA et al. (1991)
Purification and characterisation of particulate and endothelium-derived relaxing factor synthase from cultured and native bovine aortic endothelial cells
Proc Nate Acad Sci (USA) 88: 10480-10484

Pontes de Carvalho LC (1986)
The faithfulness of the immunoglobulin molecule: Can monoclonal antibodies ever be monospecific
Immunol Today 7: 33

Popovic M, Reitz MS, Sarngadharan MG et al. (1982)
The virus of Japanese T-cell leukaemia is a member of the human T-cell leukaemia virus group
Nature 300: 63-66

Popovic M, Sarin PS, Robert-Guroff M (1983)
Isolation and transmission of human retrovirus (Human T-cell Leukemia Virus)
Science 219: 856-859

Popovic M, Sarngadharan MG, Read E, Gallo RC (1984)
Detection, isolation, and continuous production of cytopathic retroviruses (HTLV-III from patients with AIDS and pre-AIDS)
Science 224: 497-500

Poulter LW, Seymour GJ, Duke O (1982)
Immunohistological analysis of delayed-type hypersensitivity in man
Cell Immunol 74: 358-369

Prang E, Stoltz C, Shabert J (1997)
The effect of glutamine on body weight and body cell mass (abstract)
Presented at the International Conference on AIDS Wasting
Fort Lauderdale, Florida. November 16-19, 1997

Prescott SM, Fitzpatrick FA (2000)
Cyclooxygenase-2 and carcinogenesis
Biochimica et Biophysica Acta 1470 (2): M69-78

Preussmann R (1983)
Public health significance of environmental N-nitroso compounds
In: Egan H, ed. Environmental Carcinogens: Selected methods of analysis.
VM. 6: N-nitroso compounds
IARC scientific publications no. 45.
Lyon, France Internal Agency for Research on Cancer, pp. 3-17

Preussmann R, Stewart BW (1986)
Carcinogenicity of nitro sure as in humans
In: Schmahl D, Kaldor JM (ed.)
Carcinogenicity of alkylating cytostatic drugs
IARC Scientific publications no. 78
International Agency for Research of Cancer, Lyon

Pryor GT, Howard, RA, Bingham CR et al. (1980)
Biomedical Studies on the effects of abused inhalant mixtures, Final Report
National Institute on Drug Abuse, Rockville U.S.

Pschyrembel W (1990)
Klinisches Wörterbuch.
256 Aufl.
De Gruyter, Berlin

Puente J, Miranda D, Gaggero A et al. (1991)
Immunological defects in septic shock.
Deficiency of natural killer cells and T-Iymphocytes
Rev Med Chil 119: 142-146

Purtilo DT, Connor DH (1975)
Fatal infections in protein-calorie malnourished children with thymolymphatic atrophy
Arch Dis Childhood 50: 149-152

R

Rabinovitch A, Guarez-Pinzon WL (1998)
Cytokines and their roles in pancreatic islet beta-cell destruction and insulin-dependent mellitus
Biochem Pharmacol 15: 55: 1139-1149

Racker E (1976)
Why do tumour cells have a high aerobic glycolysis?
J Cell Physiol 89: 697-700

Racker E, Spector M (1981)
Warburg Effect revisited: Merger of biochemistry and molecular biology
Science 23: 303-307

Raffi F, Brisseau JM, Planchon B et al. (1991)
Endocrine functions in 98 HIV-infected patients: A prospective study
AIDS 5: 729-733

Raghupathy R (1997)
Th1-type immunity is incompatible with successful pregnancy
Immunol Today 18 (10): 478-482

Ralston SH (1997)
The Michael Mason Prize Essay 1997: Nitric oxide and bone: What a gas!
Br J Rheumatol 36: 831-838

Ramshaw IA, Ramsay AJ, Karupiah G et al. (1997)
Cytokines and immunity to viral infections
Immunol Rev 159: 119-135

Rao M, Steiner P, Victoria MS et al. (1977)
Pneumocystis carinii pneumonia. Occurrence in a healthy American infant
JAMA 238: 2301-2302

Rappoport J (1988)
AIDS Inc., Scandal of the Century
Human Energy Press
San Bruno CA, USA

Rasnick D (1996)
Inhibitors of HIV protease useless against AIDS
Reappraising AIDS 4 (8): 1-4

Razzaque-Ahmed A, Blose DA (1983)
Delayed-type hypersensitivity skin testing. A review
Arch Dermatol 119: 934-945

Reddy BS, Hirose Y, Lubet R et al. (2000)
Chemoprevention of colon cancer by specific cyclooxygenase-2 inhibitor, Celecoxib, administered during different stages of carcinogenesis
Cancer Res 60 (2): 293-297

Reinherz EL, Kung PC, Goldstein G et al. (1979)
Separation of functional subsets of human T cells by a monoclonal antibody
Proc Natl Acad Sci 76: 4061-4065

Reinherz EL, Geha R, Wohl ME et al. (1981 a)
Immunodeficiency associated with loss of T4+ inducer T-cell function
NEJM 304: 811-816

Reinherz EL, Rosen FS (1981 b)
New concepts of immunodeficiency
Am J Med 71: 511-513

Remick DG, Villarete L (1996)
Regulation of cytokine gene expression by reactive oxygen and reactive nitrogen intermediates
J Leukoc Biol 59 (4): 471-475

Rene E, Jaary A, Brousse N (1988)
Demonstration of HIV infection of the gut of AIDS patients
Gastroenterol 94: A373 (Abstract)
Rey MA, Spire b, Dormont D et al. (1984)
Characterization of the RNA dependent DNA polymerase of a new human T-lymphtropic retrovirus (lymphadenopathy associated virus)
Biochem Biophys Res Comm 121: 126-133

Reynolds JV, Zhang SM, Thorn AK et al. (1987)
Arginine as an immunomodulator
Surg Forum 38: 415-418

Reynolds JV, Thorn AK, Zhang SM et al. (1988)
Arginine, protein malnutrition, and cancer
J Surg Res 45: 513-522

Richman DD, Fischl MA, Grieco MH et al. and the AZT Collaborative Working Group (1987)
The toxicity of Azidothymidine (AZT) in the treatment of patients with AIDS and AIDS-related complex
NEJM 317: 192-197

Richman DD (1990)
Zidovudine resistance of HIV (summary)
Rev Infect Dis 12 (Suppl 5): Jul-Aug 1990

Richter C (1996)
Nitric oxide and its congeners in mitochondria: Implications for apoptosis
In: Moncada S, Bagetta G (eds.)
Nitric oxide and the cell: Proliferation, differentiation and death
Portland, London

Richter C (1997 a)
Antibiotika-induzierte Schaden an Mitochondrien
Forschungsprojekt. Unveröffentliches Manuskript
Laboratorium für Biochemie I, Eidgenossische Technische Hochschule, Zürich

Richter C (1997 b)
AZT (Azidothymidin, Zidovudin)—induzierte Schaden an Blutzellen
Forschungsprojekt. Unveröffentlichtes Manuskript
Laboratorium für Biochemie I, Eidgenössische Technische Hochschule, Zürich

Rice-Evans CA, Miller NJ, Paganga G (1996)
Structure-antioxidants activity relationships of flavonoids and phenolic acids
Free Rad Biol Med 20: 933-956

Rieder MJ, Uetrecht J, Shear NH et al. (1988)
Diagnosis of sulfonamide hypersensitivity reactions by in vitro

"rechallenge" with hydroxylamine metabolites
Ann Intern Med 110: 286-289
Rieder MJ, Uetrecht J, Shear NH, Spielberg SP (1988)
Synthesis of in vitro toxicity of hydroxylamine metabolites of sulfonamides
J Pharmacol Exp Med 244: 724-728

Rieder MJ, Krause R, Bird JA, Debakan GA (1995)
Toxicity of sulfonamide-reactive metabolites in HIV-infected, HTLVinfected, and non-infected cells
J Acquir Immune Deficiency Syndr Human Retrovirol 8: 134-140

Rifkind D, Marchioro TL, Schneck SA, Hill RB (1967)
Systemic fungal infections complicating renal transplantation and immunosuppressive therapy: Clinical, microbiologic, neurologic and pathologic features
Amer J Med 43: 28-35

Rink L, Cakman I, Kircher H (1998)
Altered cytokine production in the elderly
Mech Ageing Dev 102 (2-3): 199-209

Rivier C (1998)
Role of nitric oxide and carbon monoxide in modulating the ACTH response to immune and nonimmune signals
Neuroimmunomodulation 5 (3-4): 203-213

Robbins JB (1967)
Pneumocystis carinii pneumonitis. A review
Pediatr Res 1: 131-135
Robbins JB (1968)
Immunological and clinicopathological aspects of Pneumocystis carinii pneumonitis
In: Bergma D, Good RA (ed.)
Immunologic Deficiency Disease in men
National Foundation, March of Dimes

Robert-Koch-Institut (1999)
AIDS / HIV.
Bericht zur epidemiologischen Situation in der Bundesrepublik Deutschland zum 31.12.1998. Berlin

Rocken M, Biedermann T, Ogilvie A (1997)
The role of Th1 and Th2 dichotomy: Implication for autoimmunity
Rev Rheum Engl Ed 64 (10 Suppl): 131S-137S

Rode HN, Christou NV, Bubenik O (1982)
Lymphocyte function in anergic patients
Clin Exp Immunol 47: 155-161

Roederer M, Staal FJT, Raju PA, Ela WS, Herzenberg LA (1990)
Cytokine in HIV replication is inhibited by N-Acetyl-L-Cysteine
Proc Natl Acad Sci USA 87: 4884-4888

Roederer M, Staal FJ, Osada H, Herzenberg LA, Herzenberg LA (1991 a)
CD4 and CD8 cells with high intracellular glutathione levels are selectively lost as the HIV infection progresses
Int Immunol 3: 933-937

Roederer M, Raju PA, Staal FJ, Herzenberg LA, Herzenberg LA (1991b)
N-acetylcysteine inhibits HIV expression in chronically infected cells
AIDS Res Human Retroviruses 7: 563-573

Rohde T. Ullum H, Rasmussen JP et al. (1995)
Effects of glutamine on the immune system: influence of muscular exercise and HIV infection
J Appl Physiol 79: 146-150

Rohde T, Maclean DA, Pedersen BK (1996)
Glutamine, lymphocyte proliferation and cytokine production
Scand J Immunol 44: 648-650

Roitt JM, Brostoff J, Male DK (1985)
Immunology
Gower Medical Publishing, London

Romagnani S (1991)
Human TH1 and TH2 subsets: Doubt no more
Immunol Today 12: 256-251

Romagnani S (1999)
The Th1 / Th2 paradigma and allergic disorders
Allergy 53 (46 Suppl): 12-15

Root-Bernstein RS (1993)
Rethinking AIDS.
The tragic cost of premature consensus
The Free Press, New York

Rose DP, Connolly JM (1999)
Omega-3 fatty acids as cancer chemopreventive agents
Pharmacol Therap 83 (3): 217-244

Rosenberg YJ, Anderson AO, Pabst R (1998)
HIV-induced decline in blood CD4/CD8 ratios: Viral killing or altered lymphocyte trafficking?
Immunology Today 19 (1): 10-17

Rosenthal GJ, Kowolenko M (1994)
Immunotoxicologic manifestations of AIDS therapeutics
In: Dean JH, Luster MI, Munson AE, Kimber J (eds.)
Immunotoxicology and Immunopharmacology. Second edition
Raven Press; New York (pp. 249-265)

Roth E, Mühlbacher F, Karner J et al. (1985)
Liver amino acids in sepsis
Surgery 97: 436-442

Roth VR, Kravcick S, Angel JB (1998)
Development of cervical fat pads following therapy with Human Immunodeficiency Virus type-1 protease inhibitors
Clin Infect Dis 27: 65-67

Rothman S (1962)
Remarks on sex, age, and racial distribution of Kaposi's sarcoma and on possible pathogenic factors
Acta Union Int Contra Cancer 18: 326-329

Rous P (1911)
A sarcoma of the fowl: Transmissible by an agent separable from the tumor cells.
J Exp Med 13 : 397-411

Rubin RH, Young LS (eds.) (1988)
Clinical approach to infection in the compromised host
Plenum Medical Book Company, New York, London, 2nd ed.

S

Saag MS, Kilby JM (1999)
HIV-1 and HAART: A time to cure, a time to kill
Nature Medicine 5: 609-611

Sacks DL, Lal SL, Shrivastava SN et al. (1987)
An analysis of T cell responsiveness in Indian Kalaazar
J Immunol 138: 908-913

Sagan LA (1987)
The Health of Nations.
True Causes of Sickness and Well-being
Basic Books, New York
Deutsche Ausgabe: Die Gesundheit der Nationen.
Die eigentlichen Ursachen von Gesundheit und Krankheit im Weltvergleich
Rowohlt, Reinbek bei Hamburg, 1992

Saint-Marc T, Partizani M, Poizot-Martin I et al. (1999 a)
A syndrome of peripheral fat wasting (lipodystrophy) in patients receiving long-term nucleoside analogue therapy
AIDS 13: 1659-1667
Saint-Marc T, Touraine JL (1999 b)
Reversibility of peripheral-fat wasting (lipodystrophy) on stopping stavudin therapy
Antiviral Ther 4 (Suppl 2): 31

Saito H, Trocki O, Alexander JW et al. (1987)
The effect of route of nutrient administration on the nutritional state, catabolic hormone secretion, and gut mucosal integrity after burn injury
JPEN ll: 1-7

Salk J, Bretscher PL, Salk M et al. (1993)
A strategy for prophylactic vaccination against HIV
Science 260: 1270-1272

Sanders SP (1999)
Asthma: Viruses and nitric oxide
Proc Soc Exp Biol Med 220: 123-132

Santiago E, Perez-Mediavilla LA, Lopez-Moratalla N (1998)
The role of nitric oxide in the pathogenesis of multiple sclerosis
J Physiol Biochem 54: 229-237

Saraste M (1999)
Oxidative phosphorylation at the fin de siecle
Science 283: 1488-1497

Sarngadharan MG, Popovic M, Bruck L, Schüpbach J, Gallo RC (1984)
Antibodies reactive with a human T-Iymphotropic retrovirus (HTLV—III) in the serum of patitents with AIDS
Science 224: 506-508

Sarngadharan MG, Markham PD (1987)
The role of human T-Iymphotropic retroviruses in leukemia and AIDS
In: Wormser GP (ed.)
AIDS-acquired immunodeficiency syndrome—and other manifestations of HIV infection
Noyes, Park Ridge NJ (pp. 197-198)

Sasso SP, Gilli RM, Sari JC et al. (1994)
Thermodynamic study of dihydrofolate reductase inhibitor selectivity
Biochemica et Biophysica Acta 1207: 74-79

Satoh T, Horn SSM, Shonmugarn KT (1983)
Production of nitrous oxide in Klebsiella pneumoniae: Mutants altered in nitrogen metabolism
J Bacteriol 155: 454

Sawaoka H, Tsuji S, Tsuji M et al. (1999
Cyclooxygenase inhibitors suppress angiogenesis and reduce tumor growth in vivo
Laboratory Invest 79 (12): 1469-1477

Scandalios JG (ed.) (1992)
Molecular Biology of Free Radical Scavenging Systems
Cold Spring Harbor Laboratory Press, Cold Spring Harbor NY, USA

Schafer O, Hamm-Künzelmann B, Hermfisse U, Brand K (1996)
Differences in DNA-binding efficiency of Sp1 to aldolase and pyruvate kinase promoter correlates with altered redox states in resting and proliferating rat thymocytes
FEBS Lett 391: 35-38

Schatz G, Mason TL (1974)
The biosynthesis of mitochondrial proteins
Ann Rev Biochem 43: 51-87

Schmid KO (1964)
Studien zur Pneumocystis-Erkrankung des Menschen
1. Frankf Z Pathol 74: 121-125

Schmidt HHHW, Wilke P, Evers B, Böhme E (1989)
Enzymatic formation of Nitrogen oxides from L-arginine in bovine brain cytosol
Biochem Biophys Res Communic 165: 284-291

Schooley RT, Hirsch MIS, Colvin RD et al. (1983)
Association of herpesvirus infections with T-lymphocyte subset alterations, glomerulopathy and opportunistic infections after renal transplantation
NEJM 308: 307-313

Schreeder MIT, Thompson SE, Hadler SC et al. (1981)
Hepatitis B in homosexual men: Prevalence of infection and factors related to transmission
J Infect Dis 146: 7-15.

Schreiber SL, Crabtree GR (1992)
The mechanism of action of cyclosporin A and FK 506
Immunology Today 13: 136

Schrödinger E (1967)
My view of the world
Cambridge University Press, Cambridge UK

Schupbach J, Popovic M, Gilden RV, Gonda MA, Sarngadharan MG, Gallo RC (1984)
Serological analysis of an subgroup of human T-lymphotropic retroviruses (HTLV-III) associated with AIDS
Science 224: 503-505

Schüpbach J, Haller O, Vogt M et al. (1985)
Antibodies to HTLV III in Swiss patients with AIDS and Pre-AIDS and in groups at risk for AIDS
NEJM 312: 265-270

Schwartz RH (1988)
Deliberate inhalation of isobutyl nitrite during adolescence: A descriptive study
In: Haverkos HW, Dougherty JA (ed.) (1988)
Health Hazards of Nitrite Inhalants
National Institute on Drug Abuse, Rockville U.S.

Schweizer M, Richter C (1996)
Peroxinitrite stimulate the pyrimidine nucleotide-linked Ca2+ release from intact rat liver mitochondria
Biochemistry 35: 4524-4528

Scott P, Natovitz P, Coffman RL et al. (1988)
Immunoregulation of cutaneous leishmaniasis: T cells lines which transfer protective immunity or exacerbation belong to distinct parasite antigens
J Immunol 140: 10-14

Seifter E, Rettura G, Barbul A et al. (1978)
Arginine: An essential amino acid for injured rats
Surgery 84: 224-230

Sell S, Hsu P-L (1993)
Delayed hypersensitivity and T-cell subset selection in syphilis pathogenesis and vaccine design
Immunol Today 14: 576

Semba RD, Graham NMH, Ciaffa WT et al. (1993)
Increased mortality associated with vitamin A deficiency during human immunodeficiency virus type 1 infection
Arch Intern Med 153: 2149-2154

Senn CK, Racker L (1996)
Antioxidant and redox regulation of gene transcription
FASEB J 10: 709-720

Sessa WC (1994)
The nitric oxide synthase family of proteins
J Vascular Res 31: 331-343

Shabert JK, Winslow C, Lacey JM, Wilmore DW (1999)
Glutamine-antioxidant supplementation increases body cell

mass in AIDS patients with weight loss: A randomized, double-blind controlled trial
Nutrition 15: 860-864
Shahidi H, Kilbourn RG (1998)
The role of nitric oxide in interleukin-2 therapy induced hypotension
Cancer metastasis Rev 17 (1): 119-26

Shanahan F, Leman B, Deem R et al. (1989)
Enhanced peripheral blood T-cell cytotoxicity in inflammatory bowel disease
J Clin Immunol 9: 55-64

Shaw JH, Wolfe RR (1987)
Glucose and urea kinetics in patients with early and advanced gastrointestinal cancer: The response to glucose infusion and TPN
Surgery 101: 181-186

Shear NH, Spielberg SP (1985)
In vitro evaluation of a toxic metabolite of sulfadiazine
Can J Physiol Pharmacol 63: 1370-1372

Shear NH, Spielberg Sp, Grant DM, Tang BK (1986)
Differences in metabolism of sulfonamides predisposing to idiosyncratic toxicity
Ann Intern Med 105: 179-184

Shearer GM, Bernstein DC, Tung KS et al. (1986)
A model for the selective loss of major histo-compatibility complex restricted T-cell immune response during the development of acquired immune deficiency syndrome
J Immunol 137: 2514-2521
Shearer GM, Clerici M, Sarin A et al. (1995)
Cytokines in immune regulation / pathogenesis in HIV infection
In: Chadwick O, Cardev G (eds.)
T-cell Subsets in Infectious and Autoimmune Diseases
Ciba Foundation Symposium 195.
Wiley, Chichester, 1995
Shearer GM, Clerici M (1996)
Protective immunity against HIV infection: Has nature done the experiment for us?
Immunol Today 17: 21-24

Shearer GM (1997)
Th1 / Th2 changes in aging
Mech Ageing Dev 94 (1-3): 1-5

Sheldon W (1959)
Experimental Pneumocystis Carinii infection in rabbits
Exp Med 110:110-147

Shenton J (1998)
Positively False.
Exposing the myth around HIV and AIDS
J.-B. Tauris, London-New York

Sher A, Gazzinelli RT, Oswald JP et al. (1992)
Role of T-cell derived cytokines in the down-regulation of mmune responses in parasitic and retroviral infection
Immunol Rev 127: 183-204

Shigenaga MK, Hagen TM, Ames BN (1994)
Oxidative damage and mitochondrial decay in aging
Proc Natl Acad Sci USA 91: 1071-1078
Siegel JH, Cerra FB, Coleman B et al. (1979)
Physiological and metabolic correlations in human sepsis
Surgery 86: 163-193

Sies H, Wendel A (eds.) (1978)
Function of glutathione in Liver and Kidney
Springer Verlag, Heidelberg-Berlin-New York

Sies H (ed.) (1995)
Oxidative Stress
Academic Press, Orlando Fla.

Sigell LT, Kapp FT, Fugaro GA et al. (1978)
Popping and snorting volatile nitrites: A current fad for getting high
Am J Psychiatry 135: 1216-1218

Siliprandi N, Siliprandi O, Bindoli A et al. (1978)
Effect of oxidation of glutathione and membrane thiol groups on mitochondrial functions
In: Sies H, Wendel A (eds.)
Function of Glutathion in Liver and Kidney
Springer Verlag, Heidelberg-Berlin-New York

Simopoulos AP (1999)
Evolutionary aspects of omega-3 fatty acids in the food supply
Prostagl Leucotriens Essent Fatty Acids 60 (5-6): 421-429

Singh S, Evans TW (1997)
Nitric oxide, the biological mediator of the decade: Fact or fiction?
Eur Respir J 110 : 699-707
Sinoussi F, Mandiola, L, Shermann JC (1973)
Purification and partial differntiation of the particles of murine sarcoma virus (M. MSV) according to their sedimentation rates in sucrose density gradients
Spectra 4: 237-243

Sjöholm A (1998)
Aspects of the involvement of interleukin-1 and nitric oxide in the pathogenesis of insulin-dependent diabetes mellitus
Cell Death Differ 5: 461-468

Sjoerdsma A, Golden JA, Schechter PI (1984)
Successful treatment oflethal protozoal infections with the ornithine decarboxylase inhibitor, alpha difluoromethylornithine
Trans Assoc Am Phys 97: 70

Skurrick IH, Bogden JD, Baker H et al. (1996)
Micronutrient profiles in HIV-infected heterosexual adults
J Acquir Imm Def Syndr Hum Retrovir 12: 75-80

Small CB, Kaufman A, Armenaka M, Rosenstreich DL (1993)
Sinusitis and atopy in human immunodeficiency virus infection
J Infect Dis 167: 283-290

Smith I, Howells DW (1987)
Folate deficiency and demyelination in AIDS
Lancet 2: 215
Smith KJ, Skelton HG, Drabick JJ et al. (1994)
Hypereosinophilia secondary to immunodysregulation in patients with HIV-1 disease
Arch Dermatol 130: 119-121

Smith RS, Pozefsky T, Chhetri MK (1974)
Nitrogen and amino acid metabolism in adults with protein-calorie malnutrition
Metabolism 23: 603-618

Smothers K (1991)
Pharmacology and toxicology of AIDS therapies
The AIDS Reader 1: 29-35

Snyder SH, Bredt DS (1992)
Biological roles of nitric oxide
Scientific American 266: 28-35

Sörensen PJ, Jensen MK (1981)
Cytogenetic studies in patients treated with trimethoprimsulfamethoxazole
Mutat Res 89 (1): 91-94

Son K, Kim Y-M (1995)
In vivo cisplatin-exposed macrophages increase immunostimulant-induced nitric oxide synthesis for tumor cell killing
Cancer Res 55: 5524-5527

Sonnabend JA (1989)
AIDS: An explanation for its occurrence among homosexual men
In: Ma P, Armstrong O (eds.)
AIDS and Infections of Homosexual Men
Butterworths, Boston. 2nd ed.
Souliotis VL, Valvanis C, Boussiotis VA et al. (1994)
Comparative dosimetry of O6-methyl-guanine in humans and rodents treated with procarbazine
Carcinogenesis 15: 1675-1678

Spector BD, Perry GS, Kersey JH (1978)
Genetically determined immunodeficiency disease (GDID) and malignancy
Report from the Immunodeficiency-Cancer Registry
Clin Immunol Immunopathol 11: 12-29

Spector NH, Fox BH, Kerza—Kwiatecki AP et al. (1985)
Neuroimmunomodulation
Proceedings of the First International Workshop on NIM
JWGN, Bethesda 1985

Spector NH (1988)
Neuroimmunomodulation
Gordon and Breach, Montreux

Spielberg SP, Leeder SJ, Cribb AE, Dosch H-M (1989)
Is sulfamethoxazole hydroxylamine (SMX-HA) the proximal toxin for sulfamethoxazole (SMX) toxicity?
Eur J Clin Pharmacol A 173: 04.37
Staal FJT, Roederer M, Herzenberg L, Herzenberg L (1990)

Intracellular thiols regulate activation of NF-kB and transcription of HIV
Proc Natl Acad Sci USA 87: 9943-9947

Stadler J, Schmalik WA, Doehmer J (1996)
Inhibition of cytochrome P 450 enzymes by nitric oxide
Adv Exp Med Biol 387: 187-193

Stahl F, Schnorr D, Pilz C, Dosner G (1992)
Dehydroepiandrosterone (DHEA) levels in patients with prostatic cancer, heart diseases and under surgery stress
Exp Clin Endocrinol 99 (2): 68-70

Stamler JS, Singel OJ, Loscalzo J (1992)
Biochemistry of nitric oxide and its redox-activated forms
Science 258: 1898-1902

Stamler JS (1994)
Redox signaling: Nitrosylation and related target interactions of nitric oxide
Cell 78: 931-936

Stamler JS (1995)
S-nitrosothiols and bioregulatory actions of nitrogen oxides through reactions with thiol groups
Curr Topics Microbiol Immunol 196: 19-36

Steen R, Skold O (1985)
Plasmid borne or chromosomally mediated resistance by Tu 7 is the most common response to ubiquitous use of trimethoprim
Antimicrob Agents Chemother 27: 933-937

Stein-Werblowsky R (1977)
The induction of precancerous changes in the uterine epithelium of the rat: The role of spermatozoa
Gynecol Oncol 5: 251

Stein-Werblowsky R (1978 a)
On the aetiology of testicular turn ours. An experimental study
Eur Urol 4: 57

Stein-Werblowsky R (1978 b)
On the aetiology of cancer of the prostate
Eur Urol 4: 370

Stolina M, Sharma S, Lin Y et al. (2000)
Specific inhibition of cyclooxygenase restores antitumor reactivity by altering the balance of IL-10 and IL-12 synthesis
J Immunol 164 (1): 361-370

Stone RS, Morrison JF (1986)
Mechanism of inhibition dihydrofolate reductases from bacterial and vertebrate sources by various classes of folate analogues
Biochemica et Biophysica Acta 869: 275-285

Stoner GD, Mukhtar H (1995)
Polyphenols as cancer chemopreventive agents
J Cell Biochem Suppl 22: 169-80

Strack O (1997)
Phenolic metabolism
In: Dey PM, Harborne JB (eds.)
Plant Biochemistry Academic Press, London

Strahl C, Blackburn EH (1996)
Effects of reverse transcriptase inhibitors on telomere length and telomerase activity in two immortalized human cell lines
Mol Cell Biol 16: 53-65
Strassmann G, Fong M, Kenney JS, Jacob CO (1992)
Evidence for the involment of interleukin-6 in experimental cancer cachexia
J Clin Invest 89: 1681-1684

Stringer JP (1993)
The identity of Pneumocystis carinii: Not a single protozoan but a diverse group of exotic fungi
Infect Agents Dis 2: 109-117

Stuehr DJ, Marletta MA (1985)
Mammalian nitrate biosynthesis: mouse macrophages produce nitrite and nitrate in response to Escheria coli lipopolysaccharide
Proc Natl Acad Sci (USA) 82: 7738-7742

Subbaramaiah K, Zakim D, Weksler BB, Dannenberg AJ (1997)
Inhibition of cyclooxygenase: A novel approach to cancer prevention
P.S.E.B.M.—216: 201-210

Suematsu M, Wakabayashi Y, Ishimura Y (1996)
Gaseous monoxides: a new class of microvascular regulator in the liver
Cardiovasc Res 32 (4): 679-686

Surcell H-M, Troye-Blomberg lvi, Raulie S et al. (1994)
TH1 / TH2 profiles in tuberculosis, based on the proliferation and cytokine response of blood lymphocytes to mycobacterial antigens
Immunology 81: 171-176
Sutton WL (1963)
Aliphatic nitro compounds, nitrates, nitrites, alkyl nitrites
In: Fassett DW, Irishd (ed.)
Industrial Hygiene and Toxicology. Vol. II
Interscience, New York. pp. 414-438

Svec F, Porter JR (1998)
The actions of exogenous dehydroepiandrosterone in experimental animals and humans
Proc Sac Exp Biol Med (P.S.E.B.M.) 218 (3): 174-191

Swerdlow R H (1998)
Is NADH effective in the treatment of Parkinson's disease?
Drugs and Aging 13 (4): 263-268

Szabo C, Southan GJ, Thiemermann C, Vane JR (1994)
The mechanism of the inhibitory effect of polyamines on the induction of nitric oxide syothase: Role of aldehyde metabolites
Br J Pharmacol 113: 757-766

Szmuness W (1979)
Large scale efficacy trials of hepatitis B vaccines in the USA: Baseline data and protocols
J Med Vir 4: 327-340

T

Tachibana K, Mukai K, Hiraoka I et al. (1985)
Evaluation of the effect of arginine-enriched amino acid solution on tumour growth
JPEN 9: 428-434

Tahi D (1997)
Did Luc Montagnier discover HIV? Interview with Luc Montagnier
Continuum 5 (2): 31-34

Tamir S, Tannenbaum SR (1996)
The role of nitric oxide (NO) in the carcinogenic process
Biochem Biophys Acta 1288 (2): F 31-36

Tandler B, Hoppel CL (1972)
Mitochondria: A historical review
Academic Press, New York

Tang AM, Graham NMH, Kirby AI et al. (1993)
Dietary micronutrient intake and risk of progression to acquired immunodeficiency syndrome (AIDS) in human immunodeficiency virus type 1 (HIV-1) infected homosexual men
Am J Epidemiol 138: 937-951

Tannenbaum SR, Fett D, Young VB et al. (1978)
Nitrite and nitrate are formed by endogenous synthesis in the human intestine
Science 200: 1487-1489

Tannenbaum SR, Tamir S, de Rojas-Walker T, Wishnok JS (1994)
DNA damage and cytotoxicity caused by nitric oxide
In: Loeppky RN, Michejda CJ (ed.)
Nitrosamines and Related N-Nitroso Compounds. Chemistry and Biochemistry
American Chemical Society, Washington, DC 1994

Tashiro T, Yamamori H, Takagi K et al. (1998) n-3 versus n-6 polyunsatured fatty acids in critical illness
Nutrition 14 (6): 551-553

Tayek JA (1992)
A review of cancer cachexia and abnormal glucose metabolism in humans with cancer
J Am Col Nutr 11: 445-456

Taylor BS, Alarcon LH, Billiar TR (1998)
Inducible nitric oxide synthase in the liver: Regulation and function
Biochemistry (Mose) 63: 766-781

Taylor JF, Templeton AC, Vogel CL et al. (1971)
Kaposi's sarcoma in Uganda: A clinicopathological study
Int J Cancer 8: 122

Taylor-Robinson AW, Liew FY, Severn A et al. (1994)
Regulation of the immune response by nitric oxide differentially produced by T helper type-1 and T helper type-2 cells
Eur J Immunol 24: 980-984

Temin HM, Mizutani S (1970)
DNA polymerase in virions of Rous Sarcoma virus
Nature 226: 1211-1213

Temin HM, Baltimore D (1972)
RNA-directed DNA synthesis and RNA tumor viruses
Adv Virus Res 17: 129-186
Temin HM (1974)
On the origin of RNA tumour viruse
Harvey Lect 69: 173-197

Temin HM (1985)
Reverse transcription in the eukaryotic genome: Retroviruses, pararetroviruses, retrotransposons and retrotranscripts
Mol Biol Evol 2: 455-468

Tempelton AC (1976)
Kaposi's sarcoma
In: Andrade R, Gumpert SL, Popkin GL et al. (ed.)
Cancer of the skin: Biology, diagnosis and management
Gaunders, Philadelphia

Teng SC, Gabriel A (1997)
DNA repair by recycling reverse transcripts
Nature 386: 31-32

Teng SC, Kim B, Gabriel A (1996)
Retrotransposon reverse-transcriptase-mediated repair of chromosomal breaks
Nature 383: 641-644

Termynck T, Avrameas S (1986)
Murine natural monoclonal antibodies: A study of their polyspecificies and their affinities
Immunol Rev 94: 99-112

Then RL (1993)
History and future of antimicrobial diaminopyrimidines
J Chemother 5 (6): 361-368
Then RL (1996)
Nebenwirkungen von Sulfonamid-Trimethoprim-Verbindungen
Antwortschreiben Hoffmann-La Roche Ltd., Basel, vom 09.07.1996 an die Studiengruppe für AIDS-Therapie c/o F. De Fries, im Zürich.

Thomas L (1984)
AIDS and the immune surveillance problem
In: Friedman-Kien AE, Laubenstein LJ (ed.), op. cit.

Thomsen LL, Miles DW, Happerfield Let al. (1995)
Nitric oxide synthase activity in human breast cancer
Br J Cancer 72: 41-44

Till M, Mac Donnell KB (1990)
Myopathy with human immunodeficiency virus type 1 (HIV-1) infection: HIV-Zidovudine
Ann Intern Med 113: 492-494

Tönz O, Lüthy J (1996)
Folsäure zur primären Verhütung von Neuralrohrdefekten
Schweiz Äztezeitung 77 (14): 596-572

Tokuda H, Ito Y, Kanaoka T, Yoshida O (1987)
Tumour promoting activity of extracts of human semen in Sencar mice
Int J Cancer 40: 554

Tollefsbol TO, Cohen HJ (1985)
Culture kinetics of glycolytic enzyme induction, glucose utilization, and thymidine incorporation of extended-exposure of phytohaemagglutinin-stimulated human lymphocytes
J Cell Physiol 122: 98-104

Tomita R, Tanjok K (1998)
Role of nitric oxide in the colon of patients with ulcerative colitis
World J Surg 22: 88-92

Toplin I (1973)
Tumor virus purification using zonal rotors
Spectra 4: 225-235

Tracey G, Wei H, Manogue KR et al. (1988)
Cachektin / tumor necrosis factor induces cachexia, anaemia and inflammation
J Exp Med 167: 1211-1227

Tshambalala-Msimang M (2000)
Schreiben vom 23.02.2000 an De Fries F
Studiengruppe AIDS-Therapie, Eglistr. 7, Zürich
Tel./Fax: +41/14013424 eMail: FelixDEFRIES@Bluewin.ch

Tumijama T, Lake D, Masuho Y, Hersh EM (1991)
Recognition of human immunodeficiency virus glycoproteins by natural anti-carbohydrate antibodies in human serum
Biochem Biophys Res Commun 177: 279-285

Turinsky L Gonnerman WA (1982)
Temporal alteration of intracellular Na+, K+, Ca2+, Mg2+ and PO43—in muscle beneath the burn wound
J Surg Res 33: 337-344

Turksen K, Kupper T, Degenstein L et al. (1992)
Interleukin-6: Insights to its function in skin by overexpression in transgenic mice
Proc Natl Acad Sci USA 89: 5068-5072

Turner VF (1990)
Reducing agents and AIDS: why are we waiting?
The Medical Journal of Australia 153: 502

Turner VF (1998)
Where have we gone wrong?
Continuum 5 (3): 38-44

Tyler DD (1992)
The mitochondrion in health and disease
VCH Publishers, New York

U

Uetrecht JP (1985)
Reactivity and possible significance of hydroxylamine and nitroso metabolites of procainamide
J Pharmacol Exp Med 232: 420-425

Ullum H, Gotzsche PC, Victor J et al. (1995)
Defective natural immunity: An early manifestation of human immunodeficiency virus infection
J Exp Med 182: 789-799

Ulrich R, Zeitz M, Heise W et al. (1989)
Small intestinal structure and function in patients infected with HIV: Evidence for HIV induced enteropathy
Ann Intern Med 111: 15-21

V

Vadas MA, Miller JF, Mc Kenzie IF et al. (1976)
Ly and la antigen phenotypes of T cells involved in delayed-type hypersensitivity and in suppression
J Exp Med 144: 10-19

Valdez H, Lederman MM (1997)
Cytokines and cytokine therapies in HIV-infection
AIDS Clin Rev 98: 187-228

Van Buren CT, Rudolph F, Kulkarni AD et al. (1990)
Reversal of immunosuppression induced by a protein-free diet: comparison of nucleotides, fish oil and arginine
Crit Care Med 18: S114-117

Van der Hulst RR, Van Kreel BK, Von Meyenfeldt et al. (1993)
Glutamine and the preservation of gut integrity
Lancet 341: 1363

Van der Ven AJAM, Koopmans pp, Vree TB, Van der Meer JWM (1991)
Adverse reactions to co-trimoxazole in HIV infections
Lancet 338: 431-433

Van Dijk WC, Verburgh HA, Van Rijswijk REN (1982)
Neutrophil function, serum opsonic activity and delayed hypersensitivity in surgical patients
Surgery 92: 21-27

Van Loveren H, Kato K, Meade R et al: (1984)
Characterization of two different Lyt-1+T cell populations that mediate delayed-type hypersensitivity
J Immunol 133: 2401-2411
Van Meerten E, Verwey J, Schellens JH (1995)
Antineoplastic agents. Drug interactions of clinical significance
Drug Saf 12 (3): 168-182

Van Rooijen N, Ganders A (1997)
Elimination, blocking, and activation of macrophages: Three of a kind?
J Leukoc Biol 62 (6): 702-709

Vanec J, Jirovec O (1952)
Parasitare Pneumonie., Interstitielle Plasmazellen—Pneumonie der Frühgeborenen verursacht durch Pneumocystis Carinii
Zbl. Bakt 158: 120

Vanec L Jirovec O, Lukes J (1953)
Interstitial plasma cell pneumonia in infants
Ann Pediatr 180: 1-21

Varmus H (1987)
Reverse transcription
Sci American 257: 48-54

Varmus H (1988)
Retroviruses
Science 240: 1427-1435

Veierod MB, Laake P, Thelle DS (1997)
Dietary fat intake and risk of lung cancer: A prospective study of 51452 Norwegian men and women
Europ J Cancer Prevention 6 (6): 540-549

Vergani O, Mieli-Vergani G (1996)
Autoimmune hepatitis
Ann Ital Med Int 11 (2): 119-124

Vermeulen A, Deslypere JP, Paridaens R (1986)
Steroid dynamics in the normal and carcinomatous mammary gland
J Steroid Biochem 25 (5B): 799-802

Viard JP, Rakotoambinina B (1999)
Lipodystrophic syndromes in a cohort of HIV-1 infected patients receiving HMRT with a protease inhibitor
Antiviral Ther 4 (Suppl 2): 32-33

Vigano A, Principi N, Vika ML et al. (1995 a)
Immunologic characterization of children vertically infected with human immunodeficiency virus, with slow or rapid disease progression
J Pediatr 126: 368-374

Vigano A, Principi N, Crupi L et al. (1995 b)
Elevation of IgE in HIV-infected children and its correlation with the progression of the disease
J Allergy Clin Immunol 95: 627-632

Vilette JM, Bourin P, Doinel C et al. (1990)
Circadian variations in plasma levels of hypophyseal, adrenocortical and testicular hormones in men infected with human immunodeficiency virus
Clin Endocrinol Metabol 70: 572-577

Vilmar E, Rouzioux C, Vezinet-Brun F et al.(1990)
Isolation of new lymphotropic retrovirus from two siblings with haemophilia B, one with AIDS
Lancet i: 753-757

Vincent VA, Tilders FJ, van Dam AM (1998)
Production, regulation and role of nitric oxide in glial cells
Mediators Inflamm 7 (4): 239-255

Vingerhoets J, Vanhams G, Kestens L et al. (1994)
Deficient T cell responses in non responders to hepatitis B vaccination: Absence of TH1 cytokine production
Immunol Lett 39: 163-168

Viola JP, Rao A (1999)
Molecular regulation of cytokine gene expression during the immune response
J Clin Immunol 19 (2): 98-108

Vodovotz Y (1997)
Control of nitric oxide production by transforming growth factor-beta 1: Mechanistic insights and potential relevance to human disease
Nitric oxide 1 (1): 3-17

Vogelstein B, Kinzler KW (1992)
Carcinogens leave fingerprints
Nature 355: 209-210

Volberding PA et al. (1990)
Zidovudine in asymptomatic HIV infection: a controlled trial in persons with fewer than 500 CD4-positive cells per cubic millimeter (ACTG 019)
NEJM 322: 941-949

Von Roenn JH, Armstrong D, Kotler DP et al. (1994)
Megestral acetate in patients with AIDS-related cachexia
Ann Intern Med 121: 393-399

W

Wagner DA, Young VR, Tannenbaum SR (1983)
Mammalian nitrate biosynthesis: Incorporation of 15NH3 into nitrate is enhanced by endotoxin treatment
Proc Natl Acad Sci USA 80: 4518-4521

Wakefield AE, Fritscher CC, Malin AS et al. (1994)
Genetic diversity in human-derived Pneumocystis carinii isolates from four geographical locations shown by analysis of mitochondrial V RNA gene sequences
J Chem Microbiol 32: 2959-2961

Waldholz M (1996)
Some AIDS cases defy new drug cocktails
Wall Street Journal, Oct 10 1996

Waldmann TA, Strober W, Blaese RM (1972)
Immunodeficiency disease and malignancy: Various immunologic deficiencies of man and the role of immune processes in the control of malignant disease
Ann Intern Med 77: 605-628

Waliszewski P, Molski M, Konarski J (1998)
On the holistic approach in cellular and cancer biology: Nonlinearity,

complexity, and quasi-determinism of the dynamic cellular network
J Surg Oncol 68: 70-78

Wallace DC (1997)
Mitochondrien-DNA, Altern und Krankheit
Spektrum der Wissenschaft 10: 71-80

Wallace DC (1999)
Mitochondrial diseases in man and mouse
Science 283: 1482-1488

Wang T, Marquardt C, Foker J (1976)
Aerobic glycolysis during lymphocyte proliferation
Nature 261: 702-705

Wang Z, Horowitz HW, Orlikowsky T et al. (1999)
Polyspecific self-reactive antibodies in individuals infected with human immunodeficiency virus facilitate T cell deletion and inhibit costimulatory accessory cell function J Infect Dis 180: 1072-1079

Wangensteen OH, Wangensteen SD (1979)
The rise of surgery
In: From empiric craft to scientific discipline
University of Minnesota Press, Minneapolis U.S.

Warburg O, Poesener K, Negelein E (1924)
Über den Stoffwechsel der Carcinomzelle
Biochem Z 152:309-344

Warburg O, Poesener K, Negelein E (1929)
1st die aerobe Glycolyse spezifisch für die Tumoren?
Biochem Z 203: 482-483

Warburg O (1956)
On the origin of cancer cells
Science 123: 309-314

Warburg O (1967)
The prime cause and prevention of cancer
Triltsch, Würzburg

Warren S (1932)
The immediate causes of death in cancer
Am J Med Sci 184: 610-615

Waterhouse C, Jeanpretre N, Keilson J (1979)
Gluconeogenesis from alanine in patients with progressive malignant disease
Cancer Res 39: 1968-1972
Waydhas Ch, Nast-Kolb D, Jochum M et al. (1992)
Inflammatory mediators, infection, sepsis, and multiorgan failure after severe trauma
Arch Surg 127: 460-467

Weber JN, Wadsworth J, Rogers LA et al. (1986)
Three-year prospective study of HTLV-III / LAV infection in homosexual men
Lancet i: 1179-1182

Weber J (1997)
Distinguishing between response to HIV vaccine and response to HIV
Lancet 350: 230-231

Weber R, Ledergerber W, Opravil M et al. (1990)
Progression of HIV infection in misusers of injected drugs who stop injecting or follow a programme of maintenance treatment with methadone
Br Med J 301: 1361-1365

Wegmann TG, Lin H, Guilbert L, Mosmann TR (1993)
Bidirectional cytokine interactions in the maternal-fetal relationship; is successful pregnancy a Th2 phenomenon?
Immunol Today 114: 353

Wei X, Charles JG, Smith A et al. (1995 a)
Altered immune response in mice lacking inducible nitric oxide synthase
Nature 375: 408-411

Wei X, Ghosh SK, Taylor ME et al. (1995 b)
Viral dynamics in human immunodeficiency virus type 1 infection
Nature 273: 117-122

Weigle WO (1997)
Advances in basic concepts of autommune disease
Clin Lab Med 17 (3): 329-340

Weinberg ED (1992)
Iron depletion: A defense against intracellular infection and neoplasia
Life Sciences 50: 1289

Weinhouse S (1976)
The Warburg hypothesis fifty years later
Z Krebsforsch Klin Onkol 87: 115-126

Welbourne TC, Joshi S (1994)
Enteral glutamine spares endogenous glutamine in chronic acidosis
JPEN 18: 243-246

Weller R (1956)
Weitere Untersuchungen über experimetelle Rattenpneumocystose im Hinblick auf die interstitielle Pneumonia der Frühgeborenen
Zschr f Kinderheilkunde 78: 166-176

Werner P (1996)
Otto Warburg und das Problem der Sauerstoffaktivierung
Basilisken Presse, Marburg/Lahn

Western KA, Perera DR, Schultz MG (1970)
Pentamidine isethionate in the treatment of Pneumocystis carinii pneumonia
Ann Intern Med 73: 695-702

Wever RM, Lurcher TF, Cosentino F, Rabelink TJ (1998)
Atherosclerosis and the two faces of endothelial nitric oxide synthase
Circulation 97: 108-112

White A (1998)
Children, pesticides and cancer
The Ecologist 28 (2): 100-105

WHO (1998)
Weekly Epidemiological Record 73: 373-380

Widy-Wirski RS, Berkley S, Downing R et al. (1988)
Evaluation of the WliO clinical case definition for AIDS in Uganda
JAMA 260 (22): 3286-3289

Wilder E, Smart T (1998)
Other pathogenic bacterial infections
In: Marco M, Kass S, Harrington M (eds.)
The OI Report.
A critical Review of the Treatment and Prophylaxis of HIV-related Opportunistic Infections
Treatment Action Group (TAG), New York

Wilkinson J IV, Clapper ML (1997)
Detoxication enzymes and chemoprevention
P.S.E.B.M. 216: 192-200

Willner RE (1994)
Deadly deception.
The proof that sex and HIV absolutely do not cause AIDS
Peltec Publishing Co., Inc., USA
Wilmore OW, Aulic LH (1978)
Metabolic changes in burned patients
Surg Clin North Am 58: 1173-1187

Wilmore DW (1994)
Glutamine and the gut
Gastroenterology 107: 1885-1892

Wirthmüller U (1997)
Die Methode der PCR im Routinelabor
Haemo (Bern) Juni 1997: 2-4

Wisniewski TL, Hilton CW, Morse EV, Svec F (1993)
The relationship of serum DHEAS and cortisol levels to measures of immune function in human immunodeficiency virus-related illness
Am J Med Sci 305 (2): 79-83

Witschi A, Junker E, Schranz C et al. (1995)
Supplementation of N-acetylcysteine fails to increase glutathione in lymphocytes and plasma of patients with AIDS
AIDS Res Hum Retroviruses ll: 141-143

Wolthers KC, Wisman GBA, Otto SA et al. (1996)
T-cell telomere length in HIV-1 infection: No evidence for increased CD4+ T cell turnover
Science 274: 1543-1547

Wolthers KC, Schuitemaker H, Miedema F (1998)
Rapid CD4+ I-cell turnover in HIV-1 infection: A paradigma revisited
Immunology Today 19 (1): 44-48

Wood JJ, Rodrick ML, O'Mahony JB et al. (1984)
Inadequate interleukin-2 production: A fundamental deficiency in patients with major burns
Ann Surg 200: 311-320
World Cancer Research Fund / American Institute for Cancer Research (1997)
Food, nutrition and the prevention of cancer: A global perspective
American Institute for Cancer research, Washington DC, USA

Wright DN, Nelson Rp, Ledford DF (1990)
Serum IgE and human immunodeficiency (HIV) infection
J Allergy Clin Immunol 85: 445-452

Wrong O (1993)
Water and monovalent electrolytes. In: Garrow JS, James WPT (eds.) Human Nutrition and Dietetics\ Churchill Livingstone, Edinburgh. 9th ed.

Wu G, Morris SM (1995)
Arginine metabolism: Nitric oxide and beyond
Biochem J 336 (Pt1): 1-17

X

Xie K, Deng Z, Fidler IJ (1996)
Activation of nitric oxide synthase gene for inhibition of cancer metastasis
J Leucoc Biol 59: 797-803

Y

Yakes FM, Van Houten B (1997)
Mitochondrial DNA damage is more extensive and persists longer than nuclear DNA damage in human cells following oxidative stress
Proc Natl Acad Sci USA 94: 514-519

Yegorov YE, Chemov DN, Akimov SS (1996)
Reverse transcriptase inhibitors suppress telomerase function and induce senescence-like processes in cultured mouse fibroblasts
FEBS lett 389: 115-118

Yonetani T (1998)
Nitric oxide and haemoglobin
Nippon Yallurigahu Zasshi 112: 155-160

Young I (1995)
The stonewall experiment. A gay psychohistory
Cassell, London

Young LS (1984)
Pneumocystis Carinii Pneumonia. Pathogenesis, Diagnosis, Treatment
Marcel Dekker, New York

Z

Zagury D, Bernhard J. Leonhard R et al. (1986)
Long term cultures of HTLV-III-infected T-cells: A model of cytopathology of T-cell depletion in AIDS
Science 231: 850-853
Zakowski RC, Gottlieb MS, Groopman J (1984)
Acquired immunodeficiency syndrome (AIDS), Kaposi's sarcoma, and Pneumocystis carinii pneumonia
ln: Young LS (ed.) (1984)
Pneumocystis Carinii Pneumonia: Pathogenesis, Diagnosis, Treatment
Marcel Dekker Inc., New York

Zamzami N, Hirsch T, Dallaporta B et al.(1997)
Mitochondrial implication in accidental and programmed cell death: Apoptosis and necrosis
Bioenerget Biomembran 29 (2): 185-193

Zaretsky MD (1995)
Toxicity and AIDS-prophylaxis: Is AZT beneficial for HIV+ asymptomatic

persons with 500 or more T4 cells per cubic millimeter?
Genetica 95: 91-101

ZDN—Zentrum zur Dokumentation für Naturheilverfahren e.V (1995)
Warum die HIV / AIDS-These nicht mehr langer haltbar ist raum&zeit 78: 57-62

ZDN—Zentrum zur Dokumentation für Naturheilverfahren e.V (1998)
HIV-Foto: Betrügt die Bayer-Forschung die Wissenschatt? raum&zeit 93: 84-87

Zeleniuch-Jacquotte A, Chajes V, Van Kappel et al. (2000)
Reliability of fatty acid composition in human serum phospholipids
Europ Clin Nutr 54 (5): 367-372
Zhang PC, Pang CP (1992)
Plasma amino acid patterns in cancer
Clin Chem 38: 1198-1199

Zidek Z, Marek K (1998)
Erratic behavior of nitric oxide within the immune system: Illustrative review of conflicting data and their immunological aspects
Int J Immunopharmacol 20: 319-343

Zieger TR, Young LS, Benfell K et al. (1992)
Clinical and metabolic efficacy of glutamine-supplemented parenteral nutrition after bone marrow transplantation: A randomized double-blind, controlled study
Ann Intern Med 116: 821-827

Zimmermann J, Selhub J. Rosenberg IH (1987)
Competitive inhibition of folate absorption by dihydrofolate reductase inhibitors, trimethoprim and pyrimethamine
Am Clin Nutr 46: 518-522

Zinsser H (1921)
Delayed hypersensitivity
J Exp Med 34: 495
Zisbrod A, Haimov M, Schanzer H et al. (1980)
Kaposi's sarcoma after kidney transplantation
Transplantation 30: 383

Zvibel J. Kraft A (1993)
Extracellular matrix and metastasis
In: Zen MA, Reid LM (ed.)
Extracellular matrix: chemistry, biology and pathology with emphasis on the liver
Marcel Dekker Inc., New York

Tables

Table I
The pathogenesis of AIDS according to the retroviral theory

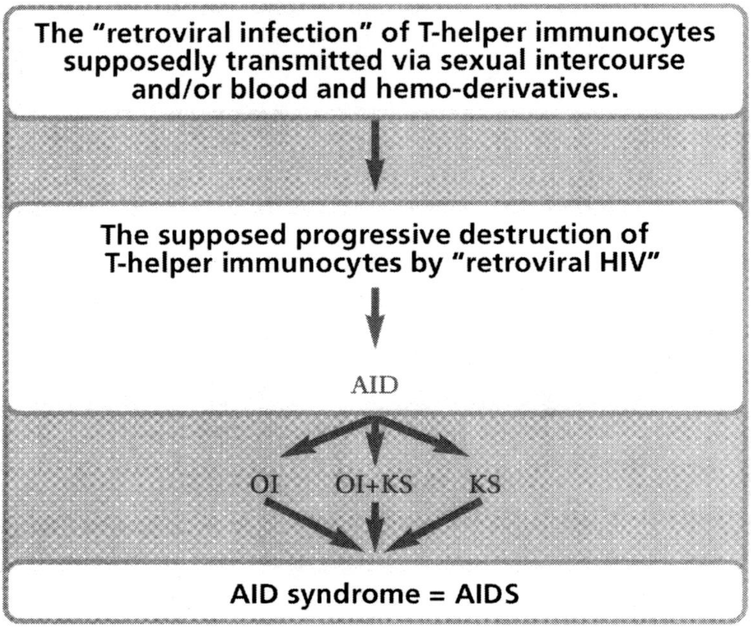

The "retroviral infection" of T-helper immunocytes supposedly transmitted via sexual intercourse and/or blood and hemo-derivatives.
The supposed progressive destruction of T-helper immunocytes by "retroviral HIV"
AID
OI
OI+KS
KS
AID syndrome = AIDS

Table II
Actual clinical manifestations observed in extreme or prolonged stress to immunocytes and/or stress to endothelial cells on the basis of various causes or a combination of causes.

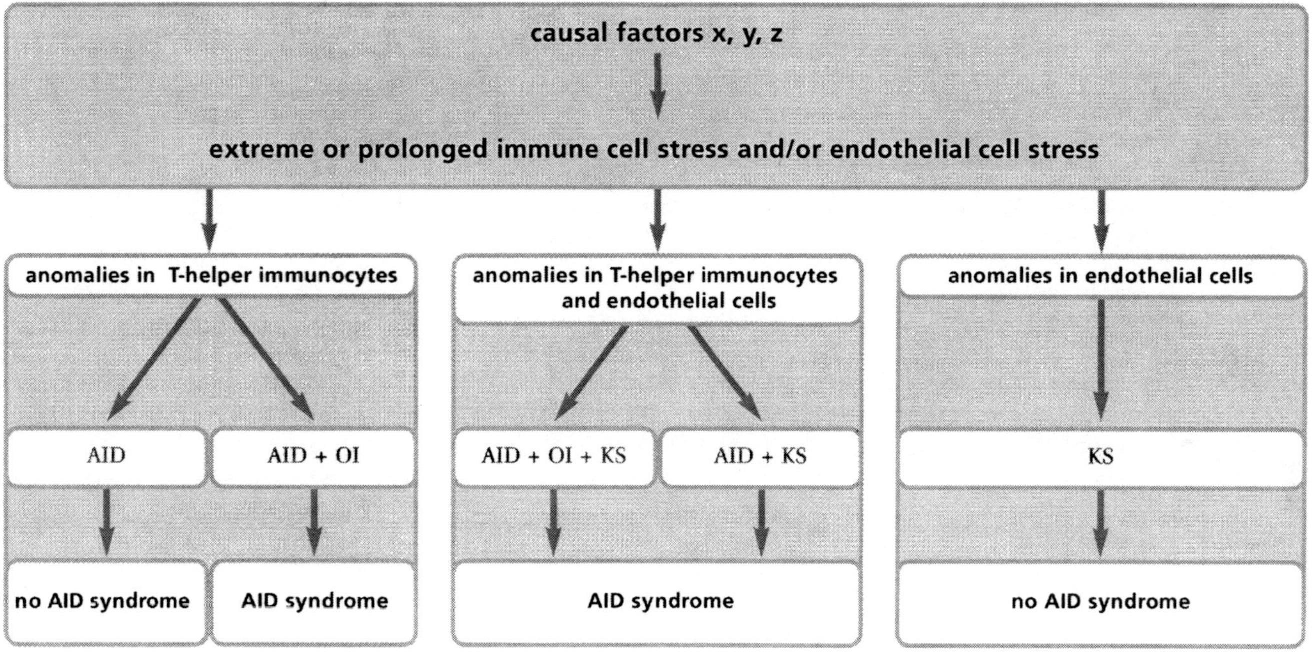

causal factors x, y, z
extreme or prolonged immune cell stress and/or endothelial cell stress
anomalies in T-helper immunocytes
AID
AID + OI
no AID syndrome
AID syndrome
anomalies in T-helper immunocytes and endothelial cells
AID + OI + KS
AID + KS
AID syndrome
anomalies in endothelial cells
KS
no AID syndrome

Table III
The double strategy of the immune response

disease factors x, y, z

↓

dependent on dosage, duration, disposition etc: imbalance in Th1-Th2 response

type-1 cytokine dominance	variable transitional forms: cytokine mixture	type-2 cytokine dominance
↓	↓	↓
Th1 dominance -DTH skin reaction ↑↑ -T-helper cells in serum ↑↑ -T-helper cell stimulation in vitro ↑↑ -B-lymphocyte activity ↓ -antibody production ↓	Th1-Th2 mixture -DTH skin reaction ↑↓ -T-helper cells in serum ↑↓ -T-helper cell stimulation in vitro ↑↓ -B-lymphocyte activity ↑↓ -antibody production ↑↓	Th2 dominance -DTH skin reaction ↓↓ -T-helper cells in serum ↓↓ -T-helper cell stimulation in vitro ↓↓ -B-lymphocyte activity ↑↑ -antibody production ↑↑
↓	↓	↓
healthy immune defense against all intracellular pathogens	Variable intracellular and extracellular immune defense	Insufficient intracellular immunity but effective extracellular (antibacterial) immunity
↓	↓	↓
possible consequences: damage to tissues and cells in the event of excessive cytokine production	Possible imbalance: temporary or permanent Th1-Th2 switch when the disease factors persist	Possible consequences: Acute infections possibly with lethal outcomes (sepsis, opportunistic infections). Chronic infections

Table IV
Diagram of the fusion between an archaeum and a proteobacterium for the formation of the nucleus and the development of proto-mitochondria (eukaryote cellular symbiosis) that took place some 2 billion years ago (Gray 1999)

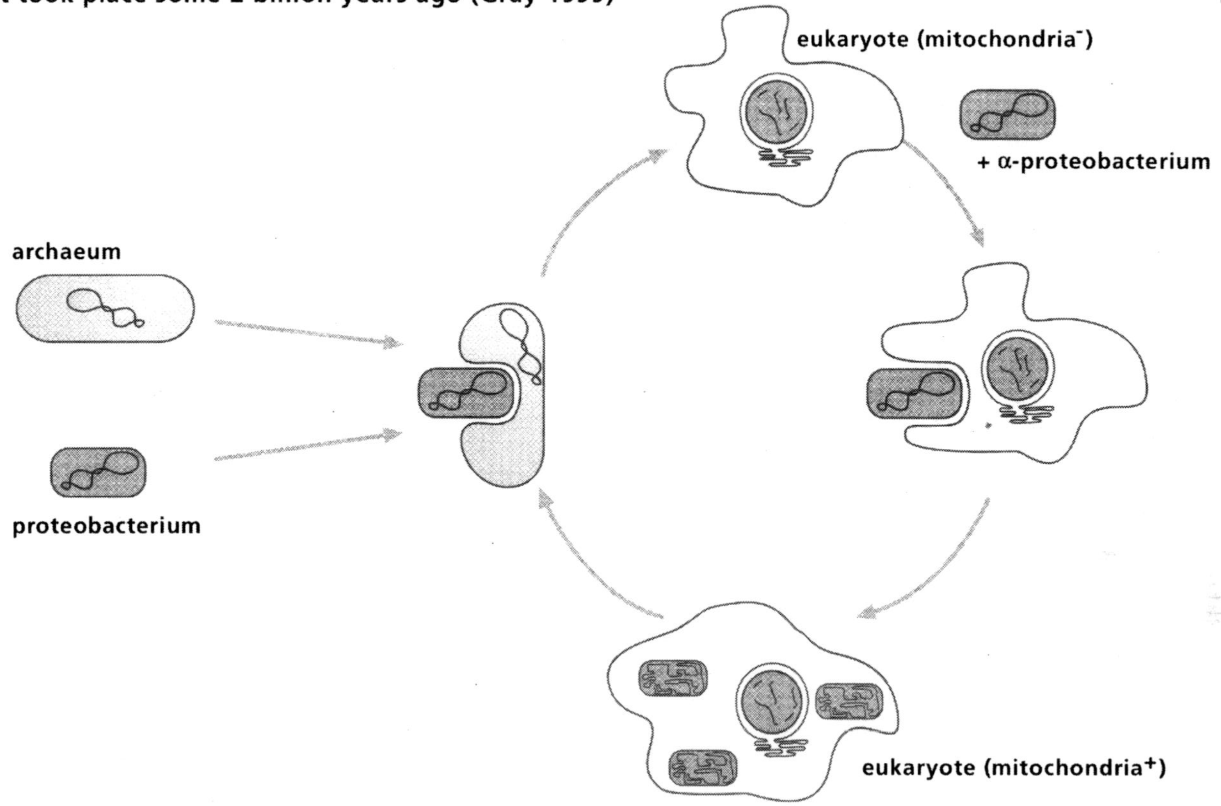
archaeum
proteobacterium
eukaryote (mitochondria⁻)
+ α-proteobacterium
eukaryote (mitochondria⁺)

Table V
The alternating switch between OXPHOS and aerobic glycolysis: physiological and pathophysiological cell models.

Cell model	Energy production	Functional state	Alternating switch	mitochondrial membrane	Cytokine profile
cell during division cycle (S stage)	predominantly aerobic glycolysis in the cytoplasm	protection against oxidative and nitrosative stress of the cell as a whole and mitochondria	intact; after division cycle and proliferation of the new mitochondria, return to OXPHOS	balanced mitochondrial membrane potential	type-1 - type-2 cytokine balance, Th1-Th2 cell balance
tumor cell caught in division cycle	high predominance of aerobic glycolysis in the cytoplasm	extreme counterregulation against oxidative and nitrosative stress, cellular dyssymbiosis	blocked; division cycle maintained despite the formation of transcripts for OXPHOS proteins	increased mitochondrial membrane potential. H+ leakage from the inner mitochondrial membrane	type-2 cytokine imbalance Th2 dominance
fetal cell before the start of the aerobic respiration	predominantly aerobic glycolysis in the cytoplasm	protection against oxidative and nitrosative stress, physiological immaturity of mitochondria	OXPHOS arrested until first breath, formation of transcripts for OXPHOS proteins prefabricated in the mitochondria	increased mitochondrial membrane potential. H+ leakage from the inner mitochondrial membrane	type-2 cytokine dominance Th2 cell dominance
adult cell (apoptosis)	inactivated OXPHOS in the mitochondria	extreme oxidative and nitrosative stress, cellular dyssymbiosis through loss of mitochondrial membrane potential	no longer possible when programmed cell death reaches the effector stage	strongly reduced mitochondrial membrane potential	type-1 cytokine dominance Th1 cell dominance

Table VI
Compensated/decompensated oxidative and nitrosative stress.

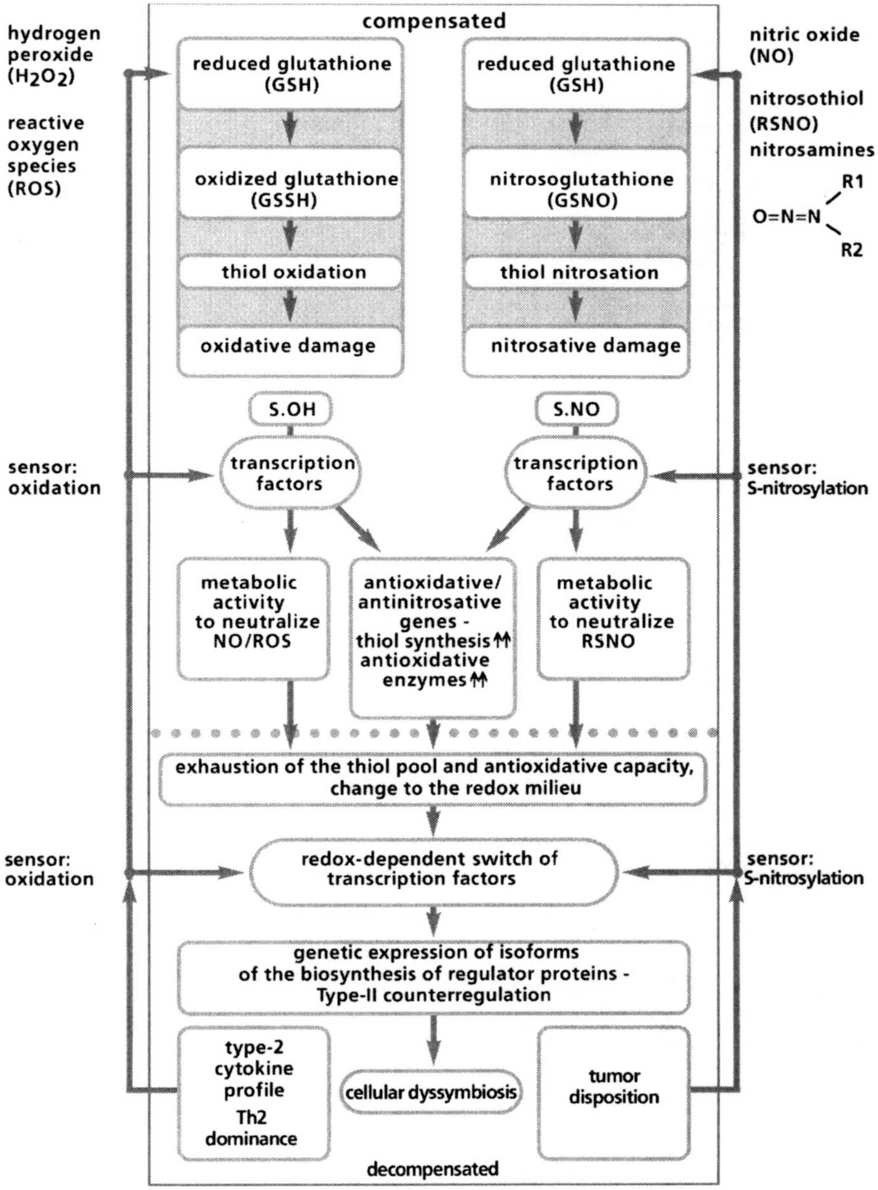
compensated
hydrogen peroxide (H_2O_2)
reactive oxygen species (ROS)
reduced glutathione (GSH)
oxidized glutathione (GSSH)
thiol oxidation
oxidative damage
nitric oxide (NO)
nitrosothiol (RSNO)
nitrosamines
O=N=N R1 R2
reduced glutathione (GSH)
nitrosoglutathione (GSNO)
thiol nitrosation
nitrosative damage
S.OH
S.NO
sensor: oxidation
transcription factors
transcription factors
sensor: S-nitrosylation
metabolic activity to neutralize NO/ROS
antioxidative/ antinitrosative genes - thiol synthesis ↑↑ antioxidative enzymes ↑↑
metabolic activity to neutralize RSNO
exhaustion of the thiol pool and antioxidative capacity, change to the redox milieu
sensor: oxidation
redox-dependent switch of transcription factors
sensor: S-nitrosylation
genetic expression of isoforms of the biosynthesis of regulator proteins - Type-II counterregulation
type-2 cytokine profile Th2 dominance
cellular dyssymbiosis
tumor disposition
decompensated

Table VII
Cellular symbiosis and dyssymbiosis subject to NO and ROS production.

T-helper immunocytes	NO	ROS	Peroxinitrite	Cellular symbiosis	Counterregulation	Antioxidative capacity	Clinical symptoms
Th1 - Th2 balance type-1 – type-2 cytokine balance	- Ca-dependent NO ↑↓ - cytotoxic NO ↑↓ only after stimulation	- O_2- ↑↓ - other ROS ↑↓	- ONOO ↑↓	- intact: - regulated alternating switch - Ca^{2+} cycling ↑↓ - mitochondrial membrane potential ↑↓	- physiological	intact: - consumption dependent on needs	Intact cell-mediated and humoral immunity
Th1 dominance type-1 cytokine profile	- cytotoxic NO ↑↑ - RSNO ↑↑ - nitrosative stress ↑↑	- O_2- ↑↑ - other ROS ↑↓ - oxidative stress ↑↑	- ONOO ↑↑ - oxidative/ nitrosative stress	cellular dyssymbiosis: - Ca^{2+} cycling ↑↑ - mitochondrial membrane potential ↓↓ - apoptosis/necrosis	- too weak	in mitochondria: - consumption ↑↑ - danger of exhaustion	- inflammatory processes - autoimmune reactions
Th2 dominance type-2 cytokine profile	- cytotoxic NO ↓↓ - RSNO ↑↑ - nitrosative stress ↓↓	- O_2- ↓↓ - other ROS ↓↓ - oxidative stress ↓↓	- ONOO ↓↓ - nitrosylation via thiol bonding	cellular dyssymbiosis: - OXPHOS ↓↓ - predominantly aerobic glycolysis	- strong - heat shock protein ↑↑ - heme oxygenase ↑↑ - ferritin ↑↑ - Cox-2, PGE2 - Bcl-2 ↑↑	plasma levels: - glutathione ↓↓ - cysteine ↓↓ - homocysteine ↓↓ - glutamine ↓ - glutamate ↑ - urea ↑	- antibodies ↑↑ - eosinophiles ↑ - DTH ↓↓ - AID, AIDS, cancer, muscular and nerve degeneration - protein catabolism in the muscles (wasting, cachexy)
inhibition of maturation Th1 - Th2 (NO > O_2-)	- Ca-dependent NO ↑↑ - cytotoxic NO after stimulation ↑↑	- O_2- ↑ - other ROS ↑ - oxidative stress ↑	- ONOO ↓ - nitrosative stress through thiol exhaustion	cellular dyssymbiosis: - DNA and protein damage in the nucleus and in mitochondria - Ca^{2+} cycling ↑↑	- variable - dependent on energy loss provoked by disruption of OXPHOS system	- thiol pool and thiol proteins in mitochondria ↓	- degenerative symptoms - susceptibility to infection - disposition to tumors - senile illnesses
inhibition of maturation Th1 - Th2 (O_2- < NO)	- Ca-dependent NO ↑ - cytotoxic NO after stimulation ↑	- O_2- ↑↑ - other ROS ↑↑ - oxidative stress ↑↑	- ONOO ↓ - oxidative stress through thiol exhaustion	cellular dyssymbiosis: - DNA and protein damage in the nucleus and in mitochondria -Ca^{2+} cycling ↑↑	- variable - dependent on energy loss provoked by disruption of OXPHOS system	- thiol pool and thiol proteins in mitochondria ↓	- degenerative symptoms - susceptibility to infection - disposition to tumors - senile illnesses

Table VIII
Clinical examples of cellular dyssymbioses as a result of Type-I overregulation or Type-II counterregulation.

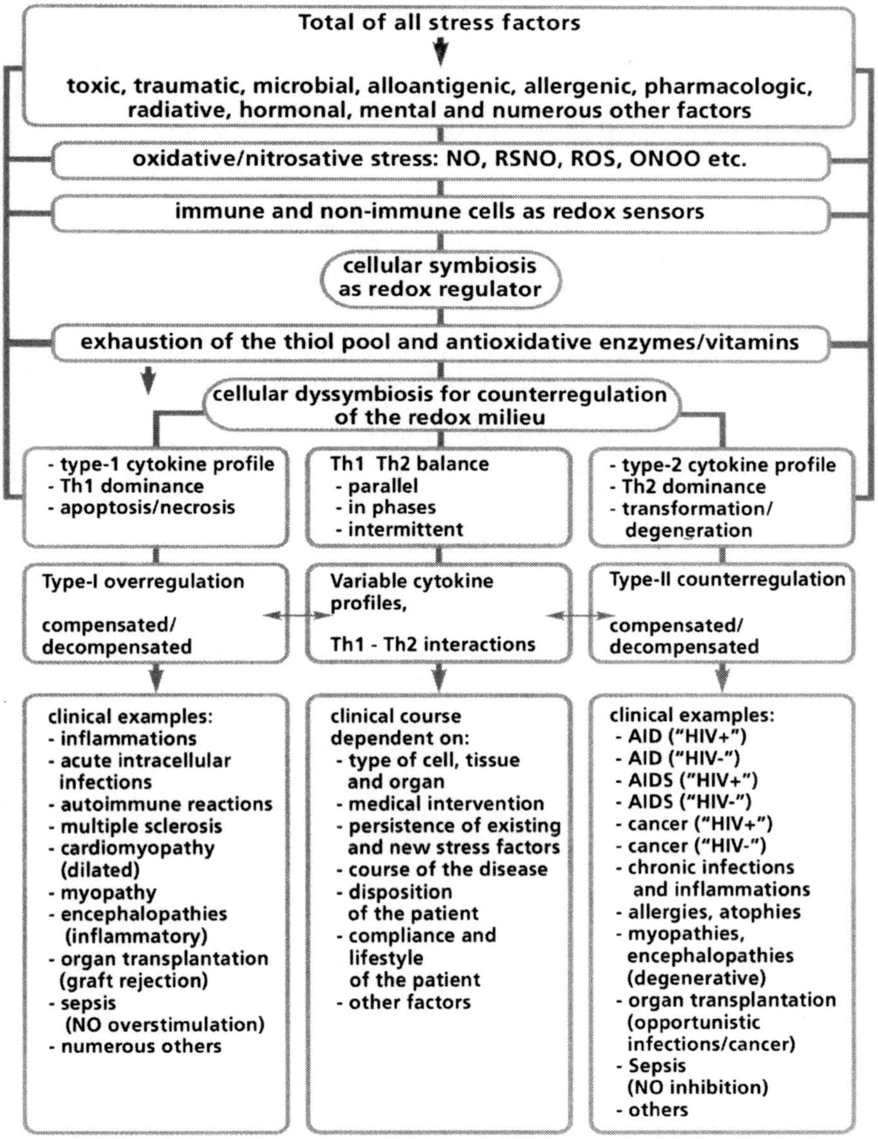

Total of all stress factors
toxic, traumatic, microbial, alloantigenic, allergenic, pharmacologic, radiative, hormonal, mental and numerous other factors
oxidative/nitrosative stress: NO, RSNO, ROS, ONOO etc.
immune and non-immune cells as redox sensors
cellular symbiosis as redox regulator
exhaustion of the thiol pool and antioxidative enzymes/vitamins
cellular dyssymbiosis for counterregulation of the redox milieu
- type-1 cytokine profile
- Th1 dominance
- apoptosis/necrosis
Th1 Th2 balance
- parallel
- in phases
- intermittent
- type-2 cytokine profile
- Th2 dominance
- transformation/ degeneration
Type-I overregulation
compensated/ decompensated
Variable cytokine profiles,
Th1 - Th2 interactions
Type-II counterregulation
compensated/ decompensated
clinical examples:
- inflammations
- acute intracellular infections
- autoimmune reactions
- multiple sclerosis
- cardiomyopathy (dilated)
- myopathy
- encephalopathies (inflammatory)
- organ transplantation (graft rejection)
- sepsis (NO overstimulation)
- numerous others
clinical course dependent on:
- type of cell, tissue and organ
- medical intervention
- persistence of existing and new stress factors
- course of the disease
- disposition of the patient
- compliance and lifestyle of the patient
- other factors
clinical examples:
- AID ("HIV+")
- AID ("HIV-")
- AIDS ("HIV+")
- AIDS ("HIV-")
- cancer ("HIV+")
- cancer ("HIV-")
- chronic infections and inflammations
- allergies, atophies
- myopathies, encephalopathies (degenerative)
- organ transplantation (opportunistic infections/cancer)
- Sepsis (NO inhibition)
- others

Table IX
The phantom "HIV"

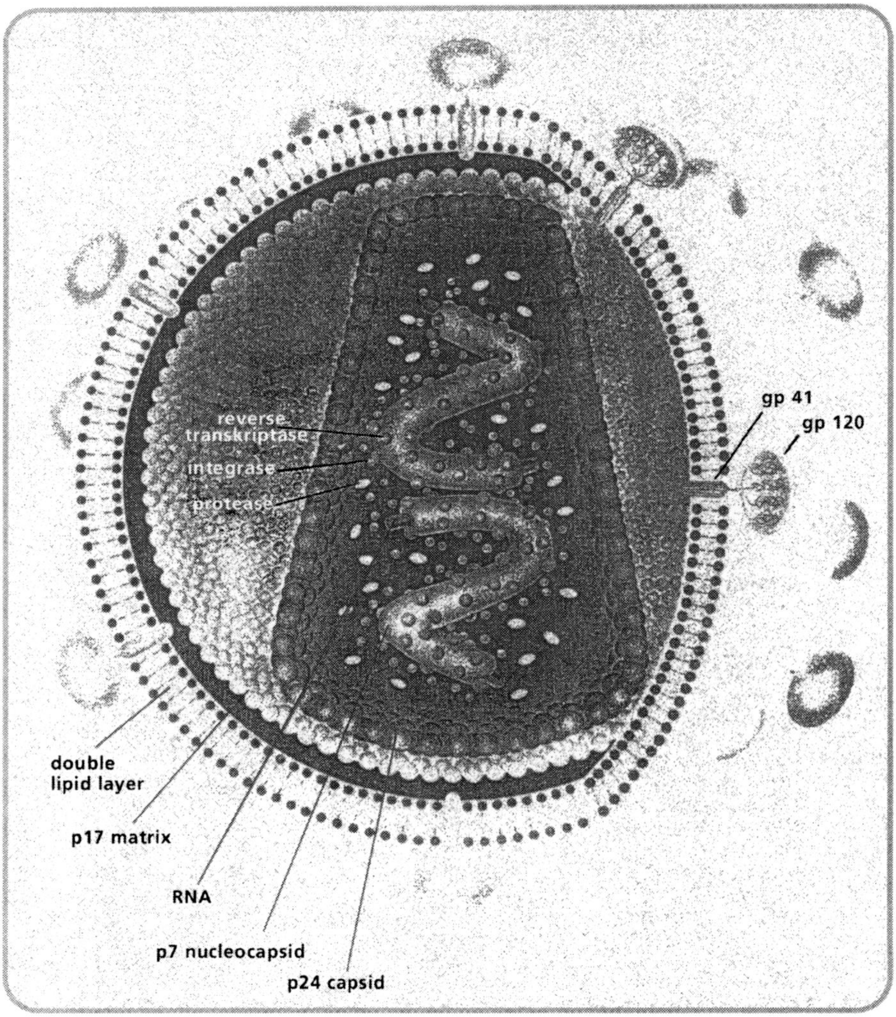

reverse transkriptase
integrase
protease
gp 41
gp 120
double lipid layer
p17 matrix
RNA
p7 nucleocapsid
p24 capsid

Virtual computerised picture of the "HI" virus based on speculative assumptions.

Table X
The experimental findings of the Montaigner team as counter-evidence to the "HIV causes AID and AIDS" theory.

Cell cultures	First stimulation of the "HIV characteristic" PHA, interleukin-2	oxidative/ nitrosative second stimulation	programmed cell death apoptosis/necrosis
A human CEM cells	Yes acute prestimulation of non-specific "HIV characteristics"	Yes PHA interleukin-2	Yes Peak of cell deaths 6 to 7 days after first acute prestimulation of non-specific "HIV characteristics", however, following second stimulation, peak of production of non-specific "HIV characteristics" of the surviving cells only after 6 to 10 days
B human CEM cells, monocytes	Yes chronic stimulation of non-specific "HIV characteristics"	Yes PHA interleukin-2	No No cell death of the surviving cells despite the continuous production of non-specific "HIV characteristics"
C human T-helper lymphocytes	Yes acute prestimulation of non-specific "HIV characteristics"	Yes PHA interleukin-2	Yes Three days after the first acute prestimulation of non-specific "HIV characteristics" and the subsequent second stimulation
D human T-helper lymphocytes	No without acute prestimulation of non-specific "HIV characteristics"	Yes PHA interleukin-2	Yes Five days after the stimulation without the first prestimulation of non-specific "HIV characteristics"

Table XI
The experimental findings of the Gallo team as counter-evidence to the "HIV causes AID and AIDS" theory.

Cell cultures	First stimulation "HIV characteristics" PHA, interleukin-2	Oxidative/ nitrosative second stimulation	Proportion of T-helper lymphocytes in the cell culture before stimulation	Proportion of T-helper lymphocytes in the cell culture after stimulation
A human T-lymphocytes	Yes acute prestimulation of non-specific "HIV characteristics" →	Yes PHA interleukin-2	34%	3%
B human T-lymphocytes	No Without acute prestimulation of non-specific "HIV characteristics" →	Yes PHA interleukin-2	34%	10%
C human T-lymphocytes	No Without acute prestimulation of non-specific "HIV characteristics" →	No without stimulation with PHA interleukin-2	34%	approx. 34%

Table XII
Diagram of the mitochondrial channels (modified schematic after Zamzani, 1996)

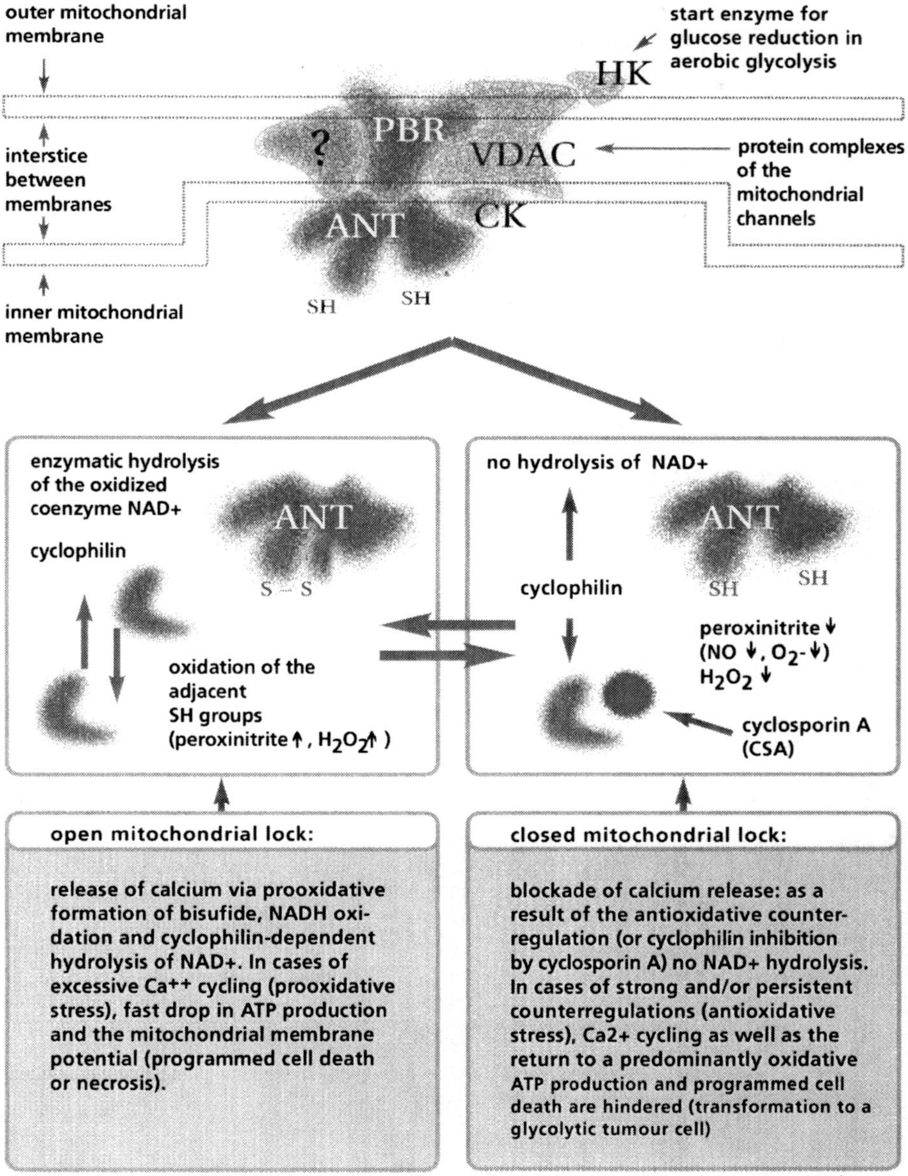
outer mitochondrial membrane
start enzyme for glucose reduction in aerobic glycolysis
HK
?
PBR
VDAC
protein complexes of the mitochondrial channels
interstice between membranes
ANT
CK
SH
SH
inner mitochondrial membrane
enzymatic hydrolysis of the oxidized coenzyme NAD+
cyclophilin
ANT
S – S
oxidation of the adjacent SH groups (peroxinitrite ↑, H_2O_2↑)
no hydrolysis of NAD+
cyclophilin
ANT
SH
SH
peroxinitrite ↓
(NO ↓, O_2- ↓)
H_2O_2 ↓
cyclosporin A (CSA)
open mitochondrial lock:
release of calcium via prooxidative formation of bisufide, NADH oxidation and cyclophilin-dependent hydrolysis of NAD+. In cases of excessive Ca++ cycling (prooxidative stress), fast drop in ATP production and the mitochondrial membrane potential (programmed cell death or necrosis).
closed mitochondrial lock:
blockade of calcium release: as a result of the antioxidative counterregulation (or cyclophilin inhibition by cyclosporin A) no NAD+ hydrolysis. In cases of strong and/or persistent counterregulations (antioxidative stress), Ca2+ cycling as well as the return to a predominantly oxidative ATP production and programmed cell death are hindered (transformation to a glycolytic tumour cell)

Table XIII
The channel rhythm in mitochondrion

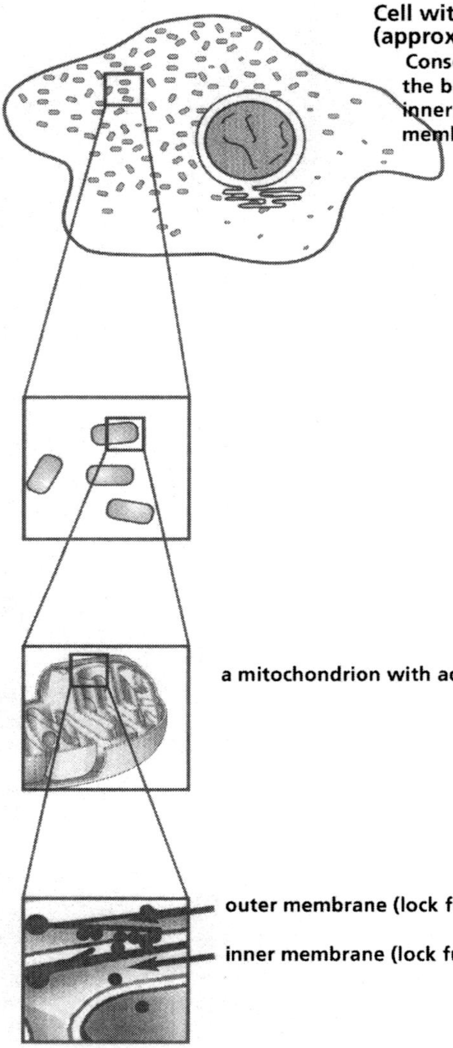

Cell with a nucleus and mitochondria (approx. 1,300 per cell).
Consequently in humans the bioenergetically active area of the inner mitochondrial membrane is nearly 100,000 m2
a mitochondrion with active DNA
outer membrane (lock function)
inner membrane (lock function)

The lock rhythm in mitochondria

Introduction and emission of gases, proteins, Ca^{2+} ions, etc. (highly simplified schematic representation).

When the locks are blocked (energy deficiency) the archaeal part of the genome acts as "proton deficiency memory" resulting in a switch to anaerobic glycolysis.

→ transformation to a tumour cells (permanent energetic provision via fermentation of glucose despite the presence of oxygen)

Table XIV
Programmed cell death in metastatic tumor cells after the transfer of a functional iNOS gene (experiment by Xie et al. 1996).

Origin and characteristics of tumor cells before manipulation	manipulation methods/ no manipulation as control	Characteristics of tumor cells without/ after manipulation	Tumor growth in naked mice without/ after manipulation
- metastatic tumor cells (mouse melanoma) - after stimulation with IL-2/LPS: → iNOS↓, iNO↓	control without manipulation	- metastatic tumor cells - iNOS↓, iNO↓ - no programmed cell death	fast growing tumor
- metastatic tumor cells (mouse melanoma) - after stimulation with IL-2/LPS: → iNOS↓, iNO↓	transmission of functional iNOS gene (transfection)	→ non metastatic tumor cells - iNOS↑, iNO↑ - programmed cell death!	slow growing tumor
- metastatic tumor cells (mouse melanoma) - after stimulation with IL-2/LPS: → iNOS↓, iNO↓	transmission of non-functional iNOS gene (transfection)	- metastatic tumor cells - iNOS↓, iNO↓ - no programmed cell death	fast growing tumor
- metastatic tumor cells (mouse melanoma) - after stimulation with IL-2/LPS: → iNOS↓, iNO↓	Transmission of a neomycin gene (transfection)	- metastatic tumor cells - iNOS↓, iNO↓ - no programmed cell death	fast growing tumor

Table XV
Programmed cell death in metastatic tumor cells after repeated injection of synthetic lipopeptides (LPS analogs) and induction of the iNOS enzyme for the synthesis of iNO (experiment by Xie et al. 1996)

Origin and characteristics of tumor cells before manipulation	manipulation method no manipulation as control	Characteristics of the tumor cells without/after manipulation
- metastatic tumor cells (mouse sarcoma) - after stimulation with IL-2/LPS: → iNOS↓, iNO↓	control test without manipulation	- metastatic tumor cells - iNOS↓, iNO↓ - no programmed cell death
- metastatic tumor cells (mouse sarcoma) - after stimulation with IL-2/LPS: → iNOS↓, iNO↓	repeated injections of synthetic lipopeptides (LPS analogs)	→ compete remission of metastatic tumour cells → iNOS↑↑, iNO↑↑ - programmed cell death!

Table XVI
Introduction of vaccinations and the decline in disease mortality.

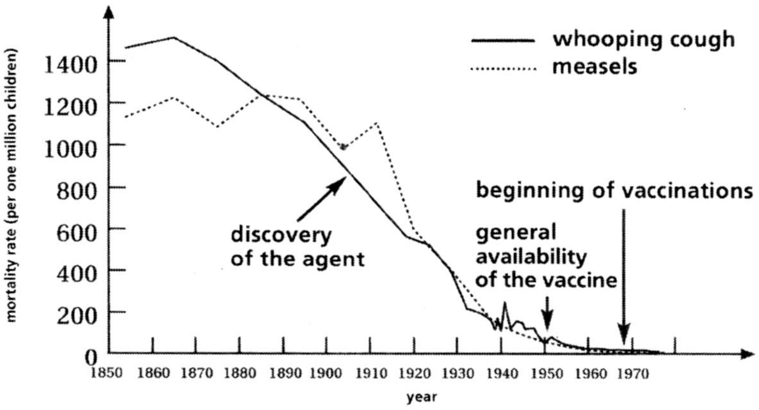
whooping cough
measels
1400
1200
1000
800
600
400
200
0
mortality rate (per one million children)
discovery
of the agent
beginning of vaccinations
general
availability
of the vaccine
1850 1860 1870 1880 1890 1900 1910 1920 1930 1940 1950 1960 1970
year

whooping cough and measels:
mortality rate of children under 15
in England and Wales

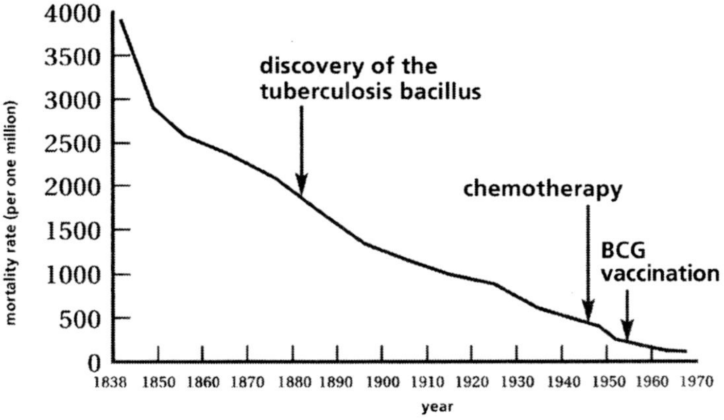
4000
3500
3000
2500
2000
1500
1000
500
0
mortality rate (per one million)
discovery of the
tuberculosis bacillus
chemotherapy
BCG
vaccination
1838 1850 1860 1870 1880 1890 1900 1910 1920 1930 1940 1950 1960 1970
year

tuberculosis of the respiratory tract:
mortality rate in England and Wales

Examples of the progressive decline in disease and mortality rates via infectious illnesses from 1838-1970 (Sagan 1992)

Table XVII

Typical laboratory findings in cumulative wasting syndrome.

indicators of Type-II counterregulation of cellular dyssymbiosis in systemic diseases ("HIV+", AIDS, cancer, sepsis, trauma, burns, surgery, Crohn's disease, ulcerative colitis, chronic fatigue, overtrained athletes, etc.)

intracellular: reduced glutathione (GSH)↓↓: measured in T4 lymphocytes or in peripheral monocytes

plasma levels (serum levels)

reduced glutathione (GSH) ↓↓
(dependent on amino acids)

Aminoacids:
cystein (cystin) ↓↓, glutamine ↓↓, arginine ↓↓

glutamate ↑↑, urea ↑↑, lactate ↑↑, glucose ↑↑, insulin ↑↑, total choline ↓

Minerals:
magnesium ↓, selenium ↓, copper ↑, zinc ↓, iron ↓, serum ferritin ↑↑

Markers for counterregulation;
prostaglandin PG E2 ↑↑, triglycerides ↑↑, beta 2-microglobulin ↑↑, neopterin, biopterin ↑↑

L-carnitin (fatty acid transportation protein) ↓↓
coenzyme Q10 (enzyme) ↓↓

Hormones
DHEA-S ↓↓
cortisol ↑(24 h saliva swab test ↑↑)
cortisol / DHEA-S ratio ↑↑

Vitamins
total carotene (precursor of vitamin A) ↓, niacin (vitamin B3) ↑, tryptophan (precursor of niacin)↓, pyridoxine (vitamin B6) ↓, folic acid ↓, vitamin B12 ↓, vitamin C ↓, vitamin E ↓

Immunocytes in peripheral blood and immunoglobulin
T4 lymphocytes (CD4 cells, T-helper immunocytes (Th cells) = Th1 and Th2 ↓↓, T4/T8 ratio (CD4/CD8 ratio) ↓↓, natural killer cells (NK cells) ↓↓, neutrophile granulocytes ↓↓, neutropenia, eosinophile granulocytes ↑↑: eosinophilia

Antibodies
certain immunoglobulins ↑↑

Skin reaction test
DTH (delayed hyper sensitivity) ↓↓, measure of the reactivity of type-1 T-helper immunocytes (Th1) in the skin on stimulation with microbial antigens

Measurement of cytokines
type-1 cytokine profile ↓↓: indicator of Th1 immunocytes, type-2 cytokine profile ↑↑: indicator of Th2 immunocytes

Bioelectrical Impedance Analysis (BIA)
body cell mass (BCM) ↓↓, fat free mass (FFM) ↓↓, total body water (TBW) ↓↓

Lightning Source UK Ltd.
Milton Keynes UK
UKOW02f1513101116
287278UK00001B/168/P

9 781436 350839